PATHOLOGY AND

UNDERSTANDING DISEASE

PREVENTION

PATHOLOGY AND

UNDERSTANDING DISEASE

PREVENTION

Steven L. Mera BA, PhD, FIBM

Faculty of Health and Social Care,
Leeds Metropolitan University

Stanley Thornes (Publishers) Ltd

First published in 1997 by:
Stanley Thornes (Publishers) Ltd
Ellenborough House
Wellington Street
CHELTENHAM
GL50 1YW
United Kingdom

97 98 99 00 01 / 10 9 8 7 6 5 4 3 2 1

A catalogue record for this book is available from the British Library

ISBN 0-7487-3178-4

Typeset by Imagelink, Huddersfield
Printed and bound in Italy by G. Canale & C. S.p. A. - Borgaro T.se - TURIN

Contents

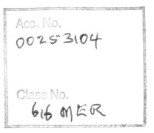

Preface

Acknowledgements
How to use the book

CONCEPTS OF HEALTH AND DISEASE

Preface

I am happy to say that after writing this book I know rather more about pathology than I thought I did at the start: my hope is that you will be in a similar position after reading it. Pathology is an exceedingly complex subject and a single-author book such as this will inevitably omit material, as well as include the occasional personal or controversial view. Where possible, I have tried to present both sides of an argument in the 'Point/counterpoint' sections, and have given my own views if I felt it appropriate.

It is possible to find pathology texts of greater length, solely devoted to the subject matter of only a single chapter in this book. My purpose is to provide a basic understanding together with an appreciation and discussion of the contemporary findings and ideas about that subject. This may have resulted in some imbalance where (as my Editor has put it) we delve deeply into the 'woodwork' in a single specialist area of a topic. I do not apologise for this, as in my experience of teaching health professionals they like to know much more about a subject than can be found in the basic texts but find the classic textbooks rather intimidating. I hope that by reading this you will understand basic pathology, be encouraged to think about and question it and feel more comfortable when the time comes to consult the specialist medical texts and journals.

It is only in a very late stage of preparation that an author gets to read his own book in its entirety. This is against a background of murmurings from the publisher, with the question 'when will that manuscript be ready?' This leads me to thank my publishers, especially Dominic Recaldin, for prolonged patience. It also leads me to some final thoughts and caveats about the book:

- It offers information about disease, prevention and treatment from a Western (European and northern American) perspective
- The conventional 'biomedical model' is pre-eminent, without perspectives from alternative and complementary medicine
- The 'biomedical model' used does not provide adequate focus on the psychosocial aspects of health and well-being

This is not to say that these perspectives have any less value than the approach taken herein, but there are better books than I could write that deal with these issues. Where appropriate, I have made recommendations for these, and other specialist books, in the reference and further reading lists at the end of each chapter.

Writing this book has, by and large, been an enjoyable experience, but not without some frustrating interludes as I tried to grapple with some issues I did not fully comprehend. I hope my attempts to clarify these matters in my own mind will make them easier for the reader to understand.

Finally, I invite your comments, particularly about areas you did not understand or any new points you think might be useful. You can write to me, or email me at merasl@aol.com.

Steven L. Mera   Leeds, September 1996

Acknowledgements

This book would not have been possible without the help of family, friends and colleagues. Pride of place goes to my family, who I now look forward to getting to know again. All my colleagues at Leeds Metropolitan University have given their help and encouragement, but special efforts were made by Trudie Silman – who encouraged the project in the first place and doggedly tried to read the unreadable. I very much appreciate the time and specialist advice given by Linda Auty, Biddy Unsworth, Alison Caswell and Mike Alexander.

Special mention and thanks are due to Tony Parker for his many excellent line drawings and patience with my inconsistency and changes of mind.

In some cases complete strangers gave illustrations for the book unhesitatingly. My thanks are due to Dr J. E. Aaron, Dr K. Waters, Eileen Padmore, Professor D.W. Purdie, Dr E. Kuipers, Dr G.J.S. Parkin, Dr U.M. Sivananthan and Dr B.J. Snow.

Invaluable advice was given by the many specialist reviewers of individual chapters. I gratefully acknowledge the comments made by Professor Gavin Reynolds, Dr Nick Francis of the Department of Histopathology, Charing Cross Hospital, Dr Kevin West, Department of Pathology, Leicester Royal Infirmary, Dr William Roche of the Department of Pathology, Southampton General Hospital, Professor D. Neary, Department of Neurology, Manchester Royal Infirmary, Dr S. Gallagher, Consultant Physician at the Southern General Hospital, Glasgow, Dr Andrew Payne, Queen Margaret College, University of Edinburgh and Dr Stephen Humphreys, Department of Histopathology, King's College Hospital. Many others remain anonymous. Their advice was a little hard to take at times but, although I might initially have thought them cruel, I came to realise that they were in fact kind. A big thank you, therefore, to all my mentors, seen and unseen, past and present, who have done so much to sharpen my work.

I am grateful to the following, who granted permission to reproduce copyright material: The Editors of *The Lancet* and *New England Journal of Medicine*, Blackwell Scientific Publishers, Churchill Livingstone and the Royal Society of Medicine. Some of the chapters are derived from material previously published under my name in *The British Journal of Biomedical Sciences* and *Medical Laboratory Sciences*, for which permission has kindly been granted.

The use of Microsoft® and Corel® clip-art is hereby acknowledged.

How to use the book

This book contains a variety of features designed to enhance the learning experience and enable readers to monitor their progress.

Learning aids

Comments

Comments appear in the margin to pick out the main theme or features in adjacent paragraphs.

Comments here relate to the next section of text

Glossary

Some of the scientific and medical terms used in the book you may not have encountered before. A brief explanation or definition of these terms will be given in the margin where appropriate.

Glossary: descriptions of medical or scientific terms appear in this format.

Point/counterpoint

Occasionally information is presented which remains controversial, usually because definitive scientific investigation is not possible, is very complicated or has not yet been completed. Experts often argue over the meaning of results and, rather than present an 'averaged' or consensus opinion, the two sides of the argument are presented as points and counterpoints. It is hoped that this will help readers to see both sides of these and other arguments.

Key points

Key point boxes are provided at intervals to reinforce the essential points of information. They consist of concise, single-line notes, much like those a tutor would use as an *aide-mémoire* when lecturing. A slightly different format is used to summarise the salient features of population studies or controlled clinical trials.

▲ **Key points**

Features of key points

▲ Concise summary of information
▲ Symbols are used in the heading to indicate population studies or controlled clinical trials

Monitoring progress

Pre-test questions

Pre-test questions are intended to ascertain your current state of knowledge, opinions or preconceptions. They are 'signposts', indicating the issues that will be discussed in the chapter. After studying the chapter you should be able to check back and see how much you have learned.

Pre-test

Review questions

Review questions appear at intervals to help you revise and assimilate the information given. Occasionally review questions attempt to tease out additional information, drawing on your experience, on information from other chapters or on wider reading of the subject. Answers are provided at the end of each chapter.

Activities

Activities draw on the skills of synthesis and analysis. Examples include case studies in which specific questions are related to problems in the history, questionnaires or collation and extrapolation of data.

1   Epidemiology

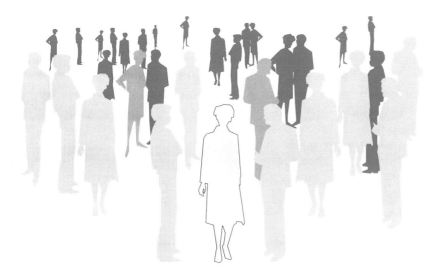

Epidemiological methods are used to investigate and monitor disease, with the aims of determining causation and limiting spread in the population. The frequency of disease is established by observational studies that determine the number of new cases arising (incidence), the number of cases in existence (prevalence) and the mortality rate. The observation of other trends occurring at the same time can give clues as to what factors might influence the cause or spread of disease. Observational data are also used to determine public health policy for preventing or treating a particular disease.

To establish cause it is necessary to investigate characteristics in individuals. One way of doing this is to establish exposure to possible aetiological agents in people with disease (cases), and compare them with people who do not have the disease (controls). An alternative approach is to identify people without disease but who have been exposed to a possible aetiological agent and compare them with people who have not been exposed. If the agent is of any importance in the disease aetiology it would be expected that more cases would appear in the exposed group than in the unexposed group.

A further investigative method is to apply some sort of intervention and measure how it affects the spread or effects of disease. The classic example of such an experimental study is the randomised controlled clinical trial used to evaluate a new treatment. Interventions designed to prevent disease such as vaccination or screening are also evaluated by epidemiological methods.

Aims of this chapter

By the end of this chapter you will have increased your knowledge of:
- ◆ The approaches used to monitor the spread of disease
- ◆ The methods used for investigating the cause of disease
- ◆ How approaches designed to prevent disease or lessen its impact can be evaluated

In addition, this chapter will help you to:
- ◆ Understand the role of observational studies in providing information about the distribution of disease, and clues about factors that influence their spread or severity
- ◆ Describe the ways in which data relating to disease frequency can be expressed and compared
- ◆ Describe the types of analytical studies and how they can be used to isolate causative agents or risk factors by their association with disease in individuals and populations
- ◆ Distinguish between case-control and cohort studies and the inherent differences in the validity of these approaches
- ◆ Understand the situations in which experimental studies can be used to confirm the relationships between causative factors and disease, or the effects of strategies designed to prevent or treat disease

Introduction

It is no accident that this book begins with a chapter on epidemiology. Without epidemiological methods we would have only a rudimentary understanding of what causes disease, how diseases are spread, and what measures can be taken to contain them. In short, it would not be possible to write a book called *Understanding Disease*, or discuss the issues implied in the subtitle *Pathology and Prevention*, without recourse to epidemiology.

What is epidemiology?

Epidemiologists are detectives on the trail of disease. The methods used help us understand how diseases evolve and spread and, in turn, this information can give clues about how particular diseases are caused. For example, malaria is usually found only in tropical climates: people in northern Europe do not develop this disease unless they have spent some time abroad. This indicates that there is something about the tropical environment that is conducive to the disease. We now know that the malarial parasite is transmitted by the malarial mosquito, and that this particular species of mosquito does not survive in cold climates.

Epidemiologists initially concerned themselves with infectious diseases that were the most prominent causes of death at the time. A classic epidemiological study was conducted by the English physician John Snow,

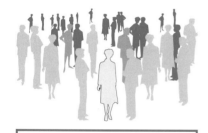

Epidemiology is the study of the incidence and distribution of diseases and conditions that influence their spread and severity

Epidemiology is used to trace the source of a disease

who found that people who suffered from cholera in the 1849 London epidemic mostly lived in the immediate area of the Broad Street pump. He established that nearly all the people who had died from cholera had consumed water from that pump. As a consequence of his investigations the pump was shut down, preventing a fresh outbreak of the disease.

Epidemic: a dramatic increase above the usual (endemic) or expected rate of occurrence of a particular disease or event in a population.

Modern epidemiologists are still involved in tracing the sources of infectious disease: finding the source of food poisoning is a common example. Even in recent times mysterious 'new' diseases have appeared for which the cause needed to be identified in order to contain its spread. One example is the finding of a previously unknown micro-organism called *Legionella pneumophila*. This was responsible for an epidemic of fatal pneumonia at an American Legion convention in Philadelphia in 1976. From this association the condition acquired the label Legionnaires' disease. We now know from epidemiological investigation of this and other outbreaks in different parts of the world that the organism has a widespread distribution, but is found particularly in standing or tepid water. Human infections are caused by inhalation of contaminated airborne water droplets, and in the original outbreak the source was traced to a contaminated water-cooled air conditioning system in the convention hotel. Recognition of the source of the organism means that measures can be taken to sterilise and monitor the water, thereby preventing further infections.

Another recently discovered infectious disease is toxic shock syndrome, a potentially fatal staphylococcal infection. Epidemiological methods were used to trace the source of the infection to tampon use by menstruating women. Perhaps of greater notoriety is the outbreak, during the late 1970s, of a disease which caused unexplained symptoms of swollen glands, high fever and fatigue in young American men. These men soon died from infection or rare cancers. We now know that the cause of their symptoms was HIV infection and that they had died from AIDS. Epidemiological methods played a fundamental part in recognising the disease for what it is, tracing its spread and mode of transmission, identifying who is at risk and the measures that should be taken to prevent further spread.

Apart from AIDS, some of the most pressing public health problems facing modern societies are the chronic diseases such as coronary heart disease and cancers. No single agent is responsible for their aetiology, and the diseases are said to be **multifactorial** in origin. With a single-cause infectious disease such as cholera, most people exposed to the aetiological agent will develop the disease unless they had built up resistance from previous exposure or immunisation. However, it is much more difficult to unravel the causes of multifactorial diseases because of the cumulative effects of the different agents involved. It becomes difficult to isolate the individual factors and to assess their relative importance in contributing to the disease.

It can be very difficult to isolate causative factors in multifactorial diseases

For example, the cause of most common cancers is a combination of genetic, environmental and behavioural factors but not all of these factors will be of the same relative importance with respect to development of the disease. In lung cancer, smoking is of fundamental importance, but not all smokers

Aetiology: pertaining to how a disease is caused.

develop lung cancer, presumably because some have a genetic protection. Things become even more difficult when trying to identify more diffuse cancer agents such as those that might be present in the diet: there is substantial variation in people's diets. Virtually everybody will be exposed to the agent at some time or other, and an agent that might be influential in causing cancer in one individual will have no effect in someone else.

Epidemiology is also used to evaluate interventions designed to prevent or treat disease, by comparing people given the intervention or treatment with others who have not received the intervention or who are left untreated. Not surprisingly, ethical problems are often associated with this approach; there are those who say that if a new and apparently effective treatment is devised it should not be withheld from those who need it but without proper epidemiological trials and analysis it is difficult to be certain how good the treatment is.

It is also necessary to determine the extent of disease so that adequate prevention or treatment strategies can be formulated and properly resourced. The principal prevention strategies that require epidemiological evaluation are immunisation and screening programmes.

These applications naturally follow each other: a disease cannot be properly prevented or treated until it is known who is affected, who is likely to be affected, and what factors are responsible for causing the disease. A variety of epidemiological methods have evolved to undertake these tasks, categorised as **observational, analytical** and **experimental** studies.

What are the methods used in epidemiology?

The first task is to acquire information about the people affected by the disease in question, at what time and where. In other words, epidemiology is the study of interactions between **time, people** and **place**. Comparisons are made in whole populations, cataloguing any variation in time or place. Next, comparisons are made in individuals, cataloguing and analysing any differences in disease or exposure to agents that might cause disease (Figure 1.1).

These seemingly straightforward tasks are not always as simple as they sound because the information available is often unreliable. Problems occur first in obtaining an accurate count of the disease frequency and secondly in being able to accurately diagnose the disease. While we may criticise the British National Health Service, it does theoretically reach everybody. In a remote corner of Africa there may not be anyone available to diagnose and report a disease – causing obvious difficulties when trying to make comparisons of disease frequencies in different parts of the world.

This is not only a problem with remote geographical areas. For example, people in the USA may not refer themselves for medical attention because of the costs involved and will therefore not be recorded. There are also geographical differences in the technology and expertise available for diagnosing disease. This can lead to relative over-recording in a certain area if a particularly enthusiastic specialist is adept at recognising a specific disease.

Observational studies provide clues about what agents might be important in the causation of disease

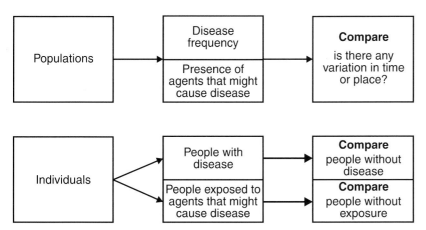

Figure 1.1 Epidemiological approaches. Epidemiological methods are used to measure differences in disease frequency, agents that might cause disease, in time or place. Population trends are used to monitor the spread of disease and to obtain clues as to why a disease spreads in a particular manner. The cause of disease, and the effects of any intervention designed to prevent or treat disease, can be established only by finding out what is going on in individuals. People with disease are compared with people who do not have the disease, and people exposed to a possibly harmful agent are compared with those who have not been exposed.

The gathering and analysis of data concerning disease frequency is known as an **observational** or **descriptive** study: you simply look at what is going on around you. Sometimes the data collected about a disease can be related to other events taking place in the same location at about the same time. In the UK cancer cases are notified to a central registry, and the cause of all deaths recorded. It is thus possible to view trends in the changing prevalence of the disease over time. The principal cause of lung cancer is now recognised as smoking, but in the 1950s this was less certain. At this time a marked increase in deaths from lung cancer among men, but not women, had been recorded. It became a matter of priority to seek an explanation for these events (Figure 1.2).

One possible explanation was provided by the observation that the per capita consumption of cigarettes had increased. Closer examination revealed that the cigarettes were consumed mostly by men – at the time it was not socially acceptable for women to smoke. Of course this did not prove that cigarette smoking actually caused lung cancer: a connection was simply made between two events. It could equally be the case that people were more exposed to industrial air pollution. Women, who were more likely at this time to remain in the home, would have been less exposed than the working man. As it turned out this was not the case, but to establish cause and effect further lines of study are necessary.

To do this properly, it is necessary to find out what is going on in individuals, using an **analytical** method (Figure 1.3). One way is to evaluate differences in people who have the disease and compare them with those who do not. In this **case-control** approach the people with lung cancer should be reasonably well

An analytical study is designed to test a hypothesis about the disease and exposure relationship

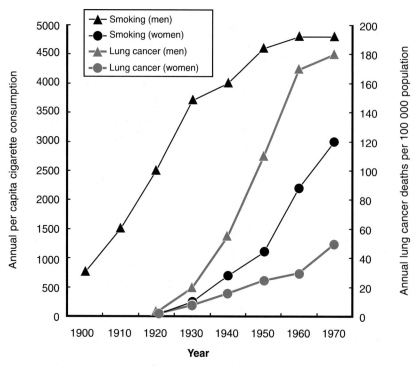

Figure 1.2 Trends in cigarette smoking and lung cancer (England and Wales). The increase in cigarette smoking since the turn of the century has been followed by an increase in deaths from lung cancer. In men, increased lung cancer deaths were most marked from the middle of the century onwards. Cigarette smoking did not become socially acceptable for women until the second world war, but this was followed by an increase in deaths from lung cancer some years later. (Data from Cairns, J. (1975) Smoking prevalence and lung cancer. *Scientific American*.)

matched with the controls for variables such as age, gender and socioeconomic group. The case-control approach works well only where agents are very influential in causing a disease: not everyone who smokes will necessarily get lung cancer; conversely some non-smokers will develop lung cancer. Essentially, the case-control approach is historical: the search is for differences in previous events between people with the disease and those who do not have the disease. It also helps to have some idea as to which previous events may be important, and this is where the connections made between trends in cigarette consumption and lung cancer made by observational studies came in useful.

An alternative approach is to observe people who are exposed to a possible harmful agent such as cigarette smoking, and wait to see what happens to them compared with people who do not smoke. If the information obtained from observational and case-control studies was correct, it could be expected that more smokers would develop lung cancer than non-smokers. In epidemiology, this approach represents another analytical method known as a **cohort** study.

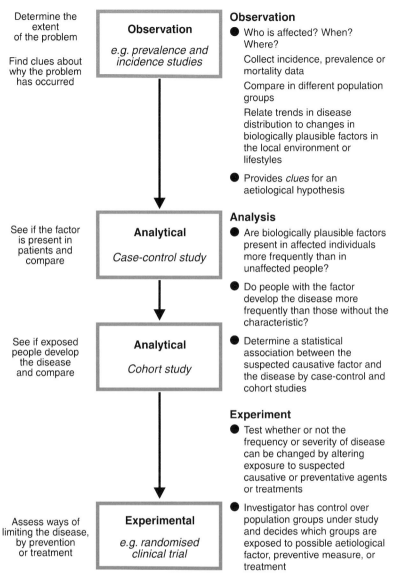

Determine the extent of the problem	**Observation** *e.g. prevalence and incidence studies*

See if the factor is present in patients and compare	**Analytical** *Case-control study*

See if exposed people develop the disease and compare	**Analytical** *Cohort study*

Assess ways of limiting the disease, by prevention or treatment	**Experimental** *e.g. randomised clinical trial*

Observation
- Who is affected? When? Where?

  Collect incidence, prevalence or mortality data

  Compare in different population groups

  Relate trends in disease distribution to changes in biologically plausible factors in the local environment or lifestyles

- Provides *clues* for an aetiological hypothesis

Analysis
- Are biologically plausible factors present in affected individuals more frequently than in unaffected people?

- Do people with the factor develop the disease more frequently than those without the characteristic?

- Determine a statistical association between the suspected causative factor and the disease by case-control and cohort studies

Experiment
- Test whether or not the frequency or severity of disease can be changed by altering exposure to suspected causative or preventative agents or treatments

- Investigator has control over population groups under study and decides which groups are exposed to possible aetiological factor, preventive measure, or treatment

Figure 1.3 The epidemiological approach. The logical sequence of epidemiology is to find out how common a disease is, or how many people die from it, and to relate this to other events going on at the same time. This gives clues as to what might be important in causing changes in incidence, prevalence or mortality. These factors can be further investigated by case-control and cohort studies. It may then be appropriate to conduct experimental studies, perhaps designed to limit exposure to causative agents and therefore prevent the disease, or to test new drugs. In practice this sequence is not necessarily followed. It is not necessary to know how many people are affected by a disease, or its cause, before a new drug is tested. At some point, however, a drug company would want to know the potential market for its product. Although there are many effective drugs that work empirically without knowing how the disease is caused, knowledge of aetiology helps in the rational design of new drugs.

▲ Key points

Observational studies

- ▲ Observation of differences in disease frequency between communities may help identify suspected causes

- ▲ Provides information to test aetiological hypotheses and substantiate clinical suspicions

- ▲ Evaluate and monitor the extent of disease

- ▲ Determine public health policy to limit spread or treat disease

Epidemiological evidence about causation is often circumstantial and incomplete, but is a guide to action

Experimental studies involve the deliberate exposure of subjects to agents or procedures that may affect the course of disease

At the end of these studies a much clearer picture of the relationship between lung cancer and cigarette smoking can be obtained, but caution is still needed before saying that smoking actually causes lung cancer. It could be that stress actually causes lung cancer and that people who are stressed may be more likely to smoke (although this is somewhat less plausible). In other words, it can be difficult to untangle events that are going on at the same time or are connected with each other. However, one more strategy, known as the **experimental approach,** is available to the epidemiologist.

There are several sorts of experimental studies. All involve exposing people or laboratory animals to agents or procedures that might cause or prevent disease or be effective in treatment. Animals are often used because it is considered unethical to use humans, although there are many who would say with some justification that it is equally unacceptable to use animals for these purposes. Leaving these issues aside, there are certain advantages and disadvantages to using animals. One advantage is that it is possible to examine the effects of agents in a controlled laboratory environment, without interference from other factors that may confound the effects on disease. It would, for example, be possible to control the diet, temperature, and living conditions of animals in ways that would be unacceptable to many human subjects. A disadvantage is that other species often respond in different ways to humans because of differences in their physiology and lifespan, so that it can be difficult to know how much reliance to place on the results.

One classic experimental study using human subjects concerned the effect of fluoride in drinking water. Dentists had observed that people with mottled teeth tended to require fewer fillings than others. It became evident that the mottling of teeth was associated with high levels of fluoride in drinking water. A wide variety of other factors could be responsible for geographic differences in tooth decay, not least of which would be sugar consumption. After all the available evidence had been examined it was decided to conduct an epidemiological experiment, in which the fluoride levels of some reservoirs would be topped-up with fluoride to match the concentrations seen in high-fluoride areas, while other low-fluoride reservoirs would be left alone. Despite the simple elegance of this study it was fraught with difficulties. One problem was that of ascertainment, in deciding who had tooth decay and needed fillings or extractions and who did not – there is a marked variation among dentists when it comes to making this decision. The other difficulty concerns the sample population: it appears that if fluoride exposure is to have any effect at all it must begin at a very early age and continue for many years. This places severe constraints on the size of the population available for comparison.

The whole issue of water fluoridation remains clouded with controversy. It may not be effective in every adult who drinks the water and there is debate about whether people should be 'force-fed', and have to pay for, things they do not necessarily want or need.

The most commonly applied experimental study is the **randomised clinical trial**. This is of absolute importance for evaluating any treatment that will be used to prevent or treat disease. When used to evaluate a treatment, a random sample of a population with the disease are given the new drug, and outcomes are compared with a control group given the old treatment or placebo.

Placebo: an inert substance or 'sham' treatment.

Observational studies

Case studies

Case studies are all about accumulating data relating to the frequency of disease in particular populations and locations. The first inkling that a new disease has evolved, or that an outbreak of disease is under way can be on a very small scale, through the description of a single interesting or unusual case, or small series of cases. These descriptions are known as **case reports** or **case series**. At this stage a simple observation has been made, and the next step is to see whether the observation has also been made in other people. This is the mechanism by which we first became aware of AIDS (see Chapter 25).

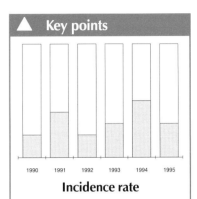

▲ **Key points**

Incidence rate

- ▲ Proportion of a defined population group developing a condition within a stated period
- ▲ Measured by longitudinal study
- ▲ Incidence rate is the total number of disease episodes regardless of whether they affect the same or different individuals

Disease frequency

The frequency of disease can be estimated in several ways. In the living it is measured either as **incidence** or **prevalence**. The incidence of a disease refers to the number of new cases that arise in a defined period of time, divided by the number of people in the population at risk. Hence a single individual who contracts the same disease twice (as a new event, not a recurrence) would be counted twice in incidence statistics. The incidence of a disease is usually expressed as cases per 100 000 population per year.

Another way of expressing the number of events is in person years, which is the product of the number of people observed and the period of observation. Hence, 10 000 people observed over a period of 1 year is equivalent, in person years, to 1000 people observed over a period of 10 years.

The prevalence of a disease is determined by a **cross-sectional** study of the population during a defined period (**period prevalence**) or a single point in time (**point prevalence**). It measures all cases of disease in existence and is usually expressed as a percentage of the number of people sampled. Incidence rates and prevalence rates will be quite different and depend on the nature of the disease. For chronic incurable diseases such as multiple sclerosis the prevalence figure will always be larger than the incidence figure, since all of those cases that were incident in previous years will accumulate and will become depleted only by death. With acute diseases that resolve quickly, the incidence figure is likely to be larger than the prevalence figure. Cross-sectional studies are also directed towards linking disease trends with the prevalence of other biologically plausible agents that could be involved in disease causation.

Cross-sectional studies provide a snapshot of events occurring in a defined time

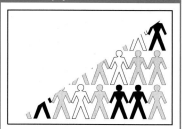
The standardised mortality ratio (SMR) is an index that adjusts for differences in population age structure

Mortality data

Mortality data can be flawed and may not reflect the true frequency of disease for several reasons. First, it is entirely feasible that a person can have a disease, say cancer, and yet die of something else, for example coronary heart disease. If the disease has a very poor survival rate, as is in the case in certain types of cancer, then the mortality figures will provide a more accurate reflection, provided the disease has been accurately identified. During life this can be difficult, and a definitive cause of death may be established only by performing post-mortem examination. However, post mortems are very rare, particularly in less developed countries.

For these reasons, it may be preferable to look at the available incidence data but this too has its pitfalls, the two main sources of error being incomplete ascertainment and misclassification. Misclassification can easily arise through errors of clinical or pathological diagnosis; in many conditions the signs or symptoms are not clear-cut or resemble other disease entities.

Adjustment and standardisation

When recording the frequency of disease it is usual to divide, or **stratify**, the population into age groups (0-9, 10-19, 20-29, 30-39 years and so on). This will give an idea of which groups of the population are liable to develop a particular disease. However, this can give a misleading impression since the various age categories will not be evenly distributed across the population (Figure 1.4). A more accurate impression for each age group will be gained by taking into account the number of people in each group (Figure 1.5).

The make-up of populations differs greatly with geographical location. For example, the age distribution of a population at a seaside town on the south coast of England will be much older than that of a cosmopolitan city such as Liverpool because people often retire to such places. Similarly, the proportion of older people in the populations of developed countries is higher than in less developed countries. Hence, the overall mortality rates for a disease such as prostate cancer (which predominantly affects older men) can appear to be different even when no real difference exists, simply because the composition of the population is different.

This problem is overcome by **standardisation**, whereby a mathematical adjustment is made so that the proportion of a particular subgroup (for example men aged 65-74) is made identical for each of the populations to be compared. The result gives the **standardised mortality ratio (SMR)** between the populations.

- A standard population is selected, to give the number of expected deaths
- Age-specific mortality rates of the two groups being compared are applied to the number in the same age groups in the standard population
- Calculation gives the number of deaths that could be expected in the standard population if the age-specific rates had prevailed
- If observed mortality in the specific population is the same as that expected the SMR will equal 100

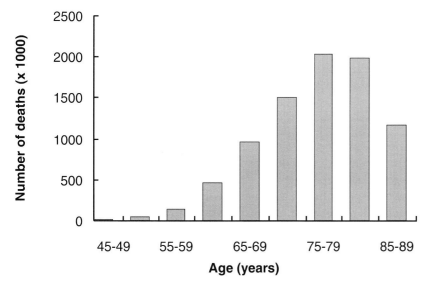

Figure 1.4 Number of deaths from prostate cancer, England and Wales, 1992. In absolute numbers, most deaths from prostate cancer occur in men aged 75-79. However this is not an accurate reflection of the risk of dying from prostate cancer, since the number of men in each age category is different. (Source: OPCS.)

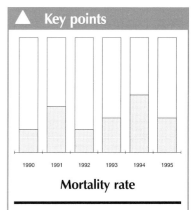

Key points

Mortality rate

▲ Form of incidence rate in which the event related to disease is death

▲ Can be calculated for any defined period of time

▲ Since few diseases are invariably fatal, mortality gives a distorted picture of disease frequency

OPCS: in England and Wales mortality statistics and, for some specified notifiable diseases, incidence data, are collated and published by the Office of Population Censuses and Surveys.

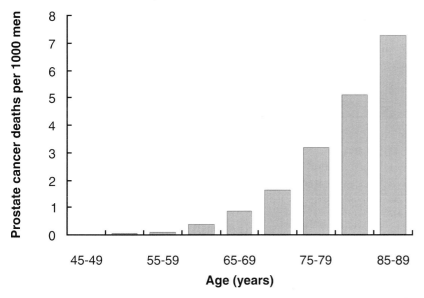

Figure 1.5 Age-adjusted death rates from prostate cancer, England and Wales 1992. When adjusted for age (by dividing the number of deaths by the number of men in each category) it becomes apparent that the risk of dying from prostate cancer increases with age. In Figure 1.4 the decline in prostate cancer deaths after age 79 is simply because there are fewer older men in the population. (Source: OPCS.)

Review question 1

Give some possible reasons why the true frequency of a disease may not be properly known.

- If mortality is high in the specific population the SMR will be greater than 100

Migration studies

The examination of disease frequency in different populations in different parts of the world can reveal useful information about the importance of environmental factors in producing disease: if a disease is common in one country but very rare in another it is reasonable to suspect that some geographically dependent environmental factors are at least partly responsible. The other possibility is that the genetic pool of the population in different countries is not the same, and it is this that contributes to differences in disease frequency. One way of sorting out the relative contributions of genetic and environmental factors is by examining what happens to disease frequency when people migrate from one country to another (Figure 1.6).

Review question 2

What do the data in Figure 1.6 suggest about the relative contributions of genetic and environmental factors in stomach, liver and colonic cancers?

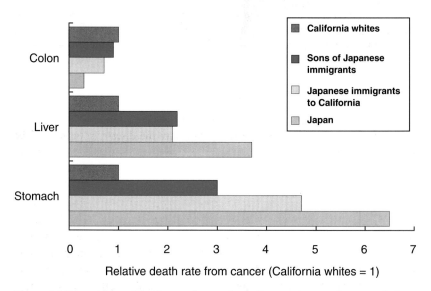

Figure 1.6 Comparison of death rates from colonic, liver and stomach cancers in host and immigrant populations.

Analytical studies

The case-control approach

The case-control approach aims to find differences in previous exposures to potential risk factors in diseased and unaffected groups of people (Figure 1.7). The method relies on the study of case notes, the use of a questionnaire or, in occupational studies, factory records.

Cases   Controls

Case-control studies compare the histories of people who have a disease with similar people who are unaffected

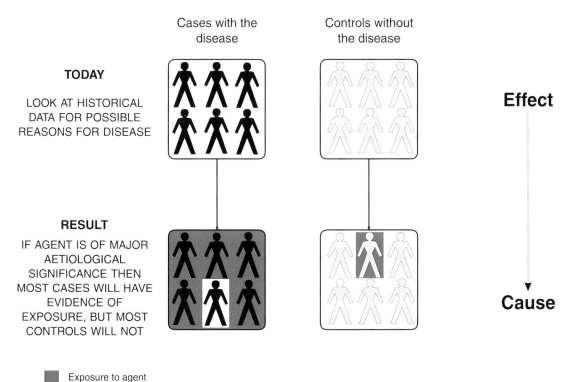

Figure 1.7 The case-control approach. In case-control studies people with a disease are compared with similar people who do not have the disease in question. The approach is essentially historical, working backwards from the effect (the disease) to try and find the cause.

Many chronic diseases exhibit a very long lag phase before exposure to an aetiological agent becomes evident as symptomatic disease. An indication of this may be seen in the observational study of the trends between cigarette consumption and lung cancer: for men no increase in deaths from lung cancer was seen until 20 or 30 years after the increase in cigarette smoking. In some circumstances later disease is related not to exposure of the affected individual, but to exposure of a parent. An example is the development of vaginal cancer in young women whose mothers had taken stilboestrol during pregnancy.

It is not surprising that when seeking data from many years previously, or data relating to parental exposure, inaccuracies creep in. The situation is compounded when the affected person has died and the information has to be supplied by proxy. The task is easier when the disease is caused by an easily identifiable agent such as cigarette smoking, although there remains a difficulty with patients who embroider the truth by seeking to avoid giving a 'bad' reply.

Sometimes a person genuinely does not know or remember that they have been exposed to causative factors. This is often the case when trying to correlate dietary factors to disease. Not only are there historical changes related to the availability and costs of foods, but there can also be changes in behaviour: a patient will very often alter a wide variety of lifestyle behaviours on receiving

> *A large study reduces the influence of chance, but not bias*

a diagnosis of a life-threatening illness. In contrast, people with serious illnesses may recall their past exposures more completely, as they have attempted to seek explanations for their condition. Control subjects who do not have the disease may find it more difficult to recall exposure accurately because it is less important and has less meaning for them. These inaccuracies are referred to as **recall bias**.

Some of these problems can be minimised by using a large sample size. This overcomes chance effects, although inherent bias will remain whatever the sample size. The sample size required is also related to the strength of the aetiological agent: a weak agent will not be revealed in a small sample.

For example, it would be necessary to take only a small sample of 1000 cases and controls to see significant differences in rates of lung cancer between smokers and non-smokers. It is now known that about 90% of lung cancer is caused by smoking, and that the prevalence of smoking in men in the UK over the past 30 years was about 30%. Therefore, if a case-control study was conducted today it could be expected that in a sample of 1000 patients with lung cancer approximately 900 would be smokers. The control group should reflect the overall prevalence of smokers, but with a slight reduction because of concentration of smokers into the case group; there should be slightly fewer than 300 smokers in a control group of 1000 people currently unaffected by lung cancer. Comparison of these data can be used to calculate the **odds ratio** for lung cancer in the two groups according to the following table:

		Disease	
		Present	*Absent*
Factor	Present	A	B
	Absent	C	D
		(A + C total cases)	(B + D total controls)

A = cases who were exposed;
B = controls who were exposed;
C = cases who were not exposed;
D = controls who were not exposed

The probability of the cases being exposed is calculated as a proportion of the total cases:

$$\frac{A}{A + C}$$

Similarly, the probability that the cases were not exposed is calculated as a proportion of the total cases:

$$\frac{C}{A + C}$$

The likelihood of exposure for the cases is calculated by dividing the probability that a case was exposed by the probability that a case was not exposed:

$$\frac{\dfrac{A}{A + C}}{\dfrac{C}{A + C}} \qquad = \qquad \frac{A}{C}$$

A similar calculation can be made for the controls, so that the likelihood of exposure is given by:

$$\frac{B}{D}$$

The odds ratio is calculated by dividing the likelihood of exposure among the cases by the likelihood of exposure among the controls:

$$\frac{A}{C} \qquad \text{divided by} \qquad \frac{B}{D}$$

The advantages of case-control studies are that they are relatively inexpensive to conduct and can be completed quickly. To examine the effects of cigarette smoking on lung cancer in a prospective cohort study (see page 19) would require a wait of 30–40 years for all the cancers to develop. It would probably also require a larger sample size to obtain statistically significant results, since only a minority of the smokers would develop lung cancer. The case-control approach is also useful for the study of rare diseases: it would take an impossibly large sample size to study a disease with a frequency of one in 1000 people by means of a cohort study.

The case-control study design is not without some drawbacks. First, questions must be asked about the accuracy of historical information. Many chronic diseases take years to develop from the original exposures to an aetiological agent, yet the case-control study seeks to discover the nature of this agent. With some agents, such as smoking, it is fairly easy for a person to remember whether he or she smoked 20 years ago, but to remember how many cigarettes were smoked daily is a little more difficult. With some other factors, perhaps agents in the diet, it can be difficult to separate out one agent from the hundreds of food items consumed. Some people may not even be consciously aware of gradual dietary changes made over decades.

There may also be problems in defining cases and controls. Very often 'cases' will be defined as people with a particular disease which was diagnosed by a certain combination of clinical and investigative procedures. There will, of course, be differences in diagnostic criteria in various centres, and over time as new diagnostic methods become available. Provided all the cases are derived from one centre, or from centres with similar facilities, at a similar

Review question 3

Calculate the odds ratio for cigarette smoking and lung cancer, given that there were 900 smokers in 1000 cases of lung cancer, and 250 smokers in a control group of 1000 people.

time, this source of bias would be small. But what of the controls? Very often controls are selected at random, or to deliberately represent characteristics of the cases (such as age, socioeconomic group or gender). They will be asked to co-operate in the study, which might consist of answering a questionnaire.

How are the controls defined as being free of the disease under investigation? A common disease such as coronary heart disease takes a long time to develop and is likely to be present in many of the controls even if it the person is unaware of it. There are very few published epidemiological studies in which control populations have been asked to submit to invasive procedures to detect asymptomatic disease, so that they can truly qualify as 'controls'. This is much less of a problem when dealing with rare diseases.

Cohort studies

A cohort study is used to detect new events (for example production of disease symptoms) that occur in a population group exposed to an agent or other characteristic over a period of time. During the study new cases of disease will arise in both the exposed and non-exposed groups: the study compares the **incidence** of disease in both groups (Figure 1.8).

The problem of bias in information recall encountered in case-control studies can be avoided in the prospective cohort approach, because there is an opportunity at the beginning of the study to record exposures as and when they occur. People destined to become cases will not know this at the outset. This can create additional problems, since all the subjects in the study are volunteers and the job of recording can become rather tedious. It may be necessary to conduct biological checks of exposure, for example by measurement of metabolites of the exposed agents in blood or urine. Whether this is possible depends on the nature of the agent sought, and there can also be a problem of compliance when it comes to getting the samples for analysis.

Prospective studies very often take a long time to complete: it is the very nature of the study that time has to elapse before disease develops. In the prospective cohort study of the relationship between cigarette smoking and lung cancer the most definitive results became available after 40 years of study. It would not be surprising if during this time some of the participants became bored with completing questionnaires and were lost to follow-up. However, sufficient time must be allowed for all the subjects who are going to develop the disease to do so.

The prospective cohort design is not suited to the study of very rare diseases, for example those with a frequency of less than one in 1000. The problem is that for statistically significant differences to be observed in exposed and non-exposed groups the sample size would have to be enormous. Notwithstanding these difficulties, the prospective cohort approach is often regarded as being more reliable than the case-control approach in the analysis of common diseases, because of the (theoretically) greater reliance that can be placed on the exposure data.

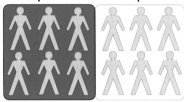

Exposed　　Unexposed

Cohort studies compare people who are exposed to a suspected aetiological or preventive agent with those who are not

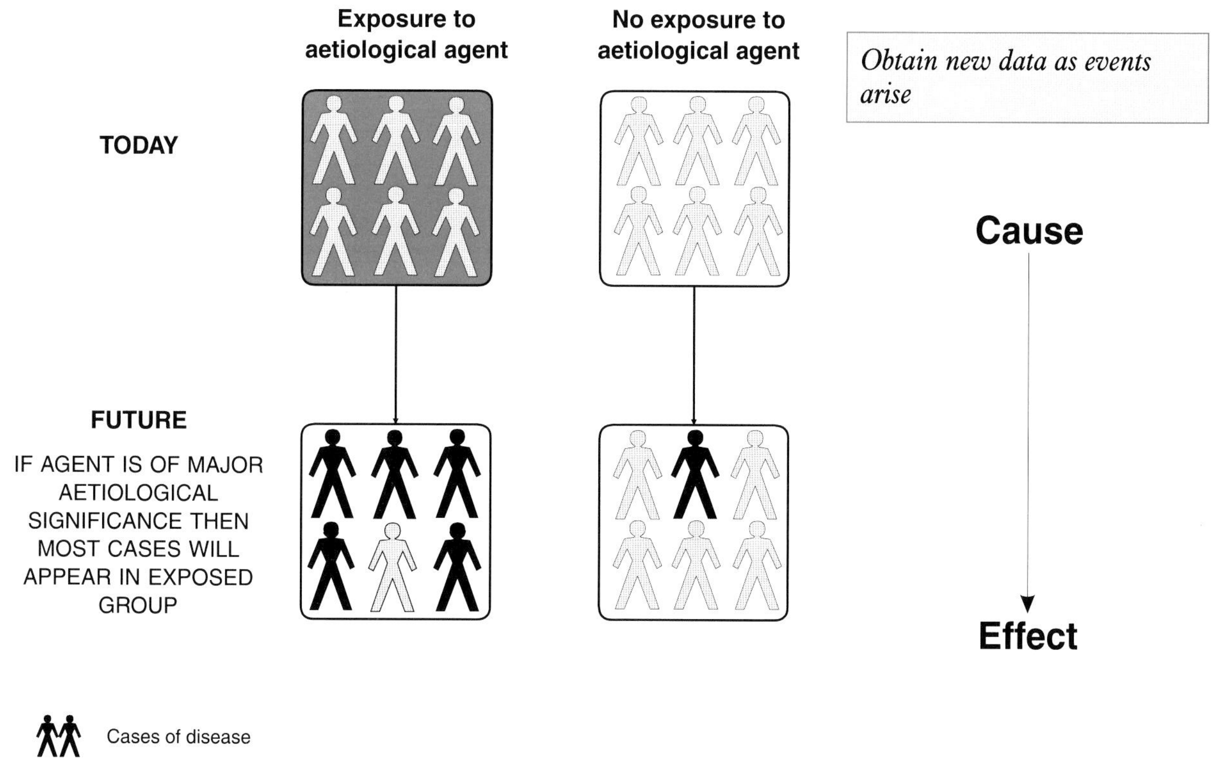

Cases of disease

Figure 1.8 In the prospective cohort study people who are exposed to a suspected aetiological agent are compared with similar people who are not exposed. The approach is one of 'wait and see', working from current exposures (cause) to future effects.

In cohort studies, calculation of the relative incidence of disease arising in the exposed and unexposed groups, or **relative risk**, is given by the formulae in the table below.

		Disease		
		Present	*Absent*	
Factor	Present	A	B	Total exposed cohort
	Absent	C	D	Total unexposed cohort

A = exposed people who develop disease;
B = exposed people who remain unaffected;
C = unexposed people who develop disease;
D = unexposed people who remain unaffected

The risk (R) of developing disease in exposed people is calculated as a proportion of the total exposed sample:

$$R \text{ (exposed)} \quad = \quad \frac{A}{A + B}$$

Similarly, the risk of developing disease in unexposed people is calculated as a proportion of the total unexposed sample:

$$R \text{ (unexposed)} \quad = \quad \frac{C}{C + D}$$

The relative risk attached to the exposure is calculated from the exposed and unexposed risk estimates:

$$\text{Relative risk} = \frac{R \text{ (exposed)}}{R \text{ (unexposed)}} \quad = \quad \frac{\dfrac{A}{A + B}}{\dfrac{C}{C + D}}$$

Table 1.1 Comparison of case-control and cohort studies

Case control studies	Cohort studies
Compare people with a disease and those without it	Compare people exposed to a suspected cause and those not exposed
Defines relative contribution of an aetiological influence to the total frequency of the disease	Defines attributable risk of developing disease following exposure
Study sequence is from effect to cause	Study sequence is from cause to effect
Allows calculation of odds ratio	Allows calculation of risk ratio
Usually retrospective, can be carried out swiftly and inexpensively	Usually prospective, expensive, may take many years for effects to develop
Useful for rare diseases	Impracticable for rare diseases
Inaccurate because of incomplete historical information and recall bias	Opportunity to record information accurately throughout study

Focus on case-control and prospective studies in lung cancer

The UK was one of the first countries to experience a rapid increase in the number of deaths attributable to lung cancer. Part of the increase was known to be because of better diagnostic methods, but by the late 1940s the increase in the deaths assumed alarming proportions. This initiated concerted studies into the possible reasons for lung cancer. The first such study, conducted by the two men widely regarded as the founders of modern-day epidemiology, Sir Austin Bradford Hill and Sir Richard Doll, began in 1948 as a case-control study in which the life histories of several hundred patients with lung cancer were compared with people who did not have the disease. At this time smoking history was only one of several possible causes investigated, although it was assumed that airborne factors were the most likely culprits (Doll originally believed the most likely reasons were the increase in motor vehicle emissions and fumes from the tarring of roads).

By 1950 it became apparent that the only single major difference between the cases and controls was cigarette smoking. Similar conclusions were reached by a parallel case-control study conducted in the USA, by Wynder and Graham (Figure 1.9; Wynder and Graham, 1950). The next step was to examine exposures to cigarette smoking by prospective studies. Again, parallel studies were established independently in the UK and the USA.

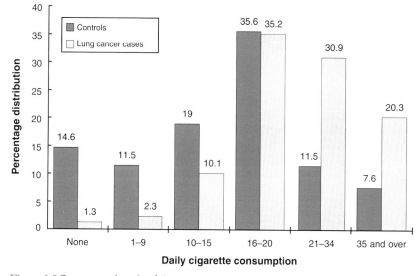

Figure 1.9 Case-control study of cigarette smoking and lung cancer in men. Comparison of lung cancer cases and controls shows that people with lung cancer are more likely to have a history of moderate or heavy smoking. Non-smokers are much more prevalent in the control group, and form a very small proportion of the patients with lung cancer. (Data from Wynder and Graham, 1950.)

The prospective study in the UK was started by Doll and Hill in 1951. Questionnaires asking for details of smoking habits were sent out to all doctors on the medical register resident in the UK. Replies were received from about three-quarters of all doctors, amounting to some 40 000 respondents (6194 women and 34 439 men). Further questionnaires were

Review question 4

What were the possible advantages and disadvantages of sending the questionnaire to all British doctors?

Review question 5

Would you expect the results after 20 years of follow-up to be very much the same as those obtained after 40 years?

sent out at regular intervals, and during the first 20 years 10 000 of the study participants had died (from all causes), as did another 10 000 over the next 20 years (Figure 1.10).

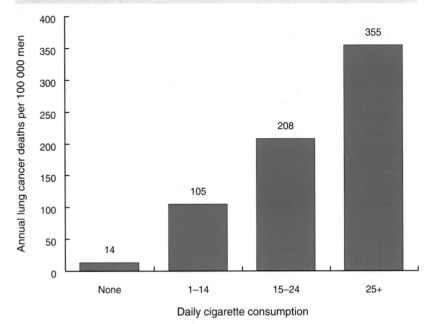

Figure 1.10 Cohort comparison of lung cancer mortality in male smokers and non-smokers. Deaths from lung cancer are more numerous in smokers than in non-smokers. Moreover, the mortality rate increases with the number of cigarettes smoked. (Data from Doll *et al.*, 1994.)

Activity 1

Data analysis

In the 40-year prospective study of mortality in relation to smoking (Doll *et al.*, 1994) the death rates were recorded for lung cancer and ischaemic heart disease, as shown in Table 1.2.

Table 1.2   Annual mortality per 100 000 men

	Non-smokers	Cigarette smokers (number of cigarettes smoked daily)		
		1–14	15–24	25 or more
Lung cancer	14	105	208	355
Heart disease	572	802	892	1025

The total exposed population (A + B) in each category is 100 000 men, as is the unexposed population of non-smokers (C + D).

1. What are the relative risk estimates for lung cancer in (a) men who

smoke 1–14 cigarettes a day and (b) men who smoke 25 or more cigarettes a day?
2. What are the relative risk estimates for ischaemic heart disease in (a) men who smoke 1–14 cigarettes a day and (b) men who smoke 25 or more cigarettes a day?
3. Why are the relative risk estimates different for (a) light and heavy smokers and (b) these two diseases?

In the 20-year prospective study of mortality in relation to smoking (Doll and Peto, 1976) the death rates shown in Table 1.3 were recorded for lung cancer and ischaemic heart disease.

Table 1.3   Annual mortality per 100 000 men

	Non-smokers	Cigarette smokers (number of cigarettes smoked daily)		
		1–14	15–24	25 or more
Lung cancer	10	52	106	224
Heart disease	717	843	973	1171

4. What are the relative risk estimates for lung cancer in (a) men who smoke 1–14 cigarettes a day and (b) men who smoke 25 or more cigarettes a day?
5. What are the relative risk estimates for ischaemic heart disease in (a) men who smoke 1–14 cigarettes a day and (b) men who smoke 25 or more cigarettes a day?
6. Explain any differences in your results.

Cause and effect

Several criteria are used for determining whether an observed association is actually instrumental in causing a disease. First, the correct **temporal sequence** must be observed: exposure to the agent must precede the development of the disease. Although it seems obvious, establishing this is not always easy. Many diseases display a long time lag before their symptoms become obvious and factors observed at the symptomatic stage of the disease are not necessarily the same as those that were present when the disease was initiated.

Probably causing most confusion is the fact that some factors can appear as a consequence of a disease. For example, evidence of infection with the Epstein–Barr virus is often found in patients suffering from rheumatoid arthritis, but this is thought more likely to arise as a consequence of the disease, due to altered immunity, rather than a causative factor.

Exposure must precede effect

> *A factor is more likely to be causal if its removal reduces the risk of disease*

Another criterion is based on the differences in disease frequency between exposed and unexposed groups. If the difference is large then greater confidence can be placed in assuming the agent is truly aetiological. This is described as the **strength of association**.

Ideally it would be best to establish a **dose–response** relationship. The risk of contracting lung cancer increases with the number of cigarettes smoked (Figure 1.11). Conversely, the risk decreases when a person stops smoking, and continues to fall the longer the person ceases to smoke (Figure 1.12). There is a dose–response relationship between the number of cigarettes smoked and the risk of death from lung cancer. Absence of a dose–response relationship does not preclude a causal relationship: some agents can exert a threshold effect above which there is no further effect.

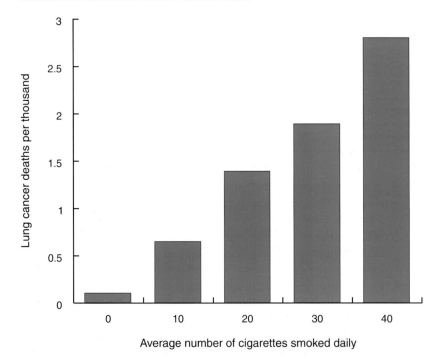

Figure 1.11 Relationship of lung cancer death rate and number of cigarettes smoked.

A further criterion is the **consistency** of the association. If researchers elsewhere record similar observations in different populations this is a good indication that the association is not spurious. Even so, caution is required because the same confounding factors can be present in different studies despite the use of different sample groups.

It also helps if there is some **coherence** across the different types of study, for example, an association observed in a case-control study design is more likely to be causative if it is also seen in cohort studies.

Finally, the relationship should be **biologically plausible**. In the case of cigarette smoking and cancer, it had already been known from animal experiments that certain chemicals behave as carcinogens and induce cancer.

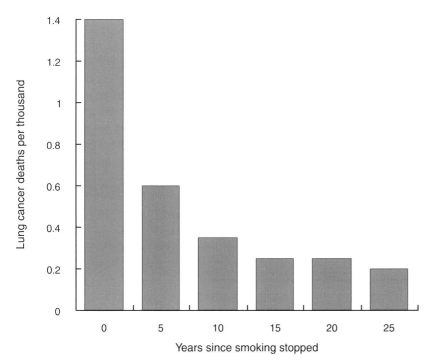

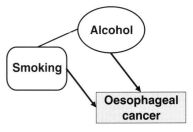

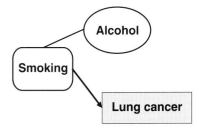

Figure 1.12 There are positive benefits in giving up smoking. After 15 years, death rates from lung cancer in ex-smokers are similar to those of people who have never smoked.

Bias: a non-random error leading to a distorted result. Usually caused by inherent differences in samples, methods of measurement, or interpretation which may apply selectively in one study group but not in another.

Statistical significance: a result is usually regarded as statistically significant if there is less than a 1 in 20 chance of a spurious association, giving a P value of <0.05 (the probability that the association is because of chance alone is less than 5 in 100). The possibility of chance association is reduced even further with P value of <0.01 (1 in 100 chance of a spurious association) but this degree of accuracy requires a much larger sample size.

Confounding: alcohol consumption and smoking are often linked, but either one, or both, of these agents can cause oesophageal cancer

No confounding: alcohol consumption and smoking are often linked, but only smoking causes lung cancer

It was then only a matter of identifying the same (or similar) agents as constituents of cigarette smoke. Other associations are plausible but more difficult to prove. For example, the reduced risk of colorectal cancer associated with fruit and vegetable consumption could be because of a wide variety of nutrient components, including 'fibre' and antioxidant vitamins present in the food. At least in this instance plausible hypotheses for the biological effects can be developed for either constituent.

Sometimes factors may display a truly significant association with a disease and yet have nothing to do with causing the disease. One commentator has pointed out that it would not be surprising if wearing *Levi 501* jeans was a statistically significant risk factor for AIDS, but this relationship is biologically implausible. The risk is there simply because young men, who form a higher risk group (in developed countries), are more likely to wear these jeans.

Even when all the above criteria are fulfilled it is necessary to consider whether an apparent causative association between an agent and disease is due to any other reason. These may be because of chance, incorrect methodology or indirect relationships involving some underlying **confounding factor**. For this reason the data are subjected to statistical analysis and the results expressed in terms of statistical significance. Although this analysis can be used to establish confidence that associations are not because of chance, no amount of statistical analysis can overcome inherent bias caused by poor methodological design, inadequate sampling or incorrect measurement. Bias

▲ Key points

Criteria for evaluation of a possible causal relationship

▲ Correct relationship in time

▲ Strength of association

▲ Consistency of association across studies in different populations

▲ Presence of a dose–response relationship

▲ Biological plausibility

▲ Coherence across various types of study

▲ Key points

Types and applications of experimental studies

Clinical trials: apply intervention to individual subjects

▲ Features random allocation of individuals into experimental (test) and control groups

▲ Evaluate drug in treatment of a disease

▲ Evaluate a prophylactic agent e.g. vaccine

▲ Evaluate a public health measure e.g. screening

Community trials (field experiments): apply intervention to communities

▲ Study a group of individuals as a whole to determine efficacy of an agent or procedure

can occur at any stage from the initial determination of cases and control groups to the analyses of results. Differences in measurement of what exactly constitutes exposure and disease or disease-free state are common sources of bias.

Sometimes a factor will become linked with a disease through its association with another factor. For example, both smoking and alcohol consumption are implicated as risk factors in certain chronic diseases. Very often these factors go hand in hand, so that the measurement of one is also a measure of the other; for example people who go to pubs are more likely to be smokers. These linked associations are known as confounding factors.

The confounding factor must independently cause the disease and not merely be associated with another exposure variable. For example, alcohol is a confounder in oesophageal cancer because both alcohol and smoking are causes of the disease. Conversely, although smoking causes lung cancer, alcohol does not and is not a confounding agent in studies of the relationship between smoking and lung cancer.

It is possible to disentangle these confounding factors by a process known as **matching**. For example, every smoker who drinks should be matched with a non-smoker who drinks. The matching of cases and controls for age and gender is almost universal, but the procedure becomes more cumbersome with each additional factor that needs to be matched: all subjects have to be screened for each of the criteria. Then, of course, it becomes impossible to assess the influence of the factor for which the subjects have been matched: what initially started as a desirable attribute may turn out to be a disadvantage.

Experimental studies

In an experimental study it is necessary to find individuals in a population who have not been exposed to the agent or procedure in question. This sample is randomly divided into two groups after matching characteristics such as age, gender, race or other factors believed to be of importance in the disease. One group is exposed to the intervention, the other group is not. Probably the most frequently used experimental study is the **controlled clinical trial**, designed to evaluate the effects of interventions which may limit the spread of disease or minimise its effects.

The purpose of a clinical trial is to weigh the effects of one type of intervention against another type or no intervention other than placebo. This method is essential for evaluating any new treatment and provides a quantitative estimate of how great or small the benefit of the new intervention is.

Primary prevention

Clinical trials are used to evaluate the effect of a preventive measure, such as a vaccine, in limiting the spread of disease. These are called **preventive** trials. These would usually be carried out in selected age groups, for example young children, who may be at particular risk of a disease. However, in **community trials** a whole community of people is subjected to an intervention, while another comparable population is not. An example is the fluoridation of water, in which the water supply of a whole community is treated with fluoride and the outcome (tooth decay) compared with another community in whom the fluoride content of the water supply remains low.

Secondary prevention

Secondary prevention measures are employed in people who are deemed to be at particular risk of developing a disease. People are identified as having an increased risk by screening (see Chapter 10). Both the screening measure (a laboratory test, for example) and any subsequent treatment or intervention must be evaluated for effectiveness. Occasionally, new screening tests or treatments should be compared, ideally by randomly subjecting one group of people to the old (or no) protocol and another group to the new protocol – in other words by a randomised controlled clinical trial.

An **intervention** trial is an evaluation of a measure designed to prevent the full development of disease in people who are deemed to be at increased risk. An example is a trial of lipid-lowering drugs in people identified by screening as hyperlipidaemic, who are at increased risk of developing coronary heart disease. The intervention can be evaluated by laboratory estimates of blood cholesterol concentrations or by differences in the incidence or mortality from coronary heart disease.

Tertiary prevention

A **therapeutic** trial is aimed at comparing an intervention designed to relieve symptoms or improve survival. At present this is probably the main application of the randomised clinical trial. Any new drug that comes onto the market must have been evaluated in this way, as must non-drug interventions such as new surgical treatments. A problem with non-drug interventions (and with some drug interventions) is that it can be difficult to conceal the type of intervention used from the patient or investigator. This is important for avoiding bias. There is still a preventive application in this type of trial: an example would be the trials of tight glycaemic control in diabetes (see Chapter 23), designed to slow down the development of further complications.

Clinical trials

There are often moral and ethical dilemmas in conducting clinical trials. If a new agent is available that is believed to greatly improve the survival prospects for a given disease, why should it not be given to all who would benefit straight away? At the same time, if the agent turns out to be not as effective as was originally believed, some people may have been deprived of the benefit of the

Primary prevention: interventions designed to prevent a disease from developing. Immunisation and risk factor modification fall into this category. Successful primary prevention reduces the incidence of a disease.

Secondary prevention: interventions designed to arrest the development of a disease that has already started, usually in an asymptomatic phase. Screening falls into this category. Successful secondary prevention reduces the prevalence of a disease.

Tertiary prevention: interventions are designed to minimise the impact of a disease, reducing suffering or disability.

The randomised clinical trial is used to determine whether a particular treatment or intervention is better than the alternatives

conventional treatment.

In some situations (for example AIDS) it seems that almost any treatment is better than nothing. In the USA drugs are only released for use after completion of large-scale studies and approval by the Food and Drug Administration (FDA). In the case of drugs that showed promise against HIV, the FDA was persuaded to relax its approval regulations, allowing drugs to be released provided they had been shown in small studies to have some effect and to be safe. The intention is that large clinical trials should be completed after the product has been placed on the market. One such drug, zalcitabine, received conditional approval after it had been shown to increase CD4 counts (see Chapter 25) in a small number of patients with AIDS. It is now known from larger trials that the drug does not substantially extend survival in patients who have AIDS. The use of ineffective drugs would be of little importance were it not for the costs and side-effects involved.

Randomisation

> *Outcomes cannot be properly evaluated if the characteristics of intervention and control groups are unequal at the outset*

An essential feature of experimental studies is randomisation. The purpose of randomisation is to make each of the intervention groups as equal as possible in all respects except for the intervention itself. With many diseases there are risk factors, both known and unknown, that will influence the development of disease and the effect of treatment. An imbalance in these factors in the intervention or control groups will markedly alter the results.

For factors that cannot be identified the solution is to allocate subjects randomly into intervention and control groups. However, this is not the best way of doing things when there are factors which are known to have an important effect on outcome. The reason is that, like tossing a coin, randomisation relies on the vagaries of chance. If a sample of 1000 eligible subjects containing 400 smokers is considered, it is quite feasible after randomisation for there to be 250 smokers in an intervention group and only 150 in the control group. If, for example, the trial is designed to assess drugs used in the prevention of myocardial infarction, this imbalance would have a marked impact on the treatment outcome.

To overcome this the important factors that can be identified are isolated before randomisation by **block stratification**, which results in several groups of subjects, for example of smokers and non-smokers, that each have to be randomised into intervention or control groups (Figure 1.13). The disadvantage of this is that the method becomes cumbersome if large numbers of known factors are to be considered. For example, in the protocol shown in Figure 1.13, the inclusion of further stratification blocks relating to low, medium, and high blood cholesterol concentrations would enormously increase the complexity of the study. At some stage a decision has to be made to randomise.

▲ Key points

Randomisation

- ▲ Major difference between clinical trials and prospective studies
- ▲ Experimental and control groups must be comparable in all respects except the factor under study, e.g. severity of disease
- ▲ Cannot match for factors which are not known – hence randomisation

Blindness

A common source of bias in analytical and experimental studies is that the

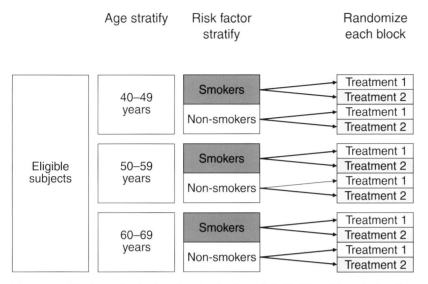

Age stratify   Risk factor stratify   Randomize each block

Figure 1.13 Block randomisation. Randomisation of all eligible subjects is aimed at producing an even distribution in each group, but chance effects could result in an uneven distribution. The purpose of block randomisation is to ensure that known risk factors that would affect the course of disease and its treatment are equally represented in the treatment groups, while allowing other, perhaps unknown, factors to be apportioned randomly. For example, two of the most important recognised prognostic factors in cardiovascular disease are age and smoking history. These should be separated before randomisation.

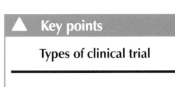

subjects or those conducting the research are aware of the purpose of the research. Hence, in a case-control study people with a disease may over-report exposure to a risk factor if they are aware of its possible association with the disease. Similarly, an observer may make greater efforts to find a change in a test group than in controls. The solution to this is **blinding**. In a **single-blind** study the participants are given no indication whether they are in the experimental or control group. In a **double-blind** study both the subjects and the observers are unaware of the allocations into experimental and control groups.

Sometimes awareness is unavoidable. For example, in a study comparing the benefits of a coronary bypass operation with those of angioplasty both the surgeon and the patient would be aware of which treatment had been given, despite randomisation of the patient to that group. In other circumstances, such as with drug treatments, attempts are made to hide this knowledge by giving a placebo or 'dummy' treatment. An advantage of giving a placebo is that it becomes possible to evaluate the true and specific effect of the intervention: some conditions can improve merely by making an intervention of any kind. This is termed the **placebo effect**.

Controlled clinical trials will be evaluated in different ways. Probably the most easily quantifiable method is to evaluate effects on survival and mortality. However, treatments also need to be evaluated for diseases that are not life-threatening, and hence measurement might be by biochemical or radiographic

Placebo effect: a clinical improvement, or side-effect, which occurs after giving an inert substance or sham treatment.

alterations, alleviation of symptoms or improvements in the quality of life. While outcome measures seek benefits arising from treatment protocols, other outcomes such as treatment complications must also be reported. There are many instances of interventions that are biologically plausible, but in which a clinical trial has been shown to worsen the lot of the patients treated. An example might be the combination of chemotherapy and radiotherapy in the treatment of small-cell lung cancers, compared with chemotherapy alone. To date no survival benefit has been shown for the combined treatment, but patients treated by this method have additional side-effects to deal with.

Prognosis

The results of therapeutic trials can be used to determine the prognosis for a patient with a given disease and treatment regimen. The most common ways of expressing prognosis are:

- As 5-year survival: the probability that a patient will survive 5 years from some well-specified point during the course of the disease
- As case fatality rate: the percentage of patients with disease who die from that disease
- As a recurrence rate: the probability of the disease recurring after a disease-free interval

Meta-analysis

Meta-analysis attempts to analyse the total evidence available for a specific disease hypothesis

Meta-analysis is increasingly used by epidemiologists to help overcome the problems of small sample size. The method combines data from a number of reported studies that examine the same question and subjects the data to statistical analysis. By combining the studies it is hoped that any inherent bias in a single study will be diluted by the other studies. Small differences or effects that were hidden in a single small study can also be revealed.

The technique is not without some problems. Very often studies will differ with respect to the eligibility of the subjects to be studied and the outcome measures sought. For example, studies aimed at assessing the influence of dietary factors and cardiovascular disease may differ by excluding smokers, or may be confined to either men or women in certain occupations. The outcome measures could be angina, requirement for medical or surgical treatment or death from myocardial infarction. The ways in which these outcome measures are assessed or diagnosed could also vary in different centres. In some respects, therefore, meta-analysis is akin to trying to add apples and oranges (both are fruit, but they are still different) and for this reason studies based on meta-analysis should be interpreted with caution.

Evaluation of reported epidemiological studies

Epidemiological studies reported in the literature are not always easy to follow, particularly in clinical trials where patients are allocated to a variety of treatment regimens and the results analysed by a series of statistical methods. The first point that needs to be clarified is the **hypothesis**. In a case-control study of the association between smoking and lung cancer the hypothesis would be 'people who have lung cancer are more likely to have a history of cigarette smoking than controls.' The question in a cohort study would be 'does exposure to cigarette smoke increase the risk of developing lung cancer?' Questions must then be asked about the cases and controls: what diagnostic criteria were used to ensure that the cases and controls were truly cases and controls? Similarly, questions need to be asked about the clinical end-points in a clinical trial. Further relevant questions are listed in Table 1.4.

Table 1.4   Evaluation of clinical trials

Trial rationale
- Is the hypothesis clearly stated? Is the hypothesis biologically plausible and consistent with previous literature?
- What are the reasons for performing the trial – in what way is the new treatment believed to represent an improvement?

Selection of subjects
- Were exclusion criteria employed? What were they, and why?
- What were the demographic characteristics and medical status of the group? How and when was disease status established?
- What was the basis of randomisation?
- How large were the intervention groups?
- How were people recruited into the study?
- Was there any matching of known risk factors?

Study methodology
- Was the study blinded?
- What were the outcome measures?
- Were all intervention groups equal with respect to prognostic factors?
- Were any complications associated with the treatment(s)?
- Were all patients kept in the originally assigned groups?
- What steps were taken to ensure that subjects complied with the treatment protocol?
- Who was lost to follow-up, and why? Did they differ from people who completed the study?
- Was the follow-up long enough? Were sufficient data presented so that conclusions can be justified?
- If results were negative, did the trial have sufficient statistical power?

Activity 2	

Epidemiological design

Laboratory studies indicate that aspirin inhibits platelet aggregation, important in the formation of atherosclerotic plaques and in the production of thrombus (see Chapter 20). These processes underlie the development of coronary heart disease. It would therefore seem feasible that if platelet aggregation is inhibited by aspirin, then various sequelae, such as angina or death from coronary heart disease, could also be reduced.

1. How would this be tested by epidemiological methods?
2. What would be the hypothesis in a case-control study design? (You may wish to refer to your answer to Question 1 before you carry on.)
3. How would you differentiate the cases from the controls?
4. How many cases and controls would you incorporate in the study?
5. What questions would you ask relating to the cases and controls?
6. What would be the hypothesis in a prospective cohort study design?
7. How would you differentiate exposed people from the non-exposed controls?
8. How many exposed and non-exposed people would you incorporate in the study?
9. How long would you need to conduct the study?
10. What outcomes would be sought and measured in each group?
11. What would be the hypothesis in a clinical trial design?
12. In a clinical trial, how would you determine who received aspirin?

ANSWERS TO REVIEW QUESTIONS

Question 1

Give some possible reasons why the true frequency of a disease may not be properly known

Estimates of disease frequency are made from incidence and prevalence data and, if life-threatening, from mortality data. Problems arise if all the true cases of disease are not brought to attention, or if the disease is not recognised for what it is. People might not seek attention for symptoms because they think they are unimportant or because they fear finding out the cause. There are also issues around the cost and availability of medical services and the possibilities for self-treatment.

Even when symptoms are reported, for many illnesses there is no obligation by medical practitioners to report the disease. In the UK, all cancers are notifiable on a regional basis. In the USA, diseases are monitored by the Centers for Communicable Diseases (CDC). When diseases are reported, accuracy depends on the sensitivity and specificity of diagnosis and the efficiency of the administrative procedures.

Mortality statistics are based on the illness a person was known to be suffering from, or the results of post-mortem examination. While this examination is more accurate, the procedure is carried out in only a minority of deaths, and these probably are an unrepresentative sample, for example the 'interesting' cases and unexpected deaths.

Question 2

What do the data suggest about the relative contributions of genetic and environmental factors in stomach, liver and colon cancers?

Death rates for stomach cancer in Japan differ markedly from those in whites living in California. The trend in immigrant Japanese is towards the rate of the Californian white population and is even more apparent when sons of immigrants are considered. This suggests a large contribution by environmental factors: as children become more integrated into the host population the differences become smaller. Similar trends are seen with liver cancer. In colonic cancer, the trend is still towards the rate of the host population, but this time the change is from an area of low incidence to one of high incidence. The most probable contributory factors are alterations to diet and general improvements in living conditions.

Question 3

Calculate the odds ratio in lung cancer cases compared with controls

The odds ratio is calculated by dividing the likelihood of exposure among the cases by that of exposure among the controls:

$$\frac{A}{C} \quad \text{divided by} \quad \frac{B}{D}$$

$$\frac{900}{100} \quad \text{divided by} \quad \frac{250}{750}$$

Odds ratio = 27.0

Question 4

What are the possible advantages and disadvantages of sending the questionnaire to all British doctors?

Possible advantages:
- Use of the medical register allowed rapid identification and recruitment of subjects
- The target group of medical practitioners could be expected by training and outlook to co-operate with a scientific investigation
- Use of the medical register minimised attrition by subjects moving away: provided the subjects still practised medicine and resided in the UK they could be traced

Possible disadvantages:
- Medical practitioners are not a representative sample of the general population with respect to gender balance and socioeconomic group. As luck would have it, this was probably not a disadvantage, since smoking is such a strong aetiological agent that it will override subtle effects contingent on socioeconomic status.

- The gender imbalance could present problems, particularly as smoking was not widely prevalent in women in 1951. This made the female sample size too small, and indeed Doll and Peto had to confine most of their analyses to men.
- The medical profession could be expected to be the first to receive information about health hazards attached to smoking. This might cause subjects to modify their behaviour, resulting in attrition of the exposed study group. This did happen, but the researchers turned this to advantage, because it became possible to examine the effects of smoking cessation on subsequent mortality.

Question 5

Would you expect the results after 20 years of follow-up to be very much the same as those obtained after 40 years?

No. The effects of smoking take many years to become manifest as symptomatic disease. It will take some years of exposure for the cells to become sufficiently damaged to undergo neoplastic transformation. The tumour cells must grow until they reach such a size, or spread far enough, to cause symptoms. This could take 20 years or longer. What should become apparent in a prospective study is that the differences between exposed and non-exposed groups will become more marked as time goes on.

Activity 1
Data analysis

1. The relative risk attached to exposure is calculated from the exposed and unexposed risk estimates:

$$\frac{\dfrac{A}{A + B}}{\dfrac{C}{C + D}}$$

Lung cancer risk in those who smoke 1–14 cigarettes daily

$$= \frac{\dfrac{105}{100\,000}}{\dfrac{14}{100\,000}}$$

$$= \frac{105}{14}$$

Relative risk =   7.5

The relative risk of lung cancer risk in those who smoke 25 or more cigarettes daily

$$\frac{355}{14}$$

Relative risk = **25.4**

2. Risk of ischaemic heart disease risk in those who smoke 1-14 cigarettes daily

$$= \frac{802}{572}$$

Relative risk = **1.4**

Relative risk of ischaemic heart disease risk in those who smoke 25 or more cigarettes daily

$$= \frac{1025}{572}$$

Relative risk = **1.8**

3. The difference in lung cancer risk for light and heavy smokers is striking. Essentially, smoking acts as a very strong aetiological agent for lung cancer and exerts a dose–response relationship.

A dose–response relationship also exists between smoking and ischaemic heart disease, but the relative risk estimates are not as high as with lung cancer. This indicates that other factors may operate in the aetiology of ischaemic heart disease, as well as cigarette smoking: in other words it is a multifactorial disease.
4. Relative risks: (a) 5.2; (b) 22.4.
5. Relative risks: (a) 1.17; (b) 1.63.
6. Relative risks for both lung cancer and ischaemic heart disease are higher after 40 years than after 20 years. This is a reflection of the very long time lag between exposure to cigarette smoke and the development of symptomatic disease.

**Activity 2
Epidemiological design**

1. Both analytical and experimental approaches would be suitable for this study. Case-control studies would give a more rapid answer. Prospective cohort and randomised controlled trials would take longer but would be more reliable.
2. The hypothesis would be along the lines of 'people with coronary heart disease are less likely to have a history of aspirin exposure'.
3. The issues here are the definitions of coronary heart disease and the controls, who should be without disease. The choices would be to look at angina

sufferers, people who have had coronary angioplasty, coronary bypass surgery or who have died from coronary heart disease. The controls could constitute people with an absence of these conditions, but this would not guarantee that all were free from coronary heart disease – the condition may still be asymptomatic.

In one study (Hennekens *et al.*, 1978) the cases were men who had died from coronary heart disease. Controls were neighbours who had not reported any symptoms of the disease.

4. Hennekens' study aimed to recruit over 1000 case-control pairs. Many of these people did not co-operate with the study and the final study population comprised 568 case-control pairs. (Be prepared for substantial drop-out rates!)

5. A variety of questions will need to be asked for matching purposes, for example age, socioeconomic group, smoking history and other risk factors pertinent to coronary heart disease, as well as the question of interest (use of aspirin). Care will be required to ensure that participants are aware of the precise nature and doses of the drugs taken, for example it could be expected that many people would report taking aspirin when in fact they had taken paracetamol.

In the case-control study of Hennekens *et al.* the cases had already died, so the researchers adopted the strategy of asking the wives about their spouse's aspirin use. With the living controls the researchers were able to ask this information directly, but just as a check on the validity of proxy information they also asked some of the control wives about their husband's use of the drug. Because this information turned out to be reasonably accurate, the researchers worked on the assumption that the information given by the case wives would also be accurate (although they did recognise this as a possible source of error). Aspirin intake was reported as daily or weekly, together with details of how many tablets were taken.

6. A suitable hypothesis would be along the lines of 'people exposed to regular aspirin use are less likely to develop coronary heart disease'.

7. The suggested hypothesis is inherently inaccurate – what exactly is meant by 'regular'? In a study conducted by Hammond and Garfinkel (1975) aspirin consumption was recorded as 'never', 'seldom' or 'often'. Since this was a prospective study, there would have been opportunities to record more accurate data than this.

8. Hammond and Garfinkel's study was based on a questionnaire given to over 1 million people, of whom 434 958 men and 558 038 women answered the question on aspirin use. Not many studies are based on such a large sample size and in fact the researchers made use of a study population enrolled for another purpose by the American Cancer Society. Hence the ambiguity over aspirin use – when the study was set up this was not believed (and remains so today) to have a major impact on incidence of cancer.

As coronary heart disease is common such a large sample size is not strictly necessary. However, this is a prospective study with no control by the researchers over aspirin intakes. Hence the study population must be large enough to accommodate all the permutations of aspirin use, so that ultimately it will be possible to compare virtually nil use and daily use with coronary heart disease outcome.

9. In the study by Hammond and Garfinkel subjects were traced for 6 years. This is not a long time in the pathogenesis of atherosclerosis and coronary heart disease. However, in practical terms, it is desirable that a therapeutic or preventive measure like aspirin should exert its effects within a short time scale.

10. The outcome measure in Hammond and Garfinkel's study was cause of death as described on death certificates. An alternative measure would be development of angina, but this would entail periodic checks of the whole study population.

11. A suitable hypothesis might be 'People randomised into a 500 mg daily aspirin group are less likely to suffer myocardial infarction than a placebo group'. It will be necessary further to define 'people' in terms of age, gender, socioeconomic group etc. It will also be necessary to define the outcome measure, perhaps as episodes of angina or death from myocardial infarction.

One of the early trials that looked at this question was published by Elwood *et al.* in 1974. Their hypothesis was that a single daily dose of aspirin would prevent reinfarction in men who had suffered a recent myocardial infarct. The outcome measure was the all-cause death rate.

12. You should not. To eliminate bias the study population must be randomised into test and placebo groups.

In the trial undertaken by Elwood and co-workers it was first necessary to establish that all subjects had previously suffered a myocardial infarction. From that point, and after excluding men who had peptic ulcer (this would be irritated by aspirin) or who were receiving anticoagulant therapy, the subjects were randomised into aspirin and placebo groups.

References

Doll, R. and Peto, R. (1976) Mortality in relation to smoking: 20 years' observations on male British doctors. *BMJ*, **ii**, 1525-36.

Doll, R., Peto, R., Wheatley, K. *et al.* (1994) Mortality in relation to smoking: 40 years' observations on male British doctors. *BMJ*, **309**, 901-11.

Elwood, P. C., Cochrane, A.L., Burr, M.L. *et al.* (1974) A randomised controlled trial of acetyl salicylic acid in the secondary prevention of mortality from myocardial infarction. *BMJ*, **i**, 436-40.

Hammond, C. and Garfinkel, L. (1975) Aspirin and coronary heart disease: findings of a prospective study. *BMJ*, **ii**, 269-71.

Hennekens, C.H., Karlson, L.K. and Rosner, B. (1978) A case-control study of regular aspirin use and coronary deaths. *Circulation*, **58**, 35-38.

Wynder, E.L. and Graham, E.A. (1950) Tobacco smoking as a possible aetiological factor in bronchogenic carcinoma. A study of six hundred and eighty four proved cases. *JAMA*, **143**, 329-36.

Further reading

Greenberg, R.S. *Medical Epidemiology*, Appleton & Lange, East Norwalk, Connecticut, 1993.

2   The causes of disease

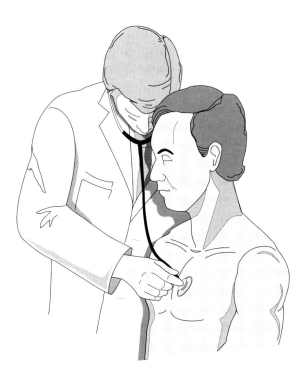

Every aspect of human function and activity is vulnerable to disruption. Ordinarily much of the disruption that accompanies everyday bodily actions is compensated by homeostatic mechanisms. There are, however, circumstances in which homeostatic mechanisms become overburdened and the consequence is temporary or permanent injury or disease.

Susceptibility to disease is determined by genetic constitution and by exposure to agents in the environment. Exposure to damaging agents is most likely to be influenced by socioeconomic group, behaviour, dietary habits and occupation. Many factors may be altered, which gives some scope for the primary prevention of certain diseases. Susceptibility for ill-health increases with age.

Aims of this chapter

By the end of this chapter you will have increased your knowledge of:

♦   The circumstances that influence susceptibility or resistance to disease
♦   The types of actions that may be taken to reduce morbidity and mortality from disease

In addition, this chapter will help you to:

♦   Understand the reasons for historical changes in the principal causes of death
♦   Discuss the relative contribution of genetic and environmental factors in causing disease
♦   Discuss the potential for reducing morbidity and mortality from specific diseases by primary and secondary prevention measures

Introduction

In most industrialised countries the principal causes of death have altered substantially since the turn of the 20th century. At that time infectious diseases such as tuberculosis, influenza and pneumonia were much more of a problem than they are today, although that is not to say that there is no room for further improvement. Currently the most pressing problems and drains on healthcare resources are the chronic diseases such as coronary heart disease and cancers. As well as representing the main causes of death they represent significant causes of continuing morbidity, even with treatment.

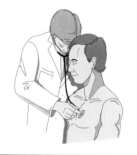

> *Most common diseases and disabilities are caused by a combination of genetic and environmental factors*

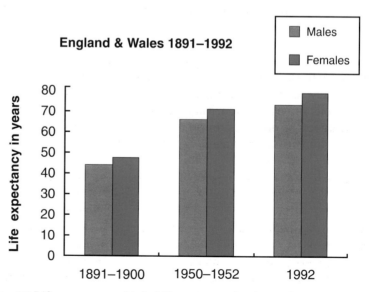

Figure 2.1 Life expectancy at birth. Life expectancy has increased dramatically over the last century. In all human populations women can expect to live longer than men. (Source: OPCS (1992) DH1 No. 16 (1891-1952), Government Actuary's Department.)

The change in the patterns of morbidity and mortality can be attributed to many reasons, the most notable of which are improvements in general living and working conditions and improvements in the availability and variety of food, together with medical advances in prevention and treatment of disease. These changes have also resulted in substantial improvements in quality of life and life expectancy (Figure 2.1) and have influenced the types of diseases people die from (Figure 2.2).

> Life expectancy: the period for which 50% of a population born in a certain year are expected to live.

Concepts of health and disease

What is health?

Perceptions of health and disease vary between individuals and professional viewpoints. Many people would define health as an absence of signs or symptoms that have recognised associations with disease. However, in many situations people believe themselves to be ill but have no measurable signs or symptoms of disease. Conversely, there are people who believe themselves to be well and have no symptoms but are found on routine check-up to have a life-threatening disease.

> *Health is a state of physical, mental and social well-being*

A more positive view of health, formulated by the World Health Organization, is that health is 'a state of physical, mental and social well-being and not merely the absence of disease or infirmity'. In other words, health is not only about physiological parameters but also about how the person feels. There are many who feel that once the balance of psychological well-being has become disrupted, then physiological changes resulting in disease are more likely to occur. A positive attitude of mind may influence not only susceptibility to disease, but also response to treatment.

Another aspect of health is that it must be maintained in a positive manner: that is, there is a limit to how much the body will 'look after itself'. If health is viewed as the capacity of the body to perform functions, then there are also ways in which functional efficiency can be increased. The most obvious example is the influence of exercise on both physiological efficiency and mental well-being. In this context there is much to be said for the expression 'if you don't use it, you lose it'.

Much disease prevention focuses on the physiological aspects of health. In these terms, much can be done to protect the body by avoidance of risk factors that increase susceptibility to disease. Hence most people are aware that smoking, excess alcohol intake and some aspects of the diet may in some ways be detrimental to health. What this does not address is the psychological motivation and desire to make positive changes. Some people perceive many of the risk factors that are capable of detrimental physiological effects as enhancing their quality of life. There are also issues of self-esteem: people who think or are told that their lives are worthless are unlikely to be concerned about a healthy lifestyle.

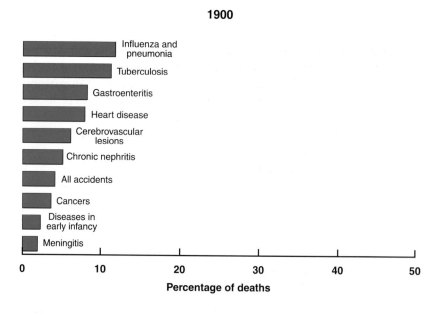

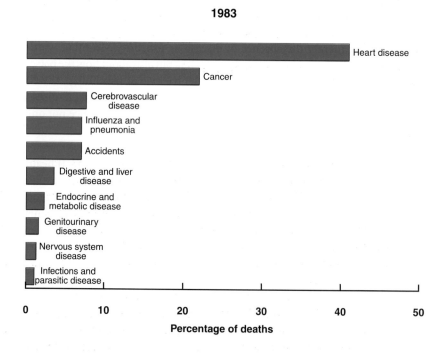

Figure 2.2 Principal causes of death, 1900 and 1983, USA. In 1900 life expectancy was shorter and the most common causes of death were acute and chronic infectious diseases such as influenza, pneumonia, tuberculosis and gastroenteritis. These conditions are now much more rare. People live longer and are more likely to die from chronic diseases such as coronary heart disease and cancer.

What is disease?

In practical terms the identification of disease is limited to something that is measurable – perceived pain, appearance of signs or symptoms or alteration in some physiological or biochemical parameter. Unfortunately, these changes often arise only in the late stages of a disease process and many people actually have disease that cannot be measured, at least by accessible techniques. In essence, all diseases result from some disturbance to cells as a result of physical or environmental insults or engendered by a genetic aberration. Essentially the disease state is the result of an inability of homeostatic mechanisms to adapt to the insult. Inadequate or excessive responses result in cellular injury. Very often the disequilibrium caused leads to disturbances in function elsewhere and may be reflected in disability, loss of growth or repair and, ultimately, impaired survival.

Disease can be viewed as a failure of adaptation

Causes of ill health

The main factors influencing disease are genetic constitution, which confers resistance or susceptibility to particular diseases, and exposure to harmful agents in the environment or associated with particular types of behaviour. When a combination of agents is influential in causing disease the condition is said to be of **multifactorial** causation. The various agents, together with any genetic predisposition for disease, are collectively referred to as **risk factors**. Some risk factors can easily be altered but others are more difficult to alter or are unalterable.

Most diseases are caused by a variety of factors that interact

Risk factor: a habit, trait or abnormality associated with an increase in susceptibility to disease.

Genetics and disease

Although many diseases can be attributed directly to some inherited genetic defect, these conditions are relatively rare. Diseases caused by agents that induce changes to the DNA of the normal cell as a sporadic event are much more common. Some segments of the genetic code are probably more liable to damage that others, and may correspond to areas in which there are individual differences in the genetic code. Hence individuals differ in their susceptibility to damage and subsequent disease, even when exposed to the same agent under comparable conditions.

Some genetic alterations, called **mutations**, are very discrete and involve only one base pair in the genetic code. This can result in inappropriate assembly of amino acids into the translated protein so that it does not function correctly. An example of this kind of disorder is sickle-cell disease, caused by the substitution of a single amino acid in the haemoglobin molecule.

Many other diseases involve more extensive alterations of the genetic code, often involving areas of a chromosome containing hundreds of genes, and even whole chromosomes. In general these alterations arise spontaneously during meiotic or mitotic cell division, and are thus not inherited in any

Mutation: a change in DNA caused by chemical or physical agents. Mutations can affect the germ cells and be passed on to the offspring, or are somatic and passed through the cell lineage by cell division.

Sickle-cell disease: a genetic disorder that results in abnormal haemoglobin in red blood cells. The cells become sickle-shaped when the oxygen concentration is low. Sickled cells block the small blood vessels, restricting blood supply to tissues.

Most genetic mutations leading to disease occur in the adult

predictable fashion. An example of this kind of abnormality is Down's syndrome (see Chapter 3).

In addition there is a wide range of common diseases in which a genetic predisposition is apparent, but over which is superimposed a number of environmental risk factors. These diseases include diabetes, coronary heart disease, hypertension and peptic ulcer. Many of these conditions show a strong familial association, but are not directly inherited in a predictable way. The inherited component has been difficult to identify, but for the disease to develop some other factor from the environment needs to be present, such as cigarette smoking, high-fat diet and stress (cardiovascular disease).

Genetic mutations can occur at any stage in the life of a cell, from the zygote to somatic cells in old people. The alterations that occur in adult life commonly become manifest as cancer. Many types of cancer, including breast cancer and colorectal cancer, are more commonly seen in particular families and are caused by a combination of genetic and environmental factors (Figure 2.3).

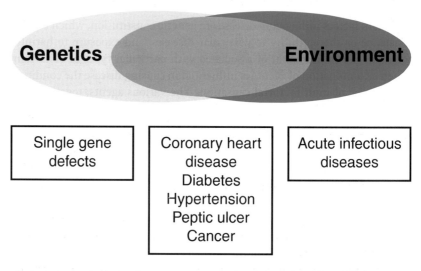

100% Inherited   **100% Environment**

Figure 2.3 The spectrum of disease. At one extreme, single gene defects are inherited and passed on to the offspring in a predictable fashion. At the other extreme there are acute infectious diseases to which almost all individuals will succumb if exposed to the aetiological agent, regardless of their individual genetic make-up. In between are many common diseases that are caused by a combination of an inherited genetic component and environmental risk factors.

Environmental and behavioural factors

Aetiological agent: a physical, chemical or biological agent that causes changes in cells that lead to disease

The most prominent determinant of health is socioeconomic status. Low socioeconomic status is accompanied by poor housing and environmental amenities, insufficient income to provide proper nutrition and unhealthy behaviours such as smoking and alcohol consumption. Another strong determinant of ill-health is age.

Some factors, such as age and family history, are impossible to alter. Others, such as cigarette smoking or alcohol consumption, can be altered and there is therefore some potential for reducing morbidity and mortality from associated diseases. The modification of these kinds of behaviour and lifestyle risk factors is referred to as **primary prevention**. There are limits as to how effective this kind of intervention can be: some risk factors are very difficult to alter in the short-term (for example, poor housing and overcrowding), others may appear easily altered but are resisted if they alter perceptions about quality of life (dietary control, for example). Also, many people (smokers, for example) take a fatalistic attitude, saying that they will have to die from something anyway. Obviously no amount of risk factor intervention will reduce deaths, but reductions in general ill-health and premature deaths (usually defined as deaths in people under the age of 65 years) can be achieved.

Another method of primary prevention is immunisation. This is limited to the prevention of infectious diseases for which vaccines are available. Probably the most eagerly awaited vaccine at the present time is one that will prevent AIDS but, although much progress has been made, this prospect is still some way off. The main problem with vaccines is that organisms often mutate, so that an immune response elicited by the vaccine is not effective if the immunised person becomes infected by the mutated organism. It is also necessary to maintain immunity by booster immunisations.

Secondary prevention aims to detect disease at an early stage before symptoms develop. The rationale is that treatment at such an early stage will be much more likely to halt progress of the disease, with the additional advantage that the treatment required could be less extensive. Effective secondary prevention strategies require establishment of an organised screening programme (see Chapter 10) in which all eligible individuals will be assessed on a regular basis. A fundamental problem with screening is persuading people to attend when they have no symptoms and therefore regard themselves as healthy.

Theoretically, secondary prevention is not as effective as primary prevention because the disease process has already started even though symptoms have not yet developed. In this sense secondary prevention can be regarded as a back-up measure once primary prevention has failed.

There are many diseases in which the risk factors are not known, cannot be altered or have little impact on pathogenesis. In these circumstances secondary prevention can improve on what can be achieved by the diagnosis and treatment of symptomatic disease. Unfortunately there are many conditions for which little can be done by either primary or secondary prevention. In these it may be possible to employ **tertiary prevention** measures. These are aimed at ameliorating the effects of disease, possibly by slowing disease progression and preventing the appearance of new symptoms.

Recent advances in treatment have met with excellent results in some hitherto chronic and life-threatening conditions (coronary heart disease and

> *Susceptibility to virtually all the common life-threatening diseases is influenced by the ways in which people live*

▲ **Key points**

Determinants of ill health

- ▲ Genetic susceptibility (family history)
- ▲ Age
- ▲ Socioeconomic group
- ▲ Behavioural factors, e.g. smoking, sexual practices, drug and alcohol abuse, response to stress
- ▲ Environmental factors (often contingent on socioeconomic group), e.g. housing, overcrowding, pollution
- ▲ Occupational factors, e.g. exposures to chemicals or ionising radiation
- ▲ Nutritional factors, e.g. nutrient-deficient diet, high-fat low-fibre diets
- ▲ General motivation, activity and exercise

Pathogenesis: processes involved in the production of disease.

some leukaemias, for example). Nevertheless, just as in the past, the most dramatic reductions in the burden of disease morbidity and mortality will be achieved by improving living conditions. This most obviously applies to the less developed countries, but it is noticeable that some sections of the population in developed countries have not benefited equally from improvements already made.

The single-cause infectious diseases that were responsible for most deaths in developed countries were relatively easy to tackle by generalised improvement in socioeconomic conditions, hygiene, sanitation and application of immunisation programmes and antibiotic therapies. Today's chronic diseases present a much more formidable problem, requiring a multifaceted approach encompassing primary prevention, secondary prevention and improved treatment. Governments in most Western countries, notably in the USA and UK, have set objectives for reducing morbidity and mortality from specific diseases, usually by implementing primary or secondary prevention measures. In the UK these objectives are set out in *Health of the Nation* key areas. In the USA, national health promotion and disease prevention objectives are encompassed by the *Healthy People 2000* initiative.

These documents are long on objectives, but are rather short on specific ways in which the objectives can be achieved, or they only reflect changes that are occurring anyway. For example, the welcome decrease in the prevalence of cigarette smoking that has occurred on both sides of the Atlantic during the past decade is certain to increase life expectancy and reduce deaths from lung cancer. It is also notable that the proven single greatest impact on health, that of socioeconomic status, is not seriously addressed. The assumption is made that there will be a 'trickle-down' effect into all strata of society as further technological advances and improvements in productivity are made. The evidence from the UK, however, does not support this effect: there has been an increasing divergence between the rich and the poor, and consequently in their expectation of health.

The *Health of the Nation* strategy for the UK is divided into five key areas:
- Coronary heart disease and stroke
- Cancers
- Mental illness
- HIV/AIDS and sexual health
- Accidents

The *Healthy People 2000* programme was implemented in the USA in 1990, with three broad goals:
- To increase the span of healthy life for Americans
- To reduce health disparities among Americans
- To achieve access to preventive services for all Americans

The priority areas addressed by *Healthy People 2000* are broadly similar to those of *Health of the Nation*, except that there are 22 categories covering not only specific disorders such as heart disease and cancers, but also targets for altering lifestyle factors and behaviours, such as physical activity and fitness, drug use and violence.

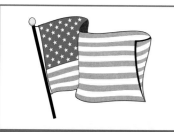

Healthy People 2000

Priority areas

1. Physical activity and fitness
2. Nutrition
3. Tobacco
4. Alcohol and other drugs
5. Family planning
6. Mental health and mental disorders
7. Violent and abusive behaviour
8. Educational and community-based programmes
9. Unintentional injuries
10. Occupational safety and health
11. Environmental health
12. Food and drug safety
13. Oral health
14. Maternal and infant health
15. Heart disease and stroke
16. Cancer
17. Diabetes and chronic disabling conditions
18. HIV infection
19. Sexually transmitted diseases
20. Immunisation and infectious diseases
21. Clinical preventive services
22. Surveillance and data systems

Socioeconomic status and health

Life expectancy increases with greater personal access to economic resources. A deprivation model of sickness holds that many of the causes or predisposing factors for disease, such as cold, dampness, filthy conditions, malnutrition, starvation and overcrowding are more prevalent among the socioeconomically disadvantaged and are accompanied by increased frequency of disease and premature death.

There is a positive and progressive association between health and socioeconomic status

These adverse conditions predispose to infections, and increase the likelihood of morbidity and mortality from long-standing illnesses such as arthritis, coronary heart disease and respiratory conditions. Every stage of life is touched by socioeconomic deprivation, from the baby *in utero* to people in old age (Figures 2.4 and 2. 5). The effects can also be very long lasting, so that the socioeconomic group status at birth remains influential throughout life, despite subsequent improvements in economic status.

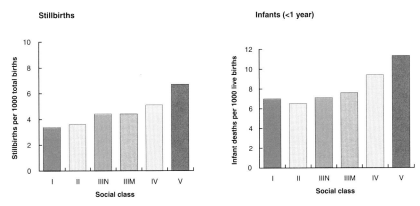

Figure 2.4 Differences in perinatal mortality with social class in England and Wales, 1988. Perinatal deaths are more frequent in lower socioeconomic groups. (Source: Delamonthe, T. (1991) *BMJ*, **303**, 1046-50.)

Housing

Intuitively, many people associate cold and damp housing conditions with excess risk of disease, particularly respiratory disorders. People in these circumstances are socially deprived and other factors such as poor diet, smoking and alcohol consumption will also be relevant in causing disease. It can therefore be difficult to untangle the impact of defective housing from the host of other circumstances surrounding these individuals. It is also difficult to alter the housing situation and directly assess the response.

Other circumstances in the home, such as air quality, very much depend on the behaviour of the occupants – respiratory symptoms in children could be caused by the effects of passive smoking rather than the damp conditions. Poor cooking facilities and incorrect use of heating appliances (usually because of lack of maintenance) can increase the concentrations of harmful carbon dioxide, carbon monoxide and nitrogen dioxide in the home. Many families

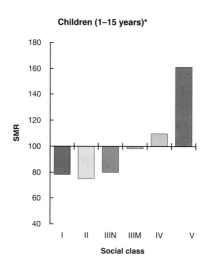

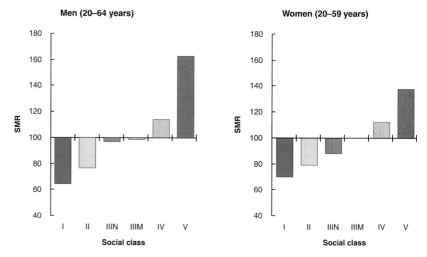

▲ Key points

Socioeconomic groups

▲ I - Professional

▲ II - Managerial and technical

▲ IIIN - Non-manual skilled

▲ IIIM - Manual skilled

▲ IV - Partly skilled

▲ V - Unskilled

Figure 2.5 Mortality rates in the UK: effect of socioeconomic class. People in the lower socioeconomic groups on average die younger than their counterparts in higher groups (SMR: the number of deaths averaged across all the groups is given the notional figure of 100. A figure above this value means that there is an excessive number of deaths). (Source: Delamonthe, T. (1991) *BMJ*, **303**, 1046-50.)

do not have the economic resources or the knowledge to identify and attend to these matters.

In addition, many people do not have a home – those sleeping rough in the streets (not an unusual sight in the large cities of Europe and north America) and families forced to live in hostels and bed-and-breakfast accommodation. The impact of these circumstances on a person's physical and mental well-being can be enormous.

Cigarette smoking and health

The most common and alterable single determinant of ill-health is smoking–it is notorious for both the range and severity of its effects. Smoking is primarily responsible for tripling the death rate from causes such as coronary heart disease and lung cancer, significantly shortening life expectancy (Figure 2.6).

> *Smoking is harmful at all levels of consumption*

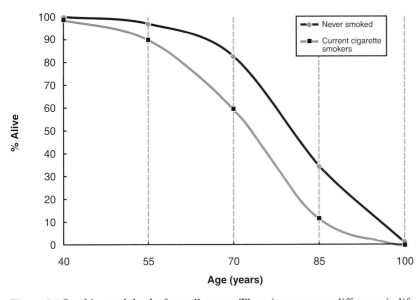

Figure 2.6 Smoking and deaths from all causes. There is an average difference in life expectancy between smokers and non-smokers of 7.5 years. (Data from Peto, R. (1994) BMJ, 309, 937-9.)

Smoking is implicated as a causative factor in a wide range of diseases, which together are responsible for most deaths in Western countries (Table 2.1). These diseases include cancers of the mouth, oesophagus, pharynx, larynx, lung, pancreas and bladder, chronic obstructive lung disease, vascular diseases and peptic ulcer. Passive smoking is thought to increase the risk of lung cancer by 10–30% and to cause respiratory complaints in children.

> *Smoking is the single most important cause of cancer*

The reason why cigarette smoking is responsible for such a wide range of diseases is probably related to the toxic chemicals within the smoke, coupled with persistent exposure. The different chemical components act on cells in different ways, causing damage to a wide range of components (Table 2.2).

> Carcinogen: chemical, physical or biological agent that is capable of inducing cancer

There are socioeconomic and gender differences in smoking habits. In the UK more than 60% of smokers belong to the manual occupational groups. Smoking is also more prevalent in the north of England, and probably contributes to the higher mortality from coronary heart disease observed in that part of the country.

Stopping smoking reduces most of the excess risk of disease, even if this is delayed until middle age. The benefits of stopping at an earlier age are greater. Targets have been set in the UK and the USA both to reduce the number of people taking up smoking and to encourage those who already smoke to stop.

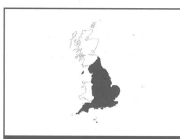

Health of the Nation

Targets on smoking

▲ Reduce the prevalence of cigarette smoking in people over the age of 16 to no more than 20% by the year 2000 (1990 prevalence was 31% of men and 28% of women)

▲ Pregnant women: reduce smoking prevalence by at least a third at the start of pregnancy

▲ Reduce the consumption of cigarettes by at least 40% by the year 2000

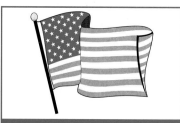

Healthy People 2000

Targets on smoking

▲ Reduce the prevalence of cigarette smoking in men and women over the age of 20 to no more than 15% from a 1987 baseline of 29%

▲ Reduce smoking prevalence in pregnant women from 25% to 10%

▲ Reduce exposure of children to cigarette smoke in the home from 39% to 20%

Table 2.1   Smoking history and cause of death (expressed per 100 000 men aged 35-69)

Cause of death	Never smoked regularly	Current cigarette smoker
Cancer		
Lung	8	196
Mouth, larynx, oesophagus	5	28
Other	109	188
Respiratory disease	9	62
Vascular disease	176	446
Other medical causes	39	81

Data from Peto, R. (1994) *BMJ*, **309**, 937-9.

Table 2.2   Properties of some of the chemical constituents of tobacco smoke

Substance	Property
Tar	Carcinogenic
Polycyclic aromatic hydrocarbons	Carcinogenic
Nicotine	Addictive drug, tumour-promoting agent
Phenol	Irritant, tumour-promoting agent
Benzopyrene	Carcinogenic
Carbon monoxide	Impairs oxygen transport and use
Formaldehyde	Toxic: cross-links and denatures proteins causing cell damage and death
Nitrosamines	Carcinogenic
Nitrogen oxides	Irritant to respiratory epithelium

A number of strategies can be used to reduce the prevalence of smoking. One obvious influence is price, which would be expected to have the most effect on people with low disposable income. However, this is the group in which smoking prevalence is highest and it is surprising how much people will sacrifice in order to continue their habit. Although price increases will undoubtedly influence some people to stop smoking, price increases will merely impose an added burden on others who are already disadvantaged.

Tobacco promotion and the use of glamorous images in association with smoking help to create the view that smoking is a socially acceptable and 'adult' pastime. In the UK controls on tobacco promotion are only voluntary, and there are still plenty of opportunities to advertise on billboards, in newspapers and magazines and by sponsorship (often involving sporting events). However, regulations require tobacco products and advertisements about them to carry warning messages about the health hazards involved.

The creation of smoke-free environments has done much to influence and reinforce public attitudes towards the view that smoking is no longer socially acceptable. In the UK smoking is banned in the workplace of all government departments and smoking is allowed only in designated zones.

Health promotion plays a vital role in achieving target reduction in smoking. The message can be put across in a wide variety of ways, including media campaigns and by personal or group education by health professionals, teachers and lay people. In the UK the current programme operated by the Health Education Authority targets teenage smoking and smoking during pregnancy mostly by means of poster and pamphlet campaigns in schools and clinics. Development work is being carried out to find the most effective ways of extending the campaign to the general adult population.

In addition to the measures aimed at the population at large, there are opportunities in which individuals can be advised of their risk. It is envisaged that much of this work will be undertaken on an opportunistic basis by health professionals working in the primary care setting. Patients will be asked routinely about their smoking habits and where appropriate given advice about stopping smoking. Nicotine replacement therapy is helpful in smokers who are motivated to stop, but who are dependent on nicotine. In highly dependent smokers regular use of nicotine gum is most appropriate, whereas less-dependent smokers may benefit from nicotine skin patches. In either type, use should be continued for up to 3 months, with a gradual withdrawal.

In the final analysis people will stop smoking only if they want to. There is a danger that by exerting pressure on smokers to stop they will feel that they are being 'got at' and their reaction may be one of defiance. Most smokers already know that their habit is harmful (Figure 2.7): the underlying reasons why they take up the habit and continue to smoke need to be addressed.

Most people take up smoking during adolescence. Probable factors leading to smoking in teenagers are peer pressure, a desire for experimentation and rebellion. At this age smoking is associated with alcohol consumption, illegal drug use, sexual experience and more general social activities. Smoking is seen as a means of enhancing self-esteem, particularly in the disadvantaged, for whom high academic and economic status is beyond reach. The number of adolescent girls taking up smoking is increasing; they often identify it as a means of keeping slim. Smokers report enhanced mood and performance and soon become psychologically and pharmacologically dependent. For both teenagers and adults smoking is very often regarded as a crutch at times of stress: it is used as a means of relaxing and coping with feelings of insecurity, depression and anger.

Although the prevalence of smoking has fallen in many developed countries, including the UK, USA and Canada (Figure 2.8), this has been accompanied by a shift in the gender and class profile. Fewer women have given up smoking, and those who have are more likely to be in the higher socioeconomic groups. This is especially true of expectant mothers (Figure 2.9).

▲ Key points

Population-based approaches to reduce the prevalence of smoking

- ▲ Price increases
- ▲ Controls on advertising and sponsorship
- ▲ Enforcement of smoke-free environments
- ▲ Health promotion programmes

▲ Key points

Approaches to encourage individuals to stop smoking

- ▲ Offer advice and information about effects of smoking
- ▲ Offer nicotine replacement
- ▲ Monitor progress with further consultations
- ▲ Set a date to stop smoking

Women make up an increasing proportion of the declining population of smokers

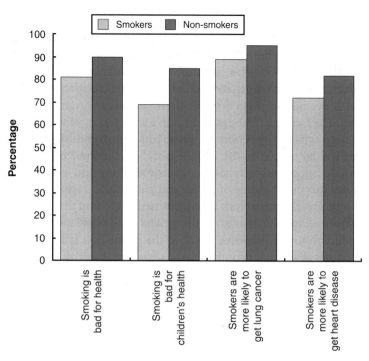

Figure 2.7 Beliefs about smoking and health. The majority of smokers and non-smokers are aware of the principal health hazards associated with smoking. Even so, there is a small tendency for smokers to be less aware of (or to deny) the risks. (Data from Graham, 1993.)

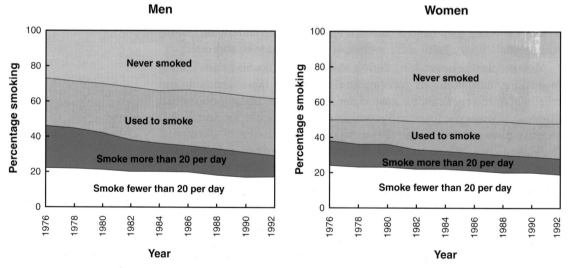

Figure 2.8 Percentage of the adult population aged 16 years and over who smoke (UK, 1976–1992). The number of male and female smokers in the UK has fallen in recent years. In men, the proportion of ex-smokers and those who have never smoked has increased. In women, the proportion of those who have never smoked remains roughly the same, and hence the reduction in smoking prevalence is because of women who have given up the habit. Men are more likely to smoke heavily (more than 20 cigarettes a day) than women. (Source: OPCS, *General Household Survey*, 1992.)

Smoking in pregnancy is associated with retardation of fetal growth and development. In turn, low birthweight is an important determinant of perinatal death. Most low birthweight babies are born to working-class mothers. In this group the prevalence of smoking is high, and the women are much less likely to stop smoking at the time of their pregnancy (Figure 2.9).

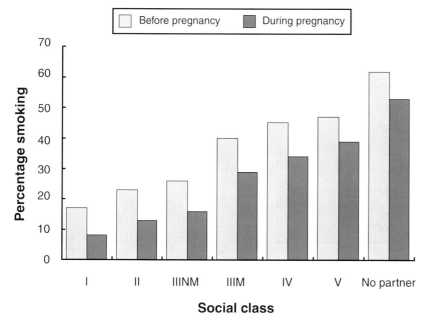

Figure 2.9 Prevalence of smoking in expectant mothers by social class. Less than 20% of women in social class I smoked before their pregnancy, compared with 47% in social class IV. About 50% of women smokers in social class I give up during pregnancy but in social class V far fewer women seem prepared to give up their habit. Mothers without a partner have the highest reported rate of smoking. (Data from White, A. *et al. Infant Feeding, 1990*, published by HMSO, London, 1992.)

Alcohol consumption

Alcohol consumption is a major cause of premature death and ill health. Although people respond in different ways because of differences in body weight or how they metabolise alcohol, in sufficient quantities all people experience adverse effects. Therefore substantial gains in health can be achieved by interventions aimed at reducing alcohol consumption in the general population. As with cigarette smoking this can be achieved through a number of mechanisms, most notably by increasing tax revenues on alcohol sales and by health education campaigns.

The principal health education message aimed at limiting alcohol consumption is by counting units of consumption. In the UK the recommended safe daily drinking limits were increased in 1995 to 2-3 units for women and 3-4 units for men. This also differs from previous advice in

There are substantial health risks in exceeding recommended limits of alcohol consumption, but low intakes can be beneficial

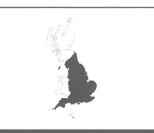

that the recommendations are in respect to daily, rather than weekly, consumption. This is to limit binge drinking which is a health and social hazard to both the drinker and other people. According to the General Household Survey (OPCS, 1992) the average consumption in the UK is below these limits (Figure 2.10), but the range of consumption would include both teetotallers and heavy drinkers. It is estimated that more than one-quarter of all men and one in 12 women regularly consume more alcohol than the (old) recommended limits. Currently the consumption of alcohol per head of population aged 15 years and over (calculated from excise returns) is about 9.0 litres a year. This represents a steady increase from the levels seen in the 1950s, although consumption has appeared to fall slightly since the late 1980s.

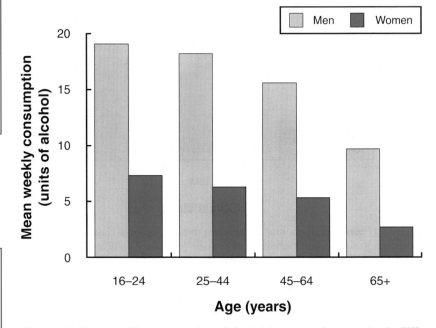

Figure 2.10 Mean weekly consumption of alcohol in men and women in the UK. Alcohol consumption is most prevalent in young men. At all ages the mean amount of alcohol consumed by women is substantially less than in men. The mean consumption for all groups is within recommended limits but the data include teetotallers and so it can be expected that a substantial number of young and middle-aged men drink significantly more than is prudent. (Source: OPCS, 1992.)

Excessive consumption of alcohol is associated with both short and longer-term behavioural and physical effects. The short-term effects include behavioural changes and hangover, and can result in deaths from poisoning, accident or violence. Long-term effects include dependence, behavioural changes and damage to various organs of the body, most notably the liver, brain and muscle.

People respond in different ways to regular and heavy alcohol consumption. In some people there will be no significant damage to the liver, while in others fatty changes are produced. The less fortunate develop alcoholic hepatitis, followed by cirrhosis and eventually liver cancer. Significant liver damage probably requires daily consumption of about 16 units of alcohol for 5 years or more. Women are more susceptible to alcoholic liver damage than men, possibly because of differences in metabolism: blood alcohol concentrations in women consuming the same amounts of alcohol as men are higher.

About 20% of heavy drinkers develop liver cirrhosis. The main complications of liver cirrhosis are portal hypertension, oesophageal varices and ascites. There is also a risk of developing hepatocellular carcinoma (liver cancer). Other cancers linked with excessive alcohol consumption are cancers of the mouth, pharynx and larynx. Alcoholics experience muscle wasting, and changes in the central nervous system can be caused by excessive consumption or alcohol withdrawal. The effects of acute intoxication include disturbances of balance, gait and speech, epilepsy and coma. Alcohol withdrawal can be accompanied by tremor of the arms and legs, delirium and epilepsy. Long-term consumption of alcohol can cause degeneration of the cerebrum and cerebellum (leading to dementia) and polyneuropathy. Heavy and persistent drinkers are at greater risk of developing long-term complications than sporadic drinkers.

Mechanisms of alcohol damage

Ethanol is the principal alcohol consumed in alcoholic drinks, but **methanol**, the main component of 'methylated spirit', consumed by 'meths' drinkers, is much more dangerous. The metabolites of methanol are formaldehyde and formic acid which are extremely toxic, causing blindness and rapid death.

Most ethanol metabolism takes place in the liver (Figure 2.11). The liver cells possess a number of enzymatic pathways for metabolising alcohol, all of which yield acetaldehyde. This substance is metabolically very active and is toxic to the liver cells. Normally acetaldehyde is rapidly oxidised by another liver enzyme, aldehyde dehydrogenase, yielding acetate, most of which leaves the liver to be metabolised by peripheral tissues, including skeletal and heart muscles to acetyl-CoA, which in turn is mostly oxidised to carbon dioxide. Acetate can also be converted to fatty acids, cholesterol and amino acids.

Some individuals, particularly those of oriental origin, have a structural defect in aldehyde dehydrogenase which means that acetaldehyde is destroyed very slowly. They display an intolerance to alcohol, with very small amounts causing facial flushing and increased heart rate.

There is some evidence that moderate consumption of alcohol can be beneficial. It is known, for example that alcohol modulates blood lipids so that the concentration of high density lipoprotein (HDL) is increased. Alcohol also affects blood clotting factors and reduces the tendency for arterial thrombosis. Together, these effects reduce the risk of coronary heart disease.

In the UK, a long-term prospective study, started in 1978, has examined the relationship between alcohol consumption and deaths in male British doctors. The data indicate that excessive consumption increases the risk of premature death, but that small amounts can actually do some good (Figure 2.12). The optimal amount in men appears to be 1-2 units a day. The current

Alcoholic hepatitis: an inflammatory condition of the liver as a response to continued cell damage and death.

Ascites: intraperitoneal accumulation of fluid. The quantity of fluid can be several litres, causing abdominal distension. A consequence of portal hypertension.

Cirrhosis: arises from the death of liver cells followed by fibrosis. The normal architecture of the liver is disrupted, causing interference to blood flow and normal functions. In most cases cirrhosis is irreversible, even after abstinence from alcohol.

Fatty liver: abnormal accumulation of fat within the liver cells – an indicator of non-lethal cell injury. In its early stages it is completely reversible.

Oesophageal varices: caused by portal hypertension. Blood flow is diverted through the coronary veins of the stomach into the submucosa of the lower oesophagus. These veins dilate and protrude directly beneath the mucosa. There is a chance that these veins will rupture, causing catastrophic blood loss.

Polyneuropathy: widespread loss of sensation caused by peripheral nerve damage.

Portal hypertension: a complication of liver cirrhosis caused by resistance in portal blood flow in the sinusoids.

Acetaldehyde: a toxic metabolite of alcohol produced in the liver. Toxicity is produced by binding with proteins, amino acids and amines, to form aldehyde adducts.

Consequences of alcohol consumption

- ▲ Acute behavioural and physical changes
- ▲ Dependence
- ▲ Liver cirrhosis
- ▲ Cancers of the mouth, pharynx, larynx, oesophagus and liver
- ▲ Damage to muscle and nervous system
- ▲ Moderate consumption associated with lower risk of death from coronary heart disease and some other causes
- ▲ Excessive consumption is associated with increased risks of death

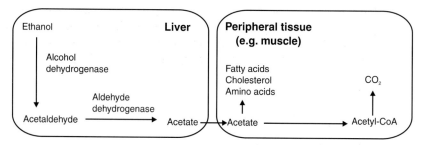

Figure 2.11 Metabolism of ethanol. In liver cells alcohol is oxidised to acetaldehyde by alcohol dehydrogenase. This highly toxic substance is metabolised to acetate by aldehyde dehydrogenase. Most of the acetate produced leaves the liver and is metabolised by the heart and skeletal muscle. The likelihood of liver damage depends on alcohol intake and the relative amounts or activities of alcohol and aldehyde dehydrogenases: most damage is mediated by accumulation of acetaldehyde.

recommendation for safe drinking is higher than this but the man who consumes 3-4 units of alcohol daily is no worse off than the teetotaller as far as long-term health risks are concerned. The rapid consumption of alcohol within the 'safe-drinking' levels would render many people unfit to drive a car.

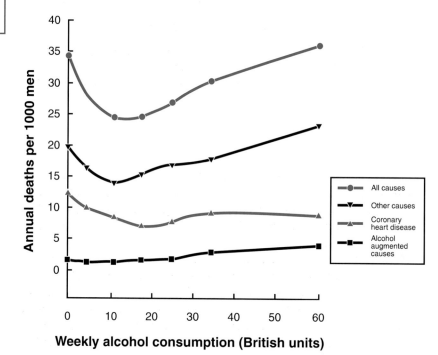

Figure 2.12 Alcohol consumption and annual deaths per 1000 men: a study of British doctors carried over 13 years. The relationship between alcohol consumption and all-cause mortality in men is a U-shaped curve, with increased risks at both very low and very high levels of consumption. Alcohol-augmented causes comprise injury, poisoning, liver disease, cancer of upper digestive tract and alcoholic psychosis. (Adapted from Doll *et al.*, 1994.)

The consumption of alcohol is very frequently accompanied by smoking: a visit to any public house or bar will confirm this association. The two agents probably act synergistically so that, for example, oral or pharyngeal cancer is much more likely to develop when both agents are present (Figure 2.13).

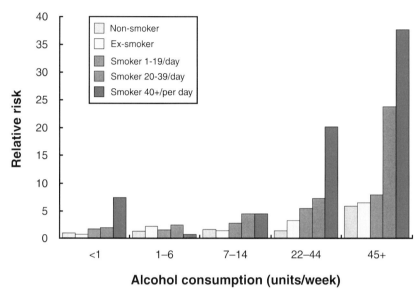

Figure 2.13 Relative risks of oral and pharyngeal cancer in men who drink alcohol and smoke cigarettes. The risk of oral and pharyngeal cancer increases with both the number of cigarettes smoked and alcohol consumed. (Adapted from Austoker, 1994.)

Body mass index (BMI): body weight (in kg) divided by the height (in metres) squared.

Obesity: the abnormal accumulation of adipose tissue throughout the body. Usually defined as a BMI in excess of 30 kg/m^2.

Obesity

A variety of disease conditions are associated with obesity. Weight reduction can prolong survival as well as reduce the impact of disabling conditions such as osteoarthritis. Although it is possible for obese people to reduce their weight to normal this can be very difficult, and 90% or more of individuals regain that weight within several years.

Studies with identical twins who have lived apart indicate that there is a genetic component to obesity. In mice, the protein product of the ob (obesity) gene, when injected, causes the animals to lose weight and to maintain the weight loss. This Ob protein, produced by fat cells, works to regulate body weight. In some mice the *ob* gene is mutated, and the lack of Ob protein means that weight gain goes unchecked. So far, no counterpart of the *ob* gene and its protein has been identified in humans, but one probably does exist.

The prevalence of obesity is increasing (Figure 2.14). It is possible that some people with a family history of obesity have inherited the equivalent of an inactive ob gene. However, in most people obesity is caused by overeating inappropriate foods and taking insufficient exercise (there is an imbalance between energy intake and energy expenditure). If most cases were inherited

Obesity increases the risk of developing chronic disabling conditions

The large increase in the prevalence of obesity indicates that most cases are caused by lifestyle factors

or caused by metabolic conditions, factors which are relatively constant, the increase in the prevalence of obesity would not be so marked. Despite the availability of drugs and other treatments the only long-term way of tackling obesity is by dietary control. For some the necessary restrictions place such constraints on their enjoyment of life that the treatment is worse than the condition, or the prospect of disease. However, there are gains for those who persevere.

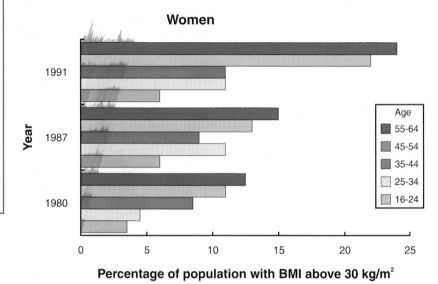

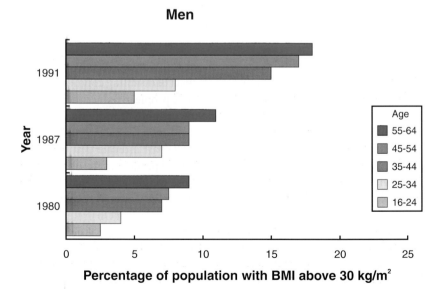

Figure 2.14 Obesity in men and women in the UK, 1980–1991. Generally, the prevalence of obesity is higher in women than in men. Obesity has become more common in most age groups. (Source: OPCS, *Health Survey for England*, 1991.)

The primary metabolic consequence of obesity is a reduced sensitivity to insulin. As a result obese individuals are much more likely to become diabetic, and to suffer the long-term consequences of diabetes such as coronary heart disease and stroke. The risk of coronary heart disease and stroke is exacerbated by the usually higher blood low-density lipoprotein (LDL) and triglyceride levels in obese people.

Further complications arise from the influence of adipose tissue in the metabolism of the sex hormones. Adipose tissue contains aromatase enzymes which convert androgens to oestrogens. Some cancers, such as endometrial cancer and breast cancer, are oestrogen-sensitive and there is evidence that the risks of these cancer types are increased in obese women. There are also differences in cholesterol loading so that the excretion pathway (synthesis of bile) becomes saturated, leading to abnormal liver function and the production of gallstones (the rather insensitive caricature of the typical patient with gallstones is 'fat, female, and forty').

Overweight also places excessive strains on the joints and there is therefore an increased tendency to osteoarthritis and back pain. One bonus is that the increased load on the bony skeleton helps to maintain bone mass so that there is some protection against osteoporosis.

Exercise

The role of exercise in improving general physical and mental well-being is increasingly being recognised, helping to overcome the negative health effects of the modern sedentary lifestyle. Historically people were much more physically active than is common in most developed countries and it is evident that the human frame is designed to be active. From the previous discussions on environmental factors and health one could be forgiven for thinking that the best strategy would be to avoid the environment and go out or do as little as possible. Unfortunately such inaction could prove disastrous.

Exercise not only helps to prevent disease but it can also enable people to overcome the effects of chronic illness more effectively. The most obvious advantages of exercise are in reducing the risk or effects of coronary heart disease, osteoporosis, obesity, hypertension and diabetes. Exercise induces measurable changes in many physiological parameters, most notably in lowering systolic and diastolic blood pressure. There are also improvements in the functional capacity of the lungs, heart and muscles and beneficial effects on the skeletal and immune systems.

The combination of exercise and modification of other risk factors can be very effective: an energy-reduced diet is easier to maintain and weight loss is concentrated on fat. The result is greater self-esteem and a boost to morale. There are, of course, some risks attached to exercise, especially if it is not introduced gradually or if the exercise is to the point of over-exertion: it is essential to know one's limits. Exercise also brings the risk of personal injury, stress fractures and joint problems. Although there have been reports of death during running and other sporting activities, often from underlying heart

Exercise can act as a catalyst for a positive approach to health and lifestyle

▲ Key points

Benefits of exercise

▲ Controls body weight
▲ Enhances mood and self-esteem
▲ Enhances cardiac performance, improves blood pressure
▲ Improves insulin sensitivity and glucose tolerance
▲ Improves blood lipid profile and risk of coronary heart disease
▲ Increases peak bone mass and maintains bone (in moderation)
▲ Improves joint function and range of movement

disease, this risk should be balanced against the undoubted improvement that proper exercise training can bring to work capacity and blood pressure.

There is evidence that physically active people outlive those who are inactive. This may be only by a few months, and people might well ask if this is worth all the effort but the main point is that exercise helps to maintain the quality of life by promoting functional independence and self-esteem. Improving health is not all about adding years to life, but adding life to the years. This concept is recognised in the American *Healthy People 2000* objectives, which were designed to offer community-based programmes and promotion for a healthy life (Figure 2.15).

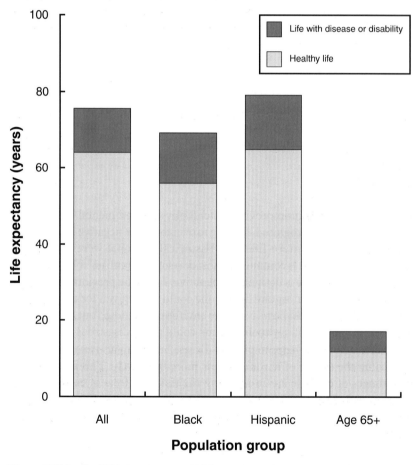

Figure 2.15 In the USA in 1990 overall life expectancy was 75.4 years, including 64 years of healthy life. For Blacks, life expectancy is reduced to 69.1 years, and includes only 56 years of healthy life. Although life expectancy for Hispanics is longer, there is no gain in years of healthy life. To a large extent these trends are probably a reflection of economic disadvantage. (Source: US Department of Health and Human Services, 1991.)

In common with modification of other risk factors, the problem with exercise is getting people to do it. This depends first on the accessibility of suitable facilities and the time needed to fit exercise into the regular lifestyle. The second factor is that of motivation: the initial sessions after some years of a sedentary lifestyle can be very discouraging. Stamina, muscle strength and joint movement can all be improved by a modest increase in activity although this is a gradual process, building over a period of many months.

The health benefits of exercise are brought about by light or moderate activity rather than by strenuous exercise. The aim is to increase calorie-burning on a regular basis, sustainable throughout the lifespan. The Healthy People 2000 recommendation is that light to moderate physical activity should be undertaken for at least 30 minutes daily. A sustained walk would meet the definition of light physical activity, but more vigorous activity (for example by engaging in sport or other fitness activities) would be needed to improve or maintain cardiorespiratory fitness.

> *The old adage that 'no pain, no gain' is not, and should not, be true*

Stress

Many people have put forward the view that the stressful nature of modern life is at least in part responsible for many present-day illnesses. Perhaps the classic example is the middle-aged man in a high-powered executive job who suddenly dies of a heart attack. Different personality types play a part in susceptibility to this disease. It is likely that stress has affected the human race from time immemorial: what has changed is the source of the stress, coupled with fewer opportunities to counter its effects because of a sedentary lifestyle.

> *Constant exposure to stress may increase susceptibility to disease*

One of the problems in examining the effects of stress on health is in defining exactly what stress is. Individual perceptions of, and responses to, possible stressful agents vary: some people thrive under pressure to meet deadlines or acquire new job skills while others become emotionally exhausted and depressed. Retrospective studies are often unreliable because stress could well be an outcome of disease rather than a cause of it. Most research has examined stress in terms of measurable life events such as bereavement, divorce or separation from children. In these studies there seems to be some relationship between adverse life events and risk of death in the short term. Certain occupations are known to involve stress, and this is reflected in suicide rates, drug or alcohol abuse. The healthcare professions have a high ranking in these statistics.

There are demonstrable physiological responses to stress, for example in the production of the 'stress' hormones adrenaline and cortisol. These changes may worsen hypertension and pre-existing cardiovascular disease. Evidence is emerging that reactions to stress are modulated by adaptive responses in the brain, and that persistent or repeated stress is more likely to have pathological consequences. Ultimately the response is an individual one, reflecting variation in personality and, presumably, neurochemistry.

These nervous and endocrine responses exert effects on the immune system. How important these effects are remain the subject of much research, but it is easy to see that any inhibition of immune responses will increase susceptibility

Adrenaline: the 'fight or flight' hormone produced by the adrenal medulla in conditions of fear or stress. Mobilises carbohydrate and fat energy stores.

Cortisol: a hormone released by the adrenal cortex, regulated by a feedback mechanism involving the hypothalamus and pituitary. Cortisol mobilises nutrient stores, increasing blood glucose levels.

Review question 1

Indicate the common diseases and conditions with which the following behavioural and lifestyle risk factors are believed to have an influence (parts of this question rely on your general knowledge and if not addressed in this chapter will be discussed in subsequent chapters).

Smoking

High-fat diet

Low-fibre diet

Low consumption of fruit and vegetables

High salt intake

High alcohol consumption

Low alcohol consumption

Multiple sexual partners

Low exercise levels

to a wide variety of diseases and impair response to treatment.

Disease: nature *versus* nurture?

While it can be said that the root of all disease is in our genes, the opportunity for genetic expression sometimes depends on the environment. Hence, when life expectancy is short because of overcrowding, malnutrition, poor hygiene and sanitation there is little opportunity for deleterious genes to become evident. As life expectancy increases chronic diseases such as non-insulin-dependent diabetes, cardiovascular disease, cancers and Alzheimer's disease become more common. Genetic factors contribute strongly to the aetiology of these conditions: sufficient time has elapsed for hitherto concealed deleterious genes to exert their effects.

It could be argued that ultimately genetic evolution is an adaptive response to the environment, although this does not occur within our own lifetime. In practical terms, the prevention and control of disease is rooted in nurture, rather than nature. With the advent of gene therapy, this state of affairs may alter but gene therapy is unlikely to become a solution for common conditions in the immediate future, or for people who happen to live in the less developed countries.

ANSWERS TO REVIEW QUESTIONS

Question 1

Indicate the common diseases and conditions with which behavioural and lifestyle risk factors are believed to have an influence

This list is not exhaustive but includes the most likely associated conditions.

Smoking	Cancers of the lung, larynx, mouth Cervical cancer Respiratory disease – bronchitis, emphysema Atherosclerosis and complications – coronary heart disease, stroke, peripheral vascular disease
High-fat diet	Obesity Coronary heart disease Colorectal cancer Breast cancer
Low-fibre diet	Coronary heart disease

	Diverticular disease
	Colorectal cancer
Low consumption of fruit and vegetables	Vitamin deficiencies, e.g. scurvy
	Coronary heart disease
	Colorectal cancer
	Stomach cancer
High salt intake	Hypertension
	Stomach cancer
High alcohol consumption	Liver cirrhosis
	Oral and pharyngeal cancer
	Hypertension
	Psychological dependence
Low alcohol consumption	Coronary heart disease
Multiple sexual partners	Sexually transmitted diseases, e.g. syphilis, gonorrhoea, hepatitis, non-specific urethritis, AIDS
	Cervical cancer
Low exercise levels	Coronary heart disease
	Obesity
	Osteoporosis

References

Austoker, J. (1994) Smoking and cancer: smoking cessation. *BMJ*, **308**, 1478-82.

Department of Health. *The Health of the Nation*, London, HMSO.

Doll, R., Peto, R., Hall, E. *et al*. (1994) Mortality in relation to consumption of alcohol: 13 years' observations on male British doctors. *BMJ*, **309**, 911-18.

Graham, H. (1993) *When Life's a Drag*, London, HMSO.

US Department of Health and Human Services (1991) *Healthy People 2000: National Health Promotion and Disease Prevention Objectives*, Boston, Jones & Bartlett.

Further reading

Fentem, P.H. (1994) Benefits of exercise in health and disease. *BMJ*, **308**, 1293-95.

Hayes, P.C. (1993) *Alcoholic Liver Disease. Baillière's Clinical Gastroenterology*, Vol. 7, London, Baillière Tindall.

Jacobson, B., Smith, A. and Whitehead, M. (1991) *The Nation's Health. A Strategy for the 1990s*, London, King Edward's Hospital Fund for London.

3   The genetic basis of disease

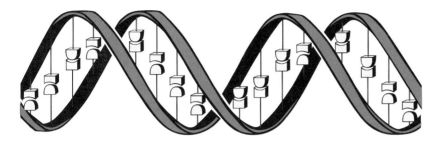

Alterations in the genetic code are found in both rare and common diseases. Genetic defects can be inherited or acquired. The inherited conditions can involve many genes present in whole chromosomes or just a small defect in a single gene, sometimes involving only one base pair.

Acquired alterations in the genetic code usually involve a number of genes. Perhaps the most commonly encountered alterations that occur in the older adult affect the growth characteristics of the cells, eventually causing cancer. These mutations are usually an outcome of injury by intrinsic or extrinsic agents. Although the mutation itself has not been inherited, the predisposition of that particular piece of the genetic code to injury can be inherited. This is why common diseases such as some cancers and coronary heart disease, though not directly inherited, appear to run in families. In these cases development of the disease will depend on exposure to other agents.

In the not-so-distant past the study of the genetic complement of cells in health and disease was limited to analysis of gross morphological changes in the chromosomes, together with biochemical techniques aimed at establishing differences in the gene products. The advent of recombinant DNA technology has allowed the production of genetic probes which can be used to detect much more subtle alterations in the genes themselves.

Pre-test

Can you list any genetic disorders?
What are the patterns of inheritance in genetic disorders?
Do genetic diseases necessarily have to be inherited?
How can genetic disorders be detected?

Aims of this chapter

By the end of this chapter you will have increased your knowledge of:
◆ The principal genetic alterations responsible for inherited and acquired diseases
◆ The methods used for identifying and analysing the genetic code
◆ How the identification of genes contributes to our ability to track disease and provide greater understanding of pathological processes

In addition, this chapter will help you to:
◆ Describe the principal methods available for the identification and analysis of genetic material and assess their advantages and limitations
◆ Describe the methods for producing genetic probes and the means by which probe and target genetic information can be visualised
◆ Evaluate the application of gene technology to our understanding of disease processes
◆ Assess the clinical applications of genetic analysis

Introduction

For conditions to be inherited a genetic defect, or **mutation**, must have originated in the egg or sperm (the **gametes** or **germ cells**). A genetic disease can be acquired at any stage of life after fertilisation, and may involve mutations in the genetic material of **somatic** cells.

Some diseases are the direct result of an inherited mutation in a single gene. Tens of thousands of **genes** control different metabolic functions in the body and, in theory, a defect could occur in any of these to cause disease. To date about 5000 disease-causing genes are known but not all have been mapped to specific chromosome locations. Less than 10% of these have been cloned and sequenced but the rate of progress in genetics is now so rapid that hardly a week seems to go by without a report appearing of a new advance.

There are fewer genetic diseases than the total number of genes, probably because of differences in gene susceptibility to damage and mutation. Cellular DNA is highly condensed by being folded in on itself and is also protected by proteins. Presumably, susceptibility to damage depends on the location and accessibility of a gene to a damaging agent. The disorders caused by single gene defects are individually very rare, but as a group they represent one of the more common types of genetic disorder. Many single gene disorders involve mutations to genes that are responsible for the production of an enzyme, although in some examples the gene is responsible for alterations in structural proteins.

Another kind of genetic disorder involves alterations to many hundreds of genes, involving either complete chromosomes or parts of chromosomes. These alterations, caused by a 'mistake' during the separation of the chromosome pairs in meiosis so that the genetic material is divided unequally ('non-disjunction'), are inherited. Large alterations to the genetic material can also occur in somatic cells, often causing the cell to become cancerous.

Genetic abnormalities cause alterations to cellular metabolism

DNA, deoxyribonucleic acid: the chemical blueprint of life. The genetic 'code' is determined by the sequence of base pairs in the DNA: adenosine, cytosine, guanine and thymine (A, C, G and T). One triplet sequence (CGA, for example) encodes a specific amino acid that, with others coded by different triplet sequences, is assembled into proteins. DNA is packaged in chromosomes in the nucleus, but is also present in mitochondria.

Gene: a segment of DNA that carries the code for making a single protein. The human genome (the genetic complement of all the chromosomes in each normal nucleated cell) comprises about 70 000 genes. Two copies of each gene are inherited, one from each parent. Only one of the gene copies is necessary to make the protein, and the other gene will be inactive.

Somatic: derived from soma, meaning 'of the body'.

Chromosome abnormalities

There are two broad categories of chromosome abnormalities, involving an alteration to the number of chromosomes or an alteration to the structure of the chromosomes. The amount of DNA is altered by these changes: there may be too much because there is an extra chromosome, or too little because a chromosome is absent. Sometimes genes are no longer in their original site in the DNA because they have been **translocated**. At the new site the gene does not function properly or alters the function of neighbouring genes. Because so much DNA is affected by chromosome abnormalities the consequences are usually very severe and may be incompatible with life. Abnormalities in the number of autosomal chromosomes usually cause multiple congenital malformations, almost invariably with mental retardation. Abnormalities of the sex chromosomes usually affect the development of genital organs and secondary sexual characteristics.

> *Alterations in the amount of chromosomal DNA cause developmental defects, often including mental retardation*

Background information: The human karyotype

The chromosome complement, known as the **karyotype**, of a normal human is 46. This comprises 22 pairs of **autosomes** and one pair of **sex chromosomes**. The complement of 46 is referred to as the **diploid** number. Half of this number, $n = 23$, would comprise the chromosome complement of a human gamete. This is referred to as the **haploid** number.

After fertilisation the zygote contains the full diploid set ($2n = 46$) of chromosomes, one of each pair having come from the mother, the other from the father. A multiple of the basic haploid set greater than diploid ($4n = 92$, for example) is known as **polyploid**. **Aneuploid** refers to chromosome numbers which are not exact multiples of the haploid set. One extra chromosome in the somatic cell ($2n + 1$) is referred to as **trisomy**. One chromosome less than normal ($2n - 1$) is referred to as **monosomy**.

Polyploid abnormalities of the zygote are not compatible with life. Some 15–20% of all conceptions are lost spontaneously, and about half of these are caused by some form of chromosomal abnormality. Triploidy ($3n = 69$) accounts for some 17% of spontaneous abortions.

Cytogenetics: analysis of chromosome abnormalities

Theoretically chromosomes can be identified in any nucleated cell but in practice it is necessary to culture the cells to obtain sufficient material and to induce cell division (mitosis) so that the chromosomes can be seen. The most accessible site of nucleated cells is the blood (leukocytes). Skin cells (fibroblasts) and fetal cells in the chorionic villus or amniotic fluid are also commonly used for cytogenetic evaluation. Cells from other sites in the body are usually less suitable for culture because of microbial contamination,

Autosome: any chromosome other than the sex chromosomes.

Chromosome: contains DNA and protein and is situated in the cell nucleus. Each chromosome has two arms, or chromatids, joined together at the centromere. The short arm of a chromosome is termed p, the long arm q. When stained, chromosomes can appear banded. The bands are allocated numbers, reading outwards from the centromere. Hence 11q13 refers to band 13 in the short arm of chromosome 11.

Sex chromosomes: determine the sex of the individual, XX in normal females, XY in normal males.

which causes the culture to fail.

During culture the cells are stimulated into division and arrested in mid-division by addition of an agent which interferes with formation of the mitotic spindle. The cells are partially lysed (to expand the chromosomes) by addition of hypertonic fluid, fixed, dried onto a glass slide and stained.

The **chromosome spread** is evaluated under the microscope, solely on the morphological criteria of chromosome number, deletions or translocations. Chromosomes are identified by their size and characteristic banding pattern when the preparations are partially digested and stained. Entirely different methods (discussed later in this chapter) are used to analyse the composition of the genes themselves.

Autosomal abnormalities

The most common autosomal abnormality is Trisomy 21 (Down's syndrome). Other more rare abnormalities include Trisomy 18 (Edward's syndrome) and Trisomy 13 (Patau's syndrome).

Trisomy 21

People with Down's syndrome have a characteristic facial appearance and are mentally retarded. They may die young although, increasingly, patients survive to the fourth or fifth decades. Down's syndrome brings an increased risk for recurrent infections, which used to be a very common cause of death in children and young adults with the abnormality. People with Down's syndrome also have an increased risk of developing acute leukaemia and, if they survive beyond the age of 40, are likely to develop Alzheimer's disease.

The incidence of Trisomy 21 in the UK is one in 650 live births. In addition there are many conceptions with this abnormality which do not survive to full term. The abnormality is strongly associated with increased maternal age. A mother who is 44 years of age or over at delivery has a one in 40 chance of delivering a child with Down's syndrome. In younger mothers (below 30 years) the incidence of Trisomy 21 is only about one in 900. Because there are so many more births to younger mothers, the greatest number of Down's syndrome children are actually born to younger mothers.

Most cases are caused by non-disjunction of chromosome 21 during meiosis (Figure 3.1). In view of the association with increased maternal age this is more likely to have occurred during formation of the egg rather than the sperm.

About 5% of cases of Down's syndrome are caused by translocation of chromosome 21 onto chromosome 14 or, occasionally, onto chromosome 22. Often one of the parents has a balanced version of the same translocation, but has only 45 chromosomes. This is called the **Robertsonian translocation** and the person is phenotypically normal because the retained combined chromosome is very large and contains virtually all the necessary genetic information. The affected child will have 46 chromosomes, one of which is a

Meiosis: a type of cell division which occurs during formation of the egg or sperm (gamete). Gametes contain half the somatic number of chromosomes.

Non-disjunction: the failure of two members of a chromosome pair to come apart during cell division, so that both are passed on to the same daughter cell.

Phenotype: the physical, biochemical and physiological characteristics of an organism.

Translocation: chromosomal rearrangement in which two different chromosomes are broken and genetic material exchanged from one to the other. In a balanced translocation the same amount of genetic material is transferred to each chromosome. In an unbalanced translocation genetic material is either gained or lost.

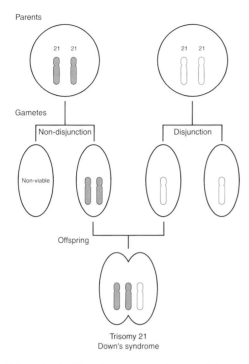

Figure 3.1 Non-disjunction in Down's syndrome. In non-disjunction a chromosome pair fails to separate, so that a gamete has two chromosome copies instead of one. Fertilisation with a normal gamete results in three copies (trisomy) of the chromosome in the somatic cells.

translocated chromosome 21 (Figure 3.2). The risk of Down's syndrome in a child is 10% when the translocation is carried by the mother and 2.5% when it is present in the father.

Non-disjunction is a purely chance event and the risk of recurrence is low. There are higher risks of producing further Down's syndrome offspring when the cause is a translocation, since a chromosomal abnormality is already present in one of the parents.

Trisomy 18

Individuals affected by trisomy 18 are mentally retarded, have a characteristic facial appearance with a prominent occiput, growth deficiency, rocker bottom feet, and heart and kidney abnormalities. Most survive only weeks or months. The incidence of trisomy 18 is about 0.12 per 1000 live births in the UK. Most cases are caused by non-disjunction, with the incidence increasing with maternal age.

Trisomy 13

Trisomy 13 causes severe mental retardation, structural abnormalities in the brain and microcephaly. Other malformations include cleft lip and palate, and

Microcephaly: small brain.

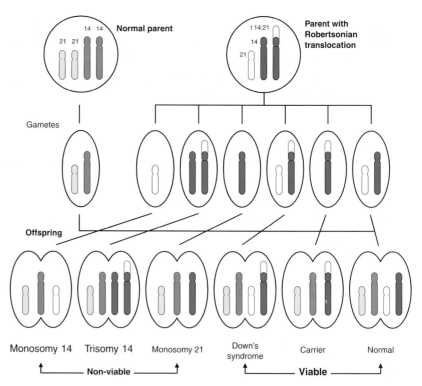

Figure 3.2 In a Robertsonian translocation most of the genetic material of two chromosomes is combined into one, so the person has a karyotype of only 45 chromosomes. The person experiences no direct ill effects, but is a carrier for more serious abnormalities because their gametes are abnormal. There are six possibilities, each gamete containing single or double copies of chromosome 14 and 21 genetic material (in the t14:21 Robertsonian translocation). Fertilisation with a normal gamete can lead to six possible combinations, including two monosomies and trisomy 14 which are not viable. Down's syndrome can arise, even though the offspring has the 'normal' complement of 46 chromosomes, because of the extra chromosome 21 genetic material present in the large t14:21 chromosome.

eye, kidney and heart defects. Most affected infants survive only hours or a few weeks. The incidence of this disorder is about 0.07 per 1000 live births. It is mainly caused by non-disjunction, and the risk of recurrence is usually low, although the condition can be caused by a translocation, which has a higher risk of recurrence.

Sex chromosome abnormalities

Turner's syndrome

A person with Turner's syndrome is female in appearance, but with short stature, broad chest and webbing of the neck. The ovaries exist only as streaks of fibrous tissue and the individual is thus infertile. In this condition one of the X chromosomes is missing; there are therefore 45 chromosomes in the karyotype, which is designated XO. The cause is meiotic non-disjunction, which most frequently occurs in the father. The incidence of Turner's syndrome in the UK is about one in 3500 female births. However, the abnormality accounts for one in 15 spontaneous abortions – in other words it is a much more frequent genetic abnormality than is suggested by the number of live cases.

Klinefelter's syndrome

Until adolescence, boys with Klinefelter's syndrome appear as normal males but individuals are infertile because of very small testes and an absence of spermatogenesis. Breast development (gynaecomastia) occurs at puberty. The condition is relatively common, accounting for about one in 500 of male births. It is caused by an extra X chromosome; the karyotype therefore consists of 47 chromosomes and is designated XXY. The extra X chromosome can be seen as a Barr body in somatic cells.

> **Barr body:** a drumstick-shaped portion of condensed chromatin in the nucleus, caused by clumping of two X chromosomes. Can be detected simply by scraping the inside of the mouth and staining the cells removed. Normal males do not have Barr bodies.

XYY syndrome

Individuals with the XYY chromosome complement (an extra copy of the Y male chromosome) appear as normal males, are usually tall in stature and are said to exhibit more aggressive behaviour than normal XY males. Very often the condition remains undetected clinically. The incidence is about one in 2000 male births.

Single gene disorders

Single gene disorders are caused by a defect in a single gene or gene group. There are clear patterns of inheritance, with the possibilities of producing further affected children, normal children or, in recessive disorders, children who by all appearances are normal but who carry the altered gene. The likelihood of passing a defective gene on to an offspring can be calculated and used to inform and counsel prospective parents with a family history of genetic abnormality. The calculations are not always precise because of the play of chance and depend on the degree of **gene penetrance** (Figure 3.3). When penetrance is incomplete the person inherits the dominant gene but does not develop the disorder or is only mildly affected. These people can still pass on the gene to produce more severely affected offspring, but the risk of severe disease is small because the low-penetrance genes tend to remain so in the offspring.

The most common single gene disorder in populations of northern European origin is cystic fibrosis. On a global scale the most common conditions are the blood disorders sickle-cell anaemia and thalassaemia.

Autosomal dominant inheritance

An autosomal dominant disorder occurs when a gene mutation exerts its full

> *A dominant disorder arises through inheritance of one copy of a defective gene*

Allele: alternative forms of a gene found at the same locus in homologous chromosomes.

Epidermolysis bullosa: a blistering skin disease. Some variants are autosomal recessively inherited, others are autosomal dominant. Caused by mutations in the genes responsible for keratin and collagen.

Heterozygous: an individual who has two different alleles of the same gene at a particular locus, one in each chromosome of the pair.

Homozygous: an individual who has two identical alleles at a particular locus, one in each chromosome of the pair.

Marfan syndrome: a connective tissue disorder caused by mutation of genes in chromosome 15 controlling synthesis of fibrillin, a component of elastic fibres. Patients are unusually tall and have abnormalities of the cardiovascular system (usually leading to aortic aneurysm), eyes and skeleton.

Neurofibromatosis type 1, von Recklinghausen's disease: disfiguring condition characterised by multiple neurofibromas (soft nodules protruding from the skin), pigmented lesions known as café au lait spots and pigmented nodules in the iris. Incidence in the UK about one in 3000. The genetic defect is in a tumour suppressor gene in chromosome 17. Type II neurofibromatosis is much more rare and is clinically and genetically distinct.

Osteogenesis imperfecta: an abnormality of type I collagen formation, causing brittle bones which fracture with minimal trauma and become deformed. There are several types of disease, ranging in severity, with dominant or recessive patterns of inheritance. There are more than 20 genes for type I collagen, distributed over 10 chromosomes.

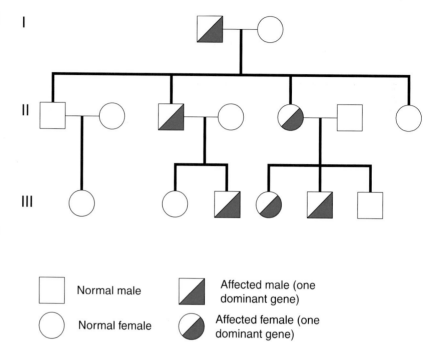

Figure 3.3 Penetrance of autosomal dominant genes. A person can inherit a dominant gene but not the associated disorder if the gene has poor penetrance. The non-penetrant gene is inherited in the usual autosomal dominant fashion and, if it has little effect in the parent, usually continues to have little effect in the offspring. Even so, it is possible to inherit a previously non-penetrant gene and be affected by the disorder.

effect on the phenotype despite the presence of a normal version of the gene, or **allele**, in the other chromosome of the pair. Autosomal dominant disorders affect male and female offspring equally. The disease trait appears in every generation and an affected individual has a parent who is affected or who at least has a non-penetrant version of the gene mutation. When one parent is affected and the other is genetically normal it can be expected that half the offspring would be normal and half would be affected. The disorder cannot be transmitted by unaffected family members who do not have the gene mutation (Figure 3.4).

Most autosomal dominant conditions are heterozygous, being produced by one affected and one normal parent. Homozygous conditions are extremely rare because this would require both parents to be affected.

Some disorders do not become apparent until later in life. An example is Huntington's disease, which usually appears only in middle age, perhaps after the individual has started a family and has already passed on the gene to the next generation.

Other examples of autosomal dominant conditions are neurofibromatosis, adenomatous polyposis coli (see Chapter 17), familial hypercholesterolaemia (see Chapter 20), Marfan syndrome, polycystic kidney disease, and some cases of Alzheimer's disease (see Chapter 26), osteogenesis imperfecta and

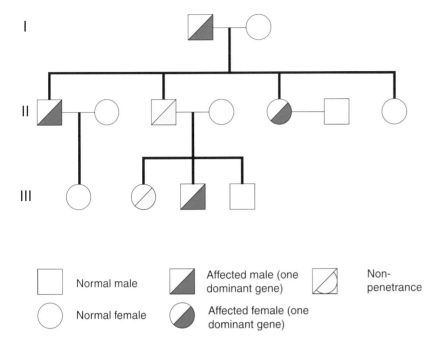

Polycystic kidney disease: cysts develop in the kidney which progressively enlarge, impairing kidney function. Patients develop chronic renal failure and hypertension. Usually asymptomatic until adulthood but can be detected in children by ultrasound examination. Gene loci occur on chromosome 16 (90% of cases) and on chromosome 2.

Normal male

Normal female

Affected male (one dominant gene)

Affected female (one dominant gene)

Non-penetrance

Figure 3.4 Autosomal dominant inheritance. Pedigree of a family with an autosomal dominant disorder. When one of the parents is affected and the other is genetically normal (row I) there is a 50% probability of having affected children (row II) (just as there are equal chances of having male or female children). The dominant gene, and the disorder, will be passed from affected individuals into every generation that follows (row III).

epidermolysis bullosa. In some cases an environmental factor may influence how severely the person is affected by the abnormal gene (for example diet in familial hypercholesterolaemia).

Autosomal recessive disorders

In autosomal recessive inheritance the parents of affected individuals are not themselves affected by the disorder but are **carriers** of the disease. The condition occurs when both healthy parents carry the same recessive gene mutation. The chances of passing both copies of the mutated gene to an affected offspring is one in four. Males and females are affected equally (Figure 3.5).

Individually, the autosomal recessive disorders are rare. The most common is cystic fibrosis (see Chapter 21), which occurs in white populations with a frequency of about one in 2500. The abnormal gene is quite common and a single copy can be found in about one in 25 people (these people are heterozygous, or carriers of the condition). A carrier for cystic fibrosis suffers no adverse effects because only one of the gene copies is mutated and the cell uses the normal gene from the other chromosome. When two mutated genes are inherited there is no choice: the cell must use a defective gene.

When an egg or sperm is formed only one chromosome of the pair is present.

▲ **Key points**

Autosomal dominant disorders

▲ Gene mutation is in one of the autosomes

▲ Males and females are equally affected

▲ Most affected people have one version of mutated gene (are heterozygotes) but it is sometimes possible to be homozygous

▲ Disorder can be passed on only by an affected parent

▲ On average 50% of offspring from an affected parent will be affected, 50% will be normal s Disorder appears in every generation

A recessive disorder can arise only by inheriting two copies of a defective gene

Carrier: a person who has a heritable gene mutation but is functionally normal. In most cases the mutant gene is recessive, and the cell uses the dominant normal version of the gene as the blueprint for translation into protein.

In a carrier of cystic fibrosis 50% of the eggs or sperm will contain the normal gene while 50% contain a mutated gene. If the carrier mates with a normal person it is impossible for affected cystic fibrosis children to be produced: only normal children or carriers can result (Figure 3.6). Cystic fibrosis arises only when a carrier or a person with the disease, mates with another carrier. (A normal person in this context is someone with two normal genes and, except for the single genetic mutation, a carrier is someone who is functionally normal.)

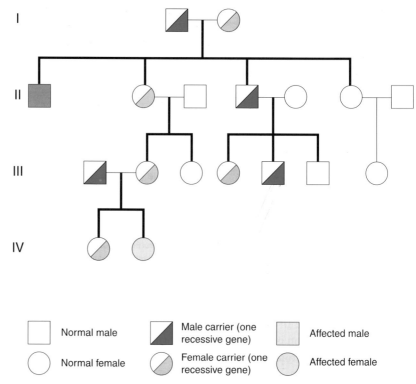

Figure 3.5 Autosomal recessive inheritance. Pedigree of a family with an autosomal recessive disorder (cystic fibrosis, for example). When both parents are carriers (row I) there is a 25% probability of having an affected child and 50% of the offspring are likely to be carriers. In this illustration the affected male (row II) is infertile. A carrier and a normal person can produce only further carriers or normal offspring. Hence a recessive disorder can skip a generation (row III). The condition reappears if a carrier has children by another carrier (row IV).

Inborn errors of metabolism

The other main autosomal recessive disorders are the **inborn errors of metabolism**. As this name suggests these involve some metabolic defect arising from deficiency of a necessary enzyme. The synthetic pathway in the cell cannot be completed and instead the precursor substances are stored. Very often the cells cannot function properly simply because of all the material stored inside them.

Lipid storage disorders

Most inborn errors of metabolism are extremely rare, or affect only specific populations. An example is Tay–Sachs disease, an autosomal recessive disorder most common in Ashkenazi Jews. It is caused by a deficiency of the lysosomal enzyme hexosaminidase A. This enzyme is normally responsible for splitting the terminal N-acetylgalactosamine residue from GM2-ganglioside (a glycolipid) (Figure 3.7) In the absence of enzyme the complete glycolipid accumulates in the lysosomes, particularly in those of the cerebral neurones and ganglion cells of the retina. The initial symptoms, apparent at 3–6 months of age, include muscle weakness but are progressively followed by blindness, convulsions and coma. Death usually follows in early childhood. Other lipid storage disorders, arising from specific enzyme deficiencies, include Gaucher's disease and Niemann–Pick disease.

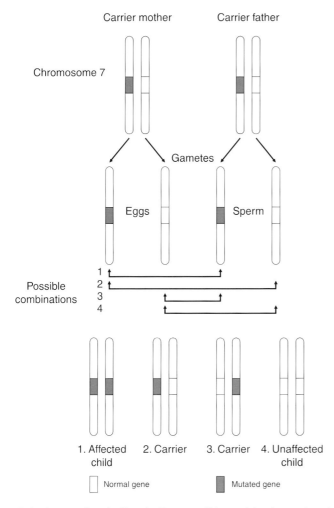

Figure 3.6 Inheritance of cystic fibrosis. Four possible combinations arise when both parents are carriers of the recessive gene for cystic fibrosis. There is a one in four chance of inheriting both copies of the defective gene, and therefore cystic fibrosis. The probability is that two of the children will be carriers.

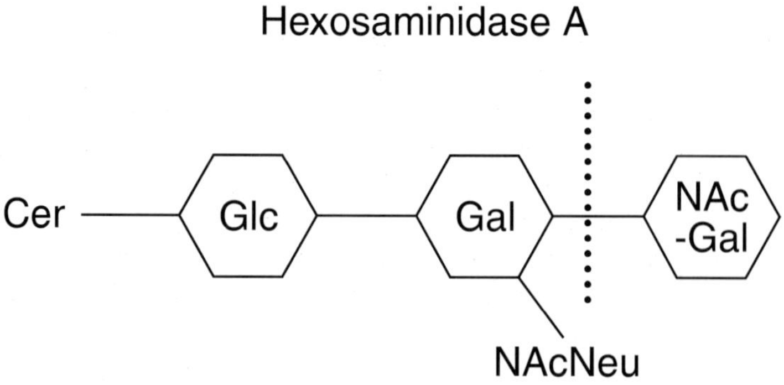

Hexosaminidase A

Figure 3.7 Ganglioside GM$_2$. Cer = Ceramide; Glc = glucose; Ga; = galactose; NAcGal = *N*-acetylgalactosamine; NAcNeu = *N*-acetylneuraminic acid.

Mucopolysaccharidoses

The mucopolysaccharidoses are single gene defect disorders caused by deficiency of lysosomal enzyme responsible for the degradation of connective tissue mucopolysaccharides (glycosaminoglycans) such as dermatan sulphate and heparin sulphate. These disorders include Hunter's syndrome (an X-linked recessive disorder) and Hurler's syndrome. Both are characterised by skeletal abnormalities, multiple organ disease and very short life expectancy.

Glycogenoses

The glycogenoses are characterised by the accumulation of glycogen in cells. The type and intracellular location of the stored glycogen, and its tissue location, vary according to the specific enzyme deficiency. The tissue location can include liver, skeletal muscle and heart muscle. When only skeletal muscle is involved (McArdle's syndrome) life expectancy is normal but patients experience painful cramps with strenuous exercise. The involvement of the liver or heart muscle (in von Gierke's or Pompe's disease, for example) is associated with early death.

Phenylketonuria

Brain damage in phenylketonuria can be largely avoided by early restriction of dietary phenylalanine

Phenylketonuria is a group of recessively inherited single gene disorders characterised by reduced ability to convert phenylalanine to tyrosine. This defect of amino acid metabolism is caused by deficiency of the enzyme phenylalanine hydroxylase. High concentrations of phenylalanine in the body cause brain damage, seizures and eczema.

Treatment is to limit the dietary intake of phenylalanine to the minimum required for normal growth. This measure should be started very early because the brain damage is irreversible. Dietary restriction must be continued throughout childhood, although it is usually safe to allow some relaxation by the time the child reaches 8 years of age. The dietary intake of protein necessary to achieve suitably low levels of phenylalanine is about one-third to one-tenth of protein intake in the normal diet. It is therefore necessary to rely on a low-phenylalanine protein substitute to ensure that the protein required for growth and the other essential amino acids are supplied. Foods with a high phenylalanine content include all types of meat, fish, cheese, eggs, bread and baked products, yeast and meat extracts and chocolate beverages. The artificial sweetener aspartame should be avoided because it consists of phenylalanine and aspartic acid. Breast milk, cows' milk and formula feeds all contain phenylalanine. A newly diagnosed baby is given a complementary feed of a low-phenylalanine protein substitute. This lowers the baby's demand for milk and suppresses lactation in the mother so that the intake of breast milk is reduced to a safe level.

Early treatment depends on early diagnosis and in the UK a relatively simple screening test is used to detect the disease routinely in all newborn babies. The method used, called the **Guthrie test**, is a microbiological procedure performed on a small heelprick blood sample and uses a special strain of *Bacillus subtilis* which requires phenylalanine for its growth (see Chapter 11).

Haemoglobin abnormalities

Abnormalities of haemoglobin structure (haemoglobinopathies) are the most common types of autosomal gene defects. They arise because of abnormal synthesis of the α or β peptide chains required for the formation of haemoglobin. There are two α-globin genes clustered in chromosome 16, while β-globin is encoded by a gene in chromosome 11. The principal inherited defects of haemoglobin synthesis are the thalassaemias and sickle-cell disease.

Haemoglobin: the molecule in red blood cells that transports oxygen around the body. The most common type, adult haemoglobin (HbA), is composed of two α and two β-globin molecules (a2β2). There is also a fetal form of haemoglobin (HbF) comprising two α and two γ-globin chains (α2γ2).

Thalassaemia

The thalassaemias arise from an absence or deficiency of α-globins or β-globins, causing incorrect assembly of haemoglobin. They are more common in Mediterranean and Asian countries and in the Middle and Far East, where carrier rates of up to 15% are found.

Thalassaemias are caused by reduced production of one or more globin chains

α-Thalassaemia

In α-thalassaemia the a-globin chain is absent or reduced. Each person has two α-globin genes, termed α1 and α2, in each of the chromosome 16 pairs, making a total of four genes. Deletion of one of the genes is completely asymptomatic. Deletion of two genes, termed the α-thalassaemia trait, is generally asymptomatic but can cause a mild haemolytic anaemia. A heterozygous individual, with only one gene copy, will have moderate haemolytic anaemia, termed **haemoglobin H disease**. In this condition, haemoglobin is formed from small amounts of α-globin together with β-globin. In the most severe form of α-thalassaemia, termed **hydrops fetalis**, no α-globin can be produced. Infants are stillborn at 28–40 weeks or die very shortly after birth (Figure 3.9).

β-Thalassaemia

In β-thalassaemia synthesis of the β-globins is defective because of mutation or deletions to the β-globin gene in chromosome 11. This is not harmful in

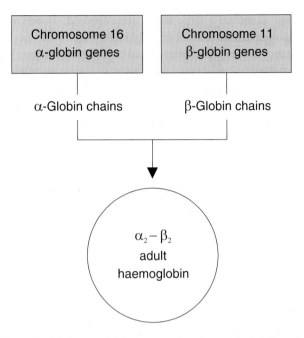

Figure 3.8 Normal adult haemoglobin is a complex of α and β-globins coded by genes in chromosomes 11 and 16.

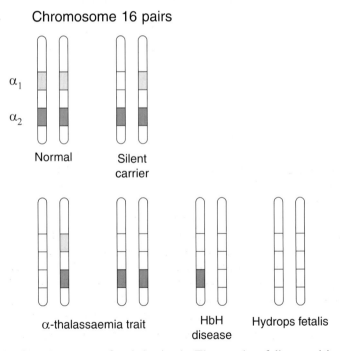

Figure 3.9 Genetic patterns of α-thalassaemia. The severity of disease arising from chromosome 16 α-globin gene deletions depends on the number of functional genes remaining. Deletion of three genes causes a moderate haemolytic anaemia, while deletion of all four genes is not compatible with extrauterine life.

the neonate because β-globins are not required for the synthesis of fetal haemoglobin (HbF) which persists in the body for some months after birth. From about 4 months of age, the loss of β-globins causes serious disabilities arising from haemolytic anaemia and tissue hypoxia. Hypoxia stimulates the proliferation of the red bone marrow in an attempt to increase red cell production and oxygen carrying capacity. This causes enlargement and distortion of the bones, leading to disfigurement of the skull and facial bones. The anaemia is so extreme that most homozygous individuals die in childhood. Heterozygous carriers of the trait are asymptomatic.

Over 150 different mutations have been identified in β-thalassaemia. Some of these occur outside the coding region of the globin genes (see page 82). Major gene deletions are unusual, and the genetic abnormalities mostly involve point mutations, small insertions, or deletions (see below). The conditions are divided into the two groups β⁰ and β⁺, depending on whether β-globin synthesis is completely absent or merely reduced.

Point mutation: change to a single base pair in DNA.

Sickle-cell disease

Sickle-cell disease is an example of how devastating the effects can be when there is a change in only one base pair in the DNA sequence. Glutamic acid is replaced by valine as the sixth amino acid in the sequence making up the b-globin components of adult haemoglobin (HbA). The altered haemoglobin in sickle-cell disease is known as HbS. In **sickle-cell trait** heterozygotes for the sickle-cell gene can synthesise both normal and sickled forms. These individuals are generally asymptomatic. When the point mutation affects both chromosomes, almost all the adult haemoglobin is in the HbS form, causing sickle-cell disease.

Sickle-cell haemoglobin polymerises when it is deoxygenated, distorting the red blood cells which take on an elongated crescent or sickle shape. Sickling is initially reversible by oxygenation, but each episode causes more membrane damage, leading to irreversible changes. Sickled red cells are easily damaged and have a lifespan of only about 7 days compared with the 120 days of normal red cells. The accelerated destruction of spent red blood cells causes haemolytic anaemia, jaundice and formation of gallstones. Because the bone marrow is working so hard to replace red cells, a trivial insult, such as a minor infection, can have a major effect and precipitate a severe **aplastic crisis**.

Sickled cells circulate very slowly compared with normal red blood cells and tend to aggregate in small vessels. The rigidity of the sickled cells contributes to the tendency of small vessels to become blocked. Cells and tissues supplied by these vessels are liable to become ischaemic or infarcted. This can occur in any organ but most commonly affects the bones, lungs, skin, kidney, brain and spleen. The course of sickle-cell disease is characterised by episodes of painful crises caused by vessel occlusion or bone marrow suppression.

Episodes of pain are usually localised to the abdomen or some part of the skeleton, and last from a few hours to a few days. More seriously, there is an increased susceptibility to infection, particularly by *Streptococcus pneumoniae*, which can cause fatal pneumonia or meningitis. Blindness is caused by retinal

Abnormal haemoglobin in sickle-cell disease leads to accelerated destruction of red blood cells

Aplastic crisis: sudden, usually temporary, cessation of bone marrow activity.

detachment and proliferative retinopathy (see Chapter 23). Children are prone to a build-up of viscous red blood cells in the spleen and liver. This can suddenly deplete the stock of red cells in the blood, causing serious anaemia and rapid onset of shock, which can be lethal.

The disease does not become evident until several months after birth because of the presence of fetal haemoglobin. Many patients die in the first few years of life but some have a relatively normal lifespan and experience only few complications. Sickle-cell disease occurs mainly in Blacks (in Africa and the USA) and also in India, the Middle East and southern Europe. About 8% of Black people in the USA carry the sickle-cell gene, but in parts of Africa where malaria is endemic the sickle gene frequency approaches 30%. This has been attributed to the slight protective effect that HbS has against the organism causing malaria.

Genetic testing for sickle-cell disease or its carrier state relies on detection of the point mutation, which changes the codon from GAG to GTC. This mutation alters the recognition site of the restriction enzyme *Mst*II. Hence the size of the restriction fragment will be altered when a β-globin gene probe is used in Southern blotting (see below). Alternatively, disease or carrier status can be determined by use of oligonucleotide probes corresponding to normal and mutated β-globin gene sequences. Each probe will hybridise only with its complementary sequence. Because a heterozygous carrier has both DNA sequences, both probes will hybridise.

X-linked disorders

X-linked recessive disorders usually become apparent in males, who have only one X chromosome. Even if they have the genetic defect, females have a normal version of the gene in the other X chromosome to counteract its effects. Females, therefore, are carriers for a condition expressed in males. Because the female carrier can transmit either of her X chromosomes to any of her offspring, on average about half of her sons will be affected and half of her daughters will be carriers (Figure 3.10).

The most common of the X-linked recessive disorders is Duchenne muscular dystrophy (incidence at birth about 0.25 per thousand males in European populations). Other examples are Becker muscular dystrophy, Haemophilia A, Haemophilia B, and fragile X syndrome (see below).

Generally the female carrier of an X-linked condition is perfectly healthy. In each somatic cell of a female one of the X chromosomes is inactivated (called **Lyonisation**, after Mary Lyons, who first described the phenomenon). This is a random process and in most carriers there will be sufficient expression of the normal gene to counteract expression of the mutant gene. In some carriers the chance inactivation favours the normal gene so that there is an imbalance of mutant gene expression. Affected women may exhibit some mild manifestations of the disorder, such as a bleeding tendency (from haemophilia gene defects) or some muscle weakness (from Duchenne muscular dystrophy gene defects). It is possible for a female to be homozygous and affected by the

Becker muscular dystrophy: a mild form of muscular dystrophy, permitting a relatively normal life. Mutation involves a different portion of the dystrophin gene than affected in the Duchenne type. The protein is not completely absent and is partly functional.

Duchenne muscular dystrophy: caused by a mutation in a large (2 million base pairs) gene in the short arm of the X chromosome coding for the protein dystrophin. Dystrophin is involved in anchoring the actin filaments (involved in muscle contraction) to the basement membrane. Poorly anchored muscle fibres tear themselves apart with the force of contraction. A progressive muscle weakness develops and the patient dies in early adulthood, often from pulmonary infection.

Haemophilia A, factor VIII deficiency: this is the most common inherited bleeding disorder, usually occurring in males but can occur in females. Incidence is between 1 in 5000 and 1 in 10 000 of the male population. Up to 30% of cases are caused by new mutations, without a family history. Clinical symptoms present with a range of severity depending on how much active factor VIII is produced and the type and position of the gene mutation. Tendency for large haemorrhage following trauma or surgical procedure. 'Wear and tear' trauma causes recurrent bleeding into the joints which can be crippling.

Haemophilia B, factor IX deficiency: follows inheritance and clinical features identical to haemophilia A but is much more rare.

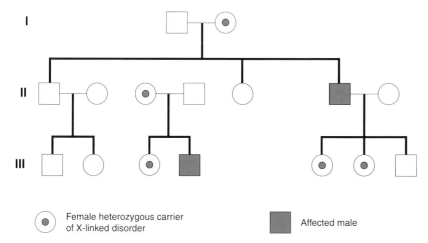

Figure 3.10 X-linked recessive inheritance. X-linked disorders can be inherited only through the female line. In the female a mutant gene in the X chromosome is balanced by a normal gene in the other chromosome and she is a healthy carrier with a 50% chance of passing the mutant gene to her offspring: female offspring will be normal or carriers, male offspring will be normal or affected by the disorder. The male does not have another X chromosome and so if he inherits the mutant gene it must be expressed. An affected father will pass the mutated gene on to all his daughters, but none of his sons.

severe disorder. This is extremely rare, requiring an affected male and a female carrier as parents.

X-linked dominant disorders are very rare. They are inherited in the same pattern as X-linked recessive disorders except that both male and female offspring who inherit the gene will be affected (there are no female carriers). Affected fathers transmit the gene only to their daughters. An example of an X-linked dominant disorder is vitamin D-resistant rickets. In this disorder there is excessive urinary excretion of phosphate and a failure of bone mineralisation.

Types of genetic mutation

In cystic fibrosis and some other single gene defects the type of mutation can take different forms: deletions, insertions and substitutions of bases in the genetic code. All of these disrupt the proper sequence of bases in the genetic code so that the wrong amino acids are assembled into the final protein. Alternatively, the alteration in coding may correspond to a stop sequence so that the final protein is truncated (Figure 3.11).

Tandem triplet expansion

Another way for diseases to be passed on from one generation to the next is by expansion of the tandem repeats that surround, or are within, a particular

▲ **Key points**

X-linked recessive disorders

▲ Gene mutation is in the X chromosome

▲ Females are carriers of the disorder and have a normal version of the gene in the other X chromosome

▲ A mutated gene inherited by a male must be expressed, because he has only one X chromosome

▲ A female carrier has a 50% chance of passing the mutated gene on to her offspring, as a carrier female or affected male

▲ An affected male will pass the mutated gene on to all his daughters, but to none of his sons

▲ Disorders include haemophilia (A and B), Duchenne and Becker muscular dystrophy and some types of colour blindness

The severity of triplet expansion disorders worsens from one generation to the next

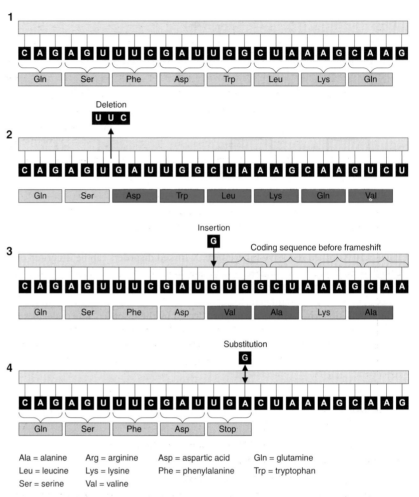

Figure 3.11 Effects of base sequence mutations on protein assembly. 1. RNA coding sequence for a hypothetical protein (for comparison with 2,3 and 4). 2. Deletion of the codon UUC causes a failure to translate phenylalanine. The removal of a single amino acid from the sequence in a protein can cause fundamental changes in its structure and activity. 3. The insertion of an additional base (guanine) causes misreading of all the downstream codons, known as a frameshift mutation. Most of the following amino acids in the protein are inappropriate, causing a failure of protein assembly or, if it is assembled, non-functional protein. A deletion of bases has a similar frameshift effect. 4. Substitution of one base for another causes the 'wrong' amino acid to be translated. In this example substitution of guanine for adenine results in a stop codon. Assembly of the protein will terminate at that point.

gene. Normally, regions surrounding genes contain between 6 and 50 repeats of a triplet sequence such as CGG (see below and Figure 3.21). At one time these repeat sequences were simply regarded as 'junk' DNA but they are now believed to play a key role in gene regulation and in the evolution of complex species.

The tandem repeats are inherited dominantly, and in most families they stay the same length from one generation to the next. In a small minority, there is a tendency for the repeats to lengthen in subsequent generations, so that eventually some segments contain more than 200 repeats. These long repeats are associated with the nervous system diseases **fragile X syndrome** and **Huntington's disease**. In these conditions the symptoms, which usually include mental handicap or weakness of voluntary muscles, worsen with each generation as the repetitive sequence becomes longer and longer. Presumably, some families may be at the upper reaches of the normal number of repeats, and further increases will cause the condition to appear in that family. In fragile X syndrome the repeated triplet comprises CGG or GCC in chromosome X. In Huntington's disease the repeats comprise CAG triplets in chromosome 4, and as the repeats lengthen the condition appears in younger people.

Fragile X Syndrome: triplet expansion disease characterised by mental retardation and presence of a non-staining site at the extremity of chromosome X (q arm) which looks as if it is about to break away.

Huntington's disease (Huntington's chorea): an inherited condition which leaves the individual unaffected until middle age. The initial signs of the disease are a lack of co-ordination similar to drunkenness. Ultimately, the sufferer becomes demented, loses physical control and suffers from wasting of body fat and muscle. The disease is fatal. There is no biochemical or anatomical abnormality that can be detected before the onset of symptoms.

Background information: DNA and RNA

DNA consists of two long strands of polynucleotides that twist around each other to form a double helix. Each nucleotide contains a molecule of deoxyribose, a phosphate group, and a purine or pyrimidine base. The two strands of polynucleotides are held together by hydrogen bonds between the bases. In DNA there are four bases – adenine, guanine, cytosine and thymine. Adenine and guanine are purines, cytosine and thymine are pyrimidine molecules.

RNA differs from DNA in two main respects:
- it comprises only a single polynucleotide chain
- the sugar molecules and bases differ: deoxyribose is replaced by ribose, and thymine bases are replaced by uracil.

These differences make the RNA molecule more susceptible to degradation than DNA, which means that the translation of proteins from the RNA template can be rapidly stopped in response to extracellular signals.

> *The form and function of all cells and organisms is specified by DNA and RNA*

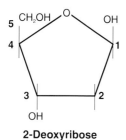
2-Deoxyribose

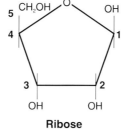
Ribose

Figure 3.12 Deoxyribose and ribose sugars have a pentose ring structure. The carbon atoms in the ring are labelled in a clockwise direction 1 to 5. Attachment of the sugars in the polynucleotide chain is at the 3' and 5' positions. At the ends of the chain, the hydroxyl group at the 3' position or a phosphate group added at the 5' position are used to determine orientation of the chain.

During assembly of the two chains of DNA a purine base will pair only with a pyrimidine base: adenine with thymine and cytosine with guanine. In the assembled DNA the two polynucleotide strands, held together at the base pairs, have opposite chemical polarities, one running 5' ➝ 3' and the other in the 3' ➝ 5' direction.

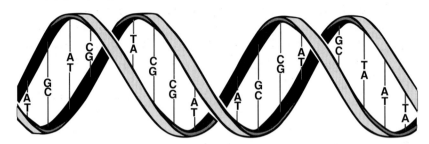

Figure 3.13 DNA consists of a double helix of two polynucleotide chains intertwined together. The chains are attached to each other by binding with complementary bases.

Nucleotide: the combination of bases, pentose sugars and phosphate groups found in DNA or RNA.

Oligonucleotide: a short chain of nucleotides manufactured synthetically or derived from DNA or RNA.

Polynucleotide: the long chain(s) of nucleotides comprising DNA or RNA.

The sequence of bases codes for amino acids in the eventual protein product, with each base triplet, or **codon** in RNA, coding for one amino acid. For example, GCC codes for alanine while AAG codes for lysine. Because the number of possible permutations of the four bases into triplet sequences (43, or 64) is greater than the number of amino acids used by humans (20), some triplet sequences code for the same amino acid. For example, leucine is coded by CUU, CUC, CUA and CUG. There are also stop sequences that signal the completion of the amino acid chain: these are UAA, UAG and UGA.

One consequence of the strict pairing between nucleotide bases is that the sequence in one strand determines the base sequence of the other. This helps to maintain the integrity of the genetic information: if one strand becomes damaged it can be accurately repaired by using the other strand as a template. This is also the basis for replication of DNA before cell division. The DNA helix is first unwound and a complementary copy of each strand is made by reading off the sequence of bases. This replication process is facilitated by **polymerase** enzymes, and for the most part is extremely accurate. However, considering the number of bases that have to be replicated, and the number of times that a cell undergoes division, it is not surprising that mutations occasionally occur. This usually has no adverse functional effect, but on occasion the result is catastrophic, depending on which gene and where in the gene the mutation has occurred.

The smallest functional unit within DNA is the gene. Each gene will code for a particular protein and may be many thousands of base-pairs (bp) in length (1 kb is 1000 bp). Because of its length, the complete DNA sequence, or **genome**, is split and packaged into discrete units, or **chromosomes**. The human cell contains 23 pairs of chromosomes of different sizes and hence different lengths of DNA, but generally each carries many hundreds of genes. Not all the base sequences in a gene code for amino acids in the final protein product. These non-coding parts of DNA are referred to as **introns**. The coding parts of the gene are referred to as **exons**.

A number of intermediary steps must be taken before any protein is produced. First there is a problem of geography; the DNA is located in the cell nucleus while the protein-replicating machinery is located in the cell's cytoplasm (see Chapter 4). The transfer of genetic information from one cell site to another is achieved by RNA, a single-stranded replica of one of the original DNA strands.

RNA is synthesised in the nucleus by a polymerase enzyme that copies, base by base, the genetic information from a small portion of the DNA, corresponding to a single gene. The two strands in DNA are known as the sense and **antisense** strands. When the antisense template is used, a new sense strand of RNA is produced. The process of producing another copy of the genetic information, this time in the form of RNA, is known as **transcription**. The genetic message is carried out of the nucleus by **messenger RNA** to the sites of protein synthesis, the **ribosomes**. At this site ribosomal RNA is synthesised from the coding sequences in the messenger template. The codons in **ribosomal RNA** are **translated** to assemble the correct sequence of amino acids.

Although all the genetic information is present in each cell, not all of it will be required by a cell at any one time, if at all. Cells translate only the genes coding for the proteins it needs for maintenance or to carry out specialised functions. This is achieved by specific recognition sequences in the DNA, which bind proteins that enable transcription or regulation. The DNA recognition sequences are often rich in adenine and thymine, as a **TATA** sequence, and are found in non-coding sequences near the gene. These are called **promoter** sequences because they bind RNA polymerase and other cofactors involved in transcription. Other DNA regulatory sequences occur in unpredictable locations along the DNA, sometimes thousands of base pairs away from the gene they influence. These form binding sites for regulatory proteins and are termed enhancers. Some enhancers drive genes in many types of cells, whereas others are active in only certain cell types, giving rise to a tissue-specific expression of the gene.

The importance of these recognition sites is illustrated when genetic mutations occur. Some patients with thalassaemia have mutations just outside the coding sequence in a promoter region. Alteration of just one nucleotide base in this area can mean that transcription from the adjacent gene does not occur, causing an absence of translated protein product (globin). In another example a fairly inactive gene is translocated to a position controlled by a strong enhancer. This occurs in the 8:14 translocation in Burkitt's lymphoma (see Chapter 23).

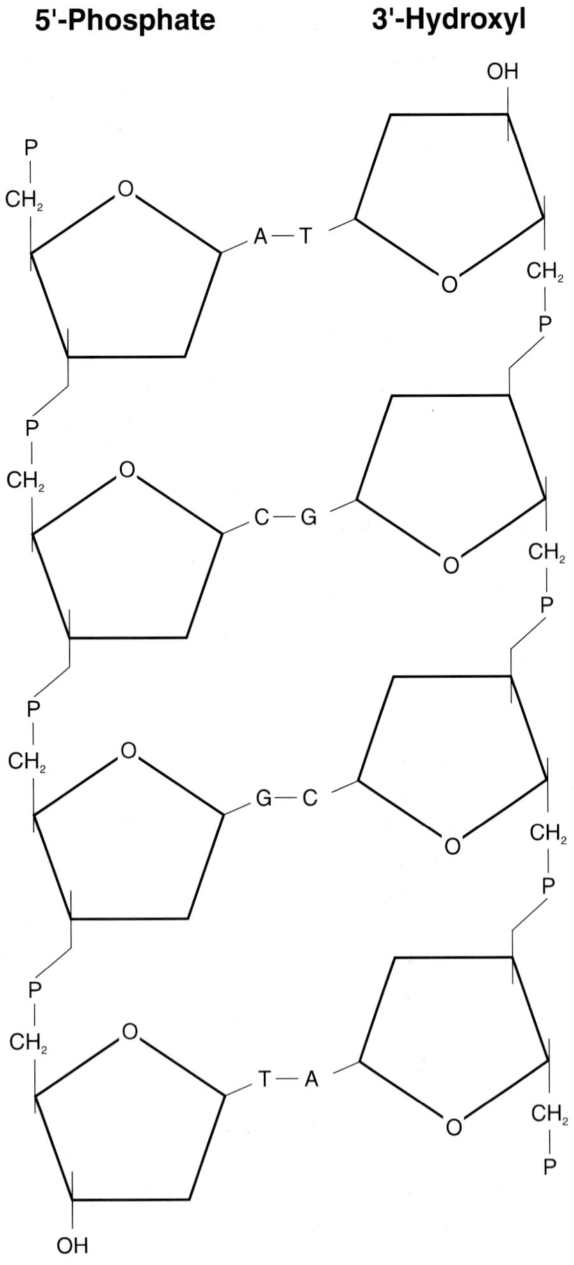

5'-Phosphate   **3'-Hydroxyl**

Figure 3.14 Diagrammatic representation of the two polynucleotide chains in DNA, one running in the 5' → 3' direction and the other 3' → 5'. P = Phosphate group.

Identification and analysis of genetic material

For many years analysis of the genetic composition of the cell was confined to the morphological analysis of chromosomes. This is in itself a powerful tool, allowing detection of chromosomal abnormalities such as Down's syndrome.

It has recently become possible to analyse the actual composition, or the base sequence, of the genetic material. The technique is very sensitive, allowing an alteration in only one base pair to be detected. It relies on using fragments of the genetic material itself, **genetic probes**, taking advantage of the property of nucleotides to combine, or **hybridise**, with their complementary series of bases.

The human genome project

Not all human genes have yet been identified. As genetic susceptibility is inherently involved in the pathogenesis of disease, alone or in combination with environmental factors, a map of the genes and their functions will probably go some way to further our understanding of complex conditions such as cancer and coronary heart disease. From this it might become possible to design and develop more logical and effective strategies for prevention and treatment.

The main difficulty is that these are mostly **polygenic** conditions – genetic susceptibility for the condition is conferred by the interaction of a large number of genes. The inheritance of these genes is difficult to follow because they are not linked together and the interaction of environmental factors is more important than in the single gene disorders. For example, even though cholesterol concentrations are determined by major genes controlling the production of apolipoproteins (see Chapter 20), their impact in an individual depends on the interaction of risk factors such as smoking, diet, amount of exercise and alcohol consumption. Other genes, such as those controlling production of angiotensin-converting enzyme (this influences predisposition for hypertension), LDL receptors and fibrinogen may assume equal significance. Moreover, their relative contribution to the final disease state will vary between individuals.

The purpose of the human genome project is to create a complete map and sequence of the human genome. The work is being carried out in genetics laboratories throughout the world, each focusing on a particular chromosomal area. By this means the complete map should eventually be assembled from the DNA sequences of many individuals. The size of the task is enormous: merely printing the names of the 3 billion base pairs would require 13 sets of the Encyclopaedia Britannica (computer buffs will know that this could be compressed into rather fewer CD-ROMs, but we are not yet as clever as cells in packing all this information into a tiny space).

The information already gathered has had a great impact on our understanding of disease. Examples are the identification of triplet expansion in Huntington's disease (in chromosome 4) and mapping of genes causing familial adenomatous polyposis (*APC* gene in chromosome 5), cystic fibrosis (CFTR gene in chromosome 7), retinoblastoma (*Rb* tumour suppressor gene in chromosome 13), some breast cancers (*BRCA* genes in chromosomes 13 and 17) and a whole series of genes in Alzheimer's disease (*APP* gene in

Only a very small proportion of the estimated 50 000 – 100 000 human genes have so far been cloned and sequenced

Gene probe: an oligonucleotide chain (synthesised, or a fragment of single-stranded DNA or RNA) used to identify a complementary sequence of bases in genetic material.

Hybridisation: the combination, under appropriate conditions of temperature and pH, of two complementary nucleotide strands. Complementary means that the correct sequence of bases must be present for the complete length of the strand, so that alanine bases will combine with guanine, and cytosine with thymine.

The human genome project will have an impact on all branches of human biology and medicine

▲ Key points

Gene mapping and sequencing

- ▲ Identification of underlying genetic predisposition is a fundamental step in understanding pathogenesis
- ▲ Allows tracing of single gene disorders
- ▲ Base sequencing allows correlation between the gene and its protein product
- ▲ Potential to advance understanding of major medical problems, for example cancer and coronary heart disease, and fundamental biological processes such as ageing

Review question 1

Why might it be helpful to know the basic genetic defect that underlies a particular disease?

chromosome 21, *S182* and *STM2/E5-1* genes in chromosomes 1 and 14, and *apoE* ε4 allele in chromosome 19). Before gene mapping the basic defects underlying these conditions were poorly understood.

Once the position of a gene is identified, base sequencing allows the composition and positions of amino acids in its protein product to be worked out. This approach, starting with mapping and cloning of the gene, followed by identification of its expressed protein, is called **reverse genetics**. As an example, in cystic fibrosis, reverse genetics methodology led to the identification of a previously unrecognised protein. By comparing the structure of the newly identified protein with other known proteins it was deduced that it is involved in the regulation of ion transport by epithelial cells (see Chapter 21).

Before gene probes became available the only way of identifying genes was by working from knowledge about the protein, using well-established biochemical techniques for identifying their sequence of amino acids. In **classical genetics** the protein must be isolated and purified. Modern protein sequencers can be used to determine the amino acid sequence and, because the genetic code is known for each amino acid, it is possible to predict the underlying gene sequence. Oligonucleotides can then be synthesised and used to probe DNA fragments. The approach becomes complicated because alternative codons exist for most amino acids and it is therefore necessary to construct an array of oligonucleotides for all the possible combinations.

Identification and analysis of DNA and RNA

Advances in the ability to localise and identify genes stem from the isolation of bacterial enzymes that can cut DNA into smaller fragments. These enzymes, called **restriction endonucleases** (restriction enzymes), act like 'molecular scissors' by cleaving the DNA into **restriction fragments**. Depending on the bacterial strain, restriction enzymes possess discrete specificities for certain base sequences in DNA, splitting the DNA into manageable bits of, say, only a few thousand base pairs.

Another fundamental feature of the techniques used to isolate and identify segments of DNA is based on the property of DNA to separate into its two component polynucleotide strands on heating. When cooled the single DNA strands combine or **anneal**, providing they contain the complementary base sequences. Many restriction enzymes split the DNA asymmetrically, leaving a single-strand overhang or **sticky end** at the site of each cut. These sticky ends allow the restriction fragment to be joined to a complementary sticky end from another DNA fragment. Typically, a fragment from human DNA will be fused with the complementary sticky ends of bacterial DNA that was cut with the same enzyme. The is the basis for producing **recombinant DNA**. As an example the enzyme *Eco*RI (from *Escherichia coli*) recognises the GAATTC sequence and cleaves it asymmetrically (Figure 3.15).

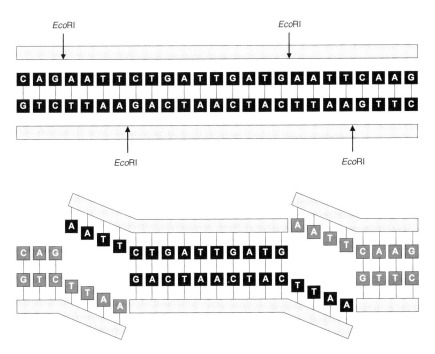

Figure 3.15 Cleavage of DNA by restriction enzymes. In this example, treatment of double-stranded DNA with the restriction enzyme *Eco*RI results in two loose or 'sticky' ends, comprising the unpaired bases AATT and TTAA.

Recombinant DNA

The first task in identifying and analysing DNA is to obtain it in sufficient quantity. Identification also depends on the production of a molecular probe, itself comprising genetic material. Both of these requirements are facilitated by recombinant DNA technology.

The sticky ends produced by restriction endonuclease cleavage allow similarly cleaved DNA from other organisms to be spliced in. All that is required is the complementary sequences of bases at the sticky ends of the two DNAs. This is achieved by using the same restriction enzyme to produce the insertion fragment and to open the host DNA. A simple enzymatic reaction can be used to mend the break in the DNA backbone. As there are more than 200 types of restriction enzyme available, a DNA break can usually be produced very close to the area of interest.

The next stage is to make more copies of the recombinant DNA. There are two principal ways of doing this: bacterial cloning and the polymerase chain reaction.

Bacterial cloning
Bacterial cloning relies on the rapid replication rate of bacteria to produce

▲ **Key points**

Plasmids

▲ Naturally occurring circular molecules of double-stranded DNA

▲ Plasmids grow and multiply within bacteria independently of the bacterial genomic DNA

▲ Contain genes that confer bacterial antibiotic resistance

▲ Antibiotic resistance is used to distinguish plasmids that contain DNA inserts from those that do not

▲ **Key points**

Insertion of DNA into plasmid

▲ Open circular plasmid DNA with restriction enzyme

▲ DNA ligase enzyme used to insert new DNA into plasmid, to produce recombinant DNA

▲ Insert within a gene coding for antibiotic resistance

▲ Introduce into bacteria

▲ Grow and plate onto medium with appropriate antibiotic

The PCR avoids bacterial cloning, and has advantages of greater sensitivity and speed

large quantities of DNA. The recombinant DNA must first be introduced into the bacteria by choosing a carrier, which will be accepted by the bacteria, as a source of the receptive DNA. The carrier usually consists of small, circular DNA molecules called **plasmids** (containing extra-chromosomal bacterial DNA), or **phages** (containing viral DNA). The type of carrier is chosen according to the size of the DNA that needs to be amplified.

Plasmids are naturally occurring extra-chromosomal elements that will grow and multiply within bacteria independently of the bacterial genomic DNA. They comprise double-stranded DNA molecules of 1–200 kb in size. As the bacteria replicate, so will the plasmids and the recombinant DNA within them. Plasmids contain unique sites recognisable by restriction enzymes and also genes that confer bacterial resistance to certain antibiotics. These genes can be spliced out of the plasmid DNA using restriction enzymes, thereby modifying the plasmid's resistance to antibiotic (Figure 3.16).

When producing recombinant DNA with plasmids, a useful strategy is to insert the new DNA in place of a gene coding for antibiotic resistance. When the plasmid-containing bacteria are cultured, those containing recombinant DNA can be readily distinguished from those with naturally occurring plasmids by differences in bacterial antibiotic resistance.

Once the bacteria with the recombinant plasmids have been isolated and grown the plasmids are harvested from the culture and the relevant DNA fragment is 'snipped out' from the recombinant molecules with restriction enzymes. A litre of bacterial cells cultured in this way can yield more copies of a specific DNA fragment than could be extracted and purified from all the cells in the entire human body.

There are other, more commercial, uses to which recombinant DNA technology can be put. One of the first applications was the production of human insulin, using *E. coli* to replicate recombinant DNA containing the normal human insulin gene. Intuitively it could be expected that human insulin would give better control of diabetes than the preparations derived from pigs and cows, but in practice the benefits are not substantial. Another product of recombinant DNA technology, human growth hormone, is a substantial improvement on the previously available product. This is because the original product was extracted from human pituitary glands, but some treated patients subsequently developed Creutzfeldt-Jakob disease and died, because of contamination with prion protein. The recombinant product avoids this risk. Other applications of the technology include the production of vaccines and antibodies in much purer forms than is possible by conventional techniques.

Polymerase chain reaction

The polymerase chain reaction (PCR) is an *in vitro* version of DNA replication, similar in principle to the processes that normally take place in dividing cells. With the help of the enzyme DNA polymerase, base sequences are read from a DNA template and nucleotides are assembled to produce a new DNA strand. The portion of DNA to be synthesised is defined by annealing primers of short oligonucleotides at each end of the target DNA sequence. The primers

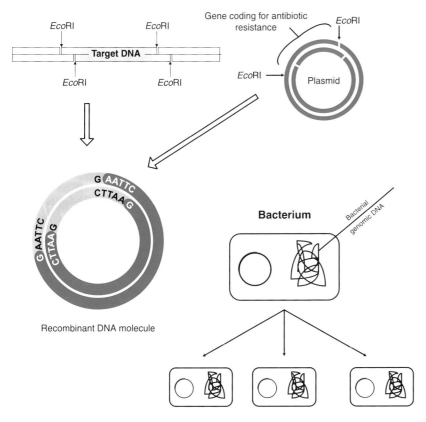

Amplification of recombinant DNA by bacterial growth

Figure 3.16 Production of recombinant DNA. A restriction endonuclease (for example *Eco*RI) is used to produce a fragment of target DNA and to splice plasmid DNA (splicing sites and resulting sticky ends are indicated by small arrows). In this example the fragment spliced out of the plasmid includes a gene coding for antibiotic resistance. The recombinant DNA plasmids will replicate inside bacteria as they divide, producing multiple copies of recombinant DNA. Bacteria containing recombinant DNA will have antibiotic resistance different from those containing unaltered plasmids, and can be distinguished on this basis. (Adapted from Rosenthal, 1994.)

effectively act as stop sequences. Large amounts of DNA can be produced in this way, to be used for biochemical analysis or as a means of synthesising DNA probes.

Two oligonucleotide primers are required, which flank the DNA fragment to be amplified. By a sequence of heat denaturation these primers can be annealed to their complementary sequences in the target DNA. The annealed primers can then be extended by the use of DNA polymerase. DNA synthesis by the DNA polymerase proceeds across the region between the primers. Since the newly synthesised product is also capable of binding primers the process can be repeated, amplifying the target DNA sequence. Successive amplification cycles double the amount of material synthesised in the previous cycle, resulting

---

▲ **Key points**

Recombinant DNA ('genetic engineering')

▲ Genes can be extracted from a DNA source and spliced into new target DNA: this is recombinant DNA

▲ Rapid proliferation of bacteria or yeasts used to generate multiple copies of recombinant DNA

▲ Provide DNA in amounts sufficient for biochemical analysis s Provides the tools for 'genetic fingerprinting'

▲ Can provide industrial quantities of pure, therapeutically important agents such as human insulin

in a logarithmic accumulation of the DNA product (Figure 3.17). The cycle can be repeated 30–35 times, producing up to a million copies of the original DNA in a matter of hours. Unfortunately, the ability of the PCR to produce large numbers of DNA sequence copies means that unless extreme care is taken there is a high risk of producing unwanted DNA from contaminating sources.

The PCR can be employed with DNA derived from any source of cells, such as blood or other body fluids. It is also possible to carry out the method on fixed paraffin-embedded tissues. This makes it possible to carry out retrospective studies, although there are limitations on the length of DNA that can be amplified in this way. The advantage of retrospective studies is that genetic changes, or infectious agents associated with disease (HIV for example), can be tracked over long periods of time.

DNA libraries

Using the gene cloning methods described it is possible to assemble a library of DNA clones that will cover the complete human genome. This of course is the aim of the human genome project: to identify the genes and base sequences within the cloned fragments. Theoretically, the whole genome can be covered by a library of 300 000 DNA clones, each of 20 000 base pairs.

An alternative is to construct partial gene libraries, for example concentrating on DNA sequences that are transcribed and used by a particular type of cell or tissue. Messenger RNA can be used for this purpose because a specialised cell transcribes (into mRNA) only those portions of the genome it needs in order to carry out its functions. For cloning purposes, it is necessary to convert the RNA into DNA with an enzyme called **reverse transcriptase** (this enzyme is used by retroviruses to incorporate themselves within host DNA). The DNA created from an mRNA template is referred to as **complementary DNA (cDNA)**. cDNA clones differ from genomic DNA clones in that they do not contain the base sequences that code for gene regulation.

Methods used in gene identification

Application of gene probes

Specific base sequences in DNA or RNA can be identified by hybridisation with complementary probes

The DNA amplified by recombination and the PCR serves as the gene library on which further studies, including gene localisation and sequencing, are undertaken. To use or examine the library requires a genetic tool or **gene probe**. The probe itself comprises single-stranded DNA, cDNA, RNA or a synthetic oligonucleotide. Under correct laboratory conditions, provided it comprises the correct complementary base sequences, the probe will hybridise to the target genetic material. Both DNA and mRNA can be analysed with gene probes.

Generally, gene probes are employed on genetic material that has been extracted from the cells and amplified. The usual procedure is to separate and

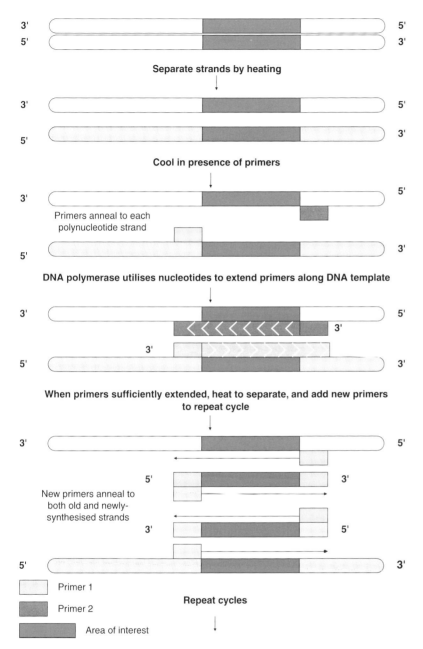

Key points

The PCR method

▲ Heat-denature DNA

▲ Add primers (usually 20 bp oligonucleotides)

▲ Cool: primers associate to complementary sequences in target DNA

▲ Add DNA polymerase: extends primer by adding further nucleotides complementary to template, across the region between primers

▲ The newly synthesised DNA strand can also act as a template and is capable of binding primers

▲ Each replication cycle doubles the amount of DNA synthesised in the previous cycle to give a logarithmic increase in DNA segments

▲ Does not require purification of cellular DNA or recombination with a carrier

▲ Amplification limited to DNA segments of less than 2000 bp

▲ Up to 1 million times amplification possible

Figure 3.17 The polymerase chain reaction. DNA is heated to separate the two polynucleotide strands in DNA. Primers that contain base sequences complementary to those at the ends of the area of interest are added to the mixture. On cooling, these anneal to each strand. The primers are extended in each direction by the addition of nucleotides and DNA polymerase. The polymerase enzyme uses the polynucleotide strand as a template, adding nucleotides. Eventually, the primers extend completely across the area of interest. A second heating cycle detaches the new polynucleotide strands from the original templates. New primers added to the mixture bind with both the old and the new polynucleotide strands, so that with repeated cycles the DNA is replicated in a logarithmic manner.

Probe labels: used to visualise hybridisation between probe and target genetic material. Radioactive isotopes (for example ^{32}P, ^{35}S, ^{125}I, ^{3}H) are detected by exposure to a photographic emulsion. Non-isotopic labels include biotin, which has an affinity for avidin and streptavidin. Avidin or streptavidin molecules are conjugated with an enzyme marker before reaction with the biotin labelled probe. The enzyme conjugate reacts with its substrate, in the presence of an acceptor dye molecule, to yield a coloured insoluble substance at the site of reaction. Alternatively, fluorescent dye markers can be used and are particularly suitable for *in-situ* hybridisation.

blot the extracted genetic material onto a solid support before starting the hybridisation. This method is known as **Southern blotting**, named after its inventor, Professor Southern (Figure 3.18). RNA can be identified in a similar way, and, in a striking example of biochemical logic, is referred to as Northern blotting. Probing for RNA sequences indicates which genes are expressed by a particular cell type, and this gives some indication of their function.

It is also possible to probe DNA or RNA in a cell or metaphase chromosome spread in its original location by *in-situ* hybridisation. The method can be employed on frozen tissue sections, cytological smears or on archival paraffin-embedded material. One application of *in-situ* hybridisation, using an array of fluorescent-labelled specific DNA probes derived from a whole chromosome is called **chromosome painting**. Binding the cocktail of probes causes the whole chromosome to fluoresce. The method is used to identify chromosomal translocations. Single probes corresponding to a specific gene locus can also be used, revealing their sites as a fluorescent spot on each chromatid. This is useful for identifying small deletions.

Restriction fragment length polymorphism analysis

Restriction fragment length polymorphisms (RFLPs) are an expression of the differences in DNA among individuals. There are so many variations in base sequence, or **polymorphisms**, particularly in the non-coding areas (introns) that we each possess our own genetic 'fingerprint'. RFLP analysis is a means of identifying these differences. The method uses restriction enzymes to cleave the DNA under investigation, which is then subjected to Southern blotting. Variations in restriction fragment lengths reflect either variations in nucleotide sequence (Figure 3.19), or variations in the numbers of tandem repeats between restriction sites (Figure 3.21).

> *Linkage analysis allows a genetic trait to be tracked in a family even when the responsible gene cannot be identified*

Variation in nucleotide sequence

A change in DNA sequence could create or destroy a restriction enzyme recognition site or alter the distance between two sites. Restriction fragment polymorphisms are inherited in a simple mendelian fashion. In an individual who is heterozygous for a particular RFLP, two restriction band patterns will be produced by Southern blotting, corresponding to the different alleles. In a homozygous individual both alleles will be identical and only one band will be revealed by Southern blotting.

> *Individual differences in DNA base sequences are reflected by altered susceptibility of the DNA to restriction endonucleases*

Variation in tandem repeats

The restriction enzyme cutting sites are not evenly distributed along the DNA molecule. Some areas, known as **hypervariable regions**, vary widely between individuals. These areas often consist of short arrays of base sequences, often repeated in tandem. These are known as **variable number of tandem repeats (VNTRs)**. They are prone to recombination at meiosis or mitosis, producing differences in the number of repeat sequences at the hypervariable loci, and different fragment sizes on endonuclease digestion. Southern blots can be

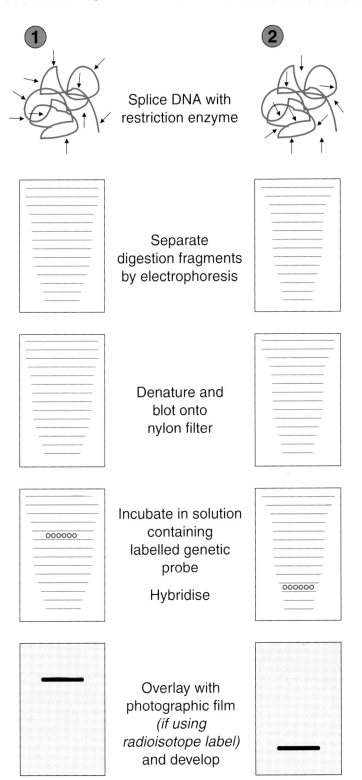

DNA is spliced into multiple fragments by digestion with a restriction enzyme.

Fragments are of different lengths according to the distribution of enzyme recognition sites along the DNA chain.

If DNA from another individual is used (column 2), cleavage will occur in different places, yielding differently sized fragments. This also happens in a single individual when DNA from the other member of a chromosomal pair is digested.

The differently sized fragments are separated by gel electrophoresis.

The separated DNA fragments are denatured in the gel with alkali, yielding single-stranded DNA. The single strand is transferred (blotted) onto another carrier medium, for example nitrocellulose or a nylon filter.

The filter is placed in a solution containing a DNA probe that is specific (complementary) for the target of interest. Hybridisation of probe and target produces a labelled DNA sequence.

Non-hybridised probe is washed away, and the filter is covered with photographic emulsion and developed. The labelled DNA sequence is revealed as a dark band on the film.

The position of the hybridised restriction fragment depends on the restriction enzyme used. Because recognition sites vary among individuals, the position of the bands will differ.

Figure 3.18 Southern blotting

Restriction fragment length polymorphism, RFLP: difference in DNA sequence revealed by different-size fragments after digestion with restriction enzymes.

Microsatellite region, variable number tandem repeat region (VNTR): identical units of up to four nucleotides repeated many times. Present throughout the genome. Their location in the genome is constant but there is individual variation in the number of repeats inherited as a typical genetic trait.

probed for these repeat sequences, permitting the visualisation of the VNTRs which occur throughout the genome. Probes for VNTRs are known as **minisatellite probes**. As the hypervariable regions are the focal area for sequence alterations the probes for these areas offer a powerful means of detecting sequence changes between individuals, providing a 'genetic fingerprint' that is unique for each individual (apart from identical twins).

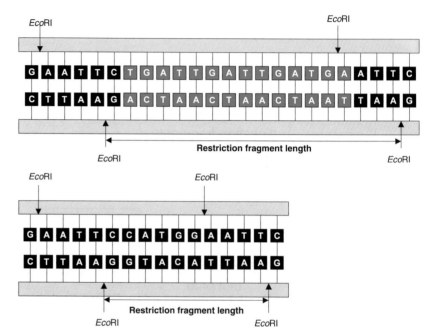

Figure 3.19 Restriction fragment length polymorphism I: variation in nucleotide sequence. In different individuals, base sequences recognised by restriction enzymes (GAATTC by *Eco*RI, for example) are separated by variable amounts of DNA. Digestion will yield fragments of different sizes. The sequences between the restriction sites are completely different in the two individuals. These differences are concentrated in non-gene areas (introns) of the DNA, and are referred to as polymorphisms.

In practice the difference in restriction fragment lengths is rather larger than implied in Figure 3.19. For example, digestion of the normal β-globin gene with the restriction enzyme *Mst*II yields two fragments of 1.1 and 0.2 kb in length. Because of substitution of a GAG enzyme digestion site by GTG only one fragment of 1.3 kb is produced by *Mst*II digestion in the sickle-cell gene (Figure 3.20).

In some cases restriction sites are closely linked with genes responsible for causing disease. Although it may not be possible to isolate and track the gene itself, it may be possible to track the associated restriction fragment and determine polymorphisms amongst family members by **linkage analysis**. Thus the restriction fragments are used as markers to follow the inheritance of an adjacent gene: the defective gene coinherits with the polymorphic site. It is not necessary to know the defects that take place within the gene itself and probes specific for those gene defects do not need to be prepared.

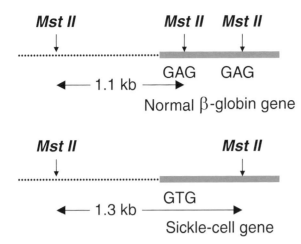

Figure 3.20 Digestion of the normal β-globin gene with *Mst*II yields two restriction fragments. Loss of a restriction site in the sickle-cell gene means that only one longer fragment is produced by *Mst*II digestion. (From Kingston, 1994.)

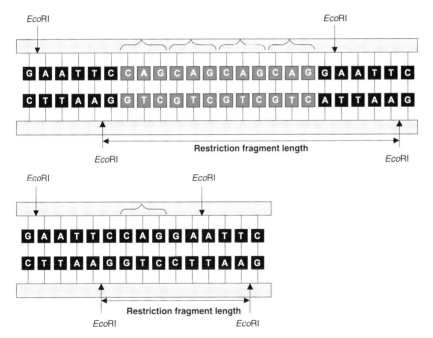

Figure 3.21 Restriction fragment length polymorphism II: variation in tandem repeats. **Top:** in this example two *Eco*RI restriction sites are separated by four CAG tandem repeats. **Bottom:** in this individual the same *Eco*RI restriction sites are separated by only one CAG sequence. Digestion of the two DNAs will yield fragments of different sizes, detectable by Southern blotting with a minisatellite probe. This method is the basis of the genetic 'fingerprinting', typically used in forensic testing of blood, semen or vaginal swabs. Tandem repeats are usually harmless, but very long sequences can cause disease. For example, normal subjects have up to 30 CAG repeats in a region of chromosome 4, but in Huntington's disease there can be 100 or more CAG trinucleotides. The severity of the disease is inversely related to the number of repeats.

▲ Key points

Restriction fragment length polymorphism (RFLP) analysis

▲ Relies on variation in DNA sequence between individuals

▲ Variation involves change in base sequence or number of tandem repeats

▲ Sequence and tandem repeat variables are polymorphisms

▲ Change in sequence at a restriction site causes alteration in restriction fragment length

▲ Alteration in number of tandem repeats between restriction sites alters size of restriction fragments

▲ In heterozygotes for RFLP, two restriction band patterns are produced corresponding to differences in each of the chromosomes of the pair

▲ Altered regions may be close to a disease locus

▲ RFLP probes used to track inheritance of associated disease locus

In every individual different-sized DNA fragments will be produced after digestion with a restriction enzyme because the sequence of bases will vary according to the 'fingerprint'. These different-sized DNA fragments can be identified by electrophoresis. By comparing the 'fingerprint' with the DNA of the parents (who will each have one copy of the normal gene together with one copy of the cystic fibrosis gene) it is possible to identify which segment of DNA is carried with the abnormal gene and which with the normal. In subsequent pregnancies, DNA from fetal cells can be compared with the 'fingerprint' pattern from each parent. It can then be determined whether the fetus is normal, a carrier, or has both copies of the gene (Figure 3.22).

Applications of genetic analysis in infectious disease and neoplasia

Detection of infective agents

Genetic methods offer advantages of speed and great sensitivity, allowing rapid identification of slow-growing organisms

Gene probing is not confined to the examination of DNA derived from humans and is of value for determining the presence of foreign DNA in a host cell. The advantage of using genetic methods is that they are much more sensitive and specific than the alternative culture or biochemical methods. Many organisms, particularly viruses, mycobacteria and some fungi have very fastidious growth requirements in culture, and some cannot be cultured at all. Sometimes growth is so slow that it may be many weeks before the organism is identified. In contrast, the PCR can be completed, and the organism identified, in hours. Another advantage is that genetic methods can be undertaken on archival material: it is not necessary to grow viable organisms. This is of value in tracking mutations in infectious organisms over time. The sensitivity of the method allows detection even when there are only small numbers of organisms.

Using *in-situ* hybridisation the genomic material of infectious organisms can be visualised in the cells themselves. For example, the method is used to establish the types of human papillomavirus (HPV) involved in pre-cancerous conditions of the cervix and to determine precisely which of the cells in smears or histological sections are infected (see Chapter 16). All these methods ultimately rely on the specificity of the gene probe. This should hybridise only with DNA sequences specific to the organism, and not to DNA in the host cell.

Neoplasia

Some of the genetic changes that occur in cancer cells are so severe that they can be seen under the microscope as deletions of parts of chromosomes, translocations or changes in chromosome number. Standard cytogenetic analysis has been very useful in demonstrating these changes, particularly in

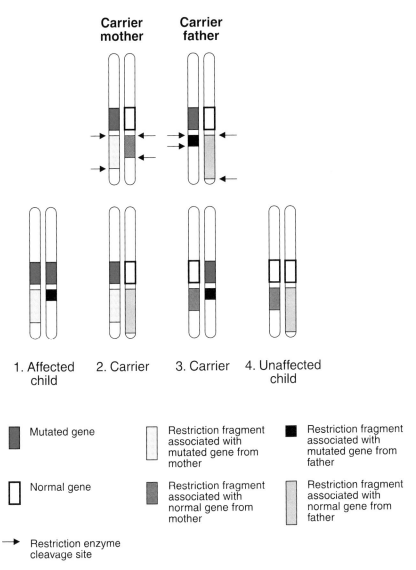

Carrier
mother

Carrier
father

1. Affected
   child

2. Carrier

3. Carrier

4. Unaffected
   child

Mutated gene

Restriction fragment associated with mutated gene from mother

Restriction fragment associated with mutated gene from father

Normal gene

Restriction fragment associated with normal gene from mother

Restriction fragment associated with normal gene from father

→ Restriction enzyme cleavage site

Figure 3.22 RFLP analysis of associated gene mutations. In a recessive genetic disorder such as cystic fibrosis an affected individual (1) will have inherited one mutated gene from the mother and one from the father. RFLP analysis relies on identifying polymorphisms associated with the affected gene rather than the gene itself. In the example shown, one of the defective genes in the affected individual is associated with a relatively long restriction fragment, while the other is associated with a short restriction fragment. RFLP analysis of the carrier parents and of other siblings can reveal which of the normal and mutated genes are associated with restriction fragments of particular lengths. For example, it can be demonstrated that the carrier sibling (3) inherited the single defective gene from the father on the basis of its associated restriction fragment. The test is used for prenatal diagnosis in subsequent pregnancies, after one affected child has already been born in the family. When the gene itself has been identified and cloned, as has happened in cystic fibrosis, it is no longer necessary to rely on this approach.

Review question 2

How feasible would it be to undertake genetic screening for diseases such as the common cancers and cardiovascular disease?

leukaemias and lymphomas. It is now possible, with gene probes, to examine some of the more subtle changes to the DNA in precancerous and cancerous cells. These often involve small deletions in tumour suppressor genes, and mutations in or around proto-oncogenes that are not visible by cytogenetic analysis. These cause alterations in the DNA sequence, or polymorphisms, which can be detected by the genetic methods of Southern blotting or polymerase chain reaction.

These techniques have shed light on the fundamental biology of many tumours, particularly those in which identifiable precursor lesions can be detected, such as the adenoma–adenocarcinoma sequence found in colorectal cancer (see Chapter 17). In addition, many of the genetic changes associated with invasive cancers have prognostic significance, adding to the accuracy of conventional tumour staging and grading methods (see Chapter 13).

Some patients with certain types of cancer, notably ovarian, breast and colorectal cancers, have a strong family history of the disease. Some rare cancer types are inherited directly, such as Wilms' tumour, retinoblastoma, neurofibromatosis and familial adenomatous polyposis. Genetic methods have not only advanced knowledge about the fundamental genetic defects in the tumours, but have also allowed affected individuals to be identified (by RFLP analysis or direct gene analysis) before they develop symptoms. This means that the individuals can be monitored closely and treated early, or even be treated prophylactically (for example, with tamoxifen to prevent breast cancer, or colectomy when the adenomas develop in familial adenomatous polyposis).

Gene therapy

In theory, recombinant DNA technology can be used to place a normal version of a gene in people who are affected by a single gene disorder. This is the so-called gene therapy. To date there remain fundamental problems in getting the new gene into all the affected cells and, once there, to stay. Even if the new genetic material can be successfully inserted into the host cells, there is no guarantee that they will switch to the production of protein encoded by that new gene fragment. The possible applications of recombinant DNA as gene therapy for cystic fibrosis are discussed in Chapter 21.

ANSWERS TO REVIEW QUESTIONS

Question 1

Why might it be helpful to know the basic genetic defect that underlies a particular disease?

The identification of genes and their proteins will stimulate the development of new therapies designed to correct these basic defects at the cellular level. This would be a significant advance on many current therapies that are designed only to mitigate the effects, rather than the cause, of the disease. One example is the current research into gene therapy, designed to correct the basic defect in the lungs of cystic fibrosis patients (see Chapter 21).

Another advantage is that it will be possible accurately to diagnose disease or assess disease susceptibility by means of DNA analysis and track patterns of inheritance. This will allow informed decisions to be made about risking pregnancy or allowing a pregnancy to continue (for severe conditions arising from single gene defects). The detection of a genetic susceptibility for a major multifactorial disease such as coronary heart disease might stimulate some people to pay greater attention to lifestyle factors that modify the risk. It is also likely that human genome sequencing will shed some light on other basic biological questions such as the genetic control of growth and development, and perhaps of greatest current interest, ageing, about which very little is known.

How feasible would it be to undertake genetic screening for common diseases such as the common cancers and cardiovascular disease?

Question 2

Inheritance of two recessive cystic fibrosis genes will invariably be accompanied by the disorder. In contrast, most of the common cancers and cardiovascular disease are polygenic (arise from the interaction of multiple genes). For most people inheritance of particular gene combinations does not necessarily mean that development of the disease condition is inevitable because they have a multifactorial aetiology. In other words, production of the disease often depends on exposure to environmental risk factors, superimposed on a genetic susceptibility. Technically it will be very difficult to screen for all the possible contributory genes and at the present state of knowledge there are probably many important genes that have yet to be identified.

Even if it were possible, the practical value of genetic screening is undermined by the non-genetic factors in the disease aetiology. In other words, screening is aimed not at detecting the disease but at detecting disease susceptibility and consequently is likely to have poor predictive value. The purpose of such screening is also questionable. Most of the risk factor interventions that can be made to alter disease susceptibility apply to everyone, whether they have a genetic risk (family history) or not.

There are, none the less, sub-groups of patients with common cancers or cardiovascular disease who have a strong genetic susceptibility and will probably develop the condition regardless of environmental influences. These patients account for about 5% of breast cancers, 1% of colorectal cancers, some ovarian cancers and a small proportion of people with cardiovascular disease (caused by familial hypercholesterolaemia). In these instances it is now fairly well understood which genes are involved, and hence screening of selected populations (people with a strong family history) will become a practical possibility. This type of screening is also useful because specific interventions can be made to improve the survival prospects, over and above measures applicable to the general population.

References

Kingston, H.M. (1994) *ABC of Clinical Genetics*, 2nd edn. London, BMJ Publishing Group.

Rosenthal, N. (1994) Tools of the trade – recombinant DNA. *N. Engl. J. Med.*, **331**, 315-17.

Further reading

BMJ (1993) *Basic Molecular and Cell Biology*, 2nd edn, London, BMJ Publishing Group.

Carman, W.F. (1991) The polymerase chain reaction. *Quart. J. Med.*, **78**, 195-203.

Emery, A.E.H. and Malcolm, S. (1995) *An Introduction to Recombinant DNA in Medicine*, 2nd edn, Chichester, John Wiley.

Housman, D. (1995) Human DNA polymorphism. *N. Engl. J. Med.*, **332**, 318-20.

Naber, S.P. (1994a) Molecular pathology – diagnosis of infectious disease. *N. Engl. J. Med.*, **331**, 1212-15.

Naber, S.P. (1994b) Molecular pathology – detection of neoplasia. *N. Engl. J. Med.* **331**, 1508-10.

Rosenthal, N. (1994a) DNA and the genetic code. *N. Engl. J. Med.*, **331**, 39-41.

Rosenthal, N. (1994b) Stalking the gene. *N. Engl. J. Med.*, **331**, 599-600.

Rosenthal, N. (1994c) Regulation of gene expression. *N. Engl. J. Med.*, **331**, 931-33.

Weatherall, D.J. (1991) *The New Genetics and Clinical Practice*, Oxford, Oxford University Press.

4 The cellular basis of disease

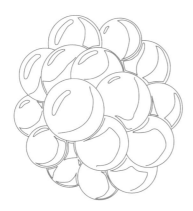

Cells are susceptible to damage by a variety of agents that arise from the external environment or as products of intrinsic cellular metabolism. Damage to cells is reflected in biochemical and morphological changes. These changes can cause the cell to behave aberrantly or cause it to die. Either eventuality can lead to disease.

Cells die in two ways. Extensive damage from external sources causes the cells to die from necrosis. This typically occurs when blood supply is suddenly cut off, as might happen in atherosclerosis and thrombosis. Necrosis of heart muscle or neurons in the brain results in heart attack or stroke.

Another mechanism of cell death is apoptosis. This normally occurs during growth and development when remodelling of tissues is required. It is an everyday event in adults, ensuring a proper balance between cell loss and cell replenishment. Sometimes failure of this 'self-destruct' mechanism, due to damage to DNA and growth regulatory proteins, leads to the development of cancer.

Extensive cell damage that results in necrosis is followed by an inflammatory reaction, intended to remove tissue debris and the cause of the original injury. The inflammatory reaction is initiated and mediated by a variety of factors that serve to dilate blood vessels and attract cells to the site of injury. Successful termination or resolution of wound healing depends on a number of factors concerning both the host response and the nature of the original injury.

Aims of this chapter

By the end of this chapter you will have increased your knowledge of:
◆ The main reasons for reversible and irreversible cell injury and the cellular adaptive responses to stressful stimuli
◆ How cellular damage or adaptive responses contribute to disease processes

In addition, this chapter will help you to:
◆ Understand the basic functions of the cell and how these are affected by injury
◆ Describe the differences between apoptosis and necrosis and discuss how apoptosis may serve as a protective mechanism in preventing disease
◆ Describe the process of inflammation and explain its purpose
◆ Discuss the role of cellular mediators of inflammation
◆ Understand the contribution of blood coagulation and other pathways in mediating inflammation
◆ Describe the various stages in the process of wound healing
◆ Describe the role of cytokines and discuss how they may contribute to disease

Introduction

In some cases the cells in a diseased tissue may be perfectly normal, but their response to abnormal stimuli has caused tissue damage and cell death. In other circumstances the cells themselves have become altered. For this to happen, some alteration to the genetic code that controls all of the cell's functions must have taken place.

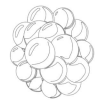

Ultimately, all diseases are caused by alterations in cells

Response to injury

Mild injury can be accommodated by cells, but can become evident as biochemical or morphological changes in cells

A number of alterations are produced when cells are injured. These may be biochemical changes, such as a switch to anaerobic respiration when oxygen is in short supply or accumulation of substances involved in cell metabolism such as lipids. Biochemical changes are often reflected by alterations in cellular appearance (morphology), although there is often considerable delay before a biochemical lesion becomes evident as altered cell morphology. Some cells adapt to their new environment by changing size and metabolic activity. Continued disruption of the normal cellular environment leads ultimately to cell death.

Background information: organisation of the cell

The cell is the smallest functional unit of the body. It is involved in a vast array of activities, directed at maintaining its own integrity and performing functions specific to the tissue of which it is part. All of these functions will at some stage involve the synthesis of macromolecules: proteins, carbohydrates, lipids and nucleic acids, activities coded for and regulated by DNA. Synthesis of macromolecules requires the availability of many metabolic intermediates that are produced in chemical reactions catalysed by enzymes. The cell's enzyme-mediated activities include the use of energy, replacement of organelles and membranes and the absorption, degradation or production of molecules and require an energy-dependent transport system. This in turn is dependent upon intact membranes and correct osmotic and fluid balance.

Under the light microscope two components of the cell are readily visible in ordinary stained preparations – the **nucleus** and the **cytoplasm**. Electron microscopy reveals that these structures are bounded by membranes, the cell membrane and the nuclear membrane. A host of other structures, or **organelles**, become visible in the cytoplasm. These include the nucleus, ribosomes, endoplasmic reticulum, Golgi complex, lysosomes, peroxisomes, mitochondria and cytoplasmic filaments. The remaining cytoplasm (without organelles) is referred to as the **cytosol**. This comprises a semi-fluid medium containing water, ions, proteins, various building-block materials such as amino acids and nucleotides, and energy materials such as glucose, glycogen and ATP.

Nucleus

Virtually all the DNA in a cell is contained within the nucleus, which is surrounded by a double membrane. Inside the membrane are the genetic coding components DNA and RNA, together with nuclear proteins. The nuclear proteins comprise a laminar protein for the nuclear membrane, structural proteins, DNA and RNA polymerases and gene regulatory proteins. All of these are synthesised in the cytoplasm and brought in through the nuclear membrane – the nuclear membrane is porous, but at the same time it is very selective regarding which molecules it allows to pass through.

The bulk of the genetic material in the nucleus is in the form of DNA, complexed with nuclear proteins called **histones**. The DNA–protein complex is referred to as **chromatin**. When the cell is not actively dividing (at interphase) a dense dark structure may be seen within the nucleus. This is the **nucleolus** and is the region in which DNA is transcribed into RNA. The newly transcribed RNA is assembled into ribosomal subunits and transported through the pores of the nuclear membrane into the cytoplasm.

Ribosomes

In the cytoplasm the ribosomal subunits are assembled into the complete ribosomes, ready for translation of the genetic message into its protein product. Ribosomes exist in the cytoplasm either as free ribosomes, or attached to the membrane of the **endoplasmic reticulum**. Different types of proteins are synthesised by ribosomes at the two sites; in general, proteins to be secreted from the cell are synthesised by membrane-bound ribosomes and proteins destined for the cell cytoplasm or nucleus are synthesised by free ribosomes.

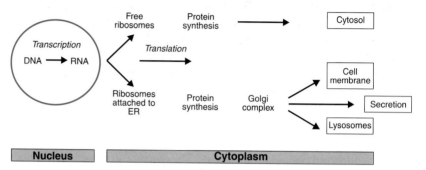

Figure 4.1 Protein synthesis in the cell. The genetic code for virtually all the proteins a cell produces is contained within nuclear DNA. When particular proteins are required the appropriate genes are transcribed to RNAs, which are assembled into ribosomal subunits and transported out of the nucleus. In the cytoplasm ribosomes exist in free form or are attached to endoplasmic reticulum. Proteins are translated from the code in ribosomal RNA. Proteins required for the cell's own purposes are synthesised by free ribosomes and exported into the cytosol. Proteins required for cell membranes, lysosomes or external secretions are sorted, assembled and packaged by the Golgi complex, and are exported in the form of secretory vesicles.

Endoplasmic reticulum

Depending upon whether or not ribosomes are attached, the endoplasmic reticulum (ER) is described as **rough** or **smooth**. It is made up of a series of membranes that enclose a network of sacs, into which newly synthesised protein is released. Various lipids (for example, phospholipids, cholesterol, ceramide) are used within the ER for the production of membranes.

One end of the endoplasmic reticulum is attached to the outer nuclear membrane. This end is covered with ribosomes (forming rough ER). Further away from the nucleus the ER becomes smooth. Portions of this become detached, creating vesicles that carry the newly synthesised protein to the **Golgi complex**.

The cholesterol required for membrane synthesis is obtained by the cell from plasma LDL. The cell uses a surface receptor protein to trap the LDL, and both the receptor and LDL are internalised at surface invaginations called **coated pits**. These pinch off the surface to form vesicles which then fuse with **endosomes**. The LDL is released from the receptor and delivered to the lysosomes. The cholesterol released by lysosomal degradation is used for membrane synthesis, while the receptor is recycled back to the cell surface.

Golgi complex

The Golgi complex is a series of flattened sacs with dilated edges. Secretory vesicles bud off from the edges either to become lysosomes or to merge with the plasma membrane, when they form part of the membrane, or pass their contents to the outside of the cell as secretions.

An important function of the Golgi complex is to sort and arrange the cell's products – most cells will be involved in the production of hundreds of different molecules for its own use or for secretion. It is also involved in the final assembly and completion of molecules. For example, addition of sugar residues (notably N-acetylglucosamine, galactose, fucose and sialic acid) to lipids and proteins, so that they may serve a variety of functions, behaving as recognition, transport or adhesion molecules.

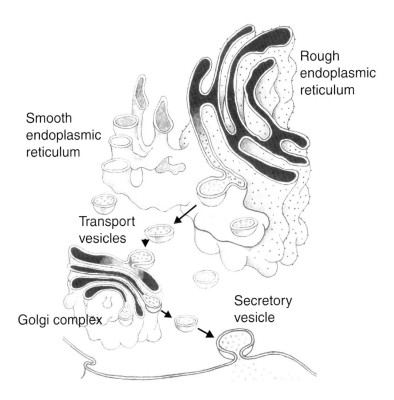

Figure 4.2 The Golgi complex. Proteins are translated from ribosomal RNA and assembled in the rough endoplasmic reticulum (top right). The newly synthesised molecules bud from the endoplasmic reticulum and migrate within transport vesicles to the Golgi complex. Transport vesicles fuse with the Golgi complex, within which the products are modified into their final form, often by the addition of sugar molecules. The products are sorted and collected within the membranes at the edge of the Golgi complex. The Golgi membranes dilate to form sacs which eventually bud off. These migrate and fuse with the cell membrane for final release from the cell.

Lysosomes

Lysosomes are packages containing enzymes and are bounded by a single membrane. The enzymes have a range of activities, which together are capable of breaking down virtually any biological macromolecule. Lysosomal enzymes include proteases, nucleases, glycosidases, lipases, phospholipases, sulphatases and phosphatases.

Lysosomes are required for breaking down unwanted macromolecules within the cell. The lysosomal enzymes are prevented from digesting cellular components that are still needed in two ways. First, the enzymes are contained within a membrane. Macromolecules that are to be broken down are presented to the lysosomes in a membrane-bound package, which fuses with the lysosome so that its contents are exposed to the lysosomal enzymes. Secondly, the enzymes are only active in the acid conditions maintained within the lysosome, and are inactive at the neutral pH of the cytoplasm.

Mitochondria

Mitochondria are similar to bacteria in size and shape. Essentially, they are the 'powerhouse' of the cell, converting nutrient energy into a form the cell can use – adenosine triphosphate (ATP) – generated by the oxidative phosphorylation of glucose, that is, by aerobic respiration. When aerobic respiration is not possible, for example due to a reduction in blood supply, the cell can survive for a limited period of time by anaerobic respiration. This involves the conversion of stored ATP into the lower energy adenosine diphosphate (ADP). If aerobic respiration cannot be restored within a short period of time the cell will die.

Mitochondria are capable of their own replication and for this purpose have their own DNA. Unlike nuclear DNA this does not contain the complete genome, only that needed to carry out its own functions. It can make some of its own proteins, but most of the proteins needed by the mitochondrion are imported from the cytosol.

Causes of cellular injury

Ischaemia, hypoxia and anoxia

Atherosclerosis is a common cause of ischaemia

Ischaemia is an insufficiency of blood supply, causing a deficit of nutrients and oxygen in the cells. Ischaemia could occur in heart muscle during exercise if it is supplied by an atherosclerotic coronary artery. **Hypoxia** refers to a deficiency of oxygen; the term **anoxia** describes a complete absence of oxygen supply.

Physical injury

Mechanical injury

Mechanical trauma causes disruption of cells, damage to blood vessels and haemorrhage. When blood leaks into connective tissues the damage caused to the surrounding cells may be minimal and the leaked red blood cells can be removed by macrophage activity. Haemorrhage may have more serious consequences; for example a blood vessel rupturing in a confined space such as the cranial cavity, as might occur in head injury, leads to a rise in intracranial pressure, cerebral ischaemia, coma or death. Some of the most common forms of serious mechanical trauma in developed countries are road accidents.

Thermal injury

Thermal injury usually arises from exposure to heat in the form of burns. High temperatures cause changes in most macromolecules (denaturation of enzymes, for example) which will affect the function and integrity of cells. The severity of a burn depends on the temperature and duration of contact and the outcome for the patient is dependent upon the depth and surface area of skin involved. First-degree burns heal rapidly without scarring, but more severe burns heal with dermal scarring (if the patient recovers). A first-degree burn involves only the epithelium and, although painful, has little systemic impact. In contrast, full-thickness burns lead to a shift in body fluids into the interstitial compartments, causing **hypovolaemic shock**. Hypovolaemia is also a consequence of water depletion, as might occur in heat exhaustion when ambient temperature is high.

Prolonged exposure to extreme cold initially results in a generalised lowering of body temperature (**hypothermia**). This causes vasoconstriction and increased blood viscosity, leading to ischaemia of the extremities and vital organs such as the brain and heart. Loss of consciousness is followed by bradycardia and atrial fibrillation.

Neonates and infants are more vulnerable to hypothermia because they have a relatively large body surface and little adipose tissue. Homeless people are likely to be exposed to the cold, particularly if wearing wet clothes. Hypothermia is a common cause of death in older people, who are often inactive, debilitated by illness and poor diet, and lack the resources to heat their homes properly. Recovery is often possible if the person is warmed but death may follow from complications of bronchopneumonia or heart failure.

Localised exposure to cold can lead to tissue freezing or **frostbite**. The cold initially causes vasoconstriction and arterial thrombosis. In a few hours tissue necrosis occurs due to ischaemia and physical damage from formation of ice crystals. Frostbite is most common in the extremities, such as the toes and fingers.

Radiation injury

Radiation is injurious because of the chemical changes that take place within cells, most notably involving DNA. Ionising radiation can directly damage

Atrial fibrillation: a common arrhythmia comprising rapid, ineffective contractions of the atria, causing irregularity of rhythm in the ventricles. The patient has a very irregular pulse.

Bradycardia: slow heart action.

Hypovolaemic shock: a shift of fluid into the interstitial spaces lowers plasma volume and blood pressure. The result is a failure adequately to perfuse organs with blood.

Hypothermia is most common in neonates and infants, older people and the homeless

DNA, but more commonly the damage is induced indirectly, by the generation of highly reactive free radicals. Cells are especially vulnerable to radiation damage when they undergo mitosis.

Chemical agents

It is good practice to handle all chemicals carefully. Not all chemicals are dangerous and probably most are either inert or harmless – indeed, many are needed by the body as nutrients. However, thousands of chemicals are hazardous and the reactions they cause in cells and tissues are numerous. Some chemicals can cause toxic effects in picogram amounts, while others may need several hundred grams before they are toxic.

Generally, chemical agents can be classified into two sorts: those which are toxic without modification, and those which become toxic after being metabolised by the body. The main effect on cells is to disrupt or cause aggregation of macromolecular components. Some chemicals interfere with enzyme activity and exert their effects rapidly. Others, described as carcinogens (see Chapter 13), initiate or promote neoplastic transformation in cells, and there is a long time lag before the effects become evident. Chemicals, particularly proteins from other species, may act as antigens and cause autoimmune reactions.

Biological agents

Micro-organisms exert a wide variety of effects on cells, producing epidermal hyperplasia and hypertrophy (warts, for example), loss of cellular constituents (cytoplasmic RNA in medullary neurons infected by poliovirus, for example) and cell death. Many bacteria produce harmful agents (toxins), some of which are lethal in extremely small quantities (botulinum toxin, for example).

Immune mechanisms

A variety of substances can initiate **allergic reactions**. In some people an immediate humoral (**anaphylactic**) hypersensitivity is caused by exposure to **allergens** such as pollen, animal hair, house mites or fungal products. Exposure to these allergens stimulates the release of vasoactive amines by mast cells, causing urticaria, rhinitis or bronchospasm (see Chapter 25).

Cell-mediated (delayed) hypersensitivity occurs some days after sensitisation to a particular substance. Such reactions are seen on exposure to certain drugs or chemicals such as dinitrochlorobenzene and phenylenediamine. Exposure of the skin causes contact dermatitis.

In **autoimmune reactions** normal or altered tissue components act as targets for the immune system. The most common autoimmune disease is rheumatoid arthritis, which involves the precipitation of antigen–antibody complexes in the joint lining (synovium), causing chronic inflammation.

Anaphylactic (Type I) hypersensitivity: specific IgE antibodies are made against allergens. The IgE antibody binds to the surface of mast cells and basophils, which are found underlying most mucosal surfaces. Cross-linking of the IgE antibodies on second exposure to the allergen causes degranulation of the mast cells. The released substances cause vasodilatation, an acute inflammatory response and tissue damage.

Delayed (Type IV) hypersensitivity: begins with the exposure of a T cell to its specific antigen. The T cell becomes activated, and on second exposure to the same antigen the T cell releases lymphokines. The lymphokines bring about vascular changes, including infiltration of lymphocytes and macrophages.

Rhinitis: inflammation of the nasal epithelium. In allergic rhinitis seromucous exudate and oedema of the submucosa cause nasal blockage.

Urticaria: raised weals in the skin ('nettle rash'). Produced by mast cell activity which results in oedema and activation of platelets and eosinophils, causing itching.

Vasoactive: substances that cause vasoconstriction (reduction in the diameter of the blood vessel lumen by contraction of smooth muscle) or vasodilatation (increase in diameter of the blood vessel lumen).
Vasoconstrictors include leukotrienes and thromboxanes, vasodilators include histamine and prostaglandins.

Genetic defects

The deleterious effects of **single gene defects** can be observed most easily in cells that carry out a specific function dependent on a single protein. Such a situation may be seen in disorders of haemoglobin synthesis, known as the haemoglobinopathies. For example, in sickle-cell disease (see Chapter 3), defective haemoglobin molecules alter the properties and shape of the red blood cells. The resultant shortened lifespan of these cells leads to haemolytic anaemia and jaundice. Other single gene defects involve the abnormal intracellular storage of metabolic precursors due to the absence of an essential enzyme in the metabolic pathway. The stored material can compromise the function of the cell or may lead to cell death.

Survivable **multiple gene defects** result in a number of different abnormalities in the phenotype, the most common of which are mental retardation and infertility.

Nutritional imbalance

The integrity of cells and tissues is affected by nutritional state, in both deficiency and excess. For example, lack of vitamins can cause serious diseases, while an excess can be toxic, particularly in vulnerable groups such as pregnant women (vitamin A can cause fetal abnormalities) and children (see Chapter 7).

Oxidative stress

Oxidative damage to cells frequently arises as a result of the generation of free radicals, a molecular species containing one or more unpaired electrons. Although they are capable of existing independently, many free radicals are extremely short lived. They very readily react with non-radicals to generate further free radicals.

> *Free radicals can cause oxidative damage to cell components*

Free radicals are generated by cell respiration and other metabolic processes, particularly inflammation, and also from exogenous sources such as radiation and cigarette smoke. In chemical formulae a superscript dot˙ represents a free radical. Free radicals can interact with a wide range of intracellular and extracellular macromolecules. It is believed that the accumulation of damaged proteins, carbohydrates, lipids and nucleic acids contributes to a range of human disorders including cancers, atherosclerosis, neurodegenerative disorders, autoimmune disease and even biological ageing.

One effect of ionising radiation in biological tissues is the production of free radicals. For example, γ rays can split water in the body to generate the hydroxyl radical $OH˙$. This is an extremely reactive radical that attacks whatever is next to it, setting up a chain reaction with generation of free radicals in adjacent molecules.

> *The most dangerous free radical is the hydroxyl ion*

The unpaired superoxide ($O_2˙$) radical is formed by the addition of one electron to a molecule of oxygen, frequently by cellular metabolism, sometimes

Antioxidant: a substance that will delay or inhibit the oxidation of an oxidisable substrate.

Respiratory burst: an enzyme-mediated event that liberates a deluge of free radicals which have potent cell-killing ability.

▲ **Key points**

Free radicals

▲ Extremely reactive chemical species with an unpaired electron

▲ Produced in cells as metabolic byproducts

▲ Produced by phagocytic cells as part of inflammatory defences

▲ Produced by action of toxic compounds

▲ Cause cell injury

▲ Caused by cell injury

as an unavoidable byproduct but also deliberately. For example, superoxide generation is unavoidable in the mitochondrial electron transport chain. The deliberate production of superoxide forms part of defensive mechanisms, mediated by inflammatory cells such as neutrophils and macrophages, as part of the **respiratory burst** intended to kill foreign organisms. The generation of these species can become counter-productive in chronic inflammation, causing damage to or destruction of host cells. Superoxide is not the principal cause of oxidative damage: the more reactive hydroxyl free radical is more dangerous, particularly if a product of its reaction, hydrogen peroxide, is not rapidly removed.

Promoters of free radical damage

Iron and copper ions are effective promoters of free radicals — encouraging formation of the hydroxyl radical that in turn is responsible for lipid peroxidation. For this reason mechanisms in the body are designed to keep these species out of harm's way. Iron is conjugated to a protein and stored in the form of ferritin, or transported as transferrin. Similarly, copper is transported in the form of caeruloplasmin. However, the metal ions can be released at the sites of tissue injury. The free ions are referred to as **pro-oxidants**.

Antioxidants

Antioxidants have the ability to prevent lipid peroxidation and to protect tissues against damage by free radicals. A variety of antioxidant mechanisms limit the availability of free radicals, including intrinsic enzymes (superoxide dismutase, glutathione peroxidase), which depend on the availability of minerals such as zinc and selenium (Table 4.1) for their action, and the antioxidant vitamins A, C and E which scavenge oxygen free radicals (Table 4.2).

Table 4.1 Intracellular antioxidants

Glutathione peroxidase	Selenium-dependent enzyme present in cytosol and mitochondria
Glutathione	General protection of free radical damage Scavenger of hydroxyl radical and singlet oxygen Reactivates some enzymes inhibited by exposure to high oxygen concentration Protects against free radical damage
Superoxide dismutase	Catalyses conversion of superoxide to hydrogen peroxide
Catalase	Removes hydrogen peroxide

Table 4.2 Dietary antioxidant vitamins and minerals

Vitamin E (α-tocopherol)	Lipid soluble; inhibits lipid peroxidation
Vitamin C (ascorbic acid)	Inhibits aqueous phase pro-oxidants Recycles vitamin E
Vitamin A (β-carotene)	Lipid-soluble radical scavenger Quencher of singlet oxygen
Zinc	Component of cytoplasmic superoxide dismutase
Manganese	Component of mitochondrial superoxide dismutase
Copper	Component of cytoplasmic superoxide dismutase Component of caeruloplasmin – converts ferrous iron to ferric (ferrous iron catalyses free radical reactions)
Selenium	Component of glutathione peroxidase

> ▲ **Key points**
>
> **Antioxidant defences**
>
> **Prevention of free radical generation:**
> ▲ Sequestration of metal ions by complexing with proteins
> ▲ Decomposition of peroxides by catalase and glutathione peroxidase
>
> **Interception of free radicals:**
> ▲ Superoxide dismutase
> ▲ α-Tocopherol
> ▲ Vitamin C

Antioxidant enzymes

The superoxide dismutases, found in mitochondria and the cytoplasm, convert superoxide to hydrogen peroxide and oxygen:

$$2O_2^{\cdot} + 2H^+ \rightarrow H_2O_2 + O_2$$

The hydrogen peroxide generated is destroyed by the enzymes catalase or glutathione peroxidase (a selenium-containing enzyme):

$$2H_2O_2 \rightarrow 2H_2O + O_2$$

If not rapidly removed the hydrogen peroxide may react with more superoxide to form the hydroxyl free radical:

$$O_2^{\cdot} + H_2O_2 \rightarrow OH^{\cdot} + O_2$$

Unfortunately, antioxidant defences are not always completely effective even in normal individuals and there is an inherited disorder in which the activity of superoxide dismutase is reduced to about 40% of normal levels. These people suffer from **amyotrophic lateral sclerosis** (motor neuron disease) at an early age.

Despite the various antioxidant mechanisms there will still be circumstances in which cells become damaged beyond recovery. Cell death induced by free radicals proceeds either as apoptosis or necrosis (see below).

The maintenance of cell integrity depends on the balance between free radical activity and antioxidant status

Lipid peroxidation

Cell membranes are particularly vulnerable to free radical attack. When OH˙ is produced adjacent to a membrane it can extract a hydrogen atom from the polyunsaturated fatty acids within the membrane. This leaves an unpaired electron on a carbon atom (that is, a carbon radical) on the fatty acid chain, which can then react with oxygen to give a peroxyl radical (fatty acid and $O_2^{\cdot}$).

Fat-soluble antioxidant vitamins are essential for controlling lipid peroxidation

Senescence: degeneration of functional capacity associated with ageing.

> ▲ **Key points**
>
> **Types of free radical damage**
>
> ---
>
> ▲ Oxidative damage to DNA
>
> ▲ Peroxidation of membrane polyunsaturated fatty acids: decreases membrane fluidity, destabilises membrane receptors
>
> ▲ Carbohydrate damage. For example, depolymerisation of hyaluronic acid results in loss of synovial fluid viscosity
>
> ▲ Oxidation of proteins such as immunoglobulins and enzymes

The resulting peroxyl radical attacks adjacent fatty acid side-chains, again to generate a new carbon radical, setting up a chain reaction. Hence the attack by one reactive free radical results in the oxidation of multiple fatty acid side-chains to lipid peroxides. This renders the membrane leaky, damages membrane proteins, and eventually results in complete breakdown of the membrane.

The hydrophobic interior of the membrane is not accessible to the enzymatic antioxidants that act in an aqueous environment and lipid-soluble antioxidants are required to prevent its peroxidation. Vitamin E (α-tocopherol) is believed to be particularly effective as an antioxidant when incorporated into the lipid layer of a membrane. It acts by scavenging intermediate peroxyl radicals, itself being converted to a radical form. The vitamin E radical is thought to be regenerated by vitamin C.

DNA oxidation

All parts of the cell are vulnerable to oxidative damage and, although chromatin is probably a good protective barrier, DNA is no exception. Oxidative damage to DNA can be repaired by enzymatic excision of the damaged area and polymerisation of replacement DNA. In some circumstances the free radical (and other) damage is beyond the capacity for repair, or errors are made, leading to accumulation of genetic mutations with time. These may contribute to senescence and other changes in the cell.

Oxidation of proteins and carbohydrates

The amino acids and peptide bonds of proteins are susceptible to free radical attack. The effects are fragmentation, altered structure and consequent functional changes. It is possible that carbohydrates are also altered by free radical oxidation, but this is not well documented.

Free radicals and disease

Exposure to free radicals is an inevitable consequence of aerobic respiration. Normally there are efficient mechanisms that can prevent or minimise any damage to cellular and tissue components. Failure or inadequacy of these mechanisms probably results in disease, most notably the chronic conditions caused by atherosclerosis, cancers and neurodegenerative diseases (see Figure 4.3). Free radicals are also generated when a cell is damaged and it therefore becomes difficult to know whether the free radicals are a cause or a consequence of disease. There is currently much interest in the role and capacity of dietary antioxidants in ameliorating damage from free radicals (see Chapter 7).

Coronary heart disease

One of the most important processes underlying the development of coronary heart disease (CHD) is atherosclerosis. According to the commonly accepted 'lipid hypothesis', most atherosclerotic plaques result from the infiltration of cholesterol, in the form of LDL, into the arterial wall. LDL is susceptible to oxidation by oxygen free radicals, whereupon it becomes damaging to cells and tissues. Normally LDL peroxidation would be minimised by dietary antioxidants such as vitamin E and vitamin C. Epidemiological studies indicate that people who had died from CHD were more likely to have had low plasma antioxidant levels, particularly if they were smokers.

Mitogens: substances that cause cells to undergo cell division.

Cancer

It is likely that free radical mechanisms often cause oxidative damage to the bases in DNA. Over time, and in concert with other agents, this could cause permanent mutations. Possible contributory factors are incomplete repair of DNA and failure of apoptosis following free radical damage. The damage to DNA could become amplified over several cell cycles, eventually causing cancer. In addition, oxidative damage to cell growth regulatory proteins can stimulate mitogenesis.

The oxidants produced by activated phagocytic cells in inflammation (neutrophils, macrophages) are responsible for free radical damage and also act as signals for mitogenesis: it is known that sites of chronic inflammation sometimes become cancerous. Epidemiological studies suggest an association between low intakes of dietary antioxidants and the development of some types of cancer (see Chapter 7), lending support to the hypothesis that free radical damage is involved at some stages of the neoplastic process.

Ageing

The free radical theory of ageing proposes that there is an increasing imbalance between pro-oxidants and antioxidant defences with age, causing acceleration of free radical-mediated tissue damage. There is some evidence that free radicals are formed at an increased rate in senescent animals, but they could just as well result from cell degeneration as be initiating or promoting factors. Animal feeding studies on the effects of ingestion of large amounts of antioxidant vitamins have produced no appreciable improvements in life expectancy. In humans, any effect could result from antioxidant inhibition of coronary heart disease or cancer.

Free radical damage has been proposed as a mechanism of ageing, but this is difficult to prove

The rate of ageing correlates with metabolic rate (see Chapter 8): animals with a high metabolic rate will generate more free radicals, which supports a role for free radicals as initiators of the ageing process. In most circumstances, however, the balance between pro-oxidants and antioxidants is maintained and, except in smokers, there are compensatory mechanisms that adequately cope with excessive free radical generation. It is likely that in most people any decline in these homeostatic mechanisms would occur relatively late in life and therefore not markedly affect overall survival.

Neurodegenerative disease

Several metabolic processes in the brain generate free radicals. Defence against oxidative damage in the brain is provided by vitamin E, vitamin C and the antioxidant enzymes catalase and glutathione peroxidase.

There is some evidence to implicate oxidative free radical damage in

Microglia: cells that function as macrophages in the brain, engulfing invading micro-organisms and dead neural tissue. The cells inhabit areas between the neurons and have a small ovoid nucleus and long thorny cytoplasmic processes.

▲   **Key points**

Conditions associated with free radical damage

- ▲ Atherosclerosis
- ▲ Cancers
- ▲ Ageing
- ▲ Rheumatoid arthritis
- ▲ Neuronal degeneration, for example Alzheimer's disease, Parkinson's disease
- ▲ Lung disease: emphysema, fibrosis
- ▲ Liver disease, for example alcoholic liver disease
- ▲ Kidney damage: microvascular and tubular injury
- ▲ Muscle damage
- ▲ Diabetes mellitus

Parkinson's disease. It is notable that the oxidation product of dopamine is itself a neurotoxin, and reductions in the levels of the protective enzyme glutathione peroxidase have been reported in Parkinson's disease. It is also notable that MPTP, which induces a Parkinson-like syndrome (see Chapter 27), is a redox chemical, probably causing neuronal damage by free radical-mediated reactions.

In another neurodegenerative disorder, Alzheimer's disease (see Chapter 26), areas of neuronal degeneration and death are accompanied by a proliferation of microglia. In culture studies these cells generate free radicals, particularly in the presence of aluminium silicate particles. The deposition of β-amyloid in the brain is also associated with Alzheimer's disease. Culture experiments have shown that this material is cytotoxic for neurons, but not in the presence of excess vitamin E, suggesting that free radical reactions are involved in β-amyloid-induced neuronal damage.

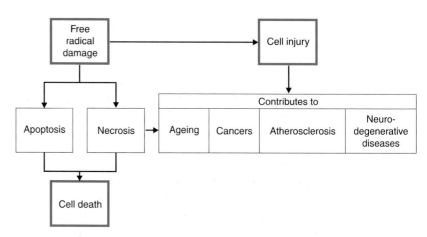

Figure 4.3 Consequences of damage by free radicals. Cell injury results when the free radical load outweighs cellular defences. This might lead to the death of the individual cell, either by apoptosis or by necrosis, when there is extensive damage affecting many cells. Persistent cell injury does not always lead to cell death – instead defects in repair may occur. Over time these cumulative defects could contribute to the ageing (senescence) of cells or adversely affect predisposition for diseases such as cancer and atherosclerosis.

Morphological and biochemical changes in cell injury

A number of alterations to cell structure resulting from injury have been observed, both nuclear and cytoplasmic. The cytoplasmic changes are associated with accumulation of lipid or water, and are reversible in the early stages. Nuclear changes are irreversible and represent the prelude to cell death.

Review question 1

Where do free radicals come from? Do they always cause damage?

Accumulation of water (cytoplasmic oedema)

The morphological appearance of cytoplasmic oedema is referred to as **cloudy swelling.** In a later stage water droplets within the cytoplasm coalesce and are seen as cloudy vacuoles. This stage is referred to by morphologists as **vacuolar degeneration** (Figure 4.4).

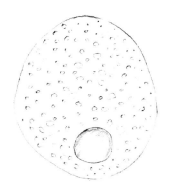 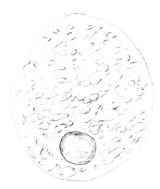

Figure 4.4 Accumulation of water. **Left**: Cloudy swelling is characterised by the accumulation of water droplets in the cytoplasm. This changes the refractive index so that when viewed under the microscope the cell appears fuzzy. **Right**: Eventually almost the whole cytoplasm becomes filled with liquid.

   The normal cell has higher potassium but lower sodium levels than the extracellular environment. This difference in tonicity is maintained by the sodium pump which requires energy in the form of ATP. When a cell becomes hypoxic, ATP levels fall because of the decrease in mitochondrial oxidative phosphorylation, leading to partial failure of the sodium pump. Potassium leaves the cell, but sodium, calcium and water enter from the extracellular fluid, causing swelling of the cell cytoplasm and contents. The ingress of calcium can be seen by electron microscopy as electron-dense deposits, usually within mitochondria.

Accumulation of lipid

Lipid accumulation in cells is referred to by morphologists as **fatty change** (Figure 4.5). Normally lipid within the cytoplasm is complexed with protein and is not stainable to any appreciable extent by fat-soluble dyes. Fatty change is characterised by the accumulation of free fatty acids as droplets within the cytoplasm. These can be stained with the fat-soluble dyes Oil red O or Sudan black. In some cases virtually all the cell cytoplasm appears to be composed of lipid as the fat droplets coalesce. Fatty change is most often seen in the liver because this is the organ most concerned with fat metabolism but it can also occur in the cells of the heart, muscle, kidney and other organs.

   In the hypoxic cell, fatty change is a consequence of reduction in the availability of ATP. This leads to detachment of ribosomes from endoplasmic reticulum and reduced protein synthesis. Proteins are essential for lipid transport out of the cell and, without them, the lipid accumulates.

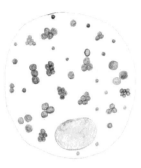 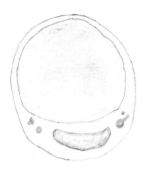

Figure 4.5 Fatty change. **Left**: Early fatty change is characterised by the appearance of discrete lipid droplets in the cytoplasm. **Right**: With persistent injury the fat droplets become larger and coalesce, eventually taking up most of the cell volume and displacing the nucleus.

Other mechanisms involved in fatty change are decreased synthesis of lipoproteins in the liver, excessive entry of fatty acids or a failure of the coupling of lipid to protein. In starvation there may be insufficient protein available to couple with the lipid or there may be excessive entry of fatty acids into the liver because the energy reserves of adipose tissue have been mobilised. If the entry of fatty acids exceeds the cell's capacity to couple them with protein, they will accumulate within the cell.

Alterations in the cell nucleus

Injury that is sufficient to cause morphological changes in the nucleus is usually catastrophic

Morphological changes in the nucleus consequent to injury take a number of forms. **Pyknosis** refers to a condensation of the nuclear chromatin. The nucleus appears smaller than normal and is more intensely stained with basic dyes. The term **karyorrhexis** is used to describe fragmentation of the nucleus. This is followed by complete dissolution of the nuclear material, known as **karyolysis**.

The initial pyknosis is believed to be caused by a fall in cellular pH. This can arise in ischaemic conditions when the cell switches to anaerobic respiration and uses its glycogen reserves to supply its energy requirements. Anaerobic respiration results in the accumulation of **lactic acid**, which cannot be completely removed unless aerobic respiration is restored.

Dissolution of cell nuclear and cytoplasmic contents is caused by release of lysosomal enzymes

The fall in pH during anaerobic respiration can damage membranes. Disruption of the lysosomal membrane causes release of highly destructive enzymes, which cause denaturation of membrane proteins surrounding the cell and its cytoplasmic organelles. In addition, lysosomal DNAases and RNAases contribute to fragmentation and lysis of the nucleus, causing cell death (Figure 4.6).

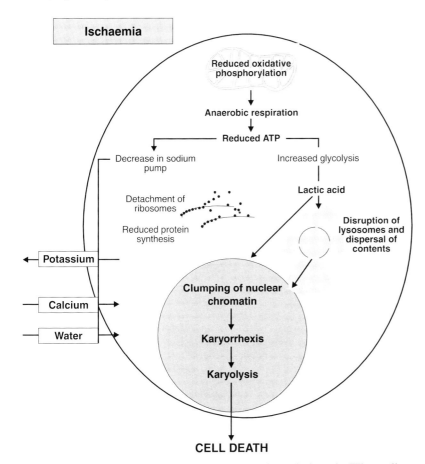

Figure 4.6 Biochemical and morphological changes due to ischaemia. When cells are starved of oxygen and nutrients aerobic respiration closes down and the cell switches to anaerobic respiration. This causes a reduction in available ATP, which may be insufficient to drive the sodium pump responsible for maintaining intracellular ionic balance. Closure of the pump results in an ingress of calcium and water, and an outflow of potassium ions. The integrity of the rough endoplasmic reticulum also relies on sodium pump activity: without it the ribosomes detach and protein synthesis ceases. A byproduct of anaerobic respiration is lactic acid; intracellular membranes are susceptible to acid attack. Disruption of lysosomal membranes will cause release of stored enzymes, which are activated by acid conditions. These enzymes will dissolve any cellular components in their path, causing the nuclear changes of karyorrhexis and karyolysis and, ultimately, death of the cell. The initial changes in ischaemia are reversible, but damage to the nucleus resulting in karyorrhexis is irreversible.

The leakage of cellular contents following the death of the cell will cause damage to adjacent cells. The amounts of enzyme released can be substantial and may be measured in the blood as a marker of cell death. For example, myocardial infarction is associated with a rise in the plasma levels of creatine kinase, lactate dehydrogenase and aspartate aminotransferase. However, these enzymes are also present in cells other than heart muscle and their release into the circulation does not necessarily indicate that cardiac damage has occurred (see Chapter 20).

Cellular adaptive responses

In conditions of partial cell injury or starvation a cell (or tissue) undergoes a number of responses to ensure its survival:
- Atrophy (reduction in cell size)
- Hypertrophy (increase in cell size)
- Induction (hypertrophy of endoplasmic reticulum)
- Hyperplasia (increase in cell number)
- Metaplasia (a change in cell type)
- Dysplasia (change in size, shape and organisation of cells)

Atrophy

Cell atrophy can result from:
- Decreased workload
- Loss of innervation
- Diminished blood supply
- Inadequate nutrition
- Loss of endocrine stimulation

In some respects atrophy can be viewed as a retreat by the cell to a smaller size to ensure survival. It can be likened to driving a car slowly in order to conserve fuel. Energy use and the number of cell structural components is reduced. In many circumstances cell atrophy is accompanied by increased numbers of **autophagic vesicles**, inside which the cellular membrane structures and organelles that are no longer required are degraded. A typical example of atrophy is seen when a limb is immobilised in a plaster cast: a reduction in muscle size follows. Some atrophic changes are associated with ageing.

Hypertrophy

When cells cannot divide their response to increased demand is to increase in size

Hypertrophy results when cells are stimulated by an increase in functional demand or by a specific hormone. The increase in the size and functional capacity of the cell is achieved by formation of greater numbers of cell organelles, including mitochondria, endoplasmic reticulum and cytoplasmic filaments. In turn the increased size of large numbers of cells causes an increase in the size of the tissue or organ as a whole.

These events can be quite normal – for example, the increased functional demand on skeletal muscle cells when athletes 'pump iron' will eventually lead to hypertrophy of the muscle mass; the growth of the uterus in pregnancy is a normal process mediated by oestrogenic hormonal stimulation of uterine smooth muscle cells.

In some circumstances hypertrophy is associated with a pathological condition. An example is the adaptive hypertrophy of heart muscle seen in patients who have increased pressure or volume load on the heart because of previous myocardial infarct or diseased cardiac valves. This response can result in a doubling of the normal weight of the heart.

Induction

Induction refers to the selective hypertrophy of ER induced by drugs or toxic agents such as phenobarbitone or carbon tetrachloride. Phenobarbitone is detoxified by an oxidase electron transport system present within the smooth ER of liver cells. The cell's adaptive response is to synthesise more smooth ER, increasing the capacity of the oxidase system to detoxify the drug. This explains the increased tolerance to the drug seen in prolonged use. Coincidentally, the capacity to detoxify other agents by oxidation is also improved. This can be a disadvantage: for example, oxidation of carbon tetrachloride results in conversion of the molecule to an extremely toxic $CCl_3^{\cdot}$ free radical.

Hyperplasia

Hormonal stimulation or increased functional demand can cause an increase in cell numbers (hyperplasia). These stimuli are common to both hyperplasia and hypertrophy, which are often seen in the same tissue. A classic example of this is oestrogen-induced growth of the uterus.

If cells can divide, they will do so when stimulated by hormones or increased functional demand

Physiological hyperplasia may be hormonally induced, for example enlargement of glandular epithelium in the female breast at puberty. A further physiological stimulus, known as compensatory hyperplasia, results from cell damage. This can be induced experimentally in the liver by partial hepatectomy. The remaining liver cells undergo increased cell division, so that the lost cells are replaced without any appreciable increase in the original size of the organ.

Pathological hyperplasia is caused by excessive hormonal stimulation. This can occur in the endometrium where hormonal imbalance can lead to bleeding and heavy menstrual periods.

Metaplasia

Metaplasia is an adaptive response to stress, in which cells of one type are substituted for those of another (Figure 4.7). This response occurs in the respiratory tract of smokers, in whom the normal simple ciliated columnar epithelium is replaced by stratified squamous epithelium. Presumably the conversion from simple to stratified epithelium offers greater protection from damage. The disadvantage is that the accompanying loss of ciliated epithelium

Metaplasia is a protective mechanism in which one cell type is replaced by another

means that mucus is not so easily cleared, causing the familiar 'smoker's cough'.

Metaplasia does not represent the conversion of a mature cell to that of another type. It is believed that a small population of immature multipotential cells within the epithelium is stimulated to produce cells of the new type by cell division. Sites of metaplasia may eventually show further morphological changes if the damaging agent is not removed: with time the cells exhibit dysplastic changes or may even become malignant.

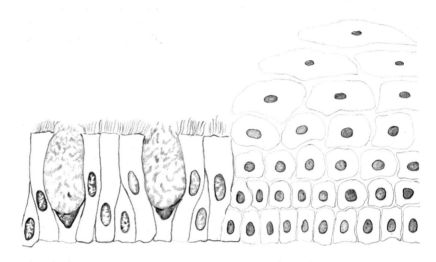

Figure 4.7 Metaplasia of respiratory epithelium. On the left of the diagram the respiratory epithelium consists of a single layer of ciliated columnar and goblet cells. The function of the goblet cells is to secrete mucus which traps particles in air and acts as a protective layer on the cell surface. Mucus is cleared by the motion of cilia. In response to repeated damage, as would occur in smokers, the cells are replaced by a thicker layer of squamous cells. On the right, the normal respiratory epithelium has been replaced by multiple layers of squamous cells.

Dysplasia

Continued stress or injury can result in a cell becoming dysplastic

Dysplasia is not strictly an adaptive response but represents an atypical proliferative response by cells in circumstances of chronic irritation or inflammation. Unlike hyperplasia, the proliferated cells are abnormal. Dysplastic cells are disorganised within the epithelium and exhibit changes in the nucleus as well as in overall size and shape. Dysplasia is most commonly encountered in the uterine cervix, where the change may be associated with infection by human papillomavirus. Dysplastic change can be regarded as a precancerous state although progression to cancer does not necessarily follow: there is ample evidence to show that dysplastic changes are reversible to normal. However, the more severe the lesion then the greater the chance of progression to cancer (see Chapter 13).

Cell death

There are limits as to how much a cell can adapt to unfavourable circumstances. In some situations it is more efficient for the damaged cells to die and be replenished by division of neighbouring cells, rather than continually to undergo repair. When cell injury is rapid and extensive, overwhelming normal function and repair capacity, the death of cells is unavoidable and uncontrolled. This process is termed necrosis. When injury is milder, perhaps as a result of normal 'wear and tear' the cell can 'elect' to die in a much more controlled manner, and is replaced by division of adjacent cells. This process is termed apoptosis.

Cells can die by accident or design

Phagocytosis: uptake of particulate matter, such as bacteria or cell debris, into macrophages. Parts of the cell membrane and cytoplasm protrude and flow around the particle to be ingested, forming a phagosome. This is engulfed within the cytoplasm and fuses with a lysosome, whereupon the contents are digested. Most phagocytic cells have the ability to move about the body.

Apoptosis

Apoptosis is also termed 'programmed cell death'. In most circumstances apoptosis is a normal cellular event: cells eventually reach the end of their useful lives and it becomes more productive to replace them by cell division than to carry on with repair. Essentially, apoptosis is a co-ordinated process, usually involving only a single cell or a small group of cells at any one time, in order to maintain the proper balance of cells in the tissue (Figure 4.8).

A balance exists between cell division and death

Examples of apoptosis may be seen during fetal development, when the webs between the fingers are removed; the formation of hollow organs such as the heart begins with a more solid structure. Apoptosis is also a normal event in fully developed tissues, particularly in sites of high cell turnover: every day millions of cells are lost and replaced by cell division in the skin, respiratory and gastrointestinal tracts.

Certain microscopic features distinguish apoptosis from the more extensive and uncontrolled loss of cells seen in necrosis. The early stages involve the enzymatic breakdown of chromatin and the collapse of the cell nucleus. In later stages the cell shrinks and is cleaved into membrane-bound clumps enclosing organelles. The membrane-bound material is recognised and engulfed by phagocytic cells (Figure 4.9).

The most striking features of apoptosis are cell shrinkage and condensation of nuclear chromatin

The precise, 'programmed' nature of apoptosis implies that the process is controlled genetically. Cell death is triggered by the appearance or loss of an external signal, leading to a cascade of events culminating in cell death. To date not much is known about the genetic control of apoptosis, but in some cells the *c-myc* proto-oncogene and *p53* tumour suppressor gene appear to play an essential role (see Chapter 15). It also seems likely that other genes, for example *bcl-2*, operate to limit the extent of cell death.

Cancers may arise if apoptosis is disabled

Cyclins: a family of molecules that form complexes and enable the cell to undergo transmission from one phase of the growth cycle to another.

The apoptotic process is probably initiated when a cell becomes marginally damaged, perhaps by internally generated free radicals. By 'electing' to die, any DNA mutations arising from the injury will not be passed on to subsequent generations of cells. This could represent an important self-defence mechanism against the development of cancer.

p53 can prolong the growth phase of the cell, allowing time for repair: if repair cannot occur, p53 invokes apoptosis

The *p53* tumour suppressor gene is responsible for producing a protein that can prevent cell division by inhibiting a class of molecules called **cyclins**.

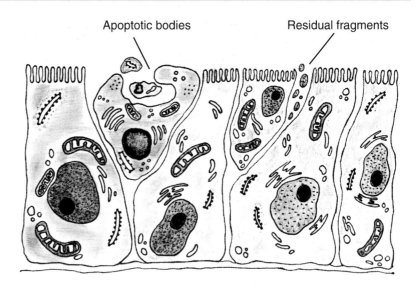

Figure 4.8 Apoptosis is the controlled death of cells without inflammation. Isolated cells in an epithelium become separated from their neighbours and split into fragments called apoptotic bodies, containing cytoplasmic organelles and sometimes nuclear fragments. The fragments are recognised by adjacent cells because of changes in membrane composition, and eliminated by phagocytosis. Occasionally the fragments degenerate extracellularly.

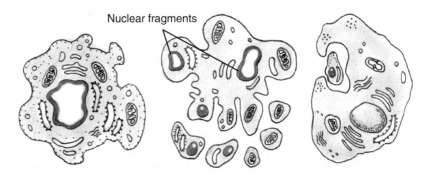

Figure 4.9 Microscopic features of apoptosis. **Left**: In the early stage of apoptosis there is an overall reduction in cell volume and distortion of shape. The nucleus becomes distorted and chromatin condenses. **Middle**: The nucleus fragments into membrane-bound segments. The cell often splits into several membrane-bound bodies each containing viable cytoplasmic organelles. **Right**: The apoptotic cell fragments are recognised by specialised phagocytic cells in the immediate environment, ingested and further degraded.

The p53 protein appears to act as a sensor of DNA damage, so that if damage is extensive cell division is inhibited and the cell dies. If the damage to DNA is only mild the cell will be allowed to attempt repair. Some cancers may arise from failure of this control mechanism. If the gene itself is damaged and can no longer produce p53 protein then cell proliferation will proceed unhindered. This allows **clones** of cells with defective DNA to accumulate (Figure 4.10). It is notable that *p53* is the most frequently mutated gene in human cancers.

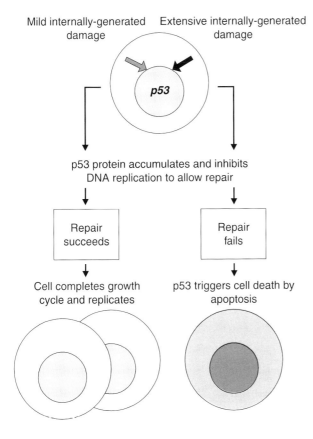

Figure 4.10 Control of cellular replication and apoptosis. When a cell becomes damaged p53 accumulates and inhibits replication so that repair can take place. If the damage is extensive and repair fails, p53 triggers cell death by apoptosis. Alternatively, if damage is only mild, accumulation of p53 leads to growth arrest and repair. The repaired cell will then complete its growth cycle and replicate. If the *p53* gene becomes damaged the apoptosis pathway is lost, so that incompletely repaired DNA is replicated and becomes fixed in daughter cell clones.

Gene and protein terminology: It is a convention for the name of a gene to be written in italic, hence *p53* (italic) refers to the gene and p53 (not italic) refers to the protein product of that gene.

It is likely that apoptosis regulates responses to a range of pathological processes, particularly those that evoke the immune and inflammatory systems. Some of the cells involved in the inflammatory response (neutrophils, for example) have only a limited capacity to break up foreign and necrotic material and once their lysosomal enzymes are exhausted the cells die, presumably by invoking apoptosis pathways. Before this, the activities of inflammatory cells are modified by a range of mediators (see p. 134) including tumour necrosis

Apoptosis is invoked in the termination of immune and inflammatory responses

Cell growth cycle: Cell division normally proceeds through a growth cycle with four distinctive biochemical phases. Most of a cell's life is spent in a resting phase, termed G_0. A series of other phases are recognisable as a cell prepares for division. The early growth phase is G_1, during which many of the enzymes necessary for DNA synthesis are produced. This is followed by the long S phase, in which the cell replicates its DNA. The cell passes through a further growth phase, G_2, immediately before division (mitosis) in the M phase.

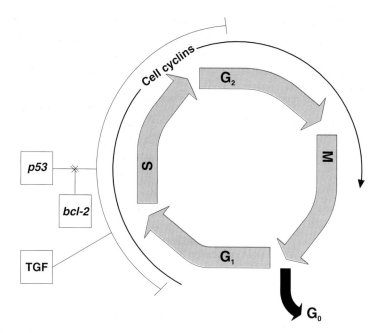

Figure 4.11 Control of the cell growth cycle. The cell cycle is driven by cyclins complexed with kinase enzymes. Progression of the cell cycle is retarded by inhibitors of the cyclin complexes, including the *p53* gene product. Expression of *bcl-2* counteracts the effects of *p53*. The cytokine TGF-β inhibits a cyclin complex that operates at an early stage in the cycle.

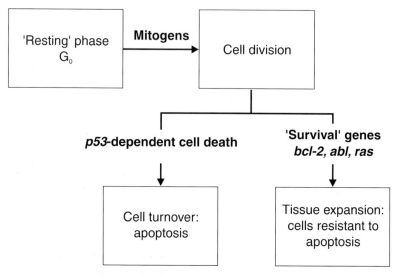

Figure 4.12 Protection from apoptosis by 'survival' genes. Cells can be rescued from apoptosis by the activities of regulating genes. When a cell becomes committed to the growth cycle (from G_0) there is an implicit commitment to apoptosis, so that cell turnover and the size of the cell population can be regulated. The crucial regulatory gene appears to be *bcl-2*, but other genes (often oncogenes or tumour suppressor genes) play a part.

factor, interferon and interleukins. Some of these act to delay the death of inflammatory cells, while others accelerate it. It is possible that defects in these control mechanisms, causing failure of apoptotic clearance of inflammatory cells, could underlie a variety of chronic inflammatory conditions (see p. 132).

Premature commitment to apoptosis is believed to cause the gradual depletion of CD4$^+$ cells that leads to AIDS (see Chapter 25). In this case binding of HIV to the CD4$^+$ receptor of uninfected cells can trigger apoptosis directly.

Many of the oncogenic viruses (see Chapter 13) interfere with apoptosis pathways. Epstein–Barr virus, human papillomavirus and hepatitis B virus are believed to cause mutations to *p53* or inactivate its protein product. These mechanisms are discussed in more detail in Chapter 16.

Necrosis

Necrosis is a term used to describe tissues in which cell death has occurred, usually because of accidental or abnormal damage. Unlike apoptosis, necrosis is not a programmed event. The cellular damage leads to disturbed osmotic balance, so that there is an influx of water and calcium. Finally, the chromatin becomes condensed and fragmented and the cell dies (Figure 4.13). The inflammatory process is involved in removing these dead cells (Figure 4.14).

> *Necrosis is a pathological event involving extensive injury and uncontrolled loss of cells*

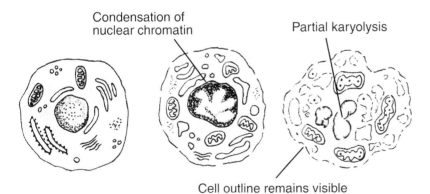

Condensation of
nuclear chromatin

Partial karyolysis

Cell outline remains visible

Figure 4.13 Necrosis. The initial cellular changes in necrosis comprise disruption of cytoplasmic organelles and condensation of nuclear chromatin. The degradative changes progress with liquefaction of cytoplasmic contents, karyorrhexis and, finally, karyolysis.

There are two main types of necrosis: **coagulative** and **liquefaction** necrosis.

Coagulative necrosis

In coagulative necrosis the outlines of the dead cells and the general tissue architecture can still be seen, but the cells have lost their nuclei and their cytoplasm is strongly acidophilic. This staining property is probably the result

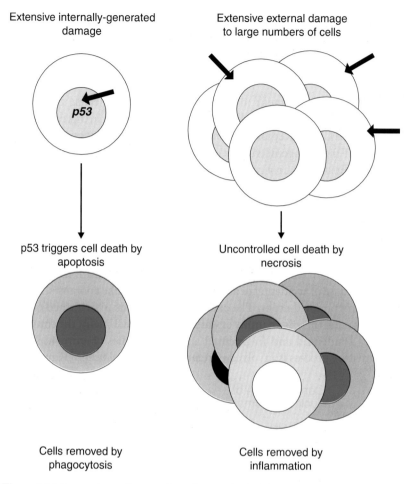

Figure 4.14 Comparison of apoptosis and necrosis. Cell death by apoptosis occurs in a co-ordinated manner, and is likened to leaves falling off a tree in autumn. In contrast, extensive damage by outside agents causes the cells to undergo unplanned death by necrosis. This would be akin to loss of leaves, or even branches, of the tree in a storm.

of protein denaturation in which previously concealed basic groups within the protein are exposed on the surface of the protein and become available for combination with acid dyes. The revealed basic groups are also believed to be responsible for **calcification**, which is often a feature of necrosis.

Coagulative necrosis causes hardening of the tissues, in much the same way as protein denaturation causes hardening when an egg is boiled. In human tissues its cause is usually severe ischaemia or chemical injury. It is the most common type of necrotic change and can occur in most tissues with the exception of brain.

Liquefaction necrosis

In contrast, a softening or even liquefying of tissue occurs in liquefaction necrosis. This type of necrosis is usually seen in the brain or is associated with focal bacterial lesions. Often caused by a brain infarct, the lesion evolves into a cyst filled with fluid and debris.

Caseous necrosis

An intermediate form between liquefaction and coagulative necrosis is known as caseous necrosis, seen in tuberculous infections. Unlike coagulative necrosis, caseous necrosis gives tissues a featureless microscopic appearance. Macroscopically the characteristic appearance is of a soft, friable, tissue debris which resembles clumps of cheese.

Fat necrosis

Fat necrosis occurs in tissues with large fat deposits or lipase enzymes, such as the female breasts and the pancreas. Lipases are released by trauma or inflammatory conditions, breaking adipose stores of tissues down into fatty acids. The released fatty acids then complex with calcium to form a calcium soap. This is seen in tissue sections as amorphous, granular basophilic deposits, surrounded by an inflammatory reaction.

Further changes in necrotic tissue

Where tissue necrosis has occurred an acute inflammatory response follows. In turn this is followed by a phase of demolition and healing. The presence of inflammatory cells, most notably neutrophils, is an important feature of necrotic tissues and is used to distinguish necrosis from the autolytic changes that take place in tissues after death.

Accumulation of substances within cells

A variety of materials can accumulate within cells as a result of altered or inadequate cellular metabolism. In some circumstances the accumulated material may compromise the normal function of the cell or cause cell death. In other cases the accumulated material makes little difference to cell function and disappears when the cause is removed. Substances accumulate within cells because:

- The substance is produced at a normal or increased rate, but cellular metabolism is insufficient to remove it
- The substance produced is a normal metabolic precursor, but the cell lacks the enzymes necessary to complete its metabolic conversion
- An exogenous substance accumulates within cells because it is resistant to degradative enzymes

Lipid

Lipid accumulation, in the form of fatty change, has already been discussed

Key points

Features of necrosis

▲ Uncontrolled loss of large numbers of cells, usually as a result of injury by exogenous agents

▲ The cells and their organelles swell due to the entry of water

▲ The cell dies as a result of irreversible changes to nuclear chromatin

▲ Dead cells are removed by inflammation

▲ Cell outlines can still be seen in coagulative necrosis

▲ In liquefaction necrosis the tissue is softened and fluid-filled cysts may be formed

▲ Leakage of lipases from dead cells break down fat stores in fat necrosis, which then become calcified

Multiple myeloma: a malignancy of plasma cells characterised by continuous synthesis of immunoglobulins; may be detectable in the urine as Bence–Jones protein.

Plasma cells: mature B cells, the antibody-secreting cells of the humoral immune response.

(p. 115). Some lipid complexes can accumulate within cells as an inherited deficiency or **lipid-storage disorder**. The best-known of these are Tay–Sachs, Niemann–Pick and Gaucher's diseases (see Chapter 3).

Protein

Protein accumulation occurs in cells of the kidney tubules when glomerular damage causes leakage of protein. The protein is reabsorbed from the glomerular filtrate by the cells lining the tubules. Protein accumulation is reversible: when the underlying cause of the proteinuria is eliminated or controlled the droplets disappear. Protein may also accumulate in plasma cells, corresponding to excess production of immunoglobulins. This occurs in multiple myeloma, and the cells contain eosinophilic cytoplasmic inclusions known as Russell bodies.

Carbohydrates

Carbohydrate accumulation can result from excessive uptake of carbohydrate by cells, such as occurs in diabetes mellitus, or may be associated with genetic disease in which a gene defect results in reduction or absence of an enzyme necessary for the metabolism of carbohydrate within the cell. In uncontrolled diabetes mellitus abnormal quantities of glucose are excreted into the urine. This is taken up by the epithelial cells of the renal tubules and stored in the form of glycogen. Glycogen also accumulates within liver cells, pancreatic cells of the islets of Langerhans and heart muscle cells.

Glycogen accumulation also occurs in the single gene defects collectively known as the **glycogen storage disorders**. In these disorders the enzyme necessary for the normal metabolism of glycogen may be lacking or an abnormal form of glycogen may be synthesised which cannot be metabolised. In either case the carbohydrate accumulates within the cell, mainly in heart muscle, liver and kidney cells. The massive deposits of carbohydrates within the cells can cause secondary injury and cell death.

Similarly, the various **mucopolysaccharidoses** involve enzyme defects leading to intracellular accumulation of carbohydrate–protein complexes. In addition to cells of the heart, liver and kidney, these complex molecules may also accumulate within neurons of the brain and in the retina. Affected individuals are usually mentally retarded and have a shortened life expectancy.

Pigments

Lipofuscin, the 'wear and tear' pigment, is associated with ageing and chronic injury

Pigments can be derived from exogenous or endogenous sources. An example of exogenous pigmentation is carbon in the lungs, and is present in most adults in developed countries where there is air pollution. Silica may also be inhaled and deposited in the lungs, particularly as a result of occupational exposure in miners and quarry-workers. Lung function is impaired because an inflammatory reaction causes the replacement of normal alveolar lung tissue by **fibrosis**. This damage is initiated by release of lysosomal enzymes from macrophages. When the silica particles are phagocytosed by these cells, hydrogen bonds are formed between the silica and the lysosomal membranes. These immobilise the membranes and cause lysosomal rupture.

The **endogenous pigments** include **lipofuscin**, haemosiderin and melanin. Lipofuscin is a protein–lipid complex also known as 'wear and tear' pigment. It is seen in the cells of the liver, brain and heart where its accumulation appears to be related to advancing age or chronic injury. In the brain, age-related accumulation of lipofuscin appears to be confined to specific sites, most notably the hippocampus. A similar age-related deposition of lipofuscin is seen in the heart: by the age of 90 years some 30% by weight of the heart muscle fibre may be composed of lipofuscin.

Lipofuscin probably represents non-degradable waste material derived from broken down membranes and other cell components, possibly because peroxidation of the lipid–protein material renders it resistant to lysosomal enzymes. Experimental induction of the pigment by a deficiency of the antioxidant vitamin E supports the theory that auto-oxidation by free radicals is involved in its production. Occasionally membranous deposits are seen in the cytoplasm. These have a characteristic whorled or 'Swiss-roll' appearance and are called **residual bodies**. These are thought to represent residual membrane debris resistant to lysosomal enzymes.

Haemosiderin is formed when there is a local or systemic excess of iron, most commonly when there is haemorrhage from a blood vessel. The released red blood cells die or are broken down by macrophages to yield haemoglobin, which in turn is converted by macrophage lysosomal enzymes into the intermediates **biliverdin** and **bilirubin** and then into haemosiderin. Haemosiderin can also be laid down in tissue if there is a systemic excess of iron; this condition is known as haemosiderosis. **Haemosiderosis** can arise in a number of circumstances, including increased absorption of dietary iron, decreased iron utilisation (in thalassaemia, for example), and increased turnover of red blood cells (in haemolytic anaemia, for example).

Normally the amount of iron in the diet far exceeds that required by the body, and the excess is not absorbed. The precise mechanisms governing the absorption of iron by the intestines are not known, but failure of these control mechanisms may lead to excessive iron absorption and storage. Large amounts of iron in the liver can damage the liver cells, causing fibrosis; this condition is called **haemochromatosis**.

Melanin pigmentation is a normal feature of the skin and, perhaps surprisingly, other sites such as the brain, the colon, ovaries and the adrenal medulla. Hyperpigmentation of the skin may result from a drug reaction or may arise from a tumour such as a benign pigmented naevus or, more seriously, malignant melanoma. These examples of hyperpigmentation appear in localised sites in the skin, but in **Addison's disease** a more general skin pigmentation occurs.

Addison's disease: an inflammatory disease in which much of the adrenal cortex is destroyed, causing reduced corticosteroid production. Normally the adrenal corticosteroids inhibit adrenocorticotrophic hormone and the structurally related melanocyte-stimulating hormone. The lack of inhibition causes melanocytes to produce melanin.

Fibrosis: the proliferation of fibrous connective tissue, or scar tissue.

Haemolytic anaemia: an anaemia caused by destruction of red blood cells. It can be caused by defects in the cell membrane, haemoglobin or intracellular enzymes. An example is hereditary spherocytosis, in which there is a functional defect in spectrin, a cytoskeletal protein that influences the shape of red blood cells and their ability to pass through small blood vessels. Extrinsic factors that can destroy red blood cells include malaria and any condition that triggers production of autoantibodies to the red blood cell surface antigens.

Inflammation

Inflammation refers to a sequence of cellular responses that are triggered by cell or tissue damage

When injury has resulted in cell death the inflammatory response is initiated to remove tissue debris and the source of injury. Inflammation can be acute or chronic. In both types, blood proteins and phagocytic cells gain access to sites of tissue damage, infection or foreign bodies. The response depends on the generation of vasoactive and chemotactic messengers that facilitate the arrival of inflammatory cells at the appropriate location.

Acute inflammation

Acute inflammation is a non-specific response aimed at the removal of injurious agents and damaged tissues

The acute inflammatory response is intended to remove extraneous and exogenous material such as micro-organisms and tissue debris, by recruitment of phagocytic cells to the site of damage. This is achieved by the combination of vascular dilation and release of **chemotactic factors** from cells and plasma during the process of blood clotting.

Early in the reaction **histamine** is released from mast cells. This causes blood vessels to dilate and increases their permeability, allowing transfer of phagocytic cells and fluid into the tissue. The whole area becomes flooded with fluid, plasma proteins and inflammatory cells. This is referred to as an **acute inflammatory exudate** and its presence is revealed by the **cardinal signs of Celsus**:

* Redness, caused by dilation of local blood vessels
* Heat, resulting from the increased blood flow
* Swelling, caused by accumulation of fluid and plasma proteins outside the blood vessels
* Pain, probably the result of increased pressure (from exudate)
* Loss of function, arising from pain and tissue swelling

Chemotaxis: a means of attracting phagocytes to a site of tissue injury by a chemical messenger system.

Exudate: protein-rich fluid which collects outside blood vessels after tissue damage which causes increased permeability of the blood vessel cell lining. Not the same as **oedema fluid**, which leaks from blood vessels because of increased pressure, e.g. back-pressure from a blocked vein.

Opsonisation: a means of enhancing phagocytosis. The molecules that are to be removed are coated with opsonins from the plasma. The opsonin-coated particle then binds with the phagocyte through a specific surface receptor. The principal opsonin is C3b, a complement component that is cleaved from C3 by some bacterial cell wall components (the alternative complement pathway) or following binding of antibody to antigen (classical complement pathway).

Plasma components

The localised ingress of fluid and plasma proteins, helps to dilute any injurious agents (for example, bacterial toxins). The fluid is drained away by the lymphatic system. Immunoglobulins and complement components of the plasma help to neutralise micro-organisms, attract inflammatory cells (chemotaxis) and promote phagocytosis (**opsonisation**).

At the wound site, the blood coagulation protein fibrinogen is converted to insoluble fibrin (see p. 134). This forms a meshwork of fine strands, plugging the wound and acting as a physical barrier.

Inflammatory cells

In acute inflammation neutrophils and macrophages are called upon to remove injurious agents and tissue debris

The first cells to arrive at the site of tissue injury are neutrophils: these phagocytose fragments of necrotic tissue (Table 4.3). Initial breakdown of the tissue into smaller fragments is achieved by the release of proteolytic enzymes from the neutrophil lysosomes. Neutrophil activity is limited because the cell is incapable of regenerating lysosomal enzymes: once the enzymes are used and phagocytosis is completed the cell degenerates and dies.

Table 4.3   Cells involved in inflammation

Cell type	Function and location	Product
Neutrophils	Phagocytic cell with membrane receptors for chemotactic messengers, normally comprise 60% of leukocytes	Enzymes and free radicals, which kill or digest micro-organisms, leukotrienes
Monocytes/ macrophages	Blood monocytes migrate into the tissues and differentiate into macrophages. Possess membrane receptors for chemotactic messengers, cytokines, growth factors. Phagocytose small and large particles	Free radicals, thromboxanes and leukotrienes
Eosinophils	Involved in allergic responses. Normally comprise 2–4% of blood leukocytes	Superoxide radical, leukotriene C_4
Mast cells	Present in connective tissues and mucosal membranes	Histamine, heparin, prostaglandins, leukotrienes, thromboxanes and chemotactic factors

The arrival of neutrophils at the site of injury is soon followed by an influx of monocytes and lymphocytes. Once at the site of injury, the monocytes differentiate into macrophages, which are able to remove tissue debris, spent neutrophils and strands of fibrin. Unlike neutrophils the macrophages are able to regenerate their lysosomal enzymes and are therefore capable of sustained activity. The lymphocytes present are a reflection of a specific immune response generated against various antigens derived from exogenous sources or released from tissue breakdown.

Acute inflammation is a balance between what is necessary to remove damaged tissues and the need to avoid additional injury to surrounding normal tissues. Almost inevitably, some further damage will result from the very process designed to deal with tissue injury. The final outcome of the inflammatory response depends on the extent of the original tissue injury, the type and persistence of the agent that caused the damage, and the capacity of specialised cells in the damaged area to proliferate. Possible outcomes are:

- Chronic inflammation, in which the injurious agent persists over an extended period of time, causing continuous tissue destruction
- Resolution, involving complete restoration of tissue architecture and function
- Healing by repair, in which the tissue is completely destroyed and lacks the ability to regenerate specialised cells.

Review question 2

How do inflammatory cells 'know' how to get to the site of injury?

Chronic inflammation

Chronic inflammation usually arises if an injurious agent is not removed by acute inflammation. Occasionally the chronic inflammatory response is implemented with no preceding acute inflammation: this usually occurs in autoimmune diseases or when the injurious agent is impervious to neutrophil breakdown.

If acute inflammation is unable to eradicate an injurious agent, further tissue damage is inevitable as a result of both the original agent and the inflammatory process itself. At the same time attempts are made to heal the lesion, but this is a continuing battle between destruction and repair.

The initial non-specific acute inflammation is supplemented by attempts to mount a specific immune response. This is reflected in the predominance of lymphocytes, rather than neutrophils and macrophages characteristic of acute inflammation. The attempts at repair are evident as fibrosis (thick bundles of collagen fibres).

The outcome of chronic inflammation depends on the balance of repeated injury and attempts at healing. The factors that aid resolution of chronic inflammation include the use of antibiotics, removal of foreign objects, and improvements in nutrition.

One particular type of chronic inflammation, with its own characteristic features, is a **granuloma**. A granuloma is distinguished by the presence of a collection of macrophages that are larger than usual and exhibit altered staining properties. To some extent they resemble epithelial cells and for this reason are given the name **epithelioid** cells. Very often the epithelioid cells are surrounded by a rim of lymphocytes. Granulomas feature in chronic infectious diseases such as tuberculosis, leprosy and syphilis. Various fungal, protozoal and parasitic infections can cause granulomas. They may also be seen as a reaction to foreign bodies such as talc, silica and beryllium.

In all these circumstances granuloma results from a failure of the inflammatory cells to eliminate the causative agent. In **sarcoidosis** no causative agent has been identified but granulomas can be produced in virtually every organ, including the lungs, lymph nodes, liver, spleen, skin and salivary glands. The condition can remain asymptomatic but most patients present with respiratory symptoms or, slightly less commonly, with fever, rash and polyarthritis. Sarcoidosis can be diagnosed by the **Kveim** test, which involves intradermal injection of a heat-sterilised suspension of sarcoid tissue from spleen or lymph nodes. In a sarcoid patient this would usually cause a nodular granuloma at the site of injection.

Resolution and repair

Cells and tissues have different capacities for regeneration. Some somatic cells, such as nerve cells and striated muscle cells, no longer possess the capacity for cell division. If injury results in the death of these cells the tissue cannot be reconstituted and scar tissue is formed. This process is known as repair.

Although the scar tissue may be adequate for maintaining the structural integrity of the tissue or organ, it cannot carry out the specialised functions of the cells that were lost.

Fortunately, most other somatic cell types retain some potential for cell division. This is an essential feature in such areas as the skin, and the respiratory and digestive tracts where cell turnover is high due to the continuous loss (exfoliation) of cells from the exposed surfaces. Provided that the initial damage has not been too extensive, complete structural and functional restoration of the tissue takes place. This process is known as resolution (Figure 4.15).

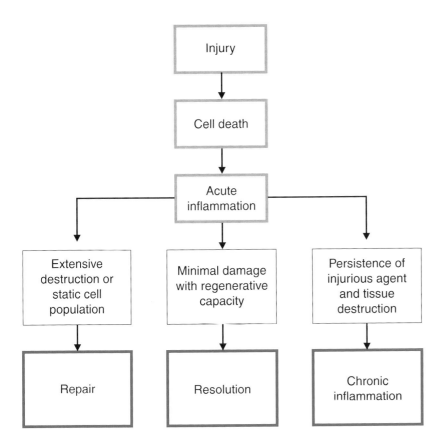

Figure 4.15 Outcomes of cellular injury. The outcome of injury involving cell death depends upon the extent of the injury and the regenerative capacity of adjacent cells. The aim is to achieve resolution so that function and morphology are restored to the state that prevailed before injury. Occasionally the injury is so extensive that there is loss of tissue architecture and hence the template for rebuilding is lost. Alternatively the neighbouring cells are unable to undergo cell division. In these instances the lesion is repaired, usually with formation of collagenous connective tissue. A further possibility is that the damaging agent is resistant to the inflammatory response necessary to clear away the agent and tissue debris. The result is chronic inflammation, which itself causes further injury in a continued and frustrated attempt to eliminate the injurious agent.

Mediators of inflammation

The inflammatory response terminates in removal of tissue debris and injurious agents by phagocytic cells. The activities of these cells are controlled by soluble chemical mediators that are produced by the cells involved in the inflammatory response, or are normal components of plasma.

Cell products as mediators of inflammation

Cell-derived mediators of inflammation are preformed and stored (apparent as microscopic cytoplasmic granules) or are synthesised when needed. The preformed substances include histamine, serotonin and lysosomal enzymes stored in mast cells, platelets, neutrophils and macrophages (Table 4.3). The newly synthesised agents include prostaglandins, leukotrienes, platelet activating factor and cytokines.

Some of the most potent mediators of inflammation are the **eicosanoids**, a group of substances derived from 20-carbon polyunsaturated fatty acids (principally arachidonic acid). Their synthesis begins with release of arachidonic acid from cell membrane phospholipids by phospholipase enzymes. This is converted in two metabolic pathways, one utilising **cyclo-oxygenases**, the other using **lipoxygenases**, to leukotriene, prostaglandin, prostacyclin and thromboxane (Figure 4.16). The initial phospholipases are inhibited by corticosteroids, which block both pathways: this is why these drugs are such potent inhibitors of inflammation. In contrast, non-steroidal anti-inflammatory drugs (NSAIDs) block only the cyclo-oxygenase pathway, and because synthesis of leukotrienes is left unblocked these drugs are less powerful (but often less dangerous).

The balance of production in the pathways can also be influenced by dietary fatty acids. High intakes of Ω-3 fatty acids (see Chapter 7) are believed to favour production of less potent inflammatory mediators by inhibition of cyclo-oxygenase pathways, in much the same way as aspirin (an NSAID).

Plasma components

Soluble plasma components synthesised by the liver form part of cascade systems that are usually activated only when there is injury. The coagulation, complement, kinin and fibrinolytic cascades all influence the inflammatory response and carry out additional specific functions. All the cascades can be activated by **Hageman factor** (Figure 4.17), which itself is activated by tissue injury, invasion by micro-organisms or, in a feedback loop, cascade products such as plasmin and kallikrein.

The blood coagulation system

Blood coagulation is fundamental in sealing the breaks caused by wounds and stemming the loss of blood. The initial event in coagulation is aggregation of platelets. Platelets are small cells 2–4 mm in diameter produced from megakaryocyte precursors in the bone marrow. When tissues are injured

---

Inflammatory mediators are produced by cells or are present as inactive precursors in plasma

Arachidonic acid: a polyunsaturated fatty acid present in large amounts in cell membrane phospholipids.

Eicosanoids: derivatives of 20-carbon chain polyunsaturated fatty acids. They include the prostaglandins, prostacyclin, thromboxanes and leukotrienes.

Platelet activating factor: causes platelets to aggregate and release their contents. Derived from basophils.

Prostaglandins: eicosanoids with a range of biological activities including inflammation, platelet aggregation, vasodilatation (lowers blood pressure), fever and as feedback inhibitors of neurotransmitter release. They also promote uterine contractions in pregnancy.

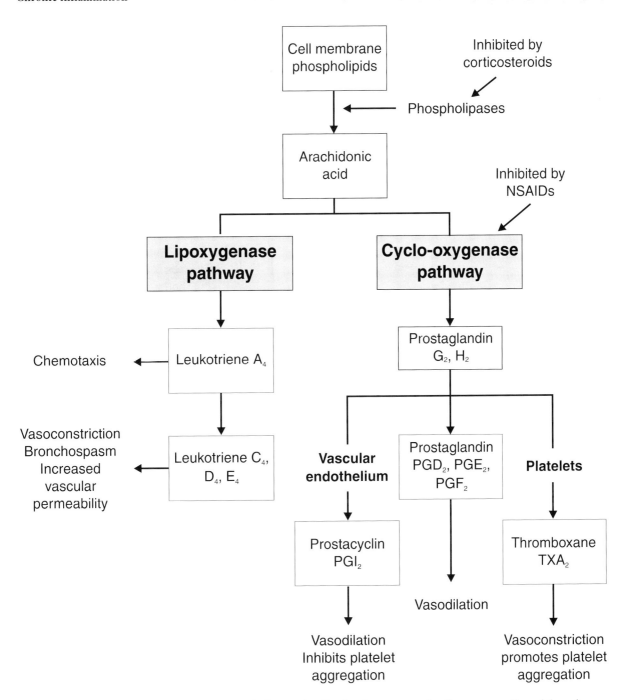

Figure 4.16 Role of arachidonic acid metabolites in inflammation. Leukotrienes, prostaglandins, prostacyclin and thromboxanes mediate the inflammatory response. They are derived from cell membrane phospholipids that are converted to arachidonic acid by phospholipase enzymes. Arachidonic acid products are synthesised along the cyclo-oxygenase or lipoxygenase pathways. The lipoxygenase pathway leads to the production of leukotrienes; prostaglandins, prostacyclin and thromboxanes are produced by the cyclo-oxygenase pathway. Platelets contain the enzyme thromboxane synthetase and can synthesise thromboxane. This enzyme is absent in vascular endothelium, which instead produces prostacyclin. Most other cells of the immune response contain the enzymes necessary to produce the other leukotriene and prostaglandin intermediates and end-products.

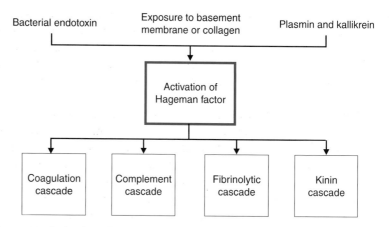

Figure 4.17 Activation of plasma cascade systems. A common denominator of plasma cascades is that they can be activated directly or indirectly by the active form of Hageman factor. Many of the active components released by these cascades are mediators of inflammation.

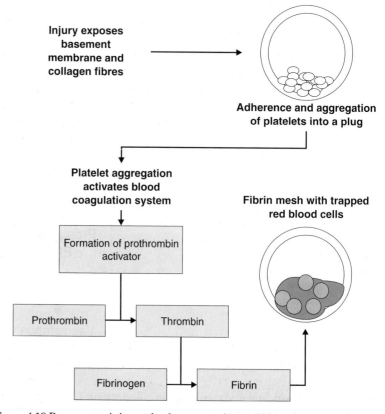

Figure 4.18 Response to injury: platelet aggregation and blood coagulation. Injury to the inside wall of a blood vessel causes exposure of subendothelial basement membrane components and collagen fibres, to which platelets adhere, in turn releasing factors and attracting further platelets to the site. The adherence and aggregation of platelets forms a plug and activates the blood coagulation system. Conversion of prothrombin to thrombin, and thence fibrinogen to insoluble fibrin, results in a thrombus.

platelets adhere to the exposed extracellular structures such as basement membrane, collagen and elastic fibres. The adhesion and aggregation of platelets cause release of their cytoplasmic constituents, most notably **serotonin** and ADP. Both of these serve to attract more platelets to the area, causing them to aggregate and release their contents so that within a minute or so a **platelet plug** is built up (Figure 4.18).

Several substances are involved in regulating platelet activity, ensuring that aggregation occurs only when needed and not, for example, in undamaged blood vessels. These include prostacyclin, a powerful inhibitor of platelet aggregation, and the thromboxanes, which stimulate platelet aggregation. A delicate balance exists between thromboxanes and prostacyclin.

Once the platelet plug has formed the next part of the process, **blood coagulation**, is activated. There are three principal components to the coagulation process. A complex **prothrombin activator** is formed, which converts the plasma protein **prothrombin** into **thrombin**, which in turn catalyses the conversion of **fibrinogen** into a **fibrin** mesh. In the intact circulatory system the fibrin mesh, containing trapped red cells, is referred to as a **thrombus**, which may occur in both arteries and veins; the term clot is usually reserved for the coagulation of blood outside the circulatory system.

The formation of the prothrombin activator is preceded by a complex cascade involving the sequential proteolytic cleavage of large protein molecules. Each of the peptides formed converts an inactive **zymogen** precursor into an active enzyme, which then acts on the next protein in the sequence. The procoagulant proteins, or **blood coagulation factors**, are numbered I to XIII. Unfortunately for students, the reaction sequence does not follow the numerical order. To complicate things further, there are two pathways of activation, termed the **intrinsic** and **extrinsic** pathways (Figure 4.19).

The intrinsic pathway is activated when blood comes into contact with a novel surface, with conversion of factor XII (Hageman factor) to its active form. The extrinsic pathway is shorter and therefore is completed more rapidly, but requires the release of an additional tissue factor by injured cells. Eventually the two pathways come together to convert prothrombin into active thrombin and thence fibrinogen into the fibrin clot. Thrombin also promotes the coagulation response by a positive feedback mechanism, and it promotes platelet aggregation.

The kinin system

The final product of the kinin system is **bradykinin**, which increases vascular permeability by making blood vessels dilate. This is an important physical property, enabling inflammatory cells to migrate through the vessel walls to the site of injury. Bradykinin is short acting because it is rapidly degraded by the enzyme **kininase**. An intermediate product in the pathway, **kallikrein**, is a potent activator of Hageman factor, thereby amplifying the original stimulus as well as the other cascade systems (Figure 4.20).

Arterial thrombus: forms at sites of vascular injury and high blood flow, such as an atherosclerotic plaque. Mostly contains platelets. presence in coronary arteries can lead to myocardial infarction. Treatments are designed to dissolve (lyse) a thrombus (for example with the fibrinolytic agent streptokinase) or to inhibit its formation (for example with aspirin).

Venous thrombus: produced by activation of blood coagulation system in areas where blood flow is very slow. Contains abundant fibrin, relatively few platelets and many trapped red blood cells. Formation can be retarded by treatment with anticoagulants (such as heparin).

Zymogen: an inactive enzyme precursor or proenzyme.

Review question 3

Why are bleeding times prolonged in (a) thrombocytopenia (decreased platelet count) and (b) severe liver disease?

The kinin system mediates inflammation, causes blood vessel dilation and initiates the fibrinolytic system

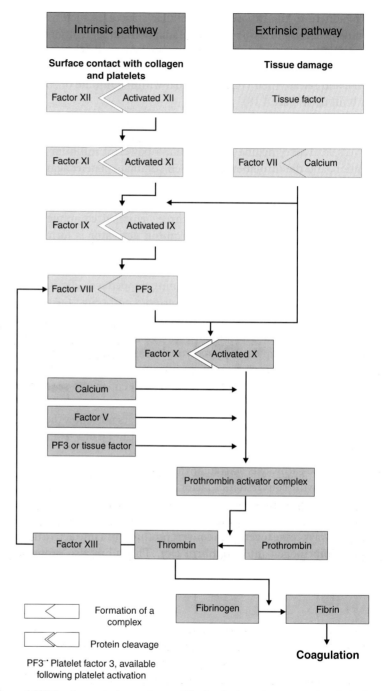

Figure 4.19 Blood coagulation pathways. The intrinsic pathway contains all the factors necessary for blood coagulation and is activated by contact between collagen and platelet surfaces. The extrinsic pathway requires the release of a lipoprotein tissue factor following injury. Both pathways operate together. The common elements of the pathways are activation of factor X and conversion of prothrombin to thrombin and fibrinogen to fibrin. At several stages of both pathways calcium ions and tissue phospholipids or lipoproteins are required as cofactors.

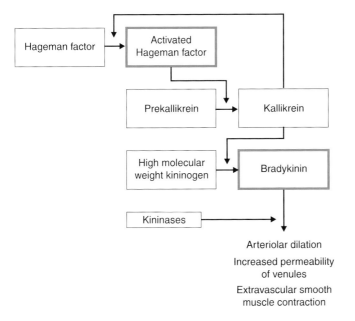

Figure 4.20 The kinin system. The active product of the kinin system, bradykinin, causes increased vascular permeability, by dilating arterioles and contracting the endothelial cells lining venules. Outside the blood vessels, bradykinin causes contraction of smooth muscle. It is a short-acting substance, degraded by kininase enzymes. An intermediate product in the cascade, kallikrein, activates Hageman factor, thereby amplifying the sequence in a feedback loop.

Endothelial cells: the cells lining blood vessels. Normally they inhibit platelet aggregation and blood coagulation, and have fibrinolytic properties. When injured these mechanisms are lost.

The fibrinolytic system

The fibrinolytic system is initiated by conversion of **plasminogen** to **plasmin**. This is achieved by the kinin cascade and by **plasminogen activator**, which is released from endothelium, leukocytes and other tissues. The end product of the fibrinolytic system, plasmin, is a protease enzyme that will lyse fibrin clots. It has other functions that are important in mediating the inflammatory system: it activates Hageman factor and cleaves the complement component C3 (Figure 4.21).

The purpose of the fibrinolytic system is to dissolve clots, but products in the cascade also mediate inflammation

The complement system

The complement system comprises a series of proteins that normally circulate in the blood in an inactive state. Two initial pathways merge into a common pathway at C3. The **classical pathway** is activated by formation of an antigen–antibody complex, whereas the **alternative pathway** is activated by the polysaccharide components of bacterial cell walls. These provide the mechanisms by which micro-organisms can be destroyed and cleared from the body (Figure 4.22).

The purpose of the complement system is to damage micro-organisms, stimulate inflammation and promote phagocytosis

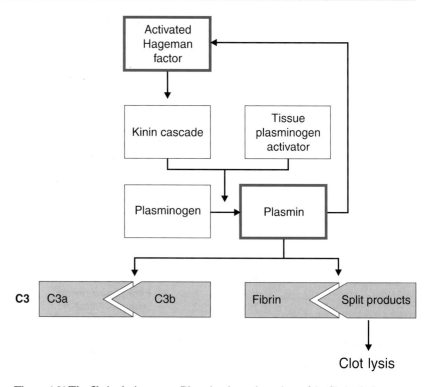

Figure 4.21 The fibrinolytic system. Plasmin, the end-product of the fibrinolytic system, has a number of activities including clot lysis, activation of C3 and activation of Hageman factor.

Wound healing

A wound can be produced in many ways, all characterised by the death of epithelial cells, a break in continuity of the tissue architecture and bleeding. Wounds represent an easy means of entry for micro-organisms, and consequently a rapid response to wound formation is needed. The first stage in this response is the formation of a fibrin clot. This is essentially an emergency repair, with the defensive role of 'plugging the gap' to control bleeding and to create a barrier against the entry of infectious organisms. Just how effective this is depends upon the extent of the wound: large irregular wounds are much more likely to become infected, to reopen, and to produce fluid exudate. The likelihood of infection also depends on the site of the wound. A wound involving the gastrointestinal, genitourinary or respiratory tracts is very likely to become infected by normal flora – these organisms are much more of a problem when present in damaged tissue and are not contained by normal borders. Extraneous infections are likely to arise from traumatic lesions.

The healing process in wounds begins with the acute inflammatory response, which usually lasts for about 3 days. As well as removing the fibrin clot, micro-organisms and tissue debris, the various inflammatory cells secrete soluble

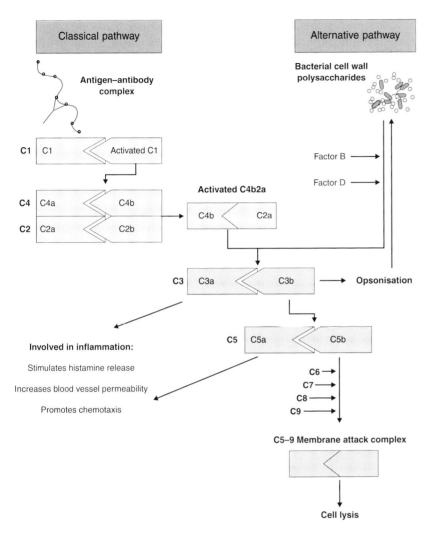

Figure 4.22 Outline of the complement system. In the classical pathway the binding of antibody to antigen activates C1. This component cleaves C4 and C2 into their component parts, which combine to form the activated C42 complex. Activated C42 splits C3 into its components C3a and C3b. Bacterial and fungal cell polysaccharides interact with the plasma proteins factor B and factor D, to split C3 in the alternative pathway. One fragment, C3a, increases vascular permeability and causes vasodilation by the release of histamine from mast cells. The other fragment, C3b, binds to bacterial cell walls and acts as an opsonin, enhancing phagocytosis by neutrophils and macrophages. C3b also combines with C42 to form a complex that splits C5 into C5a and C5b. C5a has chemotactic properties, stimulates histamine release and activates the lipo-oxygenase pathway of arachidonic acid metabolism. C5b initiates the remaining pathway in which elements of C6, C7, C8 and C9 are split and reformed to give the active membrane attack complex. This causes cell lysis.

growth factors that serve to attract other cells to the site of injury and stimulate their proliferation by cell division.

Granulation tissue comprises capillaries, fibroblasts and macrophages

▲ **Key points**

Mechanisms in wound healing

- ▲ Wound closure achieved by fibrin clot
- ▲ Tissue debris and dead micro-organisms removed by macrophage activity
- ▲ Fibroblasts and endothelial cells recruited to site of damage by chemotaxis
- ▲ Mitogenic growth factors stimulate proliferation of recruited cells
- ▲ Presence of granulation tissue comprising macrophages, fibroblasts and new blood vessels
- ▲ Wound contraction achieved by myofibroblast activity
- ▲ Represents termination of acute inflammation

Healing by primary intention takes place when the wound edges are close together

As a result of the chemotactic and mitogenic activities, fibroblasts and endothelial cells are recruited into the wound healing process, being responsible for the formation of fibrous connective tissue (mostly containing collagen) and blood capillaries, respectively. The large-scale proliferation of these cells that takes place within the fibrin matrix of the wound very much resembles an invasive process. Thus the original fibrin matrix, formed initially in the wound by blood clotting, is replaced by a new highly cellular tissue comprising macrophages, endothelial cells, fibroblasts and their products organised into blood vessels and collagen fibres. This tissue is known as **granulation tissue**, and appears within 24 hours of injury.

The process of forming new blood vessels is known as **angiogenesis**. It occurs by a budding-off process from pre-existing blood vessels. The first step is the degradation of the basement membrane to which the endothelial cell lining of the blood vessel is attached. Disruption of this membrane allows the endothelial cells to migrate, forming a capillary sprout. As the cells migrate they undergo cell division. The cells then differentiate and form basement membrane material for the new branch of the blood vessel. Initially the new vessels are leaky, allowing passage of proteins and cells into the extravascular space. Hence new granulation tissue is often oedematous.

Fibroblasts proliferate within a wound and secrete a number of connective tissue components, principally collagen, proteoglycans and fibronectin. They also acquire contractile properties similar to those associated with smooth muscle. For this reason, such activated fibroblasts are referred to as **myofibroblasts**. These contractile properties are of importance in the closure and shrinkage of the wound area.

If the amount of tissue damage is minimal, the wound healing process is said to proceed by **primary intention**. These wounds usually have minimal inflammation and scarring, the wound edges are close together, and there is no infection. Wounds with more extensive tissue loss heal by the process of **secondary intention**.

Healing by primary intention

One of the most straightforward examples of wound healing is seen in the healing of a clean surgical incision. Provided that the two opposed edges of the wound are brought closely together (for example by suturing) healing should proceed with the minimum of scarring. The incision causes the death of only a limited number of cells and structures within the skin, and this narrow space is rapidly filled with blood that forms a fibrin clot. The clot soon dehydrates to form a scab that seals the surface and provides a barrier against infection.

Within 24 hours neutrophils appear in the dermal connective tissue at the margins if the incision. The basal cells in the epidermis near the cut edge undergo division, producing epidermal thickening. These cells also grow outwards, forming epithelial spurs along the cut margins underneath the scab. The two epithelial spurs, one on each side of the incision, eventually meet so that epithelial continuity is re-established. This takes 24–48 hours.

By the third day the neutrophils have been replaced by macrophages. These cells release growth factors, stimulating the proliferation and migration of dermal fibroblasts into the area. In turn the fibroblasts secrete growth factors so that there is a co-ordinated proliferation of granulation tissue into the area.

By the fifth day, the fibrin clot has been dissolved by enzymatic and phagocytic activity of the neutrophils and macrophages, and the area is filled with granulation tissue. Vascularisation takes place by the fusion of capillary buds in the granulation tissue into continuous channels. At this stage the epidermis will have recovered to its full thickness and collagen fibres are deposited in the dermis.

During the second week the proliferation of fibroblasts and deposition of collagen continues. By this time the inflammatory infiltrate, increased vascularisation and oedema have largely disappeared. Some consolidation and remodelling of the connective tissues may now take place.

At the end of the first month the scar comprises cellular connective tissue devoid of inflammatory cells, covered by intact epithelium. It may take up to a year to complete the transformation into a relatively acellular, avascular pale collagenous scar with normal tensile strength. Dermal structures that were destroyed by the incision are permanently lost, although those that were only partially damaged may regenerate.

Healing by secondary intention

Healing by secondary intention takes place when the wound has separated edges, or when a more extensive loss of cells has occurred, for example in infarction, inflammatory ulceration, abscess formation or large surface wounds. These conditions result in a large defect that must be filled. Because so much of the normal architecture has been lost there is no template for regenerating cells to follow. Instead the area is filled by collagenous scar tissue.

Large tissue defects contain large amounts of fibrin and necrotic tissue debris that must be removed. As a consequence the inflammatory reaction is much more intense than healing by primary intention, with formation of much larger amounts of granulation tissue. A particular feature in large surface wounds is **wound contraction**, which reduces the surface area of the wound. It is mediated by myofibroblasts but depends on the wound margins remaining mobile. If this is not the case, then disfiguring scarring will result. Healing by secondary intention is characterised by the formation of large amounts of scar tissue and the process of repair is much slower than in healing by primary intention.

Factors affecting wound healing

Local and systemic factors influence the progress of wound healing. Local factors include the presence or absence of infection and foreign bodies, a good blood supply and proper co-ordination of the growth factors and cellular

---

▲ Key points

Healing by primary intention

Within 24 hours:
- ▲ Acute neutrophil response in wound margins
- ▲ Epidermis thickens at edges of cut and forms epithelial spurs
- ▲ Epidermal continuity re-established in 24-48 hours

Third day:
- ▲ Neutrophils replaced by macrophages
- ▲ Hypertrophy of fibroblasts
- ▲ Budding of capillaries
- ▲ Collagen produced at wound margins
- ▲ Epithelial thickening

Fifth day:
- ▲ Incisional space filled with granulation tissue
- ▲ Capillary buds form patent channels
- ▲ Collagen fibres bridge incision
- ▲ Epithelium recovers to full thickness

Second week:
- ▲ Continued accumulation of collagen and proliferation of fibroblasts
- ▲ Leukocyte infiltration, oedema and increased vascularity disappear

One month:
- ▲ Scar comprises connective tissue devoid of inflammatory infiltrate
- ▲ Wound site covered by intact epithelium

One year:
- ▲ Scar transformed to relatively acellular, avascular, pale collagenous tissue
- ▲ Normal tensile strength restored

Cytokines: polypeptides produced by a variety of cell types, most notably lymphocytes, monocyte/macrophages, neutrophils and endothelial cells, that influence the function of other cells. Cytokines derived from lymphocytes are referred to as lymphokines.

Second messengers: intracellular substances which alter in concentration in response to activation of cell receptors. These trigger a series of responses which ultimately cause a cellular response. The best-known second messengers include calcium ions, cyclic adenosine monophosphate and inositol triphosphate.

responses involved. Systemic factors involve the nutritional and immunological status of the patient, certain drug therapies and coexisting illnesses such as diabetes.

Local factors

Infection of the wound will delay healing. There must also be an adequate blood supply to the wound, because healing is dependent upon the formation of new blood vessels, which are themselves derived from existing vessels. Thus, any limitation to the blood flow, such as in atherosclerosis or venous abnormalities that retard drainage, will be detrimental. Healing is also impaired by the presence of foreign bodies, and chronic inflammation or granulomatous tissue will persist.

Systemic factors

Wound healing is affected by the overall nutritional state. The synthesis of new proteins, particularly collagen, may be extensive during wound healing. Any prolonged deficiency in dietary protein will therefore be deleterious. The tensile strength of the healing wound is also influenced by dietary protein, and supplementation with the sulphur-containing amino acids cystine and methionine may be beneficial. Synthesis of collagen also depends on vitamin C for the conversion of proline to hydroxyproline during formation and assembly of collagen. Wound healing requires extensive proliferation of cells, and many of the enzymes necessary for DNA and RNA synthesis are zinc-dependent. Corticosteroids delay wound healing, probably because they inhibit the inflammatory response.

Growth factors

Cell mediators with growth control functions are produced and secreted by a variety of cells. These mediators play a central role in the reconstruction or repair of the tissue. It is not difficult to imagine that aberrant production of growth factors will have profound effects on the eventual tissue architecture.

Cell responses to growth factors and inhibitors arise from binding of the peptide growth factor messenger to receptors on the cell surface. These receptors are glycoproteins that span the cell membrane. On binding of the growth factor, the intracellular domains of the receptor glycoprotein interact with cytoskeletal elements to initiate the diffusion of **second messengers**. The second messengers act on the nucleus and various cytoplasmic constituents to induce cell locomotion and differentiation.

So many growth factors have been discovered that it has been difficult to define their precise roles in wound healing and tissue regeneration. One important class of growth factors is known as the **cytokines**: nearly 100 of these peptides have been described with distinct biological activities. Each peptide possesses growth-modulating activity on certain target cells and many also influence cytoskeletal structure, chemotaxis and genetic expression, particularly of proto-oncogenes. Proto-oncogene products include the growth factors themselves and their cellular receptors. These influence wound healing by affecting cell proliferation and motility.

Sources of growth factors

The initial matrix material of wounds is fibrin, produced as a result of blood clotting. The deposited fibrin is able to induce the growth of new capillaries, which can then support new tissue. The peptide growth factors which control this process can be released into the wound in several ways.

- Some are stored in an inactive form in the cells or in the extracellular matrix. When injury occurs these are activated by physical or enzymatic disruption
- Some growth factors are delivered to the wound by the blood circulation. For example, platelet-derived growth factor and transforming growth factor are stored in platelets and released when the blood clots
- Many growth factors are elaborated by activated cells, such as macrophages, that have been attracted to the wound

The control mechanisms that occur in this process are very complex and some aspects are presently unclear. It seems likely that many growth factors work in a cascade system, with amplification and down-regulation of the preceding signals, akin to the process of blood clotting. An excess of growth stimulators, or a decrease in growth inhibitors, will lead to increased cell proliferation. The most important growth factors are those that recruit resting G0 cells into the cell cycle. The principal cytokines involved in wound healing are listed in Table 4.4.

Table 4.4 Cytokines in wound healing

Cytokine	Source	Activity
Epidermal growth factor (EGF)		Potent chemotactic agent and mitogen for epithelial cells; mitogenic for fibroblasts
Fibroblast growth factors (FGF)	Fibroblast, vascular endothelial and smooth muscle cells	Stimulates fibroblasts. Also promotes proliferation of endothelial cells and hence are important in establishing new blood vessel network
Interleukin 1 (IL-1)	Most nucleated cells	Leukocyte stimulating factor and important mediator of the immune system and inflammation. Mitogenic for fibroblasts, increases synthesis of collagen and collagenase
Platelet-derived growth factor (PDGF)	Stored in platelet α-granules and is released in blood clotting. Also	Migration and proliferation of fibroblasts, vascular smooth muscle cells and monocytes, but not endothelial or epithelial cells.

	produced by activated macrophages, endothelium, fibroblasts, smooth muscle cells, and some tumour cells	Does not stimulate DNA synthesis directly, but renders cells in G_0 or G_1 stages of the growth cycle competent to do so. A further factor is required for mitogenesis, such as plasma components, EGF or insulin
Transforming growth factor (TGF-α and TGF-β)	TGF-α produced by macrophages TGFβ is delivered to a wound by platelets	TGF-α stimulates growth of blood vessels. Binds to the EGF receptor and has similar activities to EGF TGF-β is chemotactic for macrophages. Stimulates fibroblast activity, activating collagen and fibronectin genes in these cells. Inhibits collagenase activity and deactivates macrophages. Inhibits growth of epithelial and endothelial cells
Tumour necrosis factor (TNF-α)	Monocytes, macrophages, T cells	Induces haemorrhagic necrosis in certain tumours. Also induces angiogenesis. Like IL-1, it is chemotactic and mitogenic for fibroblasts, and is believed to play a role in fibrosis and connective tissue remodelling

Cytokines in scar tissue formation

The production of scar tissue can be viewed as a result of imbalance in the cascade of growth factors and growth inhibitors that are activated within the wound. It seems likely that the cytokines of most importance in this respect are those that stimulate fibroblasts, causing secretion of collagen and hence fibrosis.

One focus of attention is macrophage-derived growth factor (MGDF), which has been implicated in the production of lung fibrosis, a cause of adult respiratory distress syndrome (see Chapter 6). This factor is a composite of several growth factors, including TNF-a, IL-1, FGF and PDGF. All of these mediators have been shown to enhance connective tissue production.

Fibronectin: a component of cell surfaces and basement membranes, involved in cell adhesion. Binds with extracellular components such as collagen, fibrin and proteoglycans.

Cytokines in tumour growth

The growth of tumours requires the participation of normal cells such as fibroblasts, endothelial cells, smooth muscle cells and probably some cells of the immune system. These are precisely the cell types that are necessary for cell proliferation in wound healing. It has been suggested that tumour growth is a very similar process to wound healing, with the exception that in normal wound healing the growth mediators are controlled and eventually stop.

Tumour cells can produce growth factors and their receptors

Many growth factors emanate from the tumour cells to induce further tumour growth, but these signals are uncontrolled. It may also be that tumour cell proliferation alters the behaviour or effect of growth inhibitors that would normally regulate the activated cells.

The possibility arises that new forms of cancer treatment could be aimed at regulating tumour growth by the manipulation of the cytokine environment. So far, most attention has focused on cytokines that either have direct inhibitory properties or will stimulate the immune and inflammatory responses to inhibit tumour cells. Most notably, these include the interferons, interleukins and tumour necrosis factor.

The interferons are of interest because they exhibit direct growth inhibition in some tumour cell lines and also enhance the cytotoxicity of natural killer and T cells. They will also induce differentiation of some leukaemic cell lines and hence have been used in the treatment of some leukaemias and lymphomas. Response rates with interferon-α have been encouraging but there are dose-related side-effects, including flu-like symptoms and leukopenia.

The interleukins are a family of peptides which modulate the activities of immune and inflammatory cells. Most trials have been conducted with interleukin-2 (IL-2), which is produced by activated T cells, causing the proliferation of other antigen-activated T cells. It also stimulates the production of the other inhibitory cytokines (TNF and interferon-γ). It is hoped that expansion of anti-tumour T cells and inhibitory agents inside a tumour will inhibit growth and improve survival. To date, IL-2 has been used for the treatment of metastatic melanoma and renal cell carcinoma, in which a response is produced in up to 30% of patients. How well this translates into improved survival is unclear because of the small size and uncontrolled nature of the trials. Treatment is associated with severe dose-limiting side-effects of fever, hypotension, adult respiratory distress syndrome, anaemia and neutropenia.

Natural killer (NK) cells: circulate in the blood and lymph. Can lyse and kill cancer cells and virus-infected cells before a specific immune response is activated. This is achieved by recognition of changes in the cell surface.

Review question 4

Why do corticosteroids impair wound healing?

Background information: cell responses to signals

All of the cellular events involved in inflammation and wound healing are mediated by chemical messengers that induce a cell to migrate, proliferate, or undertake some other particular activity. Even under normal circumstances the cellular environment is controlled by a complicated set of interactions and messages between neighbouring cells and the extracellular matrix. The messengers are usually secreted by other cells that act as single units or are organised into glands.

Several different classes of messengers exist, most notably hormones, polypeptide growth factors, eicosanoids, nitric oxide and neurotransmitters. All of these stimulate specific cell responses, and their effects are exerted only upon the appropriate cells by specific binding to receptors on the cell surface. The messengers also differ in the ways they are secreted and circulated. Hormones are produced by **endocrine** cells, and are released into the blood or lymphatic circulations. Most growth factors act much

Nitric oxide: causes vasodilation. Produced by endothelium and macrophages

Protein kinases: enzymes that activate other proteins by adding phosphate groups to them (phosphorylation). The phosphorylated proteins may be other kinase enzymes, giving a cascade of enzymes that are activated sequentially, eventually leading to a specific cellular event such as division or secretion.

more locally and are released into the extracellular matrix for action on neighbouring cells. These are known as **paracrine** mediators. Finally, the chemical **neurotransmitters** respond to a nervous impulse and bridge the synapse between a neighbouring nerve or target cell.

Hormones

There are three chemical classes of hormones: steroid, protein and small peptide. Their role is to increase or decrease cellular activity. Another way of distinguishing hormones is by their action on the target cell. The steroid hormones (for example cortisol, oestrogen and vitamin D) are lipid-soluble and freely diffuse across the plasma membrane of their target cells to bind with receptors in the cytosol or nucleus. Binding of the hormone to its receptor results in a conformational change in the receptor protein that enables it to bind at certain chromosomal sites and alter gene activity. Because of their insolubility in water, steroid hormones are carried in the blood in a complex with a carrier protein.

Water-soluble hormones interact with receptors on the surface of a cells. This stimulates the cell to release its own hormone, or triggers electrical activity. A cascade of reactions usually leads to the specific biological response, although the number of pathways leading to that response is usually quite small. Many non-steroidal hormones exert their effects by activating intracellular second-messenger pathways involving the generation of cyclic AMP (cAMP) and other molecules. These pathways allow the transmission of the message in the interior of the cell and also greatly amplify the original signal. Usually specific proteins, such as the protein kinases that phosphorylate specific target proteins, are activated, altering their activities and biological functions. These effects are reversible because the activated proteins are dephosphorylated when cAMP levels fall (the cell has efficient mechanisms for degrading cyclic AMP, so the tendency is always for the biological response to stop in the absence of renewed signals at the cell receptors).

Pharmacological modification of cell activities

Many drugs work by modifying the interactions that occur at cell receptor sites. Some actually contain or mimic the messenger itself, so that they combine with the receptors and activate the cells. These drugs are classed as **agonists**. Other drugs combine with receptors but do not activate them, thus blocking the binding of the natural messenger to the cell receptor. These drugs are described as **antagonists**.

The effectiveness of these drugs depends on how well they fit and bind to the receptor. The ability of a drug to combine with one particular type of receptor is described as its **specificity**. Hence the effect of histamine can sometimes be blocked by antihistamines that block H_1 histamine receptors

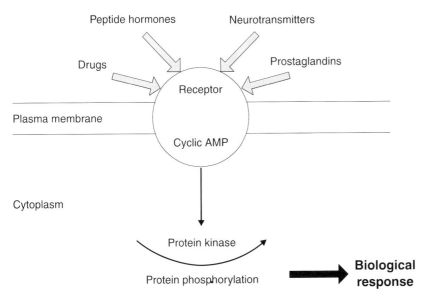

Figure 4.23 Cell signals. Cells respond to a variety of messages from the outside environment. The principal mechanism is by means of surface receptors which are specific for certain chemical messengers. Among these messengers, called ligands, are most neurotransmitters, hormones and locally generated peptides such as mediators of inflammation. Binding of a ligand causes a change in structure of the receptor. The response of the target cell is determined by the nature of the metabolic processes linked to the receptor. For example, acetylcholine stimulates contraction of skeletal muscle, but inhibits heart muscle. Very often the binding of ligand to receptor generates further intracellular chemical signals, called second messengers, which connect events in the receptor to the appropriate metabolic processes in the cell. One important second messenger, cAMP, activates protein kinase enzymes. By transferring phosphate groups from ATP to other proteins, these can activate a series of enzymes, which eventually bring about the desired cell activity.

(these antagonists are used in the treatment of allergic conditions such as hay fever), but leave H_2 histamine receptors unblocked (see Chapter 19). Conversely, anti-ulcer drugs, which block H_2 receptors, are useless in the treatment of hay fever.

ANSWERS TO REVIEW QUESTIONS

Where do free radicals come from? Do they always cause damage?

Question 1

Free radicals are inevitably generated as part of normal metabolic processes, but are eliminated by cellular enzyme and antioxidant systems. There are also physical barriers to free radical damage. For example, the nucleus is well away from the main sites of free radical generation (mitochondria) and the genetic material is protected by proteins (histones).

In the main there is a balance between cell metabolic activities and antioxidant defences, and there is no damage. The main problems occur when free radicals are generated in an uncontrolled fashion, as would happen in external (to the cell) injury. Examples are the neutrophil respiratory burst and free radicals generated by exogenous agents such as cigarette smoke or ionising radiation. These kinds of injury can overwhelm antioxidant defences as well as disrupt physical barriers.

Question 2

How do inflammatory cells 'know' how to get to the site of injury?

Tissue damage caused by trauma or infection sets off an 'alarm' by release of chemicals into the extracellular fluid. These chemicals stimulate immediately adjacent cells to release agents that cause dilation of the small blood vessels in the vicinity. Some of the released substances act as chemical messengers, attracting inflammatory cells to the site. The leaky blood vessels allow cells and fluid containing clotting factors to seep into the tissue compartment, causing oedema. Various cascade systems in the fluid become activated, releasing more chemotactic agents and hence more cells into the area. In turn, the newly arrived neutrophils and macrophages release chemotaxins. The various cell and plasma-derived factors play a number of roles in mediating inflammation and are discussed in more detail in the next section of the main text.

Question 3

Why are bleeding times prolonged in (a) thrombocytopenia and (b) severe liver disease?

Platelets promote blood coagulation. Normal adult values are 150 000–400 000/μl. Bleeding is likely to occur if the count is below 100 000 and haemorrhaging if below 50 000/μl. Conversely, an elevated count may cause increased clotting. Causes of low platelet counts are impaired production (bone marrow failure, leukaemia, aplastic anaemia, marrow infiltration by secondary cancers) or excessive destruction (autoimmune thrombocytopenic purpura, disseminated intravascular coagulation).

All the soluble blood clotting factors in plasma are synthesised by the liver. It follows that severe liver disease (alcoholic hepatitis, for example) will reduce capacity for production.

Question 4

Why do corticosteroids impair wound healing?

The principal events in wound healing are formation of a fibrin clot, its removal by fibrinolysis and the removal of tissue debris by what is essentially an acute inflammatory response. This is accompanied by a healing phase in which epithelium is regenerated and connective tissues are laid down. Corticosteroids slow down the inflammatory components of the process because they inhibit phospholipases necessary for the conversion of cell membrane phospholipids to arachidonic acid, the precursor for the most potent eicosanoid mediators of inflammation (Figure 4.15).

Further reading

Alberts, B., Bray, D., Lewis, J. et al. (1989) *Molecular Biology of the Cell*, 2nd edn, New York, Garland Publishing.

Eastman, A. (ed.) (1994) Apoptosis in oncogenesis and chemotherapy. *Semin. Cancer Biol.*, 5.

Goodman, S.R. (1994) *Medical Cell Biology*. Philadelphia, J.B. Lippincott.

Karp, J.E. and Broder, S. (1995) Molecular foundation of cancer: new targets for intervention. *Nature Med.*, **1**, 309-19.

Kovacs, E.J. (1991) Fibrogenic cytokines: the role of immune mediators in the development of scar tissue. *Immunol. Today*, **12**, 17-23.

Kumar, V., Cotran, R.S. and Robbins, S. (1992) *Basic Pathology*, 5th edn, Philadelphia, W.B. Saunders.

Peters, T.J. (ed.) (1987) *Subcellular Pathology of Systemic Disease*, London, Chapman & Hall.

Whalen, G.F. (1990) Solid tumours and wounds: transformed cells misunderstood as injured tissue? *Lancet*, **336**, 1489-92.

5   Environment and health

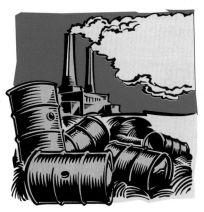

One of the most obvious environmental factors which affects health is air quality. A build-up of air pollutants may become evident as fog or smog, but invisible air pollution can be just as harmful. As might be expected, air pollution mainly affects the respiratory tract, and can cause chronic lung disease or exacerbate asthma. The effects are nearly always worse in smokers because their lungs are likely already to have some damage and they have less functional reserve.

A hazard for people in certain occupations is exposure to dusts. Both mineral and organic dusts can be dangerous, asbestos and silica being the most dangerous. Again the effects are worse in smokers, causing chronic lung disease and lung cancers.

The widespread use of pesticides and herbicides makes it inevitable that almost everybody accumulates these chemicals in their body tissues. It has been suggested that low-level exposures and storage in body tissues may be partly responsible for causing certain types of cancer but so far epidemiological studies of the possible relationship have been largely reassuring. Higher-dose exposures in manufacturing industries and at the point of use have caused some toxic side-effects, but the incidence of cancers is not notably above that of the general population.

Concerns have been expressed about the possible health risks of low-level exposure to ionising and electromagnetic radiation. Ionising radiation in high doses is undoubtedly a threat to health: the question is whether cumulative low-level exposures represent a risk. Experimental high-level exposures of animals to electric or magnetic fields does not cause adverse effects. By extrapolation, it would seem that cumulative low-level exposures would be similarly innocuous. Most epidemiological studies seem to confirm this and if there is any contribution to cancer development from exposure to electromagnetic radiation it is extremely small.

Ultraviolet radiation is undoubtedly damaging, particularly to exposed skin. It is believed to be largely responsible for the marked increase in incidence of skin cancers seen in most developed countries in the latter half of the twentieth century.

Aims of this chapter

By the end of this chapter you will have increased your knowledge of:
◆ The principal environmental hazards to health
◆ The types of disease caused by excessive exposure to hazardous environmental agents
◆ The disease risks associated with routine exposures to hazardous environmental agents

In addition, this chapter will help you to:
◆ Assess the risks to health associated with poor air quality
◆ Assess the risks to health associated with agricultural use of chemicals in the general population and in people who are occupationally exposed
◆ Understand the risks to health of ionising radiation
◆ Evaluate the role of electromagnetic radiation as a health risk
◆ Discuss the benefits that are likely to accrue from discontinuation of the use of lead in petrol

Introduction

The environment has changed dramatically in the last century because of the increases in population pressure, food production, industrialisation and transport. The changes have undoubtedly been beneficial in the sense that population growth has been accompanied by marked improvements in life expectancy and material benefits. These changes, however, have been at the expense of some environmental deterioration, affecting humans, animals and plant life.

Some aspects of environmental deterioration, such as fog and smog, are immediately apparent, but others are more insidious. Lead derived from vehicle exhaust emissions can persist in the environment for many years, and exposure in early life can impair mental development and functioning.

Since the Second World War agricultural practice has changed beyond all recognition. Fundamental to this has been the application of agrochemicals to crops and the land. The use of pesticides alone has been estimated to save up to one-third of food, cotton and other crops. In addition, the quality of food has been improved by the use of herbicides and pesticides, and prices have fallen. Another role of pesticides is in preventing disease, by controlling the organisms responsible for malaria, sleeping sickness and Weil's disease.

Air quality

In the UK the serious health consequences of air pollution came to public attention during the 'pea-souper' winter experienced by Londoners in the 1950s. These fogs were created by climactic conditions which trapped sulphur dioxide and particulate matter (pollutants emitted by industry, domestic household and power stations) in the lower atmosphere. The most notorious

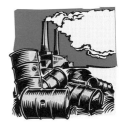

The environment plays a crucial role in altering disease trends and life expectancy

Malaria: protozoal disease caused by *Plasmodium* organisms that are parasitic in red blood cells. Transmitted to humans by the bites of infected mosquitoes.

Sleeping sickness (African trypanosomiasis): protozoal disease transmitted to humans by the bite infected tsetse flies.

Weil's disease: a spirochaete infection transmitted by water or soil contaminated with excreta of infected dogs or rodents.

fogs were experienced in December 1952. In a period of one week 4000 people died, mostly from chest infections (children) and pneumonia and heart disease (older people) (Figure 5.1). These events stimulated legislation (the Clean Air Act of 1956) aimed at establishing zones where only smokeless fuels could be used.

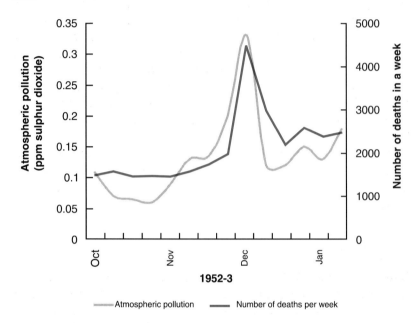

Figure 5.1 Atmospheric pollution and deaths in Greater London 1952–1953. Raised atmospheric sulphur dioxide levels in late November and early December 1952 were closely followed by increased numbers of deaths.

One consequence of the Clean Air Act was that power stations were relocated outside cities, with taller emission stacks that would disperse and dilute the emissions over a wider area. It is now recognised that this solution simply shifts the problem elsewhere, so that acid rain falls in the Scandinavian countries, destroying aquatic life and crops.

Despite legislation, air pollution is still a major problem. The source and nature of the pollutants have changed, with more frequent photochemical smogs caused by increased use of motor vehicles. Even if they do not initially cause respiratory disease, most air pollutants will exacerbate asthma (see Chapter 24) and chronic lung disease.

The main air pollutants are gases, volatile organic compounds or particulate matter:

- Sulphur dioxide
- Nitrogen oxides
- Carbon monoxide
- Ozone
- Particulate matter
- Volatile compounds (benzene, for example)

Sulphur dioxide

The winter fogs of the 1950s were caused by a combination of air pollution and a phenomenon known as temperature inversion. This occurs when calm weather prevents the mixing of air: a cold layer of air at ground level is trapped by warmer air above, preventing the dispersion of emissions from low-lying industrial and household chimneys. At that time, coal was the main source of heat and energy, causing emissions of sulphur dioxide and particulate matter such as soot. In cold moist air these combine to produce aerosols of sulphuric acid. The particulate matter is an effective carrier of the sulphuric acid droplets, ensuring that they are carried deep into the lungs. People with reduced mucociliary clearance, such as smokers and people with respiratory disease, are more vulnerable.

The acute symptoms of exposure to sulphur dioxide are bronchial irritation, bronchospasm, breathing difficulty and cyanosis. Both adults and children become vulnerable to chest infections and, in the longer term, to chronic bronchitis.

Nitrogen oxides

Nitrogen oxides include the gases nitric oxide (NO) and nitrogen dioxide (NO_2). Nitrogen oxides are produced during the combustion of fuel by the oxidation of nitrogen in air or in the fuel itself. In the UK about 45% of the total nitrogen oxide emissions are produced by motor vehicles, 35% by power stations. The main health effect is respiratory tract irritation. People who have asthma, chronic bronchitis or emphysema (Figure 5.2) are at greatest risk.

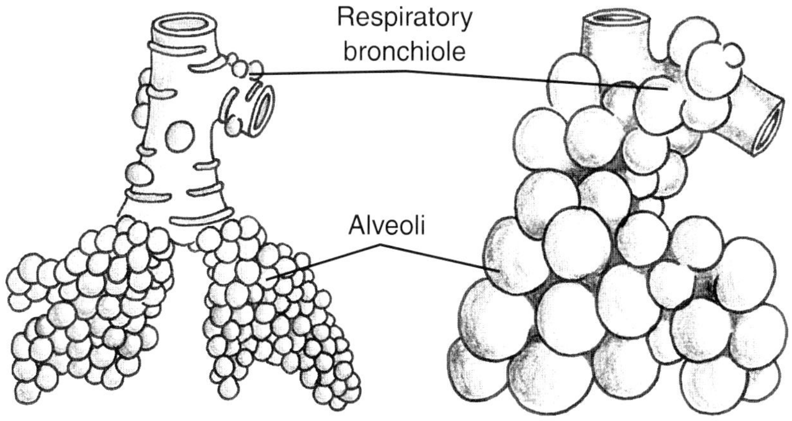

Cyanosis: blue coloration of the skin, mucous membranes and nail beds caused by inadequate oxygenation of blood. Usually a consequence of heart failure or severe respiratory disease.

Chronic bronchitis: defined as a persistent cough with production of sputum for at least three consecutive months in at least two consecutive years. Most commonly occurs in smokers and people living in smog-ridden cities.

Emphysema: permanent enlargement of air spaces in the lungs caused by destruction of their walls.

Mucociliary clearance: a mechanism for removing small particles in air. The upper respiratory tract is lined by ciliated cells and cells that secrete mucus. Particles become trapped in the mucus, which is then moved upwards by the beating action of cilia to the larynx, where it is swallowed or expelled by coughing.

Figure 5.2 Emphysema. **Left:** In the lung gaseous exchange takes place in respiratory bronchioles and alveoli, which branch from the bronchial tree like bunches of grapes. **Right:** In panacinar emphysema the respiratory bronchioles and alveoli are dilated, forming large air spaces with relatively small surface area available for gaseous exchange.

Carbon monoxide

Nowadays there are fewer fogs, but more photochemical smogs

Carbon monoxide is a product of the incomplete combustion of fossil fuels. It is emitted mostly from motor traffic, particularly petrol-engined vehicles. The gas reduces the oxygen-carrying capacity of the blood by irreversibly binding to haemoglobin, forming carboxyhaemoglobin. Exposure to carbon monoxide is likely to precipitate a heart attack in people who suffer from angina.

Ozone

Depletion of the ozone layer will increase the number of skin cancers and cataracts

Photochemical smog is commonly experienced in most major cities. It is caused by ozone, produced by the action of sunlight on volatile hydrocarbons, nitrogen oxide, sulphur dioxide and carbon monoxide, becoming trapped in the atmosphere. The major causes are motor vehicle emissions, industry and power stations. On still sunny days temperature inversion causes ozone to build up in the lower levels of the atmosphere. At low concentrations, ozone causes nausea, eye and throat irritation and headaches. Lung damage can result at high concentrations (150–200 parts per billion). The most susceptible people are asthmatics and older people, but anyone can be affected.

Ozone is beneficial to health when it is present in the upper atmosphere. Without it, humans would probably not survive for long because ozone absorbs ultraviolet light. Chronic exposure to ultraviolet radiation particularly affects the eyes and skin, causing cataracts and skin cancer.

NASA (the US space agency) estimates that a 4–5% loss of ozone occurred over the northern hemisphere in the 1980s, and a large 'hole' in the ozone layer has appeared over the Antarctic. It is predicted that ozone levels in the upper atmosphere will continue to fall. The main reason for this is believed to be the release of chlorofluorocarbons (CFCs), used as refrigerants, aerosol sprays and in various industrial applications, into the atmosphere. They are relatively inactive at ground level, but when they rise to the stratosphere they break down, generating free radicals. These free radicals catalyse the photochemical breakdown of ozone. Unfortunately, CFCs have a long half-life and, even though restrictions have been placed on their manufacture and use, the legacy of CFC damage will remain for many years.

Particulate matter

In the past coal-burning was the main source of particulate matter in the air but now diesel engines contribute about 90% of particulate emissions. Emissions from diesel engines are ten times greater than those from conventional petrol engines, and 30–70 times greater than from petrol engines fitted with a catalytic converter. The International Agency for Research on Cancer (IARC) has classified diesel engine exhaust emissions as 'probably' carcinogenic in humans.

Airborne particulates can carry acidic gases and volatile hydrocarbons into the lungs, where they may act as tumour initiators or promoters. Particulates of less than 10 µm in diameter have been associated with a range of respiratory problems including asthma and bronchitis.

Benzene

Benzene is a volatile hydrocarbon that causes leukaemia in humans. It is present in cigarette smoke and is emitted by petrol engines. The levels of atmospheric benzene are closely related to traffic density, and the build-up inside cars often reaches American maximal limits for occupational exposure to this agent.

▲ Key points

Health effects of air pollutants

Pollutant	Source	Health effects
Airborne particles	Diesel exhaust, coal burning	Carry acidic gases and volatile hydrocarbons that may be carcinogenic into the lungs
Sulphur dioxide	Fossil fuels, power stations, diesel exhaust	Bronchitis and bronchospasm, especially in asthmatics
Nitrogen oxides	Motor vehicles, power stations	Respiratory tract irritation
Carbon monoxide	Incomplete combustion of fossil fuels, tobacco smoke	Reduces oxygen-carrying capacity of blood, causes headaches and lapses in concentration, can precipitate heart attack
Ozone	Photochemical smog	Coughing, impaired lung function, eye, nose and throat irritation, aggravates bronchitis and asthma
Benzene	Petrol engine emissions	Can cause leukaemia

Reducing air pollution

The World Health Organization (WHO) air quality guidelines state maximum safe concentrations of common air pollutants. Some countries, including the USA and Japan, have mandatory air quality standards that are more stringent than the WHO guidelines; in general, the European Union directives are less stringent. At present, peak concentrations of all the main air pollutants in the UK regularly exceed WHO guidelines due to a combination of traffic congestion and temperature inversion.

Long-term improvement in air pollution will be achieved only if traffic volumes are reduced

Road traffic is responsible for the emission of virtually all carbon monoxide, and substantial proportions of carbon dioxide, nitrogen oxides, airborne particulate matter and volatile organic compounds. Catalytic converters can greatly reduce emissions of nitrogen oxides and sulphur dioxides from petrol engines, and filters will reduce emissions of particulate matter. In the UK all new cars must be fitted with catalytic converters. Although this measure will undoubtedly help by reducing engine emissions, this is largely counteracted by growth in volume of traffic.

Global warming

Carbon dioxide insulates the earth's surface. Without it, the earth would become too cold to sustain life. The main sources of carbon dioxide are animal respiration and burning of fossil fuels. Since the beginning of the industrial revolution the atmospheric concentration of carbon dioxide has increased by 25% (from about 280 parts per million to 350 parts per million). Concentrations continue to increase – and this is not helped by deforestation. Each year, the amount of tropical forest destroyed is equivalent to an area the size of Austria. Trees remove atmospheric carbon dioxide, hence removal of the trees increases the carbon dioxide levels.

The change in carbon dioxide concentration is the main reason for the 'greenhouse effect'. It is estimated that in the last 100 years the surface temperature of the earth has risen by 0.6°C, and further increases are predicted. This will probably be sufficient to change weather patterns, producing greater extremes. Although warmer weather may perhaps be welcome in the UK, elsewhere it could have damaging effects on health. One possibility is an expansion of the territory in which malaria is endemic, because of further spread and survival of the mosquito bearing the causative organism *Plasmodium falciparum*.

Occupational respiratory hazards

Most respiratory hazards encountered in the workplace involve exposures to coal, asbestos fibres, silica, isocyanates or organic dusts. The effects of these agents are compounded by smoking. The main factors which influence the ability of these materials to cause lung disease are their size, density, shape and solubility. These factors influence how easily the material can be eliminated from the respiratory tract by mucociliary clearance or phagocytosis.

Coal dust

Coal dust in the lungs can cause fibrosis, particularly if the person is a smoker

Extensive exposures to coal dust inevitably mean that small particles (2–5 mm diameter) will be retained in the bronchioles and alveoli. This deposition is referred to as **simple pneumoconiosis** and may, or may not, be accompanied by respiratory symptoms, depending on the extent of the deposition and whether the person is a smoker. Extensive exposure, particularly in smokers, is likely to lead to **progressive massive fibrosis** of the lung. This condition consists of fibrotic masses in the lung, usually several centimetres in diameter, and sometimes with a necrotic centre. The extensive disruption of lung tissue causes emphysema and damage to the airways. Not surprisingly, patients with this condition experience considerable breathing difficulties, often with a cough. The condition is progressive, and eventually patients die from respiratory failure.

Fibrosis: formation of dense collagenous connective tissue. In the lungs, fibrosis occurs within the walls (interstitial fibrosis) and is seen as a mass of enlarged air spaces separated by dense collagenous scarring.

Pleura: the serous membrane which covers the lungs.

Asbestos

Asbestos exists naturally as a fibrous mixture of silicates of iron, magnesium, nickel, cadmium and aluminium. It is extremely resistant to heat and attack by acid and alkali. Unfortunately it is also resistant to enzymatic attack by neutrophils and macrophages after it has entered the body, usually in the respiratory or gastrointestinal tracts.

Exposure to asbestos causes **asbestosis**, characterised by pleural plaques (benign collagenous thickenings of the pleura) and interstitial fibrosis of the lungs. Asbestos can be seen by histological examination of the lungs as **asbestos bodies** in the vicinity of fibrosis. These are complexes of asbestos with protein and haemosiderin (an iron-containing protein). Severe fibrosis impairs lung function and causes death because of respiratory failure. Usually quite heavy exposure to asbestos is required to produce these effects.

More ominously, exposure to asbestos can cause lung cancer and **mesothelioma** (see Chapter 14). Some studies report a ten-fold increase in the risk of lung cancer in workers occupationally exposed to asbestos. If both asbestos exposure and smoking are present the risk of lung cancer increases more than fifty-fold.

The combination of smoking and asbestos exposure substantially increases the risk of lung cancer

All the different forms of asbestos are causally related to lung cancer and mesothelioma, but the greatest risk is associated with exposure to crocidolite (blue asbestos). Crocidolite comprises long straight fibres, in contrast to chrysotile (white asbestos) which has wavy, coiled fibres that penetrate and become trapped in the lungs less readily. Although most commercial asbestos is of the chrysotile form it is usually contaminated with crocidolite.

Crocidolite is now banned in the UK and there are severe restrictions on the use of chrysotile. Asbestos was mostly used for insulation purposes and for vehicle brake linings. Workers who have been involved in its extraction, manufacture or installation are likely to have been exposed – miners, construction workers, boilermakers, workers from asbestos cement factories, shipyard workers and mechanics who had undertaken brake repairs. It is to be expected that the problems of asbestos exposure will eventually disappear in the UK, although new exposures can still arise during the demolition of buildings or replacement of old insulation.

Most studies indicate a cumulative dose–response relationship over time between asbestos exposure and relative risk of lung cancer and mesothelioma. There also appears to be a threshold dose, below which exposed people would not be expected to be at increased risk of lung cancer. This has important implications for the general population and for those living in the vicinity of buildings or factories where asbestos was manufactured or used.

Artificial mineral fibres

Most artificial mineral fibres are nothing like as dangerous as asbestos

Because of the risks attached to asbestos exposure much effort has been directed at producing substitute synthetic fibrous materials. These include rock wool, slag wool and glass wool – ceramic fibres are also being developed. Exposure to these agents is certainly not as dangerous as exposure to asbestos, but these fibres are not entirely innocuous. Initial epidemiological studies have associated exposure to rock wool and slag wool, but not glass wool, with an increased risk of lung cancer. These studies were conducted at the beginning of production when protective masks were not widely in use and further epidemiological studies are required to evaluate the risks properly.

Silica

Silica has an extraordinary ability to induce fibrotic changes in lung tissue, known as silicosis

The most common source of silica is quartz, which is present to some extent in virtually all types of rock. Workers in mines, quarries and foundries are likely to be exposed to quartz dust. Small particles of quartz can penetrate deep into the lung tissues, where they are engulfed by macrophages and neutrophils. Normally, particles taken up by these cells are incorporated into lysosomes and digested, but silica is resistant to digestion. Its crystalline structure causes the lysosomes to rupture, releasing their enzymes into the cytosol. Effectively the cell is digested from within and in the process chemotactic factors are released, attracting more neutrophils and macrophages to the site, which attempt to digest the silica. The process is accompanied by attempts at healing of the damaged tissues. Eventually macrophages predominate, surrounded by layers of collagen fibres that form a whorled fibrotic nodule.

As the disease progresses nodules fuse and replace the functional lung tissue. Clinical signs of reduced lung function are not usually apparent until the late stages of the disease, about 20 years after initial exposure. The lung changes caused by exposure to silica increase susceptibility to tuberculosis – before antibiotic therapy, tuberculosis was often a cause of death in people with silicosis.

Silica may also increase the risk of lung cancer, although this is a controversial issue and not all epidemiological studies agree. The main problem appears to be a failure to take smoking into account. Overall, silicosis probably does increase the risk of lung cancer, but the strength of association is not as great as other lung cancer risks such as smoking, or exposures to asbestos and radon.

Organic dusts

Organic dusts are a health hazard because they may carry fungal spores

Organic dusts are particles from grains, hay or straw and are often contaminated with micro-organisms, particularly fungal spores. The most probable consequence of exposure to organic dust is chronic bronchitis. Symptoms are made worse by smoking. Some people may have an allergic reaction, presenting with acute symptoms of fever, malaise, cough and breathing difficulty. This condition is known as **farmer's lung** and is caused by dust from mouldy hay, contaminated with thermophilic actinomycetes. Histological evaluation of lung biopsy in this condition shows lymphocyte infiltration and granuloma formation. Eventually the disease can proceed to extensive lung fibrosis. Most episodes of farmer's lung are transitory, improving when exposure ceases.

Isocyanate exposure

Respiratory problems arising from exposures to isocyanates are becoming more common with increasing use of these chemicals in formulations for paints, varnishes and polyurethane foam. Inhalation causes cough, wheezing and shortness of breath. Very often these symptoms are precipitated by each exposure to the agent, very much like an asthmatic reaction.

Granuloma: chronic inflammation, comprising a cluster of macrophages in the tissues. Usually caused by a persistent foreign body or infectious organism.

Thermpohilic actinomycetes: branching filamentous bacilli, originally considered to be fungi. Inhalation by sensitised individuals leads to fever, cough, malaise and breathing difficulty.

The long-term effects of isocyanate exposure include chronic obstructive airways disease

▲ **Key points**

Diseases caused by occupational exposure to airborne agents

Agent	Occupational group at risk	Possible outcome
Asbestos	Miners, construction workers, vehicle mechanics	Pleural plaques, lung fibrosis, lung cancer, mesothelioma
Silica	Miners, quarrymen, stone cutters, foundry workers	Lung fibrosis with characteristic nodules, lung cancer
Organic dusts	Farmers exposed to mouldy grains, hay or straw	Chronic bronchitis, farmer's lung, asthma
Isocyanates	Workers involved in manufacture of paints and varnishes, vehicle sprayers and finishers	Asthma, chronic obstructive airways disease

Lead

Lead is an air pollutant and contaminant of water supplies. There are two forms: organic lead and inorganic lead. At one time inorganic lead salts were widely used in the formulation of paint. Peeling paint in old houses can be a health hazard for small children who may pick at it, put it in their mouths or suck their fingers. The most commonly encountered organic compound is tetraethyl lead, which is added to petrol.

The toxic effects of lead have been documented since Roman times. Historically, the storage of food and drink in lead-glazed pottery and the conduction of water in lead pipes were responsible for most lead ingestion and

Lead affects the nervous system, blood, gastrointestinal tract, kidneys and bones

▲ **Key points**

Toxic effects of lead

▲ Headaches

▲ Tremor

▲ Irritability

▲ Coma

▲ Demyelinating neuropathy

▲ Anaemia

▲ Abdominal pain

▲ Long-term exposure to low
levels may cause impaired
mental development and
functioning in children

Calcium channels: selective pores in the cell membrane to allow transfer of ions between the cell and the outside. The open or closed state of these channels or 'gates' is controlled by an electrical potential, or by transmitter substances. The opening of calcium gates in nerve axons allows the release of neurotransmitters and hence the transfer of a chemical message from one neuron to the next.

Calmodulin: an intracellular protein that can alternately bind and release calcium, thereby providing a metabolic signal. For example, muscle contraction is mediated by calcium binding and activation of calmodulin.

consequent poisoning. Even today, domestic lead piping poses a significant risk. Lead was banned from domestic piped water systems in the UK in 1964, but there is no requirement to remove lead pipes from houses built before that date. The European safety limit in the water supply has been set at 100[t][m]g/litre. The mains water supply in all areas of the UK is well below this limit, but water from the domestic supply often exceeds the safe limit in houses with lead water pipes. This is particularly a problem in areas where the water is soft and acid, such as most of Scotland and northern England.

Lead can also be found in food, originating from airborne sources (plants become coated with lead or incorporate lead compounds washed into the soil) or solder in cans. The third main source of lead is atmospheric pollution, arising from vehicles that run on leaded petrol.

Effects of lead

The principal biological effects of lead are interference with calcium-dependent functions, but it also binds with proteins, particularly with thiol (disulphide) groups, and will denature enzymes. Lead is able to enter cells through the calcium channels and bind with calmodulin and other specific calcium-binding proteins. Calcium channels are particularly important in nerve conduction. The features of lead poisoning include seizure or coma in children and a peripheral demyelinating neuropathy, typically involving innervation of the muscles of the wrist and hand.

Most of the lead absorbed is incorporated into the bones and teeth, where it has little immediate direct effect and actually helps to limit toxicity in other parts of the body by reducing its concentration. However, the slow turnover of bone mineral ensures that elevated levels of lead can be maintained in the blood and tissues for months or years. One of the early effects of lead poisoning is anaemia, caused by interference with the synthesis of the oxygen-carrying haem molecule. Lead poisoning also produces abdominal pain or 'colic'.

Children are considered to be more sensitive to lead poisoning than adults. Because lead accumulates in the body, toxic levels may be reached only after years of low-level exposure. It is believed that chronic low-level poisoning is responsible for impaired mental development and functioning in children, evident as low IQ, learning disabilities and personality disorders.

Teratogens

A teratogen is an agent that can disrupt fetal development, causing miscarriage or the birth of a deformed child. The agent may be infectious, chemical, mechanical or nutritional.

Alcohol

Fetal alcohol syndrome: associated with mothers who regularly drink more than 30 g of alcohol a day. Characterised by growth and mental retardation. Children have a small head, small eyes and a broad nasal bridge.

The most commonly encountered teratogen is alcohol. The risk of fetal alcohol syndrome increases with total alcohol intake. The main effect is on the fetal central nervous system and therefore vulnerability extends throughout the pregnancy.

Occupational exposure to teratogens

The main occupational teratogens are lead compounds (used in the paint and battery industries) and organic solvents (commonly used in the textile and printing industries). These agents are associated with congenital malformations and childhood behavioural problems.

Teratogenic drugs

Teratogenic drugs can cause congenital malformations, especially when given in the first trimester of pregnancy (the period in which the organs are formed). The classic example is thalidomide, which was responsible for causing absent or grossly abnormal limbs. Drugs used for the treatment of manic–depressive disorders, seizure disorders, hypertension, thromboembolism and cystic acne are known to be teratogenic. Safer alternatives can usually be prescribed for pregnant women, but there are some conditions (convulsions, for example) in which it is difficult to eliminate the risks of treatment entirely. Although the drugs are associated with increased risks of congenital malformations the incidence is still low, and their use is not necessarily an automatic reason for discouraging a woman to become pregnant.

Agricultural chemicals

Herbicides

Herbicides are a heterogeneous group of chemicals used in agriculture, forestry and urban areas for the control of weeds, shrubs and broad-leaved trees. The chemicals most commonly used are phenoxyls, triazines, benzoics, carbamates, triluralin and uracils. Most research has focused on the phenoxy herbicides, particularly those containing 2,4-dichlorophenoxyacetic acid (2, 4-D) and 2,4,5-trichlorophenoxyacetic acid (2, 4, 5-T) and the chemically related chlorophenols.

> *Commercial preparations of common herbicides often contain dioxin*

   Dioxin, or tetrachlorodibenzodioxin (TCDD), has received a great deal of publicity because of numerous pollution incidents and because it was a component of 'Agent Orange' used in the Vietnam war. Of the large number of chemicals in the dioxin family, TCDD is believed to be the most toxic. A single oral dose of TCDD has an LD_{50} in guinea pigs of 6 µg/kg body weight although the toxicity varies with species, for example in hamsters the LD_{50} is nearly 2000 times the amount for guinea pigs.

LD_{50}: dose of agent needed to kill 50% of animals in a test group

   Most of the information available on dioxin toxicity for humans has been derived from occupational or accidental exposures. A study of Swedish forestry workers suggested that exposure to dioxin during herbicide spraying increased

Dioxin exposure causes acute illnesses, but there is little evidence of miscarriage, birth malformation or cancers

Chloracne: a skin condition that resembles very severe acne and causes scarring.

the risk of soft tissue sarcoma by a factor of seven and lymphoma by a factor of five but other studies in Sweden and Finland did not confirm this finding. There is some evidence for an increased risk of cancer in workers involved in the manufacture of herbicides who had been exposed to high levels of dioxin. Such high concentrations would not normally be met in the general environment. Other studies have linked exposure with cancers of the lung, colon, prostate and ovary, and with leukaemia and multiple myeloma.

There are problems in accurately determining extent of exposure to herbicides. Most farmers routinely come into contact with a wide variety of insecticides, fumigants, fertilisers, fungicides, various oils, solvents and paints necessary for the maintenance of farm buildings and machinery. It would also be unusual for workers in the manufacturing industry to be exposed to a single agent, since most manufacturers make a range of products using mixtures of different agents.

Large amounts of dioxin were accidentally released into the environment at Seveso, Italy, in July 1976. This was caused by an explosion at a chemical plant which manufactured the antibacterial compound hexachlorophene. A cloud of vapour containing dioxin was released into the air and drifted over the town. Children and adults developed nausea, headaches, diarrhoea and skin irritation. Birds fell from the sky and animals became sick or died, although no humans died. Some children developed chloracne. There was some concern that the exposure would later be reflected in birth malformations. However, over the period 1977–1982 there was no apparent increase in the frequency of malformations.

Dioxin exposure in experimental animals is associated with spontaneous abortion, and there is concern that similar effects could occur in humans. Studies in the USA have compared miscarriage rates in rural communities (where the dioxin-containing herbicide 2, 4, 5-T was used in crop-spraying) with those in urban communities. A small excess of spontaneous abortions was seen in rural areas, but there is no certainty that any of the miscarriages were in women who had been exposed to the spray. Nevertheless, the reports and public concern about the use of 2, 4, 5-T prompted its withdrawal by the manufacturers.

It should be noted that miscarriages are common: excluding elective abortions, 12–15% of known pregnancies do not come to term. It is not uncommon for a woman to have several normal pregnancies before a miscarriage and vice versa. Most identified miscarriages are attributable to maternal smoking, alcohol consumption or drug abuse. In other words, the true cause is often closer to home than some people might like to admit.

Another notorious episode in the dioxin story occurred at Love Canal, near Niagara Falls. This partly excavated canal had been used by a chemical company as a disposal facility for chemical wastes, in the assumption that the waste would be contained by the clay bed of the canal. Some 30 years later, residents nearby complained about the chemical odour from the landfill. A variety of acute illnesses was attributed to the canal and its malodorous contents and concerns were voiced about the possible long-term risks to health. Chemical analysis revealed that the site contained a cocktail of hazardous materials, including polychlorinated biphenyls (PCBs), benzene, toluene, tetrachloroethylene and dioxin. Eventually, after intense public pressure, most of the residents were relocated. Regular follow-up and screening of these families have not, so far, revealed any unusual patterns of illness, birth defects or excess cancers.

The widest and most systematic use of herbicides was in the Vietnam war, when Agent Orange was used for defoliant purposes. Agent Orange consists of a mixture of 2, 4, 5-T and 2, 4-D and is likely to contain some dioxin. Birth defects have been caused in mice by 2, 4, 5-T. In the Vietnam war there were reports that animals and children had been killed by the sprays but these reports have not been confirmed. However, not wishing to be accused of propagating chemical warfare against civilians, the military discontinued defoliant spraying in 1970.

The perception among Vietnam veterans is that Agent Orange has had a harmful effect on both themselves and their offspring. Large sums of money have been paid by the manufacturers in compensation to veterans who developed cancers and other ill-effects that were allegedly caused by exposures to Agent Orange. Soft-tissue sarcoma is believed to be caused by exposure to Agent Orange because Swedish studies have linked forestry workers who had used phenoxy herbicides with the disease. The Veterans Administration therefore launched a survey among nearly 13 500 patients who had served in Vietnam and were being treated for routine complaints in Veterans Administration hospitals. However, the prevalence of soft-tissue sarcomas in those who had served in Vietnam was not significantly different from the prevalence in those who had not.

Do herbicides represent a significant health hazard?

Point	Counterpoint
Phenoxy herbicides are likely to be contaminated with dioxin	Animal toxicity is not always a reliable indicator of toxicity in humans
Dioxin is very poisonous: LD_{50} is 6 µg/kg in guinea pigs, lower doses cause birth defects	Not all epidemiological studies agree, could represent clustering phenomenon
Exposure to spray in Swedish forestry workers has been associated with higher incidence of soft-tissue sarcomas	
Used in the Vietnam war as Agent Orange, associated with deaths in exposed civilians	Unconfirmed evidence: could be war propaganda
Vietnam veterans who developed cancers were	Cause and effect have been difficult to substantiate; Veterans

compensated by manufacturer	Administration study showed no excess risk of sarcomas in veterans
Accidental exposure to dioxin in Seveso caused widespread destruction of wildlife. Exposed children suffered nausea, headaches, diarrhoea, skin irritation and chloracne	No evidence of excess miscarriages, birth defects or cancers in exposed people
Accidental exposure at Love Canal, Niagara Falls was associated with acute illnesses	Tendency to associate illnesses with unusual events. 'Scare factor' and media coverage encourage people to complain about symptoms that might otherwise have been ignored. Long-term follow-up of relocated families suggests no excess health risks

Author's view

Herbicides are undoubtedly toxic to both plants and animals, although the risks to humans are more difficult to substantiate. The Seveso experience indicates that short-term health effects can be very severe, but the evidence is largely reassuring with respect to miscarriages, congenital defects and cancers. Accidental or occupational exposures are at relatively large doses and it is extremely unlikely that herbicide residues in or on food crops represent a substantial health risk to the consumer.

The authorities and manufacturers have often acted on the principle of 'better safe than sorry', and products have been withdrawn, although it must be said that they had very little choice in the matter because of media pressure and public furore. Rightly or wrongly, the debate has stimulated the development of new, more 'environmentally friendly' alternatives that are less persistent and break down into harmless compounds. Herbicides are needed, but we should be cautious about their use and alert to any possible dangers.

Pesticides

Pesticides have been used in one form or another for more than 100 years. The development of the chemical industry in the 1930s saw a massive expansion in the range of compounds available, many of which had greater potency and improved specificity.

Organochlorides

Normal exposures to DDT did not cause substantial harm to humans

One of the first new chemicals, introduced in the 1940s, was the organochlorine compound dichlorodiphenyltrichloroethane (DDT), a neurotoxic poison which affects the sodium channels in nerve cell membranes, causing rapid death. It is readily absorbed by insects on surface contact. Humans and other mammals do not easily absorb the chemical and hence are relatively insensitive to its effects.

Because there were no obvious dangers, DDT was used rather casually, without protective clothing – there are even stories that farm-labourers used to shake DDT down their trousers to eliminate lice and fleas. The chemical was often mixed by hand and the accidental ingestion of small amounts did not cause immediate ill-effects. Ingestion of large amounts of DDT, however, can cause minor convulsions.

Prolonged exposure to high doses of DDT (100 mg/kg body weight, or 100 parts per million) causes liver cancer in rodents. At the peak of its use in the 1960s, people were typically exposed to DDT as residues in food, at about 0.03 mg/kg body weight. It seems very unlikely that exposures of this order would be sufficient to produce liver cell changes in humans. Long-term studies of people who received heavy occupational exposures of DDT have not revealed excess morbidity or mortality. However, the International Agency for Research on Cancer (IARC) has classified DDT as 'possibly carcinogenic' to humans, in view of the fact that it can cause liver cancers in rodents.

DDT concentrates in food chains, causing depletion of some wildlife species

The use of DDT is believed to have halted a typhus epidemic in Italy at the end of the Second World War. It has also been used to control the malaria mosquito in many parts of the world. The low toxicity of DDT in mammals led to its widespread and indiscriminate use, usually to kill crop pests such as aphids, caterpillars and other insects. It was also used to dust livestock, including racing pigeons. This application led to the recognition that long-term effects are associated with DDT. Racing pigeons are preyed on by hawks, and shortly after the widespread introduction of the chemical a drastic fall in the hawk population became evident. It was discovered that DDT had accumulated in the tissues, and the birds' eggs had very thin shells that broke in the nest. Similarly, the heron population suffered a sharp decline, presumably by ingesting fish that had swum in DDT-contaminated waters.

The damage to wildlife caused some people to fear for their own reproductive capacity and that there might be even worse ill-effects. The product was eventually withdrawn in most developed countries.

There have been suggestions that DDT and other organochlorides (the PCBs) influence the development of breast cancer. There is no readily identifiable cause of breast cancer, but incidence of the disease has increased markedly in the last 50 years, at the same time as the use of pesticides has increased. The main metabolite of DDT (dichlordiphenyldichloroethylene; DDE) accumulates in adipose tissue. In the American population the average concentration of DDE in adipose tissue was about eight parts per million when measured in 1970. In 1983, average concentrations were about two parts per million, reflecting its withdrawal from use.

Initial case-control studies revealed higher adipose tissue concentrations of DDE in women with breast cancer than in controls. There were no significant differences in concentrations of PCBs. However, these studies involved only a few dozen women and suffered from the disadvantage that the measurements were made after diagnosis (it is possible that patients were

▲ Key points

Organochloride pesticides

- ▲ Act as neurotoxic poisons (DDT, for example)

- ▲ Not absorbed through human skin but are absorbed by insects

- ▲ Used to control typhus and malaria, as well as crop pests

- ▲ Prolonged oral doses causes liver cancer in rodents

- ▲ Accumulate in tissue and are concentrated by food chains

- ▲ Cause failure to breed in some wildlife species

- ▲ Controversy about possible link with breast cancer

exposed after the onset of disease).

A prospective study of women in the USA failed to show any association between DDE and breast cancer. This approach could be expected to be more reliable since the samples were collected and measured before any of the women developed breast cancer. This study was limited by small sample size, and larger prospective studies are required before firm conclusions can be drawn. From the evidence so far, it seems very unlikely that exposures to organochlorides alone are responsible for the increase in breast cancer.

Organophosphates

Thiol organophosphate derivatives are relatively non-toxic in mammals

Eventually organochlorine compounds were replaced by organophosphates. These act as substrates for cholinesterase, an enzyme responsible for eliminating the neurotransmitter acetylcholine. Normally, neurotransmitters are eliminated or reabsorbed after a nerve impulse. Without proper elimination (because organophosphate competes with the natural substrate for the enzyme) acetylcholine accumulates at the nerve endings, leading to muscle paralysis and death. Organophosphate compounds have different species specificities, so that it has been possible to develop products that have low mammalian toxicity but are highly toxic in insects. The reverse is also true: originally these compounds were developed for use as nerve gases to kill humans.

Thiol derivatives of organophosphate compounds (in which oxygen atoms are replaced by sulphur) are relatively non-toxic in humans and are metabolised by the liver without ill-effects. In insects, however, different enzymes remove the substituted sulphur atoms, yielding the original (and highly toxic) organophosphates. An example of a widely used thiocompound is malathion, which is metabolised by insects to a highly toxic compound called malaoxon.

Insecticidal preparations can produce ill-effects in humans when mishandled, usually because there is some contamination by non-specific compounds. The immediate effects of exposure to organophosphates are due to inhibition of cholinesterase, leading to symptoms in the autonomic nervous system (abdominal cramps, diarrhoea) and central nervous system (dizziness, tremor, anxiety and confusion). Symptoms usually occur within hours of exposure and disappear in a few days as new cholinesterase, is produced. There is also some evidence that high exposure can lead to a peripheral neuropathy, with symptoms of a tingling sensation and weakness, or even paralysis. In most cases the symptoms are reversible, but they may persist for some months.

The problems encountered with the older pesticides and herbicides, coupled with public pressure, have stimulated a constant search for new compounds with high specificity, low persistence and high potency. One of the new pesticides, glyphosphate, appears to fulfil these criteria and has a much higher LD_{50} than the older pesticides (Table 5.1). This compound interferes with the synthesis of aromatic amino acids in a biochemical pathway that is essential for plants but which does not exist in mammals.

Differences in animal and plant biochemical systems do not always guarantee that an agent will not be toxic to animals: the agent may simply affect a different

▲ Key points

Organophosphates

▲ Organophosphates act as substrates for cholinesterase

▲ Cause muscle paralysis and death

▲ Selective toxicity achieved because of differences in liver enzymes

▲ Thiol derivatives are relatively non-toxic to humans, but liver enzymes in insects remove the thiol groups, converting the compound to a toxic organophosphate

metabolic pathway. For example, paraquat interferes with the redox system in plant chloroplasts. The damage caused to plants cannot occur in animals, because animals cells do not contain chloroplasts but paraquat is actively taken up by the lungs, causing free radical damage, cell death and fibrosis. Fortunately, these effects occur only in large doses.

Table 5.1 Toxicity of agricultural chemicals and other agents

Compound	Use	LD_{50} (in rodents)
Parathion	Organophosphate	10 mg/kg
Malathion	Organophosphate insecticide	1.3 g/kg
Glyphosphate	Herbicide	4.3 g/kg
Paraquat	Herbicide	100 mg/kg
Botulinus toxin	Food contaminant	15 ng/kg
Soman	Organophosphate nerve gas	60 µg/kg
Paracetamol	Analgesic	5 g/kg (rats), 0.7 g/kg (humans)
Ethanol	Recreational drug	5 g/kg

The data on hazards to health associated with herbicide and pesticide use are largely reassuring – measurable effects are seen only in large accidental or occupational exposures, and these are usually of short duration. Nevertheless it is imperative that we remain vigilant about inappropriate tainting of the environment with chemical agents, whatever their type and source, and that we continue to monitor for possible effects for many years after exposure. Cancers, in particular, often take many years to develop.

It is quite natural for individuals and communities to worry about events over which they have no control. One facet of modern industrialised societies is that the control of events that affect the lives of local people is often in the hands of 'faceless' bureaucrats and multinational corporations. People could exercise more concern over events they *can* control: smoking, poor diet and lack of exercise have a far greater effect on individual health than most environmental pollutants ordinarily encountered. The main exception is air pollution and, as much is caused by vehicle use, this is not beyond individual control.

Review question 1

Why are animal experiments unreliable in determining the toxicity of a chemical?

Food irradiation

In 1986, the US Food and Drug Administration (FDA) allowed irradiation to be used for preserving grains, vegetables, fruits and spices. The process has now been approved in most industrialised countries. Paradoxically, it is the less developed countries that might most benefit from its use.

Campylobacter jejuni: a major cause of acute gastroenteritis in the UK. Symptoms begin with fever, headache and malaise, followed by diarrhoea, often with blood, and abdominal cramps. In most cases the illness is self-limiting, but can cause cholecystitis, pancreatitis or reactive arthritis.

Salmonella: infection causes a spectrum of clinical symptoms including enteric fever, enterocolitis, bone inflammation and food poisoning. It is possible to be an asymptomatic carrier: the organism is often spread by food handlers who are carriers. Transmission is by ingesting contaminated foods, particularly eggs and poultry products, or water.

Toxoplasmosis: parasitic infection transmitted by eating uncooked meat contaminated with the organism *Toxoplasma gondii.* Infection in humans takes several clinical forms. Acute infection in normal adults usually becomes apparent as swelling of the lymph glands, with or without fever. Infection can cause a febrile condition in children. Infection in early pregnancy may be asymptomatic in the mother, but can cause stillbirth or neonatal jaundice, pneumonia, encephalitis and brain damage.

Trichinosis: parasitic infection acquired by eating meat containing viable cysts of the organism *Trichinella spiralis.* In humans the parasite larvae find their way to striated muscles, causing generalised muscular aches and pains. The lungs, heart, brain and other organs can also become infected. Usually trichinosis is mild with low mortality.

Most methods of food preservation and cooking generate new molecules, some of which may be carcinogenic

Irradiation involves the exposure of foodstuffs to ionising radiation, usually from cobalt or caesium isotope sources. During the process the packaged food is placed on a conveyor belt and guided into lead-shielded chambers, where it is exposed to a specific dose of radiation. The principle is similar to that of radiotherapy (see Chapter 13): dividing or metabolising cells are more susceptible to radiation damage. High radiation doses retard spoilage and sterilise the food by killing micro-organisms and insects. If stored in the original airtight container, treated food can be kept at room temperature for years without fear of spoilage. Low doses of radiation alter biochemical reactions such as those responsible for fruit ripening or sprouting of tubers and bulbs. This works by breaking chemical bonds, thereby interfering with cell division. In a medium dose, enough bacteria are killed to delay spoilage and extend the shelf-life of the food.

Although many other methods of food preservation are available, proponents of irradiation argue that it offers advantages over the other methods. The main distinction is that irradiation preserves food without cooking it. Food-borne illness caused by *Salmonella* and *Campylobacter* in chicken and other uncooked or partly cooked meat products could be controlled by irradiation, as would trichinosis and toxoplasmosis caused by the consumption of infested pork. The method could also eliminate the need to use chemical agents as post-harvest fumigants to control mould growth and other infestations. Some of these agents are suspected carcinogens. One possible disadvantage of irradiation is that no active agent is left in the food so that unpacked foodstuffs are not protected against reinfestation.

In developed countries the problems of food spoilage are to some extent obviated by efficient methods of refrigeration and transport. This is not the case for the less developed countries. Much of the aid given to the less developed countries is as meat, grains and other plant foods. The food can be lost by spoilage or infestation even before it reaches the people who need it.

Is irradiated food safe?

No radiation remains in the food after treatment, and the food may be consumed without harm straight off the conveyor belt, although this would defeat the purpose of the process. There is little or no change in the taste of the food, although some soft fruits may be further softened by the process. Irradiation is not suitable for preserving milk because it causes changes in sulphur bonds and gives it an unpleasant taste.

Food irradiation does disrupt chemical bonds and new molecules that are toxic or carcinogenic could be created in the food, but these changes do not differ substantially from those induced by standard food preservation and cooking methods. In some cases the molecules produced by conventional food treatments are more hazardous than those induced by irradiation. For example, the carcinogens benzpyrene or benzoanthracene are produced by char-grilling meat, roasting coffee beans, boiling fats, baking bread and smoking fish, meats and cheeses. Salted foods contain a mixture of nitrosamines, which are implicated in the development of gastric cancer. All the toxicological studies so far conducted on a wide range of irradiated foods confirm the safety of the process.

Environmental radiation

In high enough doses ionising radiation undoubtedly induces cancer. Ionising radiation is emitted by the decay of radioactive elements such as uranium, thorium and plutonium. The radioactivity, in the form of X-rays, γ rays and α or β particles, interacts with atoms in their path so that they become charged, or ionised. Other, more innocuous, forms of radiation (heat, light, radio waves or microwaves) lack sufficient energy to do this and are non-ionising.

The different types of ionising radiation differ in their ability to transfer energy to other atoms – this is referred to as their linear energy transfer. The linear energy transfer ability of α particles is high and the biological effects of α particles are therefore greater than those of β particles and γ rays (this is relative – all types of ionising radiation are dangerous).

Ionising radiation has always been part of the natural environment, emanating from deposits in the earth's crust and as cosmic radiation. This background has been supplemented by the decay of radioactive rock brought to the surface by mining. The most notable applications of radioactive isotopes are in medical imaging, nuclear power installations and in atomic weapons. Most of the radiation dose a person is likely to receive during the course of a year is background radiation (Figure 5.3). For most people the risks of ill-health arising from radiation exposure are extremely small, especially when compared with the impact of much more commonly encountered risk factors (Table 5.2).

▲ Key points
Ionising radiation
▲ Emitted from unstable nuclei during radioactive decay
▲ α Particles: high-energy, positively charged particles comprising two protons and two neutrons
▲ β Particles: small positively or negatively charged electrons
▲ X-rays, γ rays: uncharged electromagnetic radiation

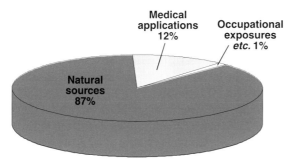

Figure 5.3 Contribution of radiation sources to annual average dose. The annual radiation dose received by the average person is mainly from background radiation emanating from natural sources. (Source: *Living With Radiation*, 4th ed, published by The National Radiological Protection Board, Chilton, 1989.)

There is still some uncertainty about the long-term effects of chronic low-dose radiation exposure. Most of what is known about the biological effects of radiation is from extrapolation of single high-dose exposures, such as those inflicted on the inhabitants of Hiroshima and Nagasaki at the end of the Second

Table 5.2 Hazards and associated risk of an individual dying in one year

Cause of death	Risk
Smoking (10 cigarettes a day)	1 in 200
All natural causes, at age 40	1 in 850
Violence or poisoning	1 in 3300
Influenza	1 in 5000
Road accident	1 in 8000
Playing football	1 in 25 000
Accident at home	1 in 26 000
Accident at work	1 in 43 500
Occupational exposure to radiation	1 in 57 000
Homicide	1 in 100 000
Lightning strike	1 in 10 000 000
Release of radiation by nuclear power station nearby	1 in 10 000 000

Source: British Medical Association, 1992.

World War. Some indication of the effects of chronic low exposures in humans can be determined from occupational exposures of people who work in nuclear power installations. There is an additional advantage in that such exposures are closely monitored by routine wearing of film badges. Studies indicate that there may be a small additional risk of leukaemias, myeloma and lung cancer, but the relative risks of Hodgkin's disease and liver cancer may be lower.

Concerns have been expressed that the Chernobyl incident in 1986 could cause an increase in the incidence of cancers in affected areas. Large amounts of radiation were released into the atmosphere as a result of the accident, especially in the immediate surroundings. Many workers at the plant received radiation doses of 250–1000 mSv (the annual dose from normal background radiation is 1–2 mSv). Some residents within a 30 km radius may have received doses of 50–60 mSv. Further afield, in Finland, the radiation dose from Chernobyl is estimated at about 0.4 mSv.

Because of the possible long-term effects of the Chernobyl accident, a European initiative has been organised to monitor the incidence of childhood leukaemia. To date there has been no evidence of increased cancer rates even in some heavily contaminated regions. The most recent evidence from Finland and Sweden similarly show negative results. However, in the more immediate environment increased rates of thyroid cancers have been found in children, with an incidence some 100 times the expected frequency. Moreover the type

To date, the most apparent physical health effect of Chernobyl is a marked increase in the incidence of childhood thyroid cancers

of thyroid cancer seen is normally rare in children and is also more aggressive than usual. These cancers became apparent some 3–5 years after the accident.

It is known that the radiation release from Chernobyl contained significant amounts of iodine-131 which, on entry into the body, becomes localised in the thyroid gland. This radionuclide has a half-life of 8 days and hence it is likely that the vulnerable period of exposure was during the first few weeks after the accident. It is possible that children are more susceptible to exposure because the thyroid gland is relatively immature, with a high proportion of proliferating cells.

There remains some concern about the possible effects of other longer-lived radionuclides such as caesium-137 (half-life 30 years) and strontium-90 (half-life 29 years). Although environmental contamination is relatively high in the Chernobyl area, regular whole body measurements have revealed that very little of these elements appears to have been transferred to the general population. The doses received are comparable with those that would be received from domestic exposure to radon by people living in Cornwall.

One surprising finding was that there was a cluster of cases of Down's syndrome (12 cases versus an expected 2–3) in Berlin within roughly 9 months of the incident. Down's syndrome has not been previously associated with radiation exposure, even in the survivors of the Japanese bombs. No excess chromosome abnormalities were reported in other regions of Europe where radiation doses were higher. It is likely that the Berlin cluster is either a chance effect or a consequence of more complete medical surveillance in the wake of Chernobyl.

Other than the thyroid cancers, for which incidence rates should now fall, it could be argued that we have 'got off lightly' as far as the physical health effects of the Chernobyl accident are concerned. Unfortunately there remains the possibility that further radiation leaks could come from material still present within the reactor site. There are also the psychological and economic costs associated with the relocation of some 4 000 000 people away from the area.

Except for nuclear accidents, probably the greatest routine risk of radiation exposure in the general population is from the indoor environment. In today's better insulated homes and commercial buildings there is a possibility that radon gas (which can rise from the ground) will, without effective ventilation, concentrate to dangerous levels. A Swedish case-control study showed that patients with lung cancer were more likely to have a history of prolonged exposure to radon (140–400 Bq/m^3) than controls. Smoking multiplies the risk.

Radon: a gas produced from the natural decay of uranium. Uranium is present in small amounts in many common rocks and minerals, including granite

The environment and leukaemia

The precise cause of leukaemia is unknown. Exposure to certain chemicals (benzene, for example) and infectious agents (particularly retroviruses) has been implicated in some types of leukaemia. Inherited genetic factors certainly play a role in altering susceptibility for the disease. The most conclusive

Viral infection, chemical exposures and ionising radiation have been implicated as causative agents in leukaemia

Leukaemia: the most common form of childhood cancer, but some forms of the disease are also common in adults. All forms of leukaemia are the result of malignant transformation of stem cells in the bone marrow. These are normally responsible for the production of blood cells.

Non-Hodgkin's lymphoma: cancer arising in the lymphatic system.

evidence for this is an association between Down's syndrome and the production of leukaemia (the relative risk is about 15). The causative agents in leukaemias probably act in a multistage process, triggering a variety of genetic alterations during maturation of the cells.

In the UK the incidence of leukaemia and non-Hodgkin's lymphoma in young people born in west Cumbria, especially in the village of Seascale, has increased. Seascale is close to Sellafield, the site of the major UK nuclear reprocessing facility. One of the first investigations of this cluster of childhood malignancies was conducted by Gardner and co-workers in 1990. Case and control data were collected for the father's occupation, together with the radiation dose received, if any, before conception of the child. This risk was compared with maternal exposure to abdominal X-rays in pregnancy and viral infection in pregnancy, Caesarean delivery, social class, parental age, family habits (eating fish or shellfish, growing own vegetables, using seaweed as fertiliser) and whether the child played on the beach or fells.

Analysis of case-control data revealed that the most significant difference between the cases of leukaemia and controls was exposure of the father to ionising radiation while he was employed at Sellafield. The risk increased if the father was exposed less than 6 months before conception (Figure 5.4). The relative risk of other radiation, such as maternal abdominal X-ray exposure in pregnancy, was calculated at about 1.5.

The subject remains controversial because the association has not been found in other human populations exposed to radiation, or in most animal studies. Further analysis of the cases has revealed that the leukaemia and lymphoma excess in Seascale is not confined to children born in the area. It follows that some factor, other than paternal exposure to radiation before conception, must have been at work in children born outside the area.

An alternative explanation, proposed by Kinlen (1993), is that the leukaemias arose from the introduction of a new (unidentified) infectious agent into the area (Figure 5.5). It is notable that many nuclear installations are located in remote geographical areas. These areas were subject to a large influx of workers and their families when the nuclear facilities were being constructed and commissioned. Before that time, population mixing in the area was relatively rare.

Kinlen's hypothesis proposes that the host community, because of its isolation, may not have been previously exposed to an infectious agent responsible for causing leukaemia and so has no immunity to that agent when it is carried into the area by the new arrivals. It is noticeable that peaks in leukaemia incidence are usually followed by a decline. This pattern could be explained by herd immunity becoming re-established. Equally, the decline could be explained by the increasingly tighter controls on radiation exposures which have been introduced over the years.

Further work by Kinlen's group of childhood leukaemia in the vicinity of military camps lends support to the hypothesis that a leukaemia agent is transmitted by population mixing. These camps were established in remote areas following the introduction of National Service in 1947. Analysis of other

Cases   Controls

Childhood leukaemia and lymphoma in west Cumbria

▲ A total of 97 cases of leukaemia and lymphoma in young people (under the age of 25 years) born and diagnosed in west Cumbria between 1950 and 1985 were compared with 1001 age- and sex-matched controls

▲ Data collected by questionnaire, hospital records and records held at nuclear plant

▲ Highest risks associated with highest paternal radiation doses before conception
Source: Gardner et al., 1990

large construction projects in remote areas (more than 20 km from a population centre) such as fossil fuel power stations, hydroelectric schemes and oil refineries, and which necessitated establishment of worker's camps for some years, also shows an excess of leukaemia in the immediate period following construction (Kinlen, Dickson and Stiller, 1995).

Herd immunity: the degree to which a community is susceptible to an infectious disease by reason of acquired immunity, either by previous infection or prophylactic immunisation.

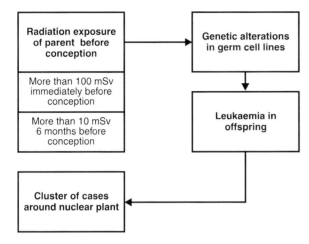

Figure 5.4 Leukaemia and radiation. The Gardner hypothesis is based on the observation that some children affected by leukaemia had fathers who had been exposed to radiation before the child's conception.

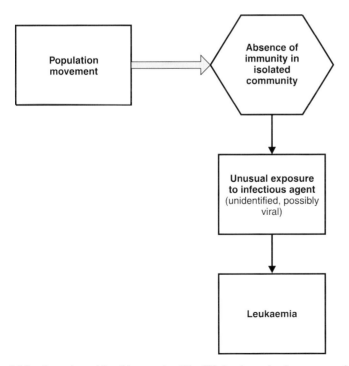

Figure 5.5 Leukaemia and herd immunity. The Kinlen hypothesis proposes that population mixing in isolated rural areas can lead to transmission of an infectious agent which causes leukaemia.

Electric and magnetic fields

> *It is unlikely that exposure to electromagnetic radiation has major adverse effects on health*

There have been fears that very low frequency electric and magnetic fields are a hazard to health. Some epidemiological studies have suggested that risks of childhood cancers may be increased, but just as many studies show no association. In one study carried out around Denver, Colorado, clusters of childhood cancers were more common near high-voltage power installations. However, the study suffered methodological problems and possible confounding factors such as passive exposure to cigarette smoke were not taken into consideration. There are also problems in accurately determining exposures to electric and magnetic fields. A later American study, conducted in Los Angeles county, more accurately ascertained exposure to electromagnetic radiation by placing recording devices within houses. Exposure to other agents, such as household chemicals and cigarette smoke, was also evaluated. This study showed no association between childhood leukaemia and exposure to electric or magnetic fields.

If electric and magnetic radiation was responsible for most childhood leukaemias the incidence should have increased greatly over the past 50 years,

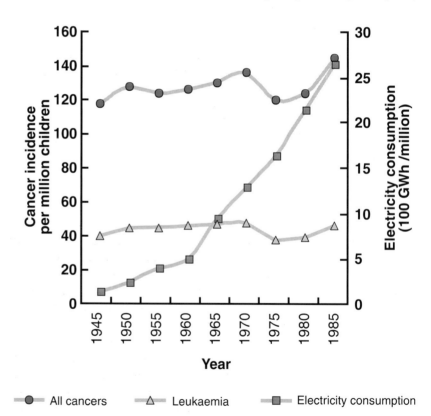

Figure 5.6 Childhood cancers and consumption of electricity. Electricity consumption in Denmark has risen dramatically over the past 50 years, but the incidence of childhood cancers, including leukaemias, has changed only slightly during this period. (Adapted from Olsen *et al.*, 1993.)

corresponding to the enormous increase in consumption of electrical power. No such increase has been demonstrated (Figure 5.6). While it can be argued that it is difficult to make historical comparisons because of changes in diagnostic criteria, it is inconceivable that an effect of the required magnitude has been missed.

Power transmission lines produce both electrical and magnetic fields (all electric currents produce magnetic fields). Magnetic fields are not easily absorbed by other objects, so that if a power line is buried in the ground its magnetic field will still be measurable on the surface. Conversely, electric fields are partially shielded by objects such as trees and buildings. Electric fields are unlike other forms of radiation such as X-rays or microwaves. X-rays have a very high energy and affect living systems because they break chemical bonds. Lower energy radiation, such as microwaves, is absorbed by molecules and produces heat but alters chemical structures only by means of the heat produced. The energy of electric and magnetic fields is much too weak to cause either heating or molecular or breakage of chemical bonds. The electric fields induced by the body's own metabolism are usually far stronger than those induced by external sources.

Although no damage comparable with X-rays or microwaves can be ascribed to electric and magnetic fields, they do have some effect on the body. Some experiments indicate that electric and magnetic fields can increase the production of enzymes involved in cell growth and may also affects various hormones – for example, the production of melatonin can be suppressed in animals by exposure to electric fields. It does not necessarily follow that these biological effects will have consequences for health but concerns have been expressed that the changes could produce an environment in which carcinogens can cause damage. However, the body has many adaptive responses and functional reserves to deal with this sort of minor imbalance.

Occupational exposure

Other epidemiological research has sought to evaluate the risks of electric or magnetic fields in the workplace. A prospective survey of New York city telephone workers showed that workers who spliced cables developed more cancers than those involved in other activities. However, even the cable splicers had lower rates of cancer than New York males as a whole. This might suggest that working in the telephone industry is a very safe occupation, but is probably a statistical aberration because of the low numbers involved.

Other occupational studies have revealed associations with leukaemias and brain tumours, but for every survey that purports to demonstrate such an association, another does not. The problem is that leukaemias and brain tumours are very rare in adults. Taken together, the studies suggest that if a positive association exists, it is very small. Even then, proof of an association is not proof of causation (see Chapter 1).

Ultraviolet radiation

The most commonly encountered risk factor for all types of skin cancer is exposure to natural and artificial forms of UV radiation

Ultraviolet (UV) radiation is the most commonly encountered risk factor for skin cancer. The main types of skin cancer are **basal cell carcinoma, squamous cell carcinoma** and **malignant melanoma**. Basal cell and squamous cell carcinomas are the most common, with malignant melanomas comprising about 10% of skin cancers. Despite their relative rarity, malignant melanomas are responsible for most deaths from skin cancer. All forms of skin cancer are increasing in incidence (Figures 5.7 and 5.8).

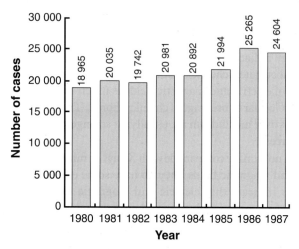

Figure 5.7 Incidence of non-melanoma skin cancers in England 1980-1987. (Source: OPCS.)

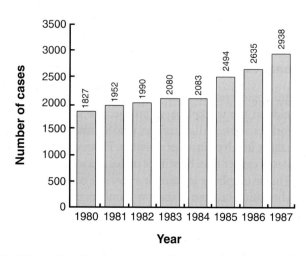

Figure 5.8 Incidence of malignant melanoma in England, 1980–1987. (Source: OPCS.)

Basal cell carcinoma: also referred to as rodent ulcer because of its capacity to erode, or 'gnaw' its way into the skin and underlying structures. It is the most common kind of skin cancer in the UK and is frequently seen on the faces of middle-aged and older people, on the sides of the nose, around the orbit or on the upper lip. The main risk factor is cumulative exposure to sunlight. Exposure to chemicals (arsenical compounds, for example) is also implicated. These cancers rarely metastasise but prompt treatment is imperative because of local invasion.

Squamous cell carcinoma: invasive cancer with an ability to metastasise, arising from keratinocytes in the epidermis or skin appendages. Found on sun-exposed (lower lip for example) or previously damaged or irritated skin. In the past it was associated with occupational exposure to soot (cancer of the scrotum in young chimney sweeps). The tumours often contain excessive amounts of keratin, giving them a crusted or cornified appearance.

While basal cell carcinomas and (to a lesser extent) squamous cell carcinoma are generally not life-threatening, they can be very disfiguring unless treated early. In contrast, the overall 5-year survival for malignant melanoma is about

50% for men and 75% for women. This improves substantially if the condition is treated early. Mortality rates for malignant melanoma have increased but not as much as incidence of the disease because of improvements in treatment and earlier presentation.

Pathology of malignant melanoma

Malignant melanomas arise from melanocytes in previously normal skin or from pigmented areas of the skin known as naevi. They may be distinguished from benign or other malignant skin lesions by the following criteria:

- Minor itch or change in sensation of pigmented area
- Lesion larger than 1 cm diameter
- Increasing size
- Irregular border
- Variation in colour: brown mixed with blue, black or grey
- Inflammation
- Bleeding or crusting

The major diagnostic signs are change in shape, size and colour.

Risk factors in malignant melanoma

A notable feature of malignant melanoma is its rapid rise in incidence in white populations all over the world. The lifetime risk of melanoma was estimated at 1 in 1500 in 1935, this had increased to 1:150 by 1985 – a tenfold increase in only 50 years. Nearly half of all cases of melanoma occur in people under the age of 40.

Malignant melanoma primarily affects white people, particularly those with light skin and fair hair. The incidence of malignant melanoma is higher in people of higher economic status and education; this is believed to be related to the fashion for tanned skin and the trend for holidays in hot climates. The British government hopes to promote sensible exposures to UV light through public information and awareness activities. Accordingly, skin cancer has been identified as a key area in the *Health of the Nation* strategy. Because of the clearly identified risk factors involved, and the marked improvements in survival made possible by early treatment, the main focus of the strategy is prevention and early recognition of the skin changes that are signs of skin cancer.

People with light skin and hair are most at risk. Skin colouring and the tendency to tan are classified as:

- Type 1 (white skin, always burns, never tans)
- Type 2 (white skin, burns easily, tans with difficulty)
- Type 3 (white skin, tans easily, rarely burns)
- Type 4 (white skin, never burns, always tans)
- Type 5 (brown skin)
- Type 6 (black skin)

Skin types 1–3 are associated with the greatest risk of malignant melanoma. A family or previous history of melanoma, history of severe sunburn and the

Malignant melanoma: arises from melanocytes, the epidermal cells responsible for the production of melanin. There are four main types which exhibit different patterns of growth. **Superficial spreading melanoma** is the most common, comprising 50% of melanomas in the UK. Tumour cells spread horizontally in the epidermis before invading the underlying dermis. This is most often seen in younger women (20–40 years), usually on the legs and lower back. In men it usually occurs on the upper and lower back. Appears as a flat lesion with variable pigmentation and irregular edges. **Nodular melanoma** grows rapidly into a well defined nodule, usually darkly pigmented but it can have little or no pigmentation or only pigmentation around the edges. Tumour grows vertically through the epidermis and dermis. Most often found in men, on the head, neck and trunk. **Lentigo melanoma** is more often seen in older women, on the face, and usually grows slowly. It is less likely to metastasise and has a better prognosis. The least common type is **acral melanoma**, which typically occurs on the palms of the hands, soles of the feet and in the area around the first toenail. This accounts for about 10% of malignant melanomas in the UK.

Melanocyte: cell of neural crest origin that, among other places, is present in the basal layer of the epidermis (in skin). Its function is to synthesise the pigment melanin and export it to the surrounding keratinocytes. Melanin serves a protective function by shielding cellular components, particularly DNA, from UV-B irradiation.

presence of many or atypical naevi are other risk factors.

Exposure to sunlight is probably not the only risk factor for malignant melanoma: it is also associated with some occupational exposures to chemicals and there are melanin-producing sites in internal organs, which, although rarely, can become malignant. In some countries melanomas most commonly arise on areas of the body that are not exposed to sunlight, such as the soles of the feet. What other factors are involved in these cases remains uncertain.

Exposure to UV

Several strands of evidence link UV exposure to risk of malignant melanoma. The incidence of malignant melanoma varies with latitude, increasing with proximity to the equator in populations with the same skin colour. Numerous epidemiological studies have indicated that risks increase substantially in people who have a history of sunburn in childhood. The importance of childhood exposure is substantiated by migration studies. For example, Australia and New Zealand are areas of high incidence of the disease. The incidence in people who emigrated to the region from less sunny climates is lower in people who were over 15 years old when they arrived than in younger immigrants.

Individual habits of sun exposure also affect the risks of contracting the disease. Other sources of UV radiation include artificial tanning devices such as sunlamps or sunbeds. Epidemiological studies demonstrate a moderate increase in risk of melanoma in sunlamp and sunbed users: the common supposition that artificial tanning serves as protection against the effects of later sun exposure is not substantiated. Relative risks range from 1.5 to 8 for all ages, increasing with frequency of sunbed use.

The incidence of malignant melanoma is 10–12 times higher in light-skinned people than in dark-skinned people in the same geographical location with similar lifestyles. This is because melanin protects the vulnerable cells situated in the basal (deepest) layer of the epidermis.

Action of UV

A cell must sustain damage to its DNA before it becomes cancerous (see Chapter 13). The principal effect of UV on DNA is to alter the nucleotide bases, leading to the formation of pyrimidine dimers and pyrimidone photoproducts. Normally these changes are recognised by the cell and repaired. The precise circumstances that cause a failure of repair are not known but could include a failure of apoptosis (see Chapter 4). It is also not entirely clear which regions of DNA are most likely to lead to tumour transformation once they become damaged, although the most obvious contenders are the proto-oncogenes and tumour suppressor genes.

Early and intermittent exposure to UV represents the greatest danger

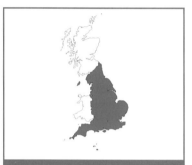

HEALTH OF THE NATION

Targets for skin cancer

▲ Halt the year-on-year increase in the incidence of skin cancer by the year 2005. Measures to achieve this might include:

▲ Increase the number of people who are aware of their own risk factors for skin cancer

▲ Persuade people at high risk to avoid excessive exposure to the sun and artificial UV sources, for themselves and their children

▲ Secure an alteration in attitude towards a tanned appearance

Genetic factors

Some people affected by malignant melanoma have a family history of the disease, although this is not a prerequisite. The genetic linkage appears to involve inheritance of naevi with a tendency towards dysplasia. Dysplastic naevi are strongly implicated as precursor lesions in melanoma.

> *Only about 10% of melanoma cases have a family history of the disease or naevus lesions*

Previous melanoma

Patients who have a skin melanoma are at increased risk of developing a further primary cancer. In one survey of patients in Scotland the prevalence of a second melanoma was about 1.2%, which represents a 200-fold increase in risk. In some patients the separate melanomas were found concurrently, but in others the time between the diagnosis of first and second tumours was up to 2 years. Some patients have been seen to present over time with five or six primary tumours.

Prognosis

The prognosis for a patient who has malignant melanoma depends on the depth of tumour invasion, measured in a histological section of the excised tumour as the **Breslow thickness**. The measurement is made from the deepest level of malignant cells up to the epidermal granular layer (Figure 5.9).

- In 1979, about 39% of treated patients had melanomas of less than 1.5 mm thick, with 93% survival at 5 years
- About 30% had melanomas 1.5–3.5 mm thick, with 67% survival at 5 years
- About 31% had melanomas thicker than 3.5 mm, with 37% survival at 5 years.

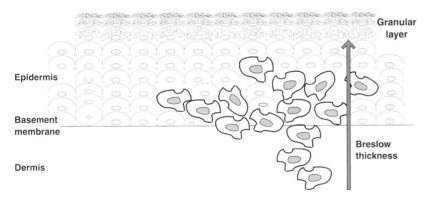

Figure 5.9 Determination of Breslow thickness in malignant melanoma. Malignant cells spread both horizontally and vertically. The Breslow thickness is measured from the base of the tumour cell deposit to the granular layer of the epidermis.

Review question 2

What actions would you advise people to take to reduce skin cancer risks?

Treatment of malignant melanoma

The treatment for malignant melanoma usually comprises a wide-margin surgical excision, often requiring skin grafting and lymph node resection. This may be supplemented with chemotherapy. Clearly, the sooner treatment is implemented the greater the chance of a successful outcome.

ANSWERS TO REVIEW QUESTIONS

Question 1

Why are animal experiments often unreliable for determining the toxicity of a chemical?

It is not always possible to extrapolate effects seen in one species to another. An example is the different LD_{50} values obtained for the same chemical in different species. Very often the difference lies in the types and amounts of liver enzymes that work to detoxify the chemical. The same is true of cancer induction: a chemical that causes tumours in a mouse may not produce tumours in a rat, and vice versa. Very often the circumstances of exposure in animals differ from those that might be encountered in humans. Typically, animals are given oral doses of the agent over a set period of time. Human exposures are usually much more haphazard and, in ordinary circumstances, do not approach the quantities necessary to induce an effect in animals.

Question 2

What actions would you advise people to take to reduce skin cancer risks?

Reducing the risks associated with skin cancer comprises primary prevention and vigilance. The main primary prevention measure is to minimise exposure to strong sunlight, particularly in the late morning and early afternoon. Clothing is usually an effective sunscreen although this will depend on the tightness of the weave. A broad-brimmed hat is good protection for the face. Sunscreens should be applied at regular intervals and after bathing. Small children and infants should be protected at all times. Sunlamps and sunbeds should be avoided.

Be on the look out for any skin changes – early diagnosis of malignant melanoma markedly improves the chances of survival. The signs are changes in size, shape or colour of pigmented skin lesions. Other signs to look out for are inflammation, change in sensation, crusting or bleeding.

References

Gardner, M.J., Snee, M.P., Hall, A.J. *et al.* (1990) Results of a case-control study of leukaemia and lymphoma among young people near Sellafield nuclear plant in West Cumbria. *BMJ*, **300**, 423–9.

Kinlen, L.J. (1993) Can paternal preconceptual radiation account for the increase of leukaemia and non-Hodgkin's lymphoma in Seascale? *BMJ*, **306**, 1718–21.

Kinlen L.J., Dickinson, M. and Stiller, C.A. Childhood leukaemia and non-Hodgkin's lymphoma near large rural construction sites, with a comparison with Sellafield nuclear site. *BMJ*, **310**, 763–8.

Olsen, J., Nielsen, A. and Schulgen, G. (1993) Residence near high voltage facilities and risk of cancer in children. *BMJ*, **307**, 891–5.

Further reading

Austoker, J. (1994) Melanoma: prevention and early diagnosis. *BMJ*, **308**, 1682-6.

Bowie, C. and Bowie, S.H.U. (1991) Radon and health. *Lancet*, **337**, 409-13.

British Medical Association. (1992) *The BMA Guide to Pesticides, Chemicals and Health*, Edward Arnold, London.

Brooks, S.M., Gochfeld, M., Hertzstein, J. *et al.* (eds) (1995) *Environmental Medicine*, Mosby, St Louis.

Fumento, M. (1993) *Science Under Siege. Balancing Technology and the Environment*, William Morrow, New York.

London S.J., Thomas D.C., Bowman J.D., *et al.* (1991) Exposure to residential electric and magnetic fields and risk of childhood leukaemia. *Am. J. Epidemiol.*, **134**, 925–6.

Morrison, H.I., Wilkins, K., Semenciw, R. *et al.* (1992) Herbicides and cancer. *J. Natl. Cancer Inst.*, **84**, 1867–1974.

Risky, R.A. *et al.* (1987) Benzene and leukaemia: an epidemiological risk assessment. *N. Engl. J. Med.*, **316**, 1044.

6   Infectious diseases

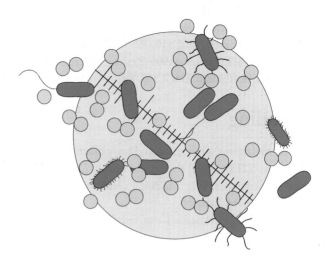

Infectious diseases are major causes of morbidity and mortality throughout the world. In developed countries, improvements in sanitation and general living conditions have reduced the burden of illness and deaths from infectious diseases. Medical advances such as vaccination and the availability of antibiotics have also had a significant impact. In the less developed countries the prevailing economic circumstances have impaired improvements in living conditions and the means to prevent or treat life-threatening infectious diseases. Diarrhoeal disease, tuberculosis, and HIV/AIDS are the most pressing public health problems in less developed countries.

Many micro-organisms inhabit the human body and cause disease only when resistance is low because of other disease states, or when natural barriers have been broken down by disease or trauma. Other micro-organisms are present in the external environment and are taken into the body through food, water, air or bodily contact.

Once inside the body micro-organisms must evade an array of defences. Some achieve this by invading the cells themselves and effectively become 'out of range' of the defence mechanisms unless the cell is destroyed as well. Other micro-organisms, staying outside cells, have greater scope to spread and multiply but are more vulnerable to specific and non-specific defence mechanisms. All infectious micro-organisms damage cells or disrupt their function, although the outcome may vary. Most infections cause necrosis but some can cause cell proliferation, albeit of abnormal cells. Most significantly, the inflammatory response to infection is often the cause of some symptoms, and can contribute to death from the infection.

Attempts to limit the spread of infectious micro-organisms by vaccination or antibiotic treatment have met with spectacular success in many cases, but genetic mutation of the organisms can render these measures ineffective.

Pre-test

- What are the most common infectious diseases in developed and less developed countries?
- How can infectious diseases be prevented?
- What are the main ways of treating infectious diseases?

Aims of this chapter

By the end of this chapter you should have increased your knowledge of:
- The types of micro-organisms responsible for causing infectious diseases
- Microbial modes of transmission, the body defences involved in resisting infection and microbial adaptation to these defences
- Interventions designed to prevent or control infection

In addition, this chapter will help you to:
- Discuss the sources of infection and how micro-organisms enter the body
- Describe the ways in which the body can defend itself against infection
- Describe the ways in which micro-organisms are adapted to evade the body's natural defences
- Discuss the rationale and application of preventive measures and treatments designed to limit the impact of infectious disease

Introduction

It is estimated that there are more micro-organisms in the human body than there are cells. For the most part the relationship is harmless and may even be advantageous; bacteria in the gut, for instance, break down indigestible food components which can then be absorbed and used. Unfortunately, in some circumstances these normally harmless micro-organisms cause damage and disease and many other micro-organisms, not normally resident in the body, attempt to invade the body, causing damage which can be life-threatening. Any invasion or abnormal growth pattern of micro-organisms which causes an adverse reaction is an **infection**.

Infectious micro-organisms are of four principal groups: **bacteria, viruses, protozoa** and **fungi**. Most of these organisms (except viruses and some protozoa) are capable of independent existence and can replicate using their own DNA and cellular systems. Although viruses contain their own genetic material in the form of DNA or RNA, they must use the DNA and other replicative machinery of the host cell to generate new copies. A further category of infectious agent are the class of proteins that cause **prion** diseases. These remain extremely rare in humans, but have attracted widespread publicity, particularly because of the possible hazards to human health posed by bovine spongiform encephalopathy (BSE).

In the developed countries infectious diseases are more likely to be seen as acute illnesses, many of which are curable with antibiotics or preventable with vaccines and hygienic measures. However, there are many infectious agents that cause chronic and incurable disease. The prime example of this is HIV.

In less developed countries diarrhoeal diseases, malaria, measles, amoebiasis, pertussis (whooping cough), schistosomiasis, tuberculosis, poliomyelitis and HIV infection are the main causes of illness and death.

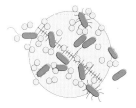

Word-wide, infectious diseases remain the most common causes of morbidity and mortality

Microbiology: the study of organisms that are microscopic in size. The smallest micro-organisms are the viruses, which can be seen only under the electron microscope. Bacteria, fungi and protozoa can all be seen under the light microscope, although special staining methods are usually required for their visualisation.

Bacterial infection

Bacteria (prokaryotes): cellular organisms containing DNA and a thick, protective cell wall. They have no distinct nucleus, their DNA being in the form of a single, circular chromosome. Additional DNA is contained within plasmids. The cytoplasm is rich in ribosomes, but membrane-bound organelles such as mitochondria and Golgi complex, which characterise eukaryote cells, are absent.

Bacteria are ubiquitous organisms. Of the many thousands of bacterial species most are harmless, but disease-causing bacteria have probably been responsible for more human deaths and disease than any other cause.

Historically, bacterial infections have been responsible for devastating effects in human populations. For example, epidemics of plague (caused by the rod-shaped bacterium *Yersinia pestis*) in the fourteenth century were responsible for reducing the population of Europe by at least a quarter. Nowadays plague is relatively rare, but bacterial infections are still a common cause of morbidity and death, mainly from respiratory and diarrhoeal diseases.

Bacteria are classified into several major types, based on their shape and staining properties. **Bacilli** are rod-shaped organisms, **cocci** are round or oval. Others, called **spirochaetes**, are curved or corkscrew-shaped. Bacteria can be separated by their staining properties with Gram's stain. **Gram-positive** bacteria have a thick external polysaccharide coating which retains the crystal violet dye used in Gram's stain, while **Gram-negative** bacteria stain pink by a relatively non-specific neutral red counterstain.

Viruses and disease

A single type of virus can produce several disease outcomes, depending on the host response and presence of cofactors

Burkitt's lymphoma: a B-cell lymphoma, endemic in Africa, affecting the jaw, ovaries and gastrointestinal tract.

Nasopharyngeal carcinoma: commonly seen in China (particularly in people of Mongolian race), Hong Kong, Philippines, Malaysia, Greenland, Malta, North Africa and Saudi Arabia. Common epidemiological features are infection with EBV, together with high consumption of salted fish and vegetables. Most tumours are anaplastic squamous cell carcinomas but up to 30% of cases are of non-squamous origin (e.g. malignant lymphomas).

Viruses: contain genetic material (DNA or RNA) packed in a protein capsule. They lack cell membranes and cytoplasm, and the machinery for synthesising macromolecules. Viruses must live within host cells.

Everyone in the world will at some time be infected by a virus, even if only that causing the common cold. Common viral infections include influenza, measles, mumps, rubella, cytomegalovirus (CMV), Epstein–Barr virus (EBV), hepatitis B virus (HBV) and human immunodeficiency virus (HIV).

There are remarkable differences in the outcomes of viral infection. Virtually everyone infected by measles becomes unwell and develops characteristic symptoms. Other viruses, such as cytomegalovirus, rarely cause symptoms (humans are the natural host for CMV) but immunosuppressed individuals may develop pneumonia and infection during pregnancy can cause fetal abnormalities. Yet other viruses produce outcomes ranging from asymptomatic carrier status to cancer.

Infections with EBV occur throughout the world, and are often asymptomatic if they occur in early childhood. Older children and young adults are more likely to become unwell, usually from infectious mononucleosis (glandular fever). In some parts of the world, various cofactors operate with a virus to cause more serious outcomes. Most notably, in African children human papillomavirus infection causes Burkitt's lymphoma, which generally follows a geographical distribution coincident with malaria. It was first believed that, like malaria, the disease was transmitted by mosquitoes but is now known that malaria is itself an important cofactor for EBV. This virus is also believed to be responsible for nasopharyngeal carcinoma (a cancer common in south-east Asia), probably in association with as yet unidentified cofactors. In addition, EBV has been incriminated as a causative factor in certain cases of Hodgkin's disease, probably acting in concert with (so far unidentified) cofactors.

Efforts are being made to develop a vaccine against EBV, with the aim of preventing Burkitt's lymphoma and nasopharyngeal carcinoma. One vaccine, derived from the virus envelope protein, has been shown to prevent EBV-associated tumours in marmosets and clinical trials in humans are currently under way.

Another viral infection that can cause different clinical outcomes is HBV. Millions of people, particularly in the less developed countries, carry the virus without experiencing any ill effect. However, in some individuals the infection causes chronic liver disease or primary liver cancer (hepatocellular carcinoma). Most carriers are infected at birth or in infancy. It is estimated that HBV carriers are 200 times more likely to die from primary liver cancer than non-infected individuals. Efforts are being made to reduce the burden of chronic liver disease and cancer by means of vaccination. An infant immunisation programme is in place in some parts of the world. Unfortunately, it is now evident that a mutant form of the virus has emerged that is not neutralised by the vaccine-induced immune response.

Other viruses do not produce such a broad range of responses. An example is HIV infection which almost invariably leads to immunodeficiency and the onset of AIDS (see Chapter 25). Although there are some long-term survivors of HIV infection who have not yet developed AIDS, for the most part the only individual variation is the time it takes for immunodeficiency to develop.

There are three types of interaction between viruses and cells. The most common is **cell death**. For example, loss of CD4+ lymphocytes is associated with HIV infection; other viral infections, such as herpes simplex and chickenpox, cause epithelial cell death, which is manifest as skin blistering or mucosal lesions. The spread of rabies and polio viruses along nerves kills the nerve cells.

A second response is **cell proliferation**. This occurs in human papillomavirus (HPV) infections, causing a wart-like overgrowth in the cervical epithelium. Viruses can also remain dormant in cells, to be **reactivated** by stress to cause cell death. Shingles is caused by reactivation of herpes zoster lying dormant in the dorsal root ganglia. The reactivated virus travels down the peripheral nerves to the skin where it causes a blistering rash. Herpes simplex behaves in a similar way, causing cold sores when it becomes reactivated.

Fungal infections

Fungi are present in the environment and as **commensals** on the skin and mucosal surfaces. Most types are not pathogenic unless the individual becomes immunosuppressed. The growth of fungi in humans can remain superficial, but some can invade deep organs and tissues – these are very difficult to eliminate and infections are very often life-threatening.

Three types of fungal organism are capable of causing disease in humans – moulds, true yeasts and yeast-like fungi. The principal fungi of pathological significance are dermatophytes (infect skin), *Candida albicans* (infects mucosal

Commensal: organism that normally inhabits the body, usually without causing disease. Extensive normal flora are found in the skin and gut.

surfaces but can cause systemic infections), *Aspergillus* species (cause lung and systemic infections), *Cryptococcus* (infects lung and brain) and *Histoplasma* (lung infections).

Moulds

Moulds grow as long filamentous structures which intertwine to form a mycelium. Examples of moulds are the dermatophytes and *Aspergillus* species. Typical conditions caused by dermatophytes are tinea (ringworm) and athlete's foot. These are treated with topical antifungal agents. More serious is **aspergillosis**, a lung infection caused by inhalation of *Aspergillus* species, which mainly occurs in immunocompromised individuals. Infection causes an allergic inflammatory reaction, leading to extensive thrombosis and necrosis once the pulmonary blood vessels have been invaded.

True yeasts

The yeasts are unicellular round or oval fungi. *Cryptococcus neoformans*, for example, causes meningitis and pulmonary infections in immunocompromised individuals. The organism is common in soils where there are bird droppings. Infections can arise from the inhalation of airborne cells. The main treatments are with amphotericin and flucytosine.

Yeast-like fungi

As their description suggests, the yeast-like fungi are similar to yeast but, under certain conditions, form long non-branching filaments. The most common example is *Candida albicans*, a commensal organism of the gut, mouth and vagina. It becomes pathogenic in individuals who are stressed, immunosuppressed or taking antibiotics, causing oral thrush, vaginitis, endocarditis and even fatal septicaemia. Candidiasis is treated with oral and topical antifungal agents such as nystatin and miconazole. Amphotericin and flucytosine are used for systemic disease.

Protozoa

Eukaryotes: all cellular organisms other than bacteria. Characterised by DNA organised into chromosomes within a nucleus, a cell or plasma membrane and membrane-bound cytoplasmic organelles.

The protozoa are single-celled **eukaryotes**. Some are free-living, but others are parasites of humans and other species. They live as intracellular parasites in a variety of cells or as extracellular parasites in the blood, intestines or urogenital system. Protozoa can reproduce asexually, which is one reason for their pathogenicity: very large numbers can be produced, particularly when host defence mechanisms are impaired.

These micro-organisms are classified by their morphology and adaptation for movement. The **sporozoa** are generally non-motile intracellular parasites and include *Plasmodium* species which inhabit red blood cells and cause malaria.

The **flagellates** move by beating one or more flagellae. These micro-organisms include *Trypanosoma*, a cause of sleeping sickness, and *Trichomonas vaginalis*, a cause of vaginitis and urethritis. The **amoebae** move by extending pseudopodia and have no fixed shape. Most notable among these is *Entamoeba histolytica*, the cause of amoebic dysentery. Another protozoan, not classified under these headings, that has assumed increasing medical importance is *Pneumocystis carinii*. This organism causes the AIDS-defining condition *Pneumocystis carinii* pneumonia (see Chapter 25).

Prion disease

Prion disease refers to the transmissible spongiform encephalopathies of animals and humans, for example, scrapie in sheep, bovine spongiform encephalopathy (BSE) in cattle (popularly known as 'mad cow disease') and Creutzfeldt–Jakob disease (CJD) and kuru disease in humans. A common feature of these conditions is the brain pathology, termed spongiform encephalopathy, in which neurons are destroyed and spaces appear in the brain tissue (microscopic vacuolation). These changes become evident as ataxia and dementia.

At one time these conditions were believed to be caused by a slow-acting virus, but it is now considered that their development involves the presence of an abnormal brain protein. The protein, termed prion protein (PrP), is coded by a single copy gene on chromosome 20 in humans. Its function is unknown, but the abnormal form of the protein (PrP^{Sc}) can transform normal cellular host protein (PrP^{C}) into abnormal protein, which then leads to the death of brain cells.

The infectivity of the disease agent has been shown by injection or dietary exposure of brain extracts from cases of spongiform encephalopathy into animals. Unlike other infectious agents prions contain no genetic material and, because the protein is naturally occurring, it elicits no immune response. The traditional approaches to controlling infectious diseases, such as vaccination or antibiotic therapy, are therefore inappropriate.

Focus on CJD and BSE

The possible relationship between human prion disease and BSE has been the subject of intense media speculation and public concern. At the time of writing most countries had banned the import of British beef and, following a series of controls to halt the use of animal remains in cattle feed and the use of offal for human consumption, a limited cull of cattle commenced in the UK. Most of these measures have been taken against a background of limited scientific evidence.

Creutzfeldt-Jakob disease

Most cases of CJD occur sporadically, with an annual incidence rate of about 1 in a million in most populations. This type accounts for 85% of cases and

---

Prion diseases are caused by an abnormal brain protein

Ataxia: lack of motor co-ordination.

Creutzfeldt–Jakob disease: a spongiform encephalopathy that usually begins in the sixth or seventh decade of life with loss of memory, progressing to dementia over the course of a few weeks. Death usually occurs within 6 months.

Kuru: a prion disease recognised in the 1950s as epidemic in some parts of Papua New Guinea. Transmitted by cannibalistic rituals involving consumption of human brain.

Prion protein: occurs naturally in all adult vertebrates but mutant forms cause death of brain cells. The protein is normally present on the surface of neurons and neuroglia but its function is not known. It is resistant to ionising and UV radiation and to protease enzymes. Infectivity of the protein can be reduced only by solvent treatment or extreme heat. The disease-related protein is believed to differ from the normal protein by a change in shape.

CJD occurs in sporadic, inherited and acquired forms

usually occurs in people who are over the age of 50, with a mean age of onset of 65 years. There is also an inherited form of CJD caused by point mutations or insertions in the prion gene. Another means of contracting the disease is injection of nervous tissue from affected individuals. This occurred in people who had been treated with growth hormone extracted from human pituitary glands from the late 1950s – until 1985, following reports of deaths of patients similarly treated in the USA. Soon after this, a genetically engineered version of human growth hormone became available, eliminating the possibility of contamination by prion protein. Other ways of contracting CJD are from corneal transplants and from use of inadequately sterilised instruments in neurosurgical procedures. The acquired form of the disease is also known as **iatrogenic CJD**.

Both the **sporadic** and iatrogenic forms of CJD are more likely to occur in genetically susceptible people. Genetic susceptibility is conferred by a polymorphism in the prion protein, with either methionine or valine present at residue 129. About 38% of Caucasians are homozygous for the methionine residue, 51% are heterozygotes and 11% are homozygotes for valine. The large majority of sporadic and iatrogenic CJD cases are in homozygotes, with more methionine homozygotes in CJD and more valine homozygotes in kuru. Presumably, the primary structure (amino acid sequence) of the prion protein is an important attribute for conversion of normal forms into the abnormal form. This will be most efficient when there is a complete match in primary structure.

The initial concern about a possible link between BSE and human prion disease arose after four cases of CJD were reported in dairy farmers in the UK. In 1995–1996 a new form of prion disease became apparent, in which the people affected were much younger (average age 27 years), the duration of illness was longer (average 13 months) and damage to brain tissues much more extensive. The initial symptoms in these new cases bore a great similarity to kuru, in which progressive ataxia and behavioural change predominate, rather than to the dementing illness of sporadic CJD. At the time of writing (mid 1996) only 14 cases of this new type of CJD referred to as **vCJD**, have been reported. Of particular concern is the possibility that these cases have been caused by exposure to BSE-infected beef.

Bovine spongiform encephalopathy

There has been an epidemic of BSE in the UK, which is believed to have originated from feed contaminated with the remains of sheep infected by scrapie. This has not been proven as a source of the disease and indeed the discontinued use of the feed has not been accompanied by as large a fall in the incidence of BSE as expected, raising the possibility of horizontal (between animals) or vertical (from cow to calf) transmission.

BSE was first identified in 1986 and several hundred thousand cattle are known to have had the disease. Early measures to control the outbreak comprised a ban on the use of animal remains in cattle feed (introduced in 1988), changing the feed type and, to protect the human population, a ban on the use of specified offal from cows (introduced in 1989). In some of the other European countries, in which BSE is much less common, the more vigorous approach to control of the disease was to cull the whole herd if a case of BSE occurred.

Currently the link between BSE and human prion disease remains tenuous. At best, epidemiological studies can yield no more than circumstantial evidence because most people have at some time in their lives been exposed to beef or beef products. None of the cases of CJD had any features suggesting excessive dietary or occupational exposure. The apparent increase in susceptibility of younger people remains unexplained.

The possibility that prion disease could spread to humans from other species can never be directly proved, because this would require the deliberate inoculation of humans with the prion agent. The scientific evidence hinges on showing the differences and similarities in prion proteins and genetics in different species. Undoubtedly, abnormal prions and disease can be introduced in experimental animals when inoculated with scrapie, BSE or CJD-infected brain tissue but the 'species barrier' must be overcome. This is evident in that only a small proportion of animals become affected, and only then after a prolonged incubation period which often approaches the life expectancy of the animal. The species barrier appears to be determined by differences in primary structures (and gene nucleotide sequence) of the prion proteins. The closer the similarity the greater the prospects for transmission.

There is no direct evidence that human prion disease can be triggered by exposure to BSE-infected meat

Different strains of prion protein exist in different species

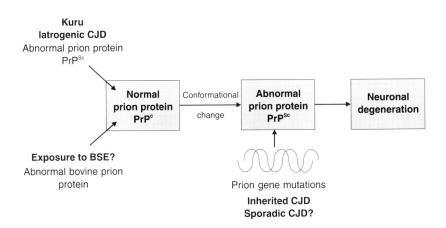

Figure 6.1 Postulated mechanisms in prion disease. The development of prion disease is believed to involve production of an abnormal prion protein (PrP^SC) or conversion of a normal protein (PrP^C) into the abnormal form. In the autosomal dominant inherited form of CJD mutations in the prion gene lead directly to the production of abnormal protein. It is possible that some sporadic cases may have been caused by similar mutations in somatic cells, occurring in later life. Exposure to abnormal prion protein in iatrogenic CJD may induce the normal protein to change conformation into the abnormal form and result in disease. The abnormal BSE prion protein may act in a similar way. This is probably a very inefficient method of conversion because of species differences in the structure of the prion proteins.

The gene nucleotide sequence for the prion protein found in cattle closely resembles that found in sheep. It would therefore not be surprising to find that cattle can be affected by scrapie-infected material. The human prion gene differs in most aspects from the bovine variant, but there are similarities, most notably in the area where human mutations, which are known to lead directly to prion disease, occur.

One way around the problem of the species barrier is to use **transgenic** animals. Transgenic mice that can express human PrP^{Sc} have not so far (after 1 year) produced PrP^{Sc} when challenged with BSE-infected material. Unfortunately, it is still too early to draw definitive conclusions because a longer incubation time than this may be necessary.

> **Transgenic:** an organism that contains genetic material artificially introduced into its genome from another species.

There is some evidence from animal studies that the species 'strain' of the original prion inoculum persists after replication in other species. Another approach, therefore, would be to type the prion protein in the vCJD cases to see if it matches that of the BSE strain. The indications are that, indeed, vCJD prion protein bears a greater similarity to BSE-extracted material than it does to the protein in sporadic CJD. These findings are based, not on any differences in the basic chemical make-up of the proteins, but on differences in their shape and consequential ability to attach to sugar molecules. Most prion proteins have two sugar molecules attached, but both vCJD and BSE prions have two attached sugar groups. Although not definitive proof, the finding supports the theory that there is a link between BSE and vCJD.

It is postulated that if vCJD is the result of BSE exposure then the condition must have been acquired during the mid-1980s when BSE became common and before the offal ban was introduced. This implies an incubation period of about 10 years or so. The shortest known incubation period for kuru is about 4.5 years, but the disease can take up to 30 years to develop. The average incubation time in recipients of contaminated growth hormone was 15 years and it is therefore possible that the 14 vCJD cases are the first sign of an impending epidemic of human prion disease in the UK.

At the time of writing it is unlikely that many health care professionals will encounter human prion disease and, apart from the economic and psychological consequences of the current concern shown by the general public and the media, it does not represent a significant public health risk. In that sense, the amount of space devoted to the topic in this book is unjustified – it is hoped that it will not be necessary to devote a whole full chapter to the subject in a future edition.

> *The provision of a safe and reliable supply of drinking water is one of the most important public health measures that can be taken*

Sources of infection

Micro-organisms enter the body through air, food, water or by contact with body secretions. The organism may exist freely in these media and be transmitted on exposure to the particular medium, or may use other biological species as **vectors** for transmission. Some infections are caused by commensal organisms, which become pathogenic because of a change in the host environment – for example, another disease that results in immunosuppression. Commensals can also become a problem when natural barriers are breached by injury or invasive pathological processes such as ulceration or malignancy.

Water-borne diseases are usually spread by the faecal–oral route – water contaminated by faecal matter from humans or animals is transferred to a new host by ingestion. Infections are more common in the less developed countries where sanitation and water treatment facilities are poor but can also be acquired from food sources such as oysters, clams, cockles and mussels which survive in polluted water and concentrate pathogens by filter feeding.

Food-borne infections can be contracted from any food that has not been preserved or isolated from potential sources of contamination. Even after thorough cooking, food is not necessarily safe unless proper hygiene precautions have been observed. Hygiene is particularly important for food handlers who have had an infection and who remain carriers.

Many kinds of organisms enter the respiratory system by inhalation of airborne droplets. Not surprisingly, the diseases they cause often involve the respiratory tract. Occasionally, symptoms in the respiratory tract are minimal, and the main impact of the infection is felt elsewhere following spread of the organism through the blood or lymphatic systems.

Organisms can be secreted in the body fluids of an infected person and spread by direct contact with those fluids. This is the mechanism by which sexually transmitted diseases are spread, but blood and blood products represent a risk if they are transfused or if contaminated needles are used.

Infectivity: ability to breach host defences.

Transmissibility: ease by which the organism can travel from its reservoir or host to a new host.

Virulence: the capacity of an organism to harm the host. This can be expressed as the number of micro-organisms necessary to cause death in 50% of individuals (the LD_{50}).

Sites of entry

All parts of the body are vulnerable to infection through bodily orifices and through the skin itself. In some infections the causative organisms remain close to the original site of entry (dermatophytes, for example) and do not spread to deeper body tissues. However, they can still be a threat to life because their spread can involve a considerable proportion of the body surface (in the respiratory tract, for example). Other micro-organisms spread throughout the body through the blood or lymphatic circulations.

Whether or not a micro-organism causes disease once it enters the body depends on several factors intrinsic to the organism and to the host. In many cases organisms enter the body and are eliminated without the host becoming aware of the event. In other circumstances entry of the organism causes an inflammatory response, evident as a slight increase in temperature and malaise and in others the organism induces acute symptoms of fever, malaise and headache, infection being followed by long-term complications. The ability of an organism to cause disease is referred to as its **pathogenicity**, and depends on the attributes of **transmissibility, infectivity, virulence** and its ability to survive in the host in the face of an array of defence mechanisms. Many bacteria possess cell wall components and capsules that enable them to resist host defences. They can also penetrate tissues by secretion of enzymes, and adhere to the tissue by means of specific glycoprotein or lipoprotein molecules (**adhesins**) that bind to receptors on host cells. Some bacteria have brush-like processes called **fimbriae** that allow them to adhere to the surfaces of other cells.

Skin infections

> *The skin is most vulnerable to infection at the site of wounds, abrasions or burns*

Superficial infections can be established on unbroken skin. This applies to various fungi (the **dermatophytes**) which can infect the keratin layer, particularly in or around the hair and nails. Some bacteria are able to gain access through hair follicles and sebaceous glands and some to bore through the skin and find their way into the blood circulation.

Protozoan infections

The blood fluke *Schistosoma*, the causative organism of **schistosomiasis** (bilharzia), swims in water and can penetrate the skin of a person who wades or swims in infested water. The fluke then enters the bloodstream and is carried to veins of the liver or bladder where it lays its eggs. From the liver and bladder it burrows to other organs, especially the gastrointestinal tract. The eggs cause inflammation and haemorrhage as they pass through the wall of the bladder or bowel. Some of the eggs are excreted in human faeces and can contaminate water supplies. After hatching in water, the organism's life cycle is completed in water snails. Schistosomiasis is very common in Asia, Africa, South America and the Caribbean, affecting up to 200 million people.

An example of a parasite that is deposited in the skin by means of an insect bite is **malaria**, caused by *Plasmodium vivax* and transmitted to the human host by the bite of an infected mosquito. Infection causes acute symptoms of chills, fever, vomiting and severe headache. The malaria parasite replicates in the liver and inside red blood cells, eventually releasing male and female sexual forms (gametocytes) into the blood. These can become lodged in the tissues, causing a granulomatous reaction. Granulomas can interfere with blood flow, leading to portal hypertension and enlargement of the spleen and liver (hepatosplenomegaly). It is estimated that malaria affects about 300 million people world-wide and kills 2–4 million people each year, most of whom are young children.

Another vector-borne disease in which an infective organism penetrates the skin is **Lyme disease**. The condition was first reported in 1975; young people living near the city of Lyme, Connecticut, developed symptoms similar to rheumatoid arthritis. The disease is caused by the spirochaete *Borrelia burgdorferi* and is transmitted by a tick, which becomes infected during its larval stage after taking a blood meal from field mice or other small animals. Lyme disease occurs in many parts of the USA, Europe and Australia. The condition first appears as a rash, which in most patients has a characteristic 'bull's-eye' appearance. This is followed by influenza-like symptoms as the rash fades. Antibiotics at this stage are very effective at limiting progression of the disease. The next stage follows weeks or months later, with neurological symptoms (facial paralysis, meningitis, encephalitis) and heart problems. Arthritis, with erosion of cartilage and bone, follows and can affect the patient for many years.

Bacterial infections

Some common bacterial infections of skin involve commensal organisms. The main culprits are *Staphylococcus aureus* and *Staphylococcus epidermidis*. These organisms can cause relatively superficial infections by invading the hair follicles. Invasion is followed by an inflammatory reaction and the formation of small abscesses or boils. These are well demarcated by a layer of fibroblasts which helps to prevent further spread of the organism. If several hair follicles are affected the abscesses merge to form a **carbuncle**. These can become necrotic in the middle which causes them to detach, leaving a large ulcer and a disfiguring scar. More serious infections can arise after the skin is cut or abraded. The greatest risk is attached to accidental wounds, but surgical wounds are not exempt from infection. So-called 'dirty' wounds are often contaminated by organisms, or their spores, that are normally present in soil and dust. The organism does not need to have invasive properties of its own, but takes advantage of the break in the physical barrier, as well as the physiological consequences of injury.

For example, the causative organism of **tetanus**, *Clostridium tetani*, has no invasive properties, and grows in a wound that is depleted of oxygen because of tissue damage. When infection occurs the organism mostly remains in its original site, but causes damage by the production of a neurotoxin. The toxin is absorbed from the site of production and is transmitted to the central nervous system by the motor nerves, causing paralysis. Initially the muscles of the jaw are affected (hence the name 'lockjaw') but muscle spasm extends to other skeletal muscles causing impaired respiration, inability to swallow and urinary retention. About 25% of patients die through respiratory failure or cardiac arrest.

Clostridium perfringens causes **gas gangrene** in dirty ischaemic wounds, but unlike *Clostridium tetani* this organism has invasive properties, producing toxins that cause further tissue damage, impairing the blood supply and maintaining anaerobic conditions.

Hospital-acquired infections

Breaks in the skin and mucosal surfaces often act as the portals of entry for hospital-acquired infections (also called **nosocomial** infections). About 10% of patients admitted for hospital treatment acquire an infection.

The condition which brought the patient to the hospital in the first place can increase their susceptibility to infection: people who are old, very young and have pre-existing disease are usually more vulnerable. Generally, the more invasive the procedures required to investigate or treat a patient the greater the risk of infection.

Staphylococci: bacteria particularly associated with the skin as commensals. Differentiated on the basis of a test for coagulase (an enzyme that clots plasma). *Staphylococcus aureus* exhibits coagulase positivity and all other staphylococci are negative. Resistance to β-lactam antibiotics is an increasing problem in combating staphylococcal infection.

Clostridium tetani: occurs in the gastrointestinal tract of humans and animals. Spores, derived from animal droppings, are often found in soil and dust. Infection is usually through a wound that in itself appears to be inconsequential. Germination of the spores is favoured by anoxia and tissue damage. Tetanus is caused by a powerful neurotoxin elaborated by the organism, producing neuromuscular blockade and muscle spasm.

Gas gangrene: *Clostridium perfringens* proliferates in subcutaneous tissues producing gas and anaerobic cellulitis (an acute spreading infection of the skin). Progresses rapidly and is fatal unless all affected tissue is excised (amputation may be necessary).

Cholera: caused by *Vibrio cholerae*, which produces a toxin that disrupts water uptake by cells lining the intestine (enterocytes). The enterocytes are undamaged, but severe dehydration can cause hypovolaemic shock and heart failure. Initial symptoms are a severe, non-bloody, watery diarrhoea. Left untreated, the mortality rate is 40–60%, but prospects are markedly improved if fluids can be replaced without delay.

Diarrhoea: abnormal faecal discharge characterised by frequent watery, loose stools. Usually results from disease or infection in the small intestine and involves increased loss of fluid and electrolytes.

Salmonella: the strain and source of salmonella can be determined by serotyping and phage typing. At one time the most common serotype in the UK was *S. typhimurium*, but the most recent rise in salmonellosis is attributable to *S. enteritidis* phage type 4. Infections were mostly caused by consumption of poultry and hens' eggs. The risk of salmonella food poisoning can be reduced by eliminating the organism at source, by careful handling at all stages in the distribution chain, and by thorough cooking.

Typhoid fever: caused by *Salmonella typhi*, producing symptoms of fever, enlarged spleen and diarrhoea. Infection spreads from the gastrointestinal tract first to the blood and lymphatics and then to other parts of the body. Because the organism survives in macrophages infections of the spleen, bone marrow, lymph nodes, liver and Peyer's patches in the gut are common. The organism is resistant to bile and survives in the gallbladder, acting as a source of reinfection of the gut. About 40% of infected individuals die if the condition is untreated.

> *Salmonellae cause diarrhoea by adhering to the gut wall and initiating inflammation*

Sources of infection may be another person in the hospital (**cross-infection**), or a contaminated piece of equipment (**environmental** infection). The most common nosocomial infections are of the urinary tract, usually arising from urinary catheterisation. Wound infections typically occur in 5–10% of surgical patients, but infection rates can be higher after operations involving the colon or limb amputation. Infections involving the blood, particularly bacterial or fungal, can be introduced by intravenous catheterisation.

Gastrointestinal tract infections

As might be expected, one of the main consequences of infection in the gastrointestinal tract is diarrhoeal disease. However, penetration of organisms through the mucosa can result in spread by the blood and lymphatics, leading to systemic effects (see Table 6.1). Occasionally, the inflammation produced in the wall of the gut in response to infection leads to ulceration and perforation. The source of infection is most commonly food and water, but commensal organisms can become a problem, particularly in the large bowel if the wall is perforated by inflammation or surgery.

Bacterial infections

The most significant life-threatening diarrhoeal diseases are **typhoid fever** and **cholera**. Typhoid fever is caused by *Salmonella typhi*, a human pathogen that does not infect or reside in other species and which is transmitted by water or food contaminated with human faeces. The organism is excreted in the faeces for many months or even years after successful treatment of typhoid fever, providing a source from which other people can become infected. Cholera is endemic in Asia and Africa, where there are an estimated 5.5 million cases and 120 000 deaths annually, and has spread to South America. In contrast, only about 70 cases have been reported in the UK in the last 20 years, and these were in people who had travelled to high-risk areas.

The most common causes of bacterial food poisoning in the UK are *Salmonella* and *Campylobacter* species. These, and other food poisoning organisms, are capable of causing disease at relatively low infective doses (about 10^2 organisms per gram of food). This is why food can so easily become a health hazard if handled. In common with infections from other sources, bacterial food-borne infections represent a hazard by direct effects of the bacteria, or by the toxins they produce.

Salmonella

Salmonella is transmitted by ingestion of contaminated food, especially egg and poultry products and water. *Salmonella* in eggs was widely believed to be caused by chicken faeces on the shell contaminating the egg when it is broken. This is probably the principal mechanism, but the organism does infect ovarian tissue in hens and can be transferred directly into the eggs. Infected humans are sources of *Salmonella*, causing new or further contamination by handling food after it has been cooked. The organism is excreted for some time after treatment, even when the patient has apparently recovered fully. About 50 000 people may be excreting salmonellae at any one time in the UK.

Ingested bacteria pass through the stomach and adhere to the epithelial cells lining the terminal small intestine, caecum and colon. They enter the epithelial cells and penetrate into the underlying lamina propria, causing inflammation. The inflammatory response mediates the release of prostaglandins which stimulate active fluid secretion, contributing to diarrhoea. Immunocompromised individuals may experience complications of acute renal failure, osteomyelitis and meningitis. Antibiotics are not needed if there are only gastrointestinal symptoms and recovery usually occurs within a week. Fluid intake should be increased to avoid dehydration. Excretion of bacteria occurs for some weeks or months after clinical recovery.

Escherichia coli: classified as enteropathogenic, enteroinvasive, enterotoxigenic and enterohaemorrhagic. Enteropathogenic *E. coli* are associated with outbreaks of diarrhoea in infants. Enteroinvasive *E. coli* can cause severe diarrhoea or dysentery but are rarely encountered. Enterotoxigenic *E. coli* cause symptoms by producing toxins, and are often responsible for 'traveller's diarrhoea' in people who have visited less developed countries, particularly in tropical areas. Enterohaemorrhagic *E. coli* cause bloody diarrhoea.

Campylobacter

Campylobacter species are among the most common causes of infectious diarrhoea in the UK. In common with *Salmonella*, the number of infections has increased substantially since the 1980s. The organism is found in the gut of wild and domestic animals. Infected poultry is the main source of transmission, although some infections have been attributed to contaminated water. Control measures include elimination of infection in broiler chickens, hygienic food preparation methods, adequate cooking and pasteurisation of milk.

Campylobacter species cause 'traveller's diarrhoea' and most cases of unreported food poisoning in developed countries

Escherichia coli

E. coli is a normal inhabitant of the human gastrointestinal tract but some strains can cause intestinal infections. The mode of transmission and pathogenicity varies with the strain of the organism, its ability to adhere and invade the mucosal surface, and the type of toxin produced.

Food-associated outbreaks of gastroenteritis caused by *E. coli* are relatively rare in developed countries, but are common in less developed countries. The main vehicles for infection are contamination by food handlers or the use of contaminated water for irrigating crops.

Historically, *E. coli* was regarded as an unusual cause of food-borne illness in developed countries. It is now recognised that one type, known as *E. coli* 0157:H7, is a cause of outbreaks and sporadic cases of haemorrhagic colitis and haemolytic uraemic syndrome in the USA and Canada. A few outbreaks have been reported in the UK and other developed countries. Transmission is by ingestion of contaminated meat or meat products (consumption of undercooked hamburgers has received wide publicity in the UK) and raw milk.

Toxins produced by some E. coli species cause haemorrhagic colitis and haemolytic uraemic syndrome

Haemorrhagic colitis: diarrhoeal disease with highly visible and copious amounts of blood in the stool, accompanied by abdominal pain.

Haemolytic uraemic syndrome: a triad of symptoms comprising acute renal failure, thrombocytopenia (platelet deficiency) and microangiopathic haemolytic anaemia (fragmentation of red cells by passage through small blood vessels occluded by thrombi).

Botulism

A very rare cause of food poisoning is botulism. The largest outbreak recorded in the UK occurred in 1989 and was associated with a contaminated batch of hazelnut puree used to flavour yoghurt. A total of 27 people were affected, one

Osteomyelitis: inflammation of the bone and bone marrow. Often caused by pyogenic (pus forming) bacteria.

of whom died.

The causative organism, *Clostridium botulinum*, produces extremely potent neurotoxins, minute amounts of which cause neuromuscular blockade. Symptoms comprise nausea, diarrhoea and vomiting, followed by neurological symptoms of blurred vision, paralysis of the pharynx and larynx and then generalised paralysis. Respiratory insufficiency may occur, and blockade of the cholinergic nervous system causes urinary retention and constipation. At one time most patients with botulism died, but survival is now more certain with prompt respiratory support and administration of antitoxin. Recovery is usually complete.

Protozoan infections

> *Intestinal protozoa are excreted as cysts in the faeces, and survive for long periods in water*

Four protozoan species cause diarrhoeal diseases in humans. These are *Giardia lamblia*, *Entamoeba histolytica* and *Cryptosporidium parvum* and *Cyclospora.*. The organisms live in many animal species and their cysts are excreted in faeces.

E. histolytica infections occur world-wide, but are more common in tropical and subtropical countries where sewage disposal systems are rudimentary and water supplies become contaminated. Infection can lead to **amoebic dysentery**. The organism adheres to the colonic mucosa, causing ulceration and the production of a watery, bloody diarrhoea containing pus and mucus. In some individuals the organism is present as a harmless commensal, living off colonic bacteria. The cysts are excreted with the faeces and can survive for some time in the external environment. Asymptomatic carriers are a source of infection for other people, particularly if they handle food. The infection can also be acquired by anal sexual activity.

Dysentery: an inflammatory disorder of the gastrointestinal tract resulting in the production of watery stools with pus, blood and mucus. Usually accompanied by abdominal pain, cramps and fever, it is caused by infection in the large intestine.

Gastroenteritis: inflammation of the gastrointestinal tract, causing symptoms of nausea, vomiting, diarrhoea and abdominal pain.

Infections with *G. lamblia* are relatively common in the USA, but are rarely seen in the UK. The organism adheres to the intestinal mucosa by means of sucking discs, disrupting water absorption and causing long-lasting diarrhoea, or **giardiasis**.

C. parvum has only recently become implicated as a causative organism of human disease. It is a very small organism and is easily overlooked. Numerous extensive outbreaks of a cholera-like diarrhoeal disease with vomiting and watery diarrhoea have been recorded in developed countries following contamination of the water supply by *Cryptosporidium* leached from agricultural land by heavy rainfall.

Cyclospora infection may be a cause of prolonged watery diarrhoea, and cases have been reported in the USA, Canada and the UK. Outbreaks have been associated with the consumption of berry fruits, particularly raspberries.

Viral infections

Viral contamination of food and water can be responsible for gastroenteritis. The causative agents include the rotaviruses, Norwalk-like virus (so named after an outbreak of gastroenteritis in a school in Norwalk, Ohio, in 1969), various other small rounded viruses (SRVs), caliciviruses, astroviruses and enteric adenovirus. Infections are seen in all parts of the world and are a major cause of death, especially in parts of Asia, Africa and South America.

Probably the most commonly encountered agents responsible for diarrhoeal disease are the rotaviruses. Under the electron microscope these viruses have a characteristic wheel-like appearance, with 'spokes' radiating from an inner core. Infection is most common in babies and infants. Viral replication in gut mucosal cells disrupts transport mechanisms, causing loss of water and electrolytes. Although the infected cells die, there is no accompanying inflammation or loss of blood.

Non-diarrhoeal diseases

A common non-diarrhoeal disease is infectious hepatitis, caused by the hepatitis A enterovirus. The virus spreads by person to person contact or by contamination of food or water. Infection causes symptoms of malaise, anorexia and nausea. Extensive damage to the liver can lead to liver failure, but this is very rare and there are usually no long-term sequelae of infection.

It is now recognised that *Helicobacter pylori* is responsible for inflammatory disorders of the stomach and duodenum which can lead to ulceration. The organism is also implicated in the causation of the most common type of stomach cancer. In some populations infection by the organism is ubiquitous, but symptoms occur in relatively few people. The various outcomes of *H. pylori* infection are discussed in Chapter 19.

Hepatitis: damage and inflammation of the liver, usually caused by viral infection although other micro-organisms can be responsible. Liver damage arising from acute viral hepatitis is reflected by raised levels of alanine aminotransferase and aspartate aminotransferase in the plasma.

Sexually transmitted infections

Another means of infection of part of the gastrointestinal tract is anal sexual activity. A variety of organisms can be transmitted in this way, to cause both local and systemic disease. The most obvious example is HIV infection. Sexually transmitted diseases are discussed in Chapter 25.

Table 6.1 Some important gastrointestinal infections

Organism	Mechanism	Symptoms	Source
Bacteria:			
Campylobacter jejuni	Infection	Diarrhoea with blood, fever, malaise, abdominal pain	Animal gastrointestinal tract, especially poultry, and milk
Escherichia coli	Infection (enteropathogenic, enteroinvasive)	Diarrhoea in infants, gastroenteritis	More prevalent in less developed countries, contaminated water used for irrigating crops, food handling
	Toxin (enterotoxigenic, enterohaemorrhagic)	Haemorrhagic colitis, haemolytic uraemic syndrome	Undercooked meat or raw milk (enterohaemorrhagic type)

Salmonella enteritidis	Infection causes inflammation in lamina propria	Diarrhoea, fever, vomiting	Animal gastrointestinal tract, especially poultry
Salmonella typhi	Organism penetrates intestinal mucosa, reaching enteric lymph nodes and spreads to other organs. Grows within macrophages	Typhoid fever, haemorrhage, perforation, toxaemia, meningitis, osteomyelitis, endocarditis	Contaminated water; person-to-person: treated patients carry the organism for months or years
Vibrio cholerae	Toxin produced after bacteria binds to enterocytes. Toxin does not damage cells but causes loss of fluid	Cholera, massive watery diarrhoea	Faecal contamination of water
Shigella	Invasion of ileum and colon causes intense inflammatory response	Dysentery	Faecal–oral route
Protozoa:			
Cryptosporidium parvum	Ingested oocytes adhere to villous enterocytes. Organism matures and reproduces beneath the cell membrane. Damage to epithelium causes diarrhoea and malabsorption	Diarrhoea, sometimes with nausea, vomiting and abdominal pain	Contamination of water by animal faeces
Entamoeba histolytica	Ingestion of cysts	Amoebic dysentery (ulceration and bloody diarrhoea), liver abscess	Contaminated water or food
Giardia lamblia	Ingestion of cysts. Multiplication occurs in jejunum, organism attaches to mucosa by sucking discs and causes intestinal obstruction	Diarrhoea and fatty stools (fat malabsorption because of obstruction)	Contaminated water, person to person spread

Viruses:			
Hepatitis A	Inflammation and damage of the liver	Fever, malaise and anorexia, followed by full recovery	Faecally contaminated water, sewage contaminated shellfish
Norwalk, SRVs		Gastroenteritis	Contaminated water, shellfish
Rotaviruses	Infection of jejunal and ileal mucosa causes loss of cells and villous atrophy	Gastroenteritis, especially in infants	Faecally contaminated food or water

Respiratory tract infections

The respiratory tract is a portal of entry for many kinds of organism that can cause both respiratory and systemic disease. The most commonly encountered infections of the respiratory tract are by rhinovirus and Coxsackie A viruses, which cause the common cold. One of the major causes of death in both developed and the less developed countries is pneumonia, most commonly caused by bacterial and viral infections. Bronchitis and influenza often predispose for pneumonia. The life-threatening systemic infections that arise from the entry of micro-organisms through the respiratory tract include measles, mumps, whooping cough and meningitis.

Pneumonia: inflammation of the substance of the lungs, characterised by cough, purulent sputum and fever. Other physical signs include pleuritic pain and rapid shallow breathing. Pneumonia can be localised, arising from the colonisation of alveolar air spaces and affecting the whole of one lobe, or diffuse, arising from the bronchi and spreading into the alveoli (termed bronchopneumonia).

Acute bronchitis

Acute bronchitis is usually caused by viral infective agents such as rhinoviruses, coronaviruses, adenoviruses and the influenza virus. The influenza virus causes most damage to the epithelium and infection increases susceptibility for secondary bacterial infections. Bacteria such as *Mycoplasma pneumoniae* also cause acute bronchitis. Secondary bacterial infections are usually caused by *Streptococcus pneumoniae* and *Haemophilus pneumoniae*.

Pneumonia

Pneumonia is caused by a variety of organisms which lead to virtually identical symptoms. Age is the main determinant of susceptibility to viral or bacterial infections. In children, pneumonia is more likely to be caused by infection with respiratory syncytial virus (RSV) or parainfluenza viruses. Any bacterial infection is probably secondary to the damage caused by the viral infection. In adults, bacterial infections are more common than viral infections.

Pneumonia caused by opportunistic infections occurs in the immunocompromised. Most notorious is *Pneumocystis carinii* pneumonia (PCP) in HIV infection (Chapter 25), although the condition can occur in malnourished children. Other opportunistic infections include *Mycobacterium avium* complex, cytomegalovirus, *Aspergillus fumigatus* and *Cryptococcus*. Malnourished individuals (usually vagrants and alcoholics) are prone to lobar pneumonia caused by *Pneumococcus* or *Klebsiella*.

Hospital-acquired pneumonia affects about 5% of all patients admitted to hospital. The risk is higher in older patients, smokers, the seriously ill, patients undergoing mechanical ventilation, patients in whom consciousness is reduced and those undergoing anaesthesia. Gram-negative organisms such as *Klebsiella*, *E. coli* and *Pseudomonas* are most likely to be responsible.

Community-acquired pneumonia is most likely to be caused by *Streptococcus pneumoniae*. *Haemophilus influenzae* infections are also commonly seen, and are more likely in children, older adults and people with chronic obstructive airways disease. *Legionella* accounts for about 5% of pneumonias, mainly in middle-aged adults.

Viral pneumonia is caused by a range of viruses, inhaled directly or reaching the lungs from the bloodstream. Respiratory syncytial virus is one of the most common causes of pneumonia in children. In children and adults influenza virus can cause severe pneumonia but, more commonly, damage to the alveolar lining cells increases susceptibility for a superimposed bacterial infection. Other viral infections causing pneumonia include measles, parainfluenza, and adenovirus. Immunocompromised patients may acquire cytomegalovirus pneumonia.

Legionnaire's disease

Legionnaire's disease was first recognised following an outbreak of pneumonia at an American Legion convention in a Philadelphia hotel in July 1976. The condition is characterised by headache, chest pain, lung congestion and high fever. It is caused by inhalation of an aerosol containing large numbers of the Gram-negative rod-shaped bacterium *Legionella pneumophila*. The bacterium has been found in many natural and artificial water environments and causes illness when a combination of factors are present:

- Specific conditions that permit growth of the organism, such as warmth and stagnant water
- Generation of aerosols containing the organism, for example in cooling towers, air humidifiers and showers
- Inhalation of contaminated aerosols by a susceptible host (smokers, older people and immunosuppressed individuals)

The organism grows inside macrophages in the lungs, which enables it to evade the body's defences. Its ability to grow intracellularly is probably important for its survival outside the body, where it has been found in several species of free-living amoebae.

Influenza

Influenza: illness starts abruptly with shivering, fever and generalised aching of the limbs, accompanied by headache, sore throat and persistent dry cough that can last for several weeks. Illness is often followed by a prolonged period of depression and lassitude, termed post-viral syndrome.

Influenza is caused by two main strains of the influenza virus, influenza A and influenza B. Influenza viruses undergo genetic changes as they spread through the host population, which means that epidemics surface regularly because of a lack of immunity. This is also why immunisation is often ineffective and new vaccines have to be developed for each strain that emerges. The virus particles bind to receptors on respiratory epithelial cells. Cytokines liberated from the damaged epithelial cells and from infiltrating inflammatory cells cause symptoms of malaise, fever and muscular aches.

Systemic diseases caused by organisms that enter through the lungs

Measles

Measles is caused by infection with paramyxovirus, transmitted in airborne droplets. The infection usually occurs in children, but the outcome of infection is quite different depending upon the nutritional state and general health of the child. In the well nourished child infection causes a temporary respiratory illness, rash, conjunctivitis and otitis media, and is serious in only a small proportion of those infected. In the malnourished child infection causes severe eye, ear, oral and gastrointestinal tract symptoms, and is a significant cause of death from pneumonia.

All measles infections cause symptoms, but the severity of illness depends on the child's general health

Mumps

Mumps is caused by an RNA paramyxovirus transmitted in airborne droplets and salivary secretions. Usually close contact is necessary, in schools or enclosed adult communities. The virus spreads systemically, growing in lymphoid tissues. It then localises in salivary and other glands, causing cell damage and inflammation. The classic sign of mumps is a painful swelling of the parotid gland. Infection can cause meningitis and encephalitis in about 10% of cases and orchitis occurs in about 20% of infected men but only rarely causes infertility.

Rubella

Rubella is caused by a single-stranded RNA togavirus that enters the body through the respiratory tract. The virus then spreads to the lymph nodes, causing lymphadenopathy, to the skin, causing a rash, and sometimes to the joints, causing mild joint pain or arthritis. In pregnant women spread to the placenta can cause fetal damage, spontaneous abortion and congenital rubella (malformations include heart defects and cataract).

Whooping cough

Whooping cough (pertussis) is caused by *Bordetella pertussis*, a Gram-negative coccobacillus. It is highly contagious and spreads by aerosol. The condition is mainly seen in childhood although no age group is exempt. Infection begins with a highly infectious catarrhal stage, with malaise, anorexia, copious nasal mucus secretion and conjunctivitis. A paroxysmal stage follows, characterised by bouts of coughing. The 'whoop' of the cough is more common in younger children, caused by forcing air through the respiratory lumen blocked by mucus and oedema. Complications are relatively uncommon but can include pneumonia, cerebral anoxia and convulsions.

Meninges: the membranous covering of the brain, consisting of three layers. From the outside, the layers are the dura mater, arachnoid and pia mater.

Meningitis

Meningitis refers to inflammation of the meninges and is most often caused by infectious agents. A range of bacterial, viral and fungal organisms can be responsible for meningitis. Many of the bacterial agents originate in the throat or lower respiratory tract and are either carried asymptomatically or cause local infections. The factors which influence invasion of the blood and meninges are poorly understood, but a common feature is a polysaccharide capsule that increases resistance to host defences. Immunocompromised patients (with AIDS, for example) are at greater risk of meningitis, often caused by the more unusual bacterial and fungal organisms.

Meningitis is subdivided into **leptomeningitis** (inflammation arising in the subarachnoid space) and **pachymeningitis** (inflammation arising in the dura). Leptomeningitis is most often caused by the blood-borne spread of infectious micro-organisms. Pachymeningitis usually arises from the direct spread of infection through the middle ear, mastoid, nasal sinuses or dural venous sinuses. Infectious agents can also enter through skull fracture.

Bacterial meningitis is life-threatening and requires urgent treatment

The three main categories of leptomeningitis are acute purulent, lymphocytic and chronic and granulomatous. **Acute purulent** meningitis is usually caused by bacterial infection. In neonates the organism is most likely to be *E. coli*, *Streptococcus* or *Listeria monocytogenes*. In children *Haemophilus influenzae* and *Neisseria meningitidis* are likely agents. Adults may be infected with *N. meningitidis*, *S. pneumoniae* (type 3) or *L. monocytogenes*. Infection causes malaise with severe headache, neck stiffness, photophobia, fever and vomiting. Severe inflammation causes secondary thrombosis in superficial blood vessels, leading to cerebral ischaemia. Obstruction of the drainage of cerebrospinal fluid (CSF) by inflammation leads to hydrocephalus. Left untreated, all forms of meningitis caused by bacterial infection are lethal. Even with treatment mortality rates are about 15% and survivors may have permanent neurological damage.

Viral meningitis is the most common and recovery is usually complete

Lymphocytic meningitis is usually caused by viral infection and is self-limiting. **Chronic and granulomatous** meningitides may be a consequence of tuberculosis, syphilis, Lyme disease or infection by *Cryptococcus neoformans*. In this condition severe chronic inflammation leads to fibrosis of the meninges and obstruction of CSF drainage. Vascular damage leads to infarction and cranial nerve lesions.

Focus on tuberculosis

Tuberculosis is endemic in less developed countries but incidence is increasing in Europe and North America

In recent years there has been a resurgence in the prevalence of tuberculosis in developed countries. The disease remains a major problem in less developed parts of the world. Contributory factors for the increase in prevalence are a decline in living standards in certain sectors of the population, relative ineffectiveness of Bacille Calmette-Guérin (BCG) vaccination, a lack of adequate population surveillance, development of drug resistance and accompanying HIV infection.

Epidemiology

Each year about three million people die from tuberculosis, mostly people in the less developed countries. Historically, tuberculosis was a significant problem in the now developed countries, responsible for up to a quarter of deaths in Europe.

Tuberculosis is essentially a disease of poverty. As improvements in social conditions were made in the developed countries the number of deaths from the disease began to decline, independently of new treatments and preventive measures. To the present day, less crowding and better ventilation remain the goals of public health efforts to control tuberculosis.

Until recently it was believed that the virtual eradication of tuberculosis in developed countries was a realistic goal, but the rapid decline seen from the beginning of the century up to about the mid-1980s has halted. A rise in incidence in both the UK and the USA is probably caused by increased homelessness in the inner cities, a rise in poverty and failure of control measures such as BCG vaccination. Coupled with these changes in social conditions is an emerging problem of drug resistance.

Between 1987 and 1993, notification rates for tuberculosis in London increased from 21 per 100 000 people to 31.5 per 100 000. The increase was most marked in inner-city areas with high proportions of immigrants and unemployed people, notification rates exceeding 65 per 100 000 in some parts of east London. In 1993 the average number of notifications per year in England and Wales was just under 6000 (Figure 6.2). These figures are probably an under-estimate, because some cases will not have been identified and notified. In some inner-city areas of the USA, incidence has risen to 150 per 100 000 people, typically in the homeless, HIV-infected and immigrant populations.

The increase in notifications has been accompanied by a change in the prevalence of non-respiratory tuberculosis. The increase has been particularly apparent in large conurbations, with rates in rural areas continuing to decline. It is unclear whether the increase in non-respiratory infections reflects a true rise, or represents an increase in reporting because of the appointment of specialists to new posts in communicable disease control.

Tuberculosis has always been a serious problem among immunocompromised patients and it is no surprise that there is a correlation between tuberculosis and HIV infection. It is estimated that in Africa more than half of HIV-infected people are also infected with *Mycobacterium tuberculosis*.

> *Tuberculosis occurs wherever there is poverty, malnutrition and poor housing*

Pathology

Tuberculosis is usually acquired by inhalation of *M. tuberculosis*. The organism has a tough waxy outer coat and can survive for long periods in dry conditions. Transmission may therefore be by means of aerosols in expired air or inhalation of household dusts. The coating also renders the organism resistant

> *Tissue damage in tuberculosis is mostly caused by an inflammatory reaction that results in granuloma formation*

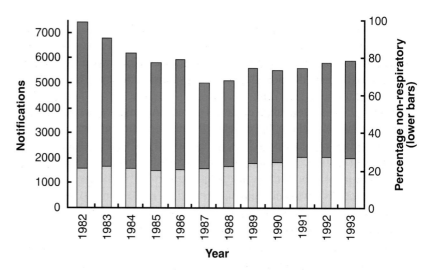

Figure 6.2 Tuberculosis notifications in England and Wales have risen since the mid-1980s. Non-respiratory tuberculosis accounted for 21% of notifications in 1987, but had increased to 27% in 1993. (Data from Hayward, A.C. and Watson, J.M. (1995) *CDR Review*, 5, R29–33.)

Tuberculosis is suppressed by the immune response and by connective tissue formation around the granuloma

Granulomatous lesions can be dormant for many years or may be reactivated to cause secondary tuberculosis

to destruction by natural defence mechanisms. This is compounded by the fact that the organism survives within phagocytic cells.

No toxins are produced by the tuberculosis mycobacteria, most of the tissue damage being caused by the inflammatory response to infection. **Primary tuberculosis** refers to the initial infection in the lungs. The organisms will be engulfed by alveolar macrophages. Macrophages containing intracellular mycobacterial antigens are recognised by T lymphocytes, which produce a variety of cytokines that attract more macrophages to the site of infection. This inflammatory response is relatively ineffective and, with time, the infected macrophages spread along the lymphatics until they reach the hilar lymph nodes. Most patients manage to contain the infection at this stage as small primary lesions or **tubercles** in the lung and hilar lymph nodes which do not progress.

The tubercle comprises granulomatous tissue with a central area of necrosis. The necrotic centre has a cheesy, or **caseous**, consistency. In most people the tubercles heal by deposition of collagen around the periphery, which effectively walls off the tubercles, and the patient experiences no symptoms or further progression, even though macrophages within the tubercle still contain viable bacteria.

If cell-mediated immunity is inadequate the condition progresses or lesions are reactivated after a period of dormancy. Reactivation of tuberculosis may be precipitated by poor nutrition, age or immunosuppression. Reactivated infection is called **secondary tuberculosis**. Secondary tuberculosis may also be acquired by additional exposure to an environmental source of the pathogen. This kind of infection usually occurs at the apex of the lung and results in a necrotic lesion surrounded by a granulomatous inflammatory response. The destruction of lung tissue leads to large cavities. In common with primary tuberculosis the necrotic lesion is eventually surrounded by a thick wall of connective tissue which contains the micro-organisms. The lesion may cause no further problems or may eventually be reactivated.

Some people are unable to mount an adequate initial immune response and the infection takes a much more rapid course. The condition, called **miliary tuberculosis,** is characterised by loss of weight, cough and loss of vigour, caused by dissemination of tubercle bacilli in the bloodstream. Infection may involve the rest of the lung, meninges, spleen, liver and bone marrow and without treatment is invariably fatal (Figure 6.3).

> *Miliary tuberculosis is caused by blood-borne spread of organisms*

Tuberculosis can lead to bronchopneumonia by the erosion of an infected lymph node into a bronchus. The caseous material, containing live organisms, passes down the bronchi and bronchioles, seeding new areas of infection in the lower portions of both lungs. Large caseous granulomas are then formed in the lower lobes.

Other types of mycobacteria also cause a chronic granulomatous inflammatory response, but the pattern of infection in the body differs. One example is leprosy, caused by *Mycobacterium leprae,* which is primarily an infection of the skin but which causes a granulomatous reaction similar to that of tuberculosis. In contrast, the increasingly common *Mycobacterium avium complex* infections seen in patients with AIDS does not always elicit a marked granulomatous response because the immune response is largely inactivated. Instead, the organism proliferates widely. In the less severely immunocompromised infection follows a course similar to that of pulmonary tuberculosis.

> *Tuberculous bronchopneumonia is caused by bronchial spread of mycobacteria from caseous lymph nodes*

Prevention and control of tuberculosis

In the UK, diagnosis and effective chemotherapy remain the cornerstone of tuberculosis control. Because tuberculosis is spread from person to person, contact tracing plays an important part in controlling spread of the disease. This usually involves screening of close family members and occasionally close contacts at work or school. Screening is by chest X-ray and **tuberculin testing.** Adults with HIV infection, and children in contact with a family member who has tuberculosis, will be given prophylactic isoniazid treatment and vaccinated with an isoniazid-resistant strain of BCG.

The standard treatment for tuberculosis is a combination of rifampicin, isoniazid and pyrazinamide. Routine BCG vaccination (see Chapter 11) is given to children at risk, although some health authorities in inner city areas have adopted a policy of vaccinating all tuberculin-negative schoolchildren aged 10–14 years.

Tuberculin testing: used for contact tracing and to determine who should receive BCG vaccination. The agent used in the Mantoux test is a purified protein derivative of *M. tuberculosis.* Intradermal injection of the agent elicits a cell-mediated immune response with induration and inflammation of the skin at the injection site. In children a positive tuberculin test is taken as evidence of infection, and treated. A negative test is repeated 6 weeks later, and BCG vaccine given if the test remains negative.

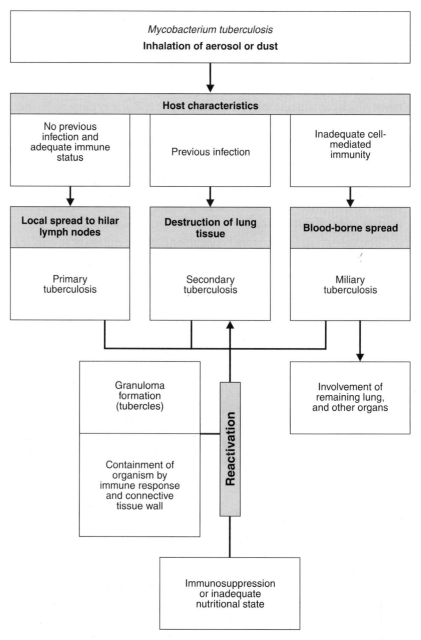

Figure 6.3 The outcome of infection by tubercle bacilli depends on whether a person has previously been infected and the adequacy of cell-mediated immune responses. In most people, first infection will result in primary tuberculosis, with containment of the organism within granuloma surrounded by a thick connective tissue wall. Suppression of the immune response by illness or poor nutritional state allows the organism to escape and reactivate the pathological process (secondary tuberculosis). Secondary tuberculosis can also be caused by further exposure to the mycobacterium in the environment. People who have a poor immunological status on first exposure to the organism may succumb to progressive miliary tuberculosis, involving other organs by blood-borne spread.

Human defences against infection

A variety of host responses prevent micro-organisms from entering the body, and eliminate them once inside. In turn, micro-organisms have evolved mechanisms designed to thwart these host responses – for example, by entering cells where they become inaccessible to non-specific (and many specific) defences. Some micro-organisms (viruses) are even able to incorporate themselves into the host cell's genome. Very often these infections remain dormant for many years, but can be reactivated at any time, usually when resistance is low because of other disease conditions. Although the strategy of 'hiding' inside cells is effective in ensuring survival of the micro-organism it does not allow great opportunity for large growth in numbers. Other micro-organisms living outside cells have far greater opportunities for growth, but are more vulnerable to host defences.

Non-specific defences

Just as the types and activities of micro-organisms are many and varied, so are the host defences that are used to dispel them from the body. The first lines of defence are the physical barriers of the skin and mucus secretions. Mucus is used to trap bacteria and wash them away, aided in the respiratory tract by ciliary motion. Unfortunately, some micro-organisms have evolved strategies to avoid removal, usually by producing adhesion molecules which bind firmly to the epithelial surfaces. Adhesion enables *H. pylori* to persist in the stomach and metaplastic duodenum (see Chapter 19). Other micro-organisms (*Pneumococcus*, for example) resist clearance by interfering with the motion of cilia. Some micro-organisms can even secrete enzymes to help them penetrate the skin or mucous membranes.

Another non-specific body defence system is the secretion of an enzyme called **lysozyme** (not to be confused with the intracellular enzymes present in lysosomes). This is present in body secretions such as saliva and tears, and helps to break down the cell wall of Gram-positive organisms.

Once inside the body, the organism needs a source of nutrition, which it can obtain simply by diverting nutrients and oxygen intended for host cell metabolism to its own use. However, the human body possesses systems that can limit the availability of essential components to microbes. A notable example is iron, which is transported or stored in the body complexed with protein (transferrin, for example) which restricts its availability to invading micro-organisms.

Micro-organisms that manage to break through the physical and chemical barriers will encounter a non-specific inflammatory response. Very often inflammation will be induced by the microbe forcing its way through the membrane, after coming into contact with cells that recognise and present antigens to other cells of the inflammatory and immune systems.

Lysozyme: an antimicrobial enzyme present in secretions such as tears and saliva, capable of breaking down the polysaccharide cell wall of susceptible bacteria.

Macrophages: cells that originate in the bone marrow, circulate in the blood as monocytes, and enter the connective tissues. They are concentrated in the lungs (alveolar macrophages), liver (Kupffer cells) and line the lymph node sinusoids where they filter out foreign or degraded material by ingesting it (phagocytosis).

Peritonitis: inflammation of the peritoneal cavity usually secondary to inflammatory gastrointestinal disease leading to perforation of the gut. Less commonly seen as a primary infection in patients with liver cirrhosis.

Toxic shock syndrome: systemic infection caused by *Staphylococcus aureus*. Associated with tampon use by healthy women, in whom proliferation of the organism, and generation of exotoxins, occurs around the neglected or retained tampon. Infection can originate at other body sites, with other staphylococcal species, in both men and women.

Review question 1

What features are required by micro-organisms to infect and survive in the human body?

Specific responses

Micro-organisms that succeed in evading the non-specific defences encounter a more specific response perpetrated by the immune system. This is in two forms, **humoral** or **cell-mediated** immunity. The humoral response involves the production of specific antibodies which will combine with components in the microbe's cell wall, or with its soluble products, to form antigen–antibody complexes. These antigen–antibody complexes evoke an inflammatory response by binding and activating complement components which serve to attract inflammatory cells to the site (see Chapter 4). Some of the activated complement components have proteolytic activity and can attack the antigen. Most micro-organisms are able to resist this kind of attack, either by isolating the bound complement component to a small portion of its membrane or by producing an antibody against it.

Cell-mediated immunity relies on activation of macrophages, or direct killing, by cytotoxic lymphocytes (CD8+ T cells). Cell-mediated immunity is usually invoked when the infective agent is carried within cells, such as in viral infections, tuberculosis and leprosy.

Spread of infection

Once in the body micro-organisms spread and proliferate. Local spread occurs, particularly if the organism is able to produce locally damaging agents such as exotoxins. They may gain access to the lymphatic and blood systems and spread freely or within cells. Swelling of the lymph nodes reflects generation of an immune response, but can also be caused by infection. The carriage of bacteria in the blood is referred to as **bacteraemia**. Some organisms will grow in the blood circulation, causing **septicaemia**. This can lead to **endotoxic shock** or, if Gram-negative organisms cause the infection, **toxic shock syndrome**, both of which are potentially fatal.

Spread and growth also occur in other tissue fluids and cavities, such as the peritoneum and pleura, causing peritonitis and pleural infections. Some viruses, such as herpes simplex and rabies viruses, spread along nerves.

Mechanisms of pathogenicity

The germ theory of disease in the 1880s helped to establish medicine as a scientific rather than empirical discipline. The theory is based on four fundamental concepts, known as **Koch's postulates**:
- The microbe must be present in every case of the disease
- The microbe must be isolated from the diseased host and grown in culture
- The disease must be reproduced when a pure culture is introduced into a non-diseased susceptible host
- The microbe must be recoverable from an experimentally infected host.

Koch's postulates have been fulfilled for the vast majority of known infectious organisms but there are some notable exceptions, mainly because of a failure to culture the organism. This applies to many viruses, *Rickettsia*, *Treponema pallidum* (causes syphilis) and *Mycobacterium leprae*. Other organisms can be cultured but do not always cause disease and, conversely, not all cases of the disease have evidence of the organism. This applies to the association of *H. pylori* with peptic ulcer (see Chapter 19). Nevertheless, the establishment of Koch's postulates provides a basic framework for the scientific investigation of infectious disease.

Factors predisposing to infection

Some human pathogens do not infect other species, or infect only closely related primates (for example measles, typhoid, hepatitis B). In humans, genetic factors and related pathologies influence both resistance and susceptibility for infection. Perhaps the best known example of a protective genetic factor is the sickle-cell gene, which confers resistance to malaria (see Chapter 3). On infection with the malarial parasite the mutated haemoglobin in the sickle cell forms fibres which cause the cell to collapse, effectively slowing growth of the parasite.

In contrast, the pathological changes that take place in the lungs of people with cystic fibrosis favours the growth of micro-organisms. In the population at large it is probable that genetic polymorphisms modulate the effectiveness of the immune response for dealing with infection. Certainly immunosuppression, as a consequence of other disease processes or drug therapy, increases the susceptibility for infection.

Toxins

Bacteria can produce **exotoxins** that directly cause cell and tissue damage and **endotoxins** that cause systemic disease.

Exotoxins

Exotoxins are proteins that are actively secreted into the surrounding area, often causing extensive cell and tissue damage. Some exotoxins are enzymes, such as hyaluronidase, collagenase, DNAase and streptokinase, which will attack local tissues and facilitate the spread of the micro-organism. Other enzymes, such as lecithinases and phospholipases, damage or kill cells by attacking the membrane. Some toxins find their way into cells, where they interfere with metabolic processes. Notable examples of this type are diphtheria and cholera toxins.

In many cases it is the toxin, rather than the bacteria themselves, that causes the disease. The body can produce antibodies to toxins, called **antitoxins**, which provide protection from future infection. In addition, the body can be stimulated to produce antibodies against chemically modified exotoxins, called

toxoids. The modified agent can no longer cause damage, but antibodies produced against it are also active against the original toxin. Toxoid vaccination is effective for the prevention of diphtheria and tetanus.

Endotoxins

Endotoxic shock syndrome comprises fever, vascular collapse and shock

Endotoxins are part of the outer lipopolysaccharide component in the cell wall of Gram-negative micro-organisms. Their effects become apparent when the bacteria die and undergo lysis, thus releasing the endotoxin. Antibiotic treatment that effectively kills Gram-negative micro-organisms may initially cause a worsening of symptoms because of endotoxin release. All endotoxins cause similar symptoms, but some are more potent than others. Symptoms include fever, weakness, and, in some cases, shock. These systemic effects are related to inflammatory processes which induce vasodilation, intravascular coagulation, endothelial damage and capillary leakage (Figure 6.4).

A most notable endotoxin is **tumour necrosis factor** (TNF), released by macrophages carrying out phagocytosis of bacteria. Extensive damage to the blood vessels in this way leads to a loss of fluid from the blood, causing hypotension, adult respiratory distress syndrome and multiple organ failure. The most potent endotoxins are found in *E. coli*, *Proteus* and *Pseudomonas aeruginosa*.

Pyogenic organisms

Some bacteria induce a particularly vigorous acute inflammatory response, resulting in tissue destruction and the formation of **pus**. These **pyogenic** bacteria contain factors in their cell walls that attract neutrophils, which release enzymes when they die, causing liquefaction of the tissues. The resultant semi-liquid exudate, or pus, contains dead tissue, live and dead neutrophils, live and dead bacteria and plasma fluid.

Type III hypersensitivity

Antigen–antibody complexes in excessive amounts can cause tissue damage

Type III hypersensitivity reactions are provoked by the local release of antigens in conditions to which the individual has already mounted an antibody response. This might occur when antibiotic treatment is given, causing a sudden and large increase in microbial antigens. Large quantities of antigen–antibody complexes are formed which remain local or may circulate. Wherever the complexes become trapped, tissue damage occurs by complement activation.

Type IV hypersensitivity

Organisms resistant to macrophage activity induce a chronic granulomatous inflammatory reaction

Type IV hypersensitivity is based on the activities of CD4+ helper T cells, and does not involve antibody production. When these cells come into contact with antigen they release soluble factors that attract and activate macrophages. Occasionally, micro-organisms are encountered that are relatively resistant to

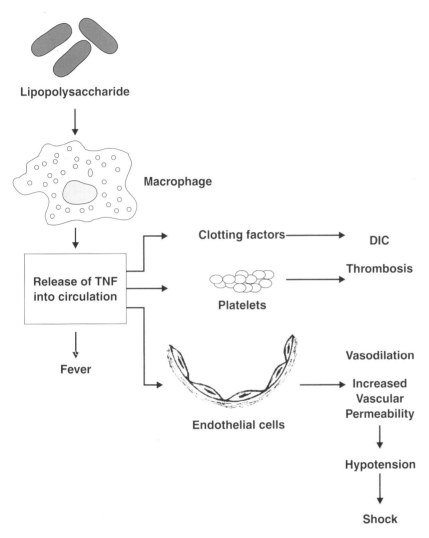

Lipopolysaccharide

Macrophage

Release of TNF into circulation

Clotting factors → **DIC**

Thrombosis

Platelets

Fever

Vasodilation

Increased Vascular Permeability

Endothelial cells

Hypotension

Shock

Adult respiratory distress syndrome: caused by damage to the pulmonary vascular endothelium or the alveolar epithelium, for example, by major trauma, septicaemia or inhalation of toxic fumes or smoke. In septicaemia, the endotoxin activates the endothelium and neutrophils, releasing neutrophil enzymes. Enzymatic disruption of membranes causes haemorrhage into the alveoli. In an organisation phase the lungs are congested, with impaired ventilation caused by interstitial fibrosis and thickening of the alveolar walls.

Disseminated intravascular coagulation: produced by activation of the blood coagulation system in small vessels throughout the body. Causes include septicaemia, disseminated malignancy, transfusion reactions, and some obstetric conditions. The clinical presentation varies from no bleeding at all to widespread haemorrhage in the mouth, nose and venepuncture sites because of consumption of clotting factors and platelets elsewhere. Treatment is by transfusion and control of the underlying cause.

Vascular shock: the blood volume is normal but poor circulation results from extreme vasodilation. This reduces peripheral resistance, so that blood pressure falls rapidly and is inadequate for tissue needs

Figure 6.4 Endotoxic shock syndrome. The lipopolysaccharide cell walls of many Gram-negative bacteria stimulate a range of responses in the infected host. Foremost among these is the release of massive amounts of tumour necrosis factor (TNF) by macrophages. This stimulates the endothelium to release nitric oxide, causing vasodilation, and activates the blood coagulation system. The principal clinical features are fever, disseminated intravascular coagulation (DIC), thrombosis, hypotension and vascular shock.

macrophage activity, and the antigenic stimulus persists. The continued, and ineffective, stimulus of macrophages causes morphological changes in the cells, which appear as flattened **epithelioid** cells and which may fuse to form **giant** cells. Together these cells are characteristic of a granuloma. The organisms that induce a granulomatous response include *M. tuberculosis*, *M. leprae* and *Treponema pallidum*.

A type IV hypersensitivity reaction can cause extensive necrosis in some

▲ Key points

Bacterial infections

- ▲ Gram-positive bacteria produce exotoxins that directly cause cell and tissue damage

- ▲ Gram-negative bacteria produce endotoxins that cause systemic disease

- ▲ Toxins can functionally impair cells without causing death

- ▲ Bacterial products may induce acute inflammation, chronic inflammation or hypersensitivity reactions

Review question 2

List the mechanisms by which micro-organisms cause cell and tissue damage

tissues. These areas of necrosis, termed **gummas,** are surrounded by a chronic inflammatory reaction. This typically occurs in advanced syphilis; gummas form in the liver, bones and testes. Syphilis also causes damage to cerebral tissues and the cardiovascular system.

Prevention of infectious disease

At the turn of the century the principal causes of death in developed countries were infectious diseases such as influenza, tuberculosis and pneumonia. These conditions have been replaced by chronic diseases such as coronary heart disease and cancers (although pneumonia remains a frequent cause of death, often complicating other conditions). Much of this change can be ascribed to improvements in social and economic conditions, but an important contribution has been made by the application of comprehensive vaccination programmes.

In developing countries the situation is entirely different and, world-wide, infectious diseases still represent the principal causes of death, particularly in infants. The greatest toll is from acute respiratory infections, followed by diarrhoeal diseases and malaria. Most of these conditions are preventable by vaccination, and again taking a global view (economics permitting), this strategy offers the greatest potential for reducing morbidity and premature deaths in the human population.

The aim of vaccination is to stimulate the immune system to respond to an innocuous version of a pathogenic bacterium or virus. The innocuous version should be similar to the pathogenic organism so that the response is effective. The pioneering work in this area was carried out by Edward Jenner, who used a cowpox virus as a vaccine against smallpox. The two viruses bear certain similarities, but the disease produced by cowpox is far less dangerous than smallpox. The principle of using a related pathogen to induce immunity has been carried forward to the present – for example in the vaccines designed to protect children against rotavirus infection, which can cause fatal diarrhoea. There are, however, a number of other approaches to preparing vaccines.

Killed whole micro-organisms and chemically modified toxins

A relatively simple procedure is to use killed whole micro-organisms. This approach is used in the preparation of vaccines against influenza, pertussis (whooping cough) and polio.

Alternatively, a vaccine can be prepared using chemically modified toxins: in many cases it is the toxin produced by the organism, rather than the organism itself, that causes tissue damage and disease. Hence it is often beneficial to 'prime' the immune system so that it can inactivate the toxin. This is the basis of vaccines used for diphtheria and tetanus vaccination.

Attenuated micro-organisms (live vaccines)

In some situations killing the micro-organism denatures their proteins, so the immune response provoked is effective only against the altered protein and not the native organism. An alternative approach is to use live micro-organisms that have been weakened, or **attenuated**, and are therefore much less virulent than those encountered in the wild state. This gives the immune system time to mount an effective response. Attenuated live micro-organisms are used in the oral polio vaccine and the combined vaccine against measles, mumps and rubella (MMR). Attenuation is usually achieved by growing the organism in culture for a long time.

Subunit vaccines

Some people are slow to mount an effective immune response to the attenuated organism, enabling it to recover and behave in a virulent manner. This problem can be overcome by using incomplete micro-organisms that are not viable; usually by extracting protein subunits from the cell wall or viral envelope. These subunit vaccines are now used to protect against some types of meningitis, pneumonia and hepatitis B.

> ### ▲ Key points
>
> #### Types of vaccine
>
> ▲ Similar but less pathogenic organism, e.g. cowpox to protect against smallpox
>
> ▲ Killed whole organism, e.g. use of influenza, injectable polio vaccine
>
> ▲ Chemically modified toxin, e.g. diphtheria, tetanus
>
> ▲ Attenuated micro-organisms, e.g. oral polio vaccine, MMR vaccine
>
> ▲ Molecular subunits: use incomplete micro-organisms, e.g. hepatitis B, pneumococci, *Haemophilus*, meningococci

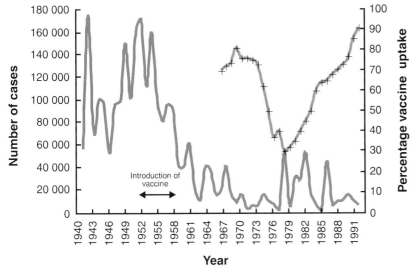

Figure 6.5 Correlation between vaccine uptake and incidence of whooping cough in England and Wales, 1940–1992. There is a close correlation between vaccine uptake and whooping cough cases. Shortly after the introduction of a vaccine (in the early 1950s) the number of cases fell sharply. The late 1970s were characterised by reduced vaccine uptake and incidence of whooping cough rose. More recently, vaccine use has increased and the incidence of whooping cough is currently low. (Adapted from Parton, R. (1994) *J. Med. Microbiol.*, **41**, 149–67.)

Although many forms of vaccine have been and remain extremely effective against their respective targets (Figure 6.5), nature very often has a way of ensuring their obsolescence by mutation, producing new strains of organism. New vaccines are being developed all the time and improvements made to the vaccines that are available – the current typhoid vaccine is unreliable and the BCG vaccine is only partly effective against tuberculosis.

Prophylactic treatment

Another means of preventing infection is to give antibiotics to people who are at particular risk of acquiring infection. One such measure, used in North America, is to give isoniazid, an antibiotic used in the treatment of tuberculosis, to children below the age of 5 who are household contacts of adults with infectious pulmonary tuberculosis.

This measure has been considered for use in less developed countries but the antibiotic must be taken for 6–12 months and when the course is finished the person is again at risk. Given the prevalence of pulmonary tuberculosis in some less developed countries, the risk of reinfection after therapy is great. In effect isoniazid therapy would have to be given throughout life, at a financial cost that cannot be supported in many less developed countries.

Antimicrobial therapy

Antimicrobial therapies take advantage of biochemical and structural differences in microbial and mammalian cells

The principle behind antibiotic drug therapy (chemotherapy) is **selective toxicity**. This means that an agent should interfere with the metabolism of the organism without causing serious adverse effects in the host, taking advantage of differences in cell structure and metabolism. Some organisms, particularly viruses, are difficult to attack because they are inaccessible inside cells: to eliminate the virus the cell must be killed – assuming that the agent is selective for infected cells.

Many antimicrobial agents are naturally produced by micro-organisms, produced to achieve selective growth advantages in competition with others. A typical example is penicillin, which was first discovered because some culture plates became contaminated with a mould which inhibited bacterial colonisation. Modern antimicrobial agents are often versions of the natural products that have been chemically modified to enhance their potency or are synthetic analogues.

Penicillins

The first penicillin (benzylpenicillin) was discovered in 1928 by the British bacteriologist Alexander Fleming, and its derivatives remain among the most important antibiotics today. The penicillin acts both by killing bacteria and by inhibiting their growth. It is mainly effective against Gram-positive bacteria such as pneumococci, streptococci, gonococci, meningococci, leptospirae and gangrene-causing clostridia.

Penicillins derive their antimicrobial properties from their β-**lactam ring** structure, which interferes with the final assembly and cross-linking of the bacterial cell wall. Some organisms are resistant to penicillin, producing an enzyme **penicillinase** that is capable of breaking the β-lactam ring. Many Gram-negative bacilli are intrinsically resistant to the action of penicillin because the outer phospholipid layer of their cell wall prevents access of the drug. Some broad-spectrum penicillins such as amoxycillin and ampicillin are more hydrophobic and are able to pass through the outer lipid layer of the membrane, overcoming this problem. Another semi-synthetic penicillin, methicillin, is active against penicillinase-producing staphylococci, although some organisms may be resistant. These derivatives are produced by chemically altering penicillin precursors.

Inhibitors of protein synthesis

This group of drugs can selectively inhibit bacterial protein synthesis and includes the tetracyclines, the aminoglycosides (gentamicin, for example), chloramphenicol and erythromycin. The drugs work by binding to cell ribosomes (the site of protein synthesis) and either inhibiting their activity or causing production of non-functioning proteins. Their selective activity is based on differences in ribosomal structure between mammalian and bacterial cells.

Inhibitors of nucleic acid synthesis

The selective toxicity achieved by inhibitors of nucleic acid synthesis is derived from differences in folate availability between bacteria and mammalian cells. Folates are involved in the synthesis of purines and pyrimidines and some amino acids. Mammals take up folate from the diet, but bacterial cells must synthesise it themselves. It is therefore possible to interfere with the bacterial synthesis of folate, usually by inhibiting enzymes in the metabolic pathways. The **sulphonamides** work in this fashion but are not widely used because of their toxicity – their main use today is in the treatment of urinary tract infections.

Antifungal agents

Most common fungal infections are superficial, but systemic infections can occur in immunocompromised patients. Unfortunately, the few agents available are toxic to human cells. This is acceptable for topical application (e.g. nystatin treatment of *Candida albicans*), but limits their use in the treatment of systemic infections.

The first-line antifungal agents are amphotericin and flucytosine. Amphotericin reacts with the ergosterol constituent of the fungal cell wall (similar to cholesterol in human cells), forming pores through which essential cell constituents are lost. Ergosterol is not a major constituent of human cells, which is why the drug has selective toxicity for fungi. However, adverse effects are very common, comprising fever, chills and nausea, and long-term therapy

Review question 3

What main trends in the prevalence of infectious diseases have accompanied changes in living conditions and technological advances in developed countries? Which infections have declined and which have assumed greater prominence?

often causes kidney damage.

Flucytosine causes fewer side-effects than amphotericin, but it has a narrow spectrum of anti-fungal activity and resistance can develop during therapy. The agent is converted by the fungal cells, but not by human cells, into fluorouracil which inhibits DNA synthesis.

Antiviral agents

There are relatively few effective antiviral agents. This reflects the difficulty of targeting an agent that is inside host cells without destroying both the infected and the uninfected host cells. The main antiviral agents inhibit nucleic acid synthesis. One such agent, **acyclovir**, inhibits a DNA polymerase enzyme used in the replication of herpes simplex (causes genital herpes and systemic infections in the immunocompromised) and varicella zoster (causes cold sores). Probably the best known of all the antiviral agents is AZT (zidovudine). This agent is used exclusively for HIV, which it inhibits by binding and blocking the activity of reverse transcriptase. This enzyme is needed by the virus to synthesise DNA. Other, newer, agents are currently undergoing clinical trials (see Chapter 25).

Some antiviral agents work by blocking the passage of the virus into the cell. This includes amantadine, which blocks the entry of influenza B viruses, but which is probably not as effective as influenza vaccines.

Antibiotic resistance

Micro-organisms are able to evade the activities of antibiotic agents in several ways. Resistance may be either innate or acquired. An organism may have **innate** resistance usually because it has structural features or enzyme activities that prevent access of or disrupt the antibiotic. When bacteria that were once sensitive to an agent become resistant they have **acquired** resistance. This implies that genetic changes take place within the bacteria. The genes that code for antibiotic resistance usually reside within **plasmids**, small, extrachromosomal circles of DNA. Plasmids can be transferred from one bacterium to another, conferring new antibiotic resistance. Very often a process of selection occurs, in which sensitive organisms are rapidly eliminated by the antibiotic, leaving the more resistant organisms to multiply.

Viral resistance to treatment

Most viral infections resolve spontaneously because of successful cell-mediated attack and the main goal of antiviral therapy is to speed up elimination of the virus. Viruses acquire resistance to therapeutic agents in several ways – one is actually beneficial to the patient, because the viral adaptation results in reduced virulence. An example of this is the response of some herpes simplex strains to acyclovir, which causes mutations in the viral gene for thymidine kinase.

Viral resistance is a particular problem in immunocompromised patients. Many strains of herpes simplex, herpes zoster and cytomegalovirus become resistant to acyclovir in patients with AIDS. These patients may be helped by treatment with foscarnet, a direct inhibitor of viral DNA polymerases.

ANSWERS TO REVIEW QUESTIONS

What features are required by micro-organisms to infect and survive in the human body?

Question 1

Micro-organisms must first get into the body and evade its non-specific protective mechanisms. All the orifices and tracts offer suitable portals of entry, as does the skin if damaged or bitten. The immediate task is to gain a foothold, first by attaching to the epithelium, then (but not necessarily) penetrating the epithelium. Many micro-organisms can avoid being washed away by attaching themselves to the epithelium by producing specific adherence proteins.

Penetration and spread into connective tissues are facilitated by secretion of enzymes. The attachment alone can stimulate an immune response and host defences will also be mobilised against any micro-organisms that penetrate and spread beyond the epithelium. Organisms can resist these defences by virtue of their structure, by taking up residence inside cells or by producing toxins active against inflammatory cells. Toxins, by causing cell damage and death, can also help to optimise the conditions for growth (e.g. for anaerobic organisms). Some of the enzymes produced by micro-organisms are also effective against mediators of inflammation, thereby blocking a co-ordinated host response.

List the mechanisms by which micro-organisms cause cell and tissue damage

Question 2

- **Local invasion** by production of enzymes which destroy connective tissues.
- **Persistence** by adhesion, resistance to phagocytosis (cell wall or capsule components) or intracellular growth induces a sustained inflammatory response which causes tissue damage and ulceration.
- **Toxins** create tissue damage or aerobic conditions suitable for growth.
- **Spread** can cause septicaemia, coagulation and toxic shock, as well as damage to distant organs.
- Continued **evasion** turns an acute inflammatory response into chronic inflammation. Proteolytic enzymes released by inflammatory cells are relatively non-specific and attack the host cells as well as invading micro-organisms.

Question 3

What are the main trends in the prevalence of infectious diseases that have accompanied changes in living conditions and technological advances in developed countries?

Various human activities and lifestyles can influence the risk of infection and, although changes in these conditions can reduce the overall infection rate, other types of infection assume greater importance. Most notably, improvements in general living conditions and sanitation have had a marked impact on the overall morbidity and mortality from infectious diseases.

Plague is now virtually unknown in developed countries and until recently incidence of tuberculosis was declining. Other risks have assumed increased importance. Changes in food production and the increasing popularity of ready-prepared meals, particularly in conjunction with 'cook–chill' systems, has increased the likelihood of food-poisoning by micro-organisms such as *Listeria* and *Salmonell*a. The introduction of canning has provided the anaerobic circumstances for growth of *C. botulinum*, although the risks are much smaller than was previously the case with other food spoilage or contaminating organisms.

The routine use of antibiotics in medicine has resulted in emergence of antibiotic-resistant bacteria. These represent a particular hazard to hospitalised patients. The use of immunosuppressive therapy (in transplant patients, for example) has resulted in increased opportunistic (often fungal or protozoal) infections in people with reduced resistance. This category extends to people infected with HIV.

Even perceived improvements in the environment have brought about new hazards. The use of air conditioning and water cooling systems has provided a new reservoir for the growth and spread, by aerosol, of *Legionella*. Breakdown of water filtration systems and overuse of supplies has led to the transmission of animal infections, causing diarrhoeal and other infections including cryptosporidiosis, giardiasis, and leptospirosis. The development of tampons has improved the daily lives of millions of women, but (rarely) these too can cause disease.

The change in sexual habits that has occurred over the past 50 years has brought about a large increase in sexually transmitted diseases. The increase in travel and the frequency at which many people undertake journeys results in exposures to microbiological hazards which would not normally be encountered and for which the individual has built up no natural resistance. Even the keeping of pets, especially exotic species, can expose people to micro-organisms that they would not normally encounter.

Further reading

Eley, R. (ed.) (1992) *Microbial Food Poisoning*, Chapman & Hall.

Mims, C.A., Playfair, J.H.L., Roitt, I.M. *et al*. (1993) *Medical Microbiology*, Mosby, St Louis.

Waites, W.M. and Arbuthnott, J.P. (eds) (1991) *Foodborne Illness: A Lancet Review*, Edward Arnold, London.

7   Diet and disease

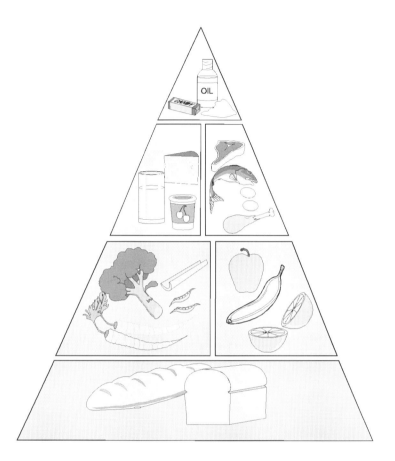

Diet is one of the most important public health problems of the world, usually because of deficiency or, more likely in developed countries, because of excess. In developed countries coronary heart disease, stroke, cancers and osteoporosis are common causes of disability and death. All of these diseases are multifactorial in aetiology, and there is some potential for preventing and ameliorating them by dietary manipulation.

Dietary factors can influence the pathological processes of atherosclerosis and thrombosis. The influence of the diet on cancers is less certain, but dietary fibre and antioxidant vitamins and minerals are believed to have some protective effect. Availability of calcium and vitamin D are important for building peak bone mass and minimising bone loss in osteoporosis.

There is some evidence that dietary factors can help to minimise the symptoms of disease. Most notably, the inflammatory process in rheumatoid arthritis can be modified by adding fish and evening primrose oils to the diet, although these effects are relatively small compared with standard pharmaceutical treatments.

Pre-test

- **What do you regard as a healthy diet?**

- **What health effects might arise from too much sugar in the diet?**

- **What health effects might arise from too much animal fat in the diet?**

- **Why is consumption of fruit and vegetables important to health?**

Aims of this chapter

By the end of this chapter you will have increased your knowledge of:
▲   The dietary components essential for health
▲   Circumstances in which dietary deficiency or excess leads to disease
In addition, this chapter will help you to:
▲   Describe the types of nutrients found in foods and their role in maintaining health
▲   Understand the effects of over- and under-nutrition
▲   Evaluate the role of dietary fibre in the prevention of disease
▲   Understand the differences in the types of fat and evaluate their role in the development of coronary heart disease and cancer
▲   Evaluate the usefulness of antioxidant vitamins and minerals in the prevention of disease

Introduction

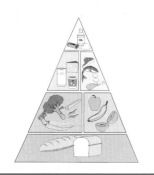

Nutritional status affects our predisposition to disease

'We are what we eat', 'An apple a day keeps the doctor away' and 'Eat your greens' are well-worn phrases that were originally based on intuition rather than scientific fact. As is often the case with medical folklore, scientific investigation has revealed that there is at least a germ of truth underlying these assertions.

The principal causes of death in developed countries – coronary heart disease (CHD), cancers and stroke – are all influenced by the diet and the diet is a main determinant of other significant causes of illness and disability such as osteoporosis, obesity, diabetes, constipation, dental caries and cataracts. Evidence is also emerging that dietary components can help to control the symptoms and severity of other common diseases, particularly inflammatory diseases such as rheumatoid arthritis.

Diet exerts its effects on health in a variety of ways. In some conditions, for example scurvy and rickets, dietary deficiency is the fundamental cause of the disease. It is possible to reverse the condition by replenishment of the deficient nutrient, but this is not always possible because of intervening secondary effects. However, in the more commonly encountered diseases of industrial countries, for example coronary heart disease and some cancers, dietary components form part of a multifactorial aetiology, which makes it much more difficult to isolate and correct the factor responsible.

The mechanisms by which dietary components exert their effects range widely, modulating the mediators of inflammation, changing blood lipid profiles and antioxidant metabolism, and even influencing human fertility. Dietary components influence or cause pathological mechanisms in two ways, through deficiency or through excess.

Because of the time scale involved in the pathogenesis of most chronic diseases, diet may not be seen as a factor in disease for many years – there is evidence that nutrition and consequent low growth rates *in utero* can influence development of diseases such as cardiovascular disease in adult life. This fact causes difficulties in conducting case-control studies: a study of the influence of dietary factors on disease may need to go back 20 years. There is therefore considerable scope for inaccuracy: after all, some people have difficulty remembering what they ate last week, let alone 20 years ago. Prospective cohort studies offer the opportunity to collect more reliable information, but can take many years to complete.

As a consequence of these difficulties the focus of dietary advice has changed over the years to take into account new epidemiological data and results from experimental studies. Initially we were advised to limit our sugar consumption to help prevent dental caries, reduce weight and control diabetes. Then came the advice to consume unsaturated fats rather than saturated fats. Nowadays it is recognised that overall fat intakes should be reduced, and that monounsaturates and the fish oils should be favoured. There is increasing evidence that the consumption of fresh fruit and vegetables is of fundamental importance to health, for their fibre, antioxidant vitamin and mineral contents which are now known to be influential in the predisposition for coronary heart disease and a variety of cancers – Mama's exhortations to 'eat your greens' were justified.

▲ Key points
Influence of dietary factors
▲ Deficiency can be the single cause of some diseases
▲ Component of multifactorial aetiology, for example CHD and cancers
▲ Influences recovery, for example wound healing
▲ Good diet is important in primary disease prevention
▲ Influences response to treatment
▲ Dietary constituents can be used as drugs: chemoprevention, treatment

Dietary reference values

In the UK recommendations for the intake of various dietary components are published by the Department of Health as reference values. These dietary reference values (DRVs) recognise that individual dietary needs differ because of variation in genetic constitution, age and metabolic requirements. The nutrient values are indicative only and are given in several forms:

- The reference nutrient intake (RNI) is the amount that is sufficient, or more than sufficient, for 97% of the population
- Most people's needs are lower than that indicated by the RNI: an estimated average requirement (EAR) will be adequate for most of the population
- A small minority (3%) of people have low needs, given as the lower reference nutrient intake (LRNI)

Energy requirements

Energy is the ability to do work. In body cells, energy is used in the form of ATP, which is generated from the oxidation of carbohydrates, fats and protein ingested as food. These food components are also broken down and used to build new carbohydrates, fats and proteins as required by the body.

Energy is required for cell growth and maintenance

The main body store of energy is in the form of fat, a highly concentrated energy source with each gram of fat able to provide 9 kilocalories (kcal) energy. Carbohydrates provide around 4 kcal/g, but stores are small, principally comprising glycogen in liver cells and glucose in blood. Protein (muscle for example) can be used as an energy source but is not generally used in the short term.

The energy required by a person depends on a large number of factors, including age, gender, body size, ethnic group and expenditure. More energy will be required during pregnancy, lactation, growth and convalescence.

Protein

Virtually all cell structures and products incorporate protein

Proteins are polymers of amino acids. Humans are able to synthesise some amino acids from other food sources, but there are twelve (the essential amino acids) that we cannot make and hence must obtain directly from the diet. Larger amounts of protein are required during growth and development for building new tissues: babies, pregnant women and lactating mothers need plentiful supplies.

Table 7.1 Estimated average protein requirements

Age (years)	Average weight (kg)	EAR (g daily)
1–3	12.5	11.7
11–14 (males)	43.0	33.8
11–14 (females)	43.8	33.1
15–18 (males)	64.5	46.1
15–18 (females)	55.5	37.1
19–50 (males)	74.0	44.4
19–50 (females)	60.0	36.0
Over 50 (males)	71.0	42.6
Over 50 (females)	62.0	37.2
Pregnancy (RNI)		Add 6
Lactation (RNI)		Add 11

The adult daily RNI for protein is 0.75 g/kg body weight, but infants under a year old need twice this amount and neonates even more. Protein should form at least 10% of the adult food intake, and in affluent societies this is easily achieved, usually by consumption of meat, fish and dairy products. In less developed countries it is more usual to obtain protein from cereal sources, which not only makes the diet very bulky but may be lacking in some essential amino acids.

There are concerns that excessive consumption of protein is a risk factor for osteoporosis, and that increased glomerular filtration rates caused by high protein consumption may contribute to further damage in patients with renal disease.

On a global scale, there is a lack of sufficient high-quality protein. In the less developed countries the lack of protein is often accompanied by energy deficiency, resulting in **protein-energy malnutrition**. Protein-energy malnutrition can be a problem in any patient who is severely ill, especially those with cancer, dementia, gastrointestinal disease, sepsis, trauma or renal disease. Other significant causes of protein-energy malnutrition are anorexia nervosa and bulimia.

Protein-energy malnutrition has a number of clinical consequences, of which susceptibility to infection is most common because the immune system is depressed. In prolonged and nearly total starvation, such as arises at times of famine or war, the clinical conditions of **marasmus** and **kwashiorkor** can be seen.

The term marasmus is applied when body weight falls below 60% of normal. It is characterised by an emaciated appearance, muscle wasting, and loss of body fat. The hair is thin and dry, and loses its pigmentation. The affected person is more susceptible to severe bacterial and viral infections, particularly tuberculosis and gastroenteritis. It is often found in children in less developed countries in periods of famine, but is an increasing problem in older people.

Kwashiorkor is most commonly seen in a child who been displaced from breast feeding by a new baby, and who has been weaned on a diet with a very low protein content, such as cassava. The child is apathetic, lethargic and has severe anorexia. There is generalised oedema and the abdomen is distended because of liver enlargement (hepatomegaly). This is caused by a failure to transport lipids out of the liver, because of the absence of protein.

The treatment for both marasmus and kwashiorkor involves correction of fluid and electrolyte abnormalities, provision of protein and energy supplements and control of infection. The current practice is to concentrate initially on energy replacement, providing adequate, rather than large, amounts of protein.

> *Protein-energy malnutrition is accompanied by vitamin deficiency and lack of immune function*

Carbohydrates

Most sugar is usually ingested in the form of sucrose, which is a **disaccharide** (two sugar units joined together) of glucose and fructose (two **monosaccharides**). Disaccharides are broken down by digestion and absorbed as monosaccharides.

It is usual to classify sugars as either **intrinsic** or **extrinsic**. Intrinsic sugars are naturally incorporated into the cellular or fibrous structure of foods; extrinsic sugars, such as honey or refined sugar, are not incorporated. There are no adverse health effects associated with intrinsic sugars, but extrinsic sugars contribute to dental caries, and their intake has indirect effects arising from a lack of 'fibre' (see below).

Starches are polymers of sugar molecules held together in straight or branched chains. All are plant-derived, and are most commonly found in potatoes and other root vegetables, rice and cereals. In the uncooked state starch is insoluble in water. Heating in water causes starch granules to swell,

> *Carbohydrate intake is usually in the form of starch, sugars, and non-starch polysaccharides*

Complex carbohydrates: residues of dietary starch and fibre that cannot be digested in the small intestine. They are broken down (fermented) by bacterial enzymes in the colon, yielding short-chain fatty acids, acetic, propionic and butyric acids and gases, some of which provide essential nutrition for the bacterial flora of the gut.

Dietary fibre: indigestible plant cell-wall material.

Non-starch polysaccharide: 'crude fibre' (plant lignins and cellulose) which is not metabolised and excreted in the stool, and hemicelluloses and soluble polysaccharides that are resistant to digestion but which are fermented by colonic bacteria.

Starch: water-soluble polymer of glucose, amylose and amylopectin. Rapidly hydrolysed by digestive enzymes to short chains of glucose. Not all starch is broken down and some 'resistant starch' enters the colon where it behaves as dietary fibre.

forming a sol. Cooked and uncooked starches have different physiological properties (affecting blood glucose and insulin levels), and cooked starch is more easily digestible than uncooked starch.

Non-starch polysaccharides (NSPs) are complex polymers that usually make up the cell walls of plants and are classed as 'dietary fibre'. They comprise insoluble cellulose and soluble components such as pectins, glucans and gums. Insoluble NSPs are found particularly in whole-grain cereals such as wheat maize and rice. A significant proportion of the NSPs in oats, barley and rye are soluble. Vegetables are lower in total NSP than cereals, and contain roughly equal proportions of soluble and insoluble forms.

Foods rich in NSP are typically bulky with low energy density, and will therefore induce a feeling of fullness without excessive calorie consumption: diets low in NSP tend to be high in fats and sugar. NSPs are believed to impair the absorption of a variety of dietary components including sugars and fats. Consequently, there has been much interest in whether the consumption of NSPs can be beneficial in limiting diseases in which fats could represent a risk factor, most notably coronary heart disease and some cancers.

The fermentation of complex carbohydrates by colonic bacteria influences the stool bulk, its water-holding capacity and rate of transit through the gut. Large amounts of fermentable NSPs encourage bacterial growth, contributing to the stool bulk (normally bacteria comprise at least a third of the stool bulk). A further consequence of fermentation is that the gut contents become more acid. This limits the growth of *Bacteroides* and *Clostridium* species in the gut which are believed to generate carcinogens or tumour-promoting substances. Water held by the NSPs has a diluent effect, which, together with the more rapid transit, minimises exposure to any carcinogenic substances that may be present in food. These mechanisms may reduce the risk of colorectal cancer (see below).

Glucose metabolism

Meals of comparable digestible carbohydrate content result in different blood glucose levels. This has led to the concept of the **glycaemic index**, which compares the post-prandial response of different types of carbohydrate with standard glucose.

Table 7.2   Glycaemic index of some common foods

Food	Glycaemic index
Glucose	100
Wholemeal bread	72
Porridge oats	49
Baked beans	40
Lentils	29

The modulation of blood glucose levels by incorporating complex carbohydrates such as those in porridge oats and lentils into food is of value for diabetics who need to control their blood sugar levels. There is evidence that some complex carbohydrates, such as those in oat products, lower plasma insulin responses. This can be of value in the control of diabetes, by evening-out wide swings in blood glucose and insulin levels.

Diet and dental caries

Tooth decay and gum disease are caused by the accumulation of dental plaque. Bacteria in the plaque secrete a sticky material to which food particles become attached. Sugar in the food is used by the plaque bacteria as an energy supply, but the bacterial metabolism produces acid which attacks the tooth enamel. The consequence of prolonged acid attack is a cavity in the tooth, or **dental caries**.

Dietary sugar is the most important determinant of tooth decay

The production of dental caries is influenced by the presence of plaque and bacteria and the ability of the enamel to resist acid attack. A key factor in tooth decay is poor oral hygiene. Once plaque is removed by brushing and flossing it takes 24 hours for the bacteria to re-establish their colonies in the plaque and acid production during this time is markedly reduced. A combination of plentiful dietary sugar and poor oral hygiene that allows a build-up of plaque ensures bacterial survival. Genetic factors affect the quality of the enamel and its resistance to decay. An important environmental factor is the availability of fluoride.

The potential to cause tooth decay depends on the type, amount, frequency and retentiveness of the sugar or starch

Sugar in any form is potentially damaging to teeth. The critical factor is probably the length of time the teeth are exposed to the sugary food, and in this respect toffees or lozenges are potentially more damaging than a can of fizzy drink. The frequency of sugar consumption has a very strong influence on the development of dental caries. It makes little difference whether the sugar is in the form of sucrose, maltose, glucose or fructose, but lactose and galactose are not as damaging. Other carbohydrates, particularly processed starches, represent a hazard because they are quickly broken down to their component sugars (maltose and glucose) by salivary amylase. Cooked starchy foods such as potatoes, rice and bread are broken down less rapidly.

Foods that are acid in their own right, such as soft drinks and pickles, can cause loss of enamel and dentine. The difference between this kind of acid attack and the acid produced in dental caries is that the latter is focal, more concentrated and more persistent. Some foods are said to be anti-cariogenic, containing factors that protect against dental caries; these include milk and cheese. Milk proteins and fats may exert a buffering effect. Calcium and phosphate in the milk are required for remineralisation and diffuse through the plaque and inhibit demineralisation. A further effect of eating hard cheese is that it stimulates the flow of saliva. Saliva is alkaline and will neutralise and wash away acid produced in the plaque, causing a rise in pH (Figure 7.1).

Dental plaque: a sticky film that covers the surface of teeth. Plaque contains acid-secreting bacteria, particularly *Streptococcus mutans*.

Enamel: the mineral coating of the tooth, comprising calcium and phosphate crystals within a protein matrix. It is one of the hardest minerals known and protects the underlying dentine and pulp from acid attack and physical trauma. Enamel is relatively soft in children but hardens with age.

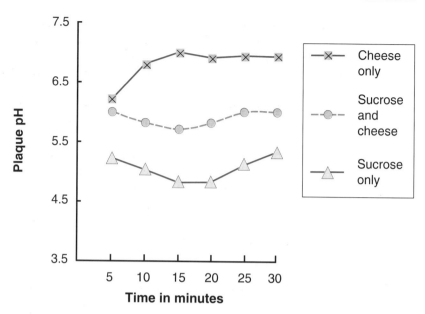

Figure 7.1 The influence of food on plaque pH. Food combinations modify the plaque pH response. Sucrose alone causes a rapid fall in pH below the critical level of 5.5. When cheese is eaten after sucrose the fall in pH is not so marked, probably because of increased saliva production. (Data adapted from Jensen, M.E. and Schachtele, C.F. (1983) *J. Dent. Res.*, **62**, 889 and Silva, M.F. de A. *et al.* (1986) *Caries Res.*, **20**, 263–9.)

Fluoride

Fluoride is the most effective means of protecting teeth from decay. The element becomes incorporated into the tooth enamel as fluorapatite. This material forms a stable lattice that is more resistant to dissolution by bacterial acids.

Table 7.3   Tooth decay and water fluoridation

Year	Fluoridated DMF score (Birmingham)	Non-fluoridated DMF score (Dudley)
1967	4.88	5.19
1970	2.63	5.07
1980	1.22	3.45

Data from Anderson, R.J., Bradnock, G. *et al.* (1982) *J. Dent. Res.*, **61**, 1311–16.

Fluoride toxicity is associated only with heavy accidental or occupational exposures

The value of fluoride in prevention of tooth decay is illustrated by epidemiological studies comparing areas where the water supply is high in fluoride with other areas where the concentration is low. One such study compared the levels of tooth decay in the Northfield area of Birmingham with those in the town of Dudley. Fluoride was added to the water supply for parts of Birmingham in 1964, whereas the Dudley supply remained non-fluoridated. The DMF score (decayed, missing or filled teeth) among 5-year-old children fell markedly in Birmingham and remained consistently lower than in children from Dudley. There was a less dramatic fall in DMF score for the Dudley children during the period of study, and the comparison shows that fluoridation can reduce tooth decay in children by about 50% (Table 7.3). Similar findings have been reproduced around the world, regardless of race, climate or social conditions.

High concentrations of fluoride cause tooth mottling. Very high levels, usually caused by occupational exposure, can cause bone fluorosis, with ossification of the ligaments and fusion of the spine. The acute toxic dose is 1–5 mg/kg body weight, and levels in excess of 15 mg/kg can be fatal. The typical daily intakes of infants and children where the water is fluoridated is in the order of 0.12 mg/kg body weight. An adult weighing 60 kg, drinking 1.5 litres of fluoridated water and ingesting 2 g of fluoride in food would have a daily exposure of 0.05 mg/kg body weight. There is therefore a considerable margin of safety before toxic effects are likely, even in areas where fluoride concentration in the water supply is high.

A fluoride concentration of 1 ppm in water is believed to confer optimal protection against dental caries, without causing mottling of teeth. Only about 10% of the British population receives a water supply that, naturally or artificially, is at or above this level but despite this there has been an overall trend towards reduced prevalence of tooth decay in children in the UK (Figure 7.2).

▲ **Key points**

Avoidance of dental caries

▲ Regular inspection of teeth by a dentist

▲ Regular brushing and flossing to remove plaque

▲ Avoid sugary foods, particularly those that persist in the mouth and adhere to plaque

▲ Avoid frequent or continuous eating

▲ Combination of foods in a mixed meal reduces impact of single components

▲ Use fluoride toothpaste

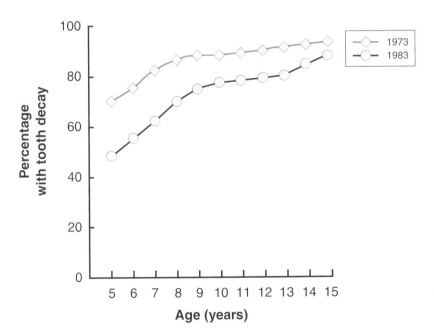

Figure 7.2 Trends in tooth decay (England and Wales, 1973-1983). Tooth decay (measured as decayed, missing or filled permanent teeth) is declining in England and Wales. (Source: OPCS.)

Review question 1

What factors might have influenced the decline in tooth decay illustrated in Figure 7.2 and Table 7.3 (including the Dudley children)?

Non-starch polysaccharides and coronary heart disease

Studies in human subjects have shown that blood lipid levels can be modulated by high doses of guar gum or pectin, although insoluble fibre such as wheat bran has an inconsistent effect. Of more immediate relevance for most individuals is the finding that oat bran and legumes have cholesterol-lowering effects: hence the current claims by advertisers that porridge and oat-based cereals are good for you.

The mechanism of action is unclear: it may be that NSPs bind to cholesterol and bile acids in the small intestine, thereby preventing their reabsorption. The bound cholesterol would instead be excreted, depleting the overall cholesterol pool. An alternative hypothesis arises from the effects of NSPs on blood insulin levels, which in turn may decrease cholesterol synthesis in the short term. Finally, the soluble NSPs are fermented by bacteria in the colon. One of the end products, propionate (a short-chain fatty acid), is known to inhibit cholesterol synthesis in the liver.

There is little evidence that NSP consumption actually has any impact on deaths from CHD. Ideally the proof will come from randomised controlled trials, but the one trial that has so far been completed indicates that there is no effect.

Non-starch polysaccharides and cancer

One of the earliest examples of epidemiological observation concerning dietary fibre and disease was the work of Denis Burkitt, who suggested that a deficiency of fibre could lead to the development of colorectal cancer and a variety of other chronic degenerative diseases. One of the problems in untangling the effects of the diet on cancer is that changes to one component will often be accompanied by concomitant alterations elsewhere. For example, increased fibre intake from fruit and vegetable sources will be accompanied by increased intake of antioxidant vitamins and minerals. Is the effect caused by the fibre, or the antioxidants? High-fibre diets are often relatively low in fat, and it may be that any benefits are due more to the relative absence of detrimental factors such as saturated fat or various carcinogens and tumour promoters than to the high amounts of fibre.

Low stool weight is associated with an increased risk of colonic cancer. An increase in average intakes of dietary NSPs from the current UK average of 13 g/day to 18 g/day would increase stool weight by about 25%. In addition, the short-chain fatty acids produced by the fermentation of polysaccharides are believed to be protective against colonic cancer. Usually our food contains more starch-containing polysaccharides than NSPs and a substantial proportion of the starch escapes digestion in the small intestine, so that short-chain fatty acids are produced in the colon. However, there is evidence that high-starch diets can reduce the rate of cell division of the gut epithelium and hence the risk of malignant transformation. It seems likely that soluble fibre from starchy foods is just as effective as, if not more than, the NSPs (insoluble fibre) in protection against colonic cancer.

A variety of case-control studies have examined fibre intake in patients with colorectal cancer. Meta-analysis of 13 such studies suggests that the risk of colorectal cancer is inversely related to intake of dietary fibre. There are also some indications that consumption of NSPs may help to reduce the risk of breast cancer but not all the epidemiological studies agree, and any benefit is very small.

Adverse effects of NSPs

It has been postulated that high intake of fibre may be detrimental because fibre reduces the amount of minerals available for absorption by acting as an ion exchanger, binding cations such as calcium, iron, copper and zinc. This binding is probably on to uronic acid or phytate residues. However, there is little direct evidence for mineral deficiency in people who usually consume diets high in NSPs, unless their mineral consumption is marginal anyway, even in older people, who should take care not to rely on phytate-rich foods.

Fat

Dietary fats are **triglycerides**, consisting of three fatty acid molecules attached to a backbone molecule of glycerol. The distinction between one fat and another is largely because of the nature of the fatty acids they contain. There are dozens of fatty acids, differing in chain length and degree of saturation.

Not all fatty acids can be synthesised by the body and the **essential fatty acids**, which are needed to manufacture cell membranes, participate in cholesterol metabolism and to synthesise prostaglandins, thromboxane and leukotrienes, must be obtained from the diet. The two essential fatty acids in humans are linoleic acid (C18:2, n-6) and α-linolenic acid (C18:3, n-3). Other physiologically important fatty acids, namely arachidonic (C20:4, n-6), eicosapentaenoic (C20:5, n-3) and docosahexaenoic (C22:6, n-3) acids, can to a limited extent be synthesised in the tissues from linoleic and α-linolenic acids.

It is estimated that the typical British diet provides around 40% of total energy intake from fat, with saturates alone contributing 16%. This is too much, contributing to obesity, coronary heart disease and a host of other adverse health effects. The greatest health risks are believed to be associated with high intake of saturated acids. The so-called Mediterranean diet contains fewer saturated fats, with a larger proportion of monounsaturates and polyunsaturates. Epidemiological studies indicate that this kind of diet is associated with a reduced risk of coronary heart disease. It is also believed that the risk of some cancers may be increased with high intakes of saturated fat, but these data are not so well substantiated.

Leukotrienes: substances derived from 20-carbon polyunsaturated fatty acids involved in inflammatory process (increase vascular permeability or are chemotactic for inflammatory cells).

Prostaglandins: a group of substances derived from 20-carbon polyunsaturated fatty acids that mediate a range of metabolic processes (inflammation for example).

Thromboxanes: a group of substances derived from 20-carbon polyunsaturated fatty acids that mediate vasoconstriction and platelet aggregation.

Dietary fatty acids are saturated, cis-monounsaturated, trans-monounsaturated or polyunsaturated

*The **Health of the Nation** target is to reduce saturated fat intake to 35% by the year 2005*

Table 7.4   Dietary reference values for fat

Fat	Average for population
Saturated fatty acids	No more than 10% of total dietary energy
Cis-monounsaturates	12% of total dietary energy
Cis-polyunsaturates (PUFA)	6% of total dietary energy from a mixture of n-3 and n-6 PUFA
Trans fatty acids	No more than 2% of dietary energy
Total	No more than 35% of energy derived from food

A chemical shorthand has been used for the structures given, omitting carbon and hydrogen atoms. For example:

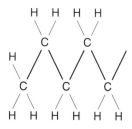

Is represented as:

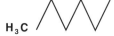

The double bonded structure

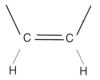

Is represented as:

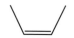

Fewer hydrogen atoms are attached to carbons involved with double bonds. Oxidation of the molecule removes double bonds and replaces them by single bonds, with additional hydrogen atoms

Figure 7.3

Background information: Saturated and unsaturated fatty acids

The fatty acids are long-chain hydrocarbons, terminating with a carboxyl (COOH) group at one end and a methyl (CH₃) group at the other. Fatty acids are either saturated or unsaturated, depending on the attachment of hydrogen atoms to carbon in the chain, and consequently the presence or otherwise of double bonds. If the chain is saturated with hydrogen atoms (two hydrogen atoms attached to each carbon) there will be no double bonds and the molecule is a **saturated** fatty acid.

The nomenclature for fatty acids gives an indication of the length of the hydrocarbon chain and the number of double bonds it contains: an 18:2 fatty acid is 18 carbon atoms long and contains two double bonds. A zero after the colon (for example 18:0) indicates that the fatty acid is saturated.

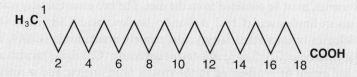

Figure 7.4 A saturated fatty acid (stearic acid, 18:0, found in lard and cocoa butter)

If a hydrogen atom is missing the carbon will link with its adjacent carbon atom by a double bond, giving an **unsaturated** fatty acid. If only one double bond is present then the molecule is a **monounsaturated** fatty acid (MUFA). There are two types of monounsaturated acid, called *cis* and *trans* according to the molecular arrangement of the double bond. Physiologically, it is believed that *trans* fatty acids behave in a similar way to saturated fats: with the exception of the double bond itself their chemical structures are very similar.

Unsaturated fatty acids are classified on the basis of the location of the first double bond (counted from the methyl end of the fatty acid molecule)

– for example n-3 or n-6.

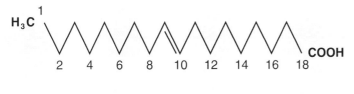

Counting from this end gives nine carbons before the double bond is reached (n-9). In some texts the carbon atoms are labelled from the carboxyl (COOH) end

Figure 7.5 *Trans*-monounsaturated fatty acid (elaidic acid, 18:1, n-9)

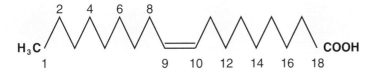

Figure 7.6 A *cis*-monounsaturated fatty acid (oleic acid 18:1, n-9, found in olive oil)

Polyunsaturated fatty acids (PUFAs) contain two or more double bonds. The polyunsaturated fatty acids comprise two classes: ω-3 (n-3) and ω-6 (n-6).

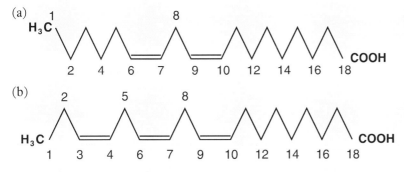

Figure 7.7 Types of PUFA (a) n-6 (linoleic acid, 18:2); (b) n-3 α-linolenic acid, 18:3)

The physical properties of the fatty acids differ according to chain length and degree of saturation: longer chain and saturated fats have higher melting points than short-chain or unsaturated fats. Manufacturers often oxidise polyunsaturated vegetable oils in order to make margarine solid at room temperature because the number of hydrogen atoms increases as the double bonds are removed – hence the term 'hydrogenated vegetable oil'. Unfortunately, oxygenation also very often alters the molecular configuration producing the less desirable *trans* forms.

Vitamins

Vitamins are organic compounds essential for many metabolic functions

Most vitamins are not produced by the body or are produced in insufficient amounts so they must be obtained from dietary sources. The specific functions of certain vitamins became known after studying people who had developed disease as a consequence of deficiency. The absence of a vitamin from the diet gives rise to both general and more specific symptoms. The general effects are lethargy, malaise and, in children, growth retardation. The specific symptoms differ according to which vitamin is deficient (Table 7.5).

Fat-soluble vitamins (A, D, E and K) can be stored by the body. These are usually carried around the body in association with lipoproteins, such as those present in chylomicrons and very-low-density lipoprotein (VLDL) particles. The **water-soluble vitamins** (C and the B complex) are not stored in the body.

Excessive amounts of vitamins can produce untoward effects such as diarrhoea, nausea, loss of co-ordination and rashes. The fat-soluble vitamins are more dangerous because toxic levels can build up. Much of the current research on the role of vitamins is focused on the so-called ACE antioxidant vitamins (vitamins A, C and E) which have the potential to protect against the development of CHD and cancer.

Table 7.5   Properties of vitamins (excluding ACE vitamins)

Vitamin	Function	Disease/symptoms of deficiency	Toxicity	Sources
Vitamin B1 (thiamine)	Metabolism of carbohydrates, lipids and alcohol	Beriberi – neuropathy. In alcoholics presenting signs can also include dementia, ataxia (lack of motor co-ordination) and sight problems	None	Cereals and grains. Removed by milling of rice and flour
Vitamin B_2 (riboflavin)	Cellular oxidative processes – release of energy	Mouth sores, a red inflamed tongue, and skin lesions. Deficiency is rare in developed countries	None	Dairy products, offal, meat and vegetables, milk. Destroyed by ultraviolet light
Niacin (nicotinic acid and nicotinamide)	Part of nucleotide coenzymes NAD and NADP: involved in oxidation and reduction reactions for energy production	Pellagra – a triad of dermatitis, diarrhoea and dementia. Rare, except in people who rely almost wholly on a diet of maize. Mild cases respond well to vitamin B complex, but dementia is often permanent	Nicotinic acid is toxic in large doses	Plants, meats, offal and fish. Can also be synthesised from dietary tryptophan (in milk and eggs)
Vitamin B_6 (pyridoxine)	Metabolism of amino acids, including conversion of tryptophan to nicotinic acid. Formation of haemoglobin	Therapy with isoniazid (antibiotic used to treat tuberculosis) leads to deficiency: vitamin B_6 now given concurrently with the drug. Dietary deficiency is extremely rare	High doses can lead to (reversible) sensory neuropathy	Meat and fish, eggs, whole cereals and some vegetables

Vitamin B$_{12}$ (cobalamins)	Recycling of folate enzymes necessary for DNA synthesis	Pernicious anaemia: failure of red blood cell maturation. Absorption depends on availability of intrinsic factor secreted by stomach parietal cells: deficiency in autoimmune disease (parietal cell antibodies). Deficiency can lead to neurological damage because the vitamin is required for nerve myelination	None	Virtually all animal products, but not green plants. Vegetarians may need supplements. Pernicious anaemia is treated by intramuscular injections of hydroxycobalamin
Folic acid (folate)	Coenzymes in reactions typically involving single-carbon transfers during synthesis of purines, pyrimidines, glycine and methionine	Megaloblastic anaemia (failure of red blood cell maturation). Glossitis (inflammation of the tongue). Requirements increase during pregnancy. Neural tube defects can be avoided by folic acid supplements before conception and in early pregnancy	Toxic in large doses	Liver, yeast extract and green leafy vegetables
Biotin	Metabolism of lipids, carbohydrates and the breakdown of branched amino acids.	Dermatitis, reversible by injection of biotin. Deficiency is very rare	None	Cereal, grains, yeast products, liver, legumes
Vitamin K (phylloquinone menaquinone)	Fat-soluble cofactor necessary for the synthesis of clotting factors and function of proteins involved in calcium homeostasis	Severe deficiency leads to a bleeding disorder: can cause intracranial haemorrhage Babies are born with low liver reserves of this vitamin: deficiency can occur spontaneously in neonates or as the more common late-onset form at 3–8 weeks in babies who have only been breast-fed. Deficiency is unlikely after first few months of life because of synthesis by gastrointestinal flora	None	Phylloquinone is found in green leafy vegetables, certain legumes, some vegetable oils; menaquinones are synthesised by bacteria in the gut

Antioxidant vitamins and minerals

The best-recognised antioxidant vitamin is vitamin E. Because it is lipid soluble it plays a substantive role in preventing the peroxidation of membrane lipids. Vitamin C acts as an antioxidant in the aqueous environment (the cytoplasm, for example), quenching free radicals such as the air pollutants ozone and nitrogen oxides in the respiratory tract. It also plays a role in regenerating vitamin E. Retinol (vitamin A) and β-carotene have been shown to have antioxidant properties *in vitro*, but whether this is an important property *in vivo* is still controversial.

Generally there are some uncertainties about the importance of free radical damage in multifactorial disease processes and how effectively these can be modified by antioxidants. For these reasons the current nutrient reference values for the ACE vitamins in particular do not reflect the much higher dietary

> *Antioxidant vitamins and minerals can limit the potentially damaging effects of free radicals*

intakes (as supplements) that have been used in some intervention studies aimed at preventing CHD or cancer.

Other important antioxidants are the flavonoids, which are notably present in red wine. These are believed to be influential in producing the 'French paradox' of low CHD mortality despite high fat consumption. Some people might consider it unfortunate that as yet there are no EAR or DRV recommendations for red wine flavonoids.

Vitamin A

> *Deficiency of vitamin A leads to eye damage*

Vitamin A is a lipid-soluble vitamin obtained from the diet in precursor form or as the vitamin itself. There are a number of precursors, called **carotenoids**, by far the most significant in the Western diet being β-carotene, which is obtained from fruit and vegetables. Because of its lipid solubility vitamin A can be transported in the body only with other lipoproteins (for example in chylomicrons or in VLDL) or as a complex with a specific binding protein.

Carotenoid precursors are converted to **retinol** by oxygenase enzymes in the intestinal lumen and in mucosal cells (enterocytes). Dietary carotenoids and retinol are absorbed by the enterocytes, and most are converted to retinyl esters. These are transported in chylomicrons to the peripheral cells or to the liver for processing and storage. When required, the stored retinol ester is re-converted to retinol and is released into the plasma in combination with a retinol-binding protein, also synthesised by the liver. Not all absorbed carotenoids are converted to retinol; some are instead transported in the lymph to peripheral tissues (Figure 7.8).

The biologically active metabolites of retinol include **retinal** (also called retinaldehyde) and **retinoic acid**. Retinal acts as a visual pigment, retinoic acid acts as an intracellular messenger and modulates cell differentiation.

Table 7.6　Vitamin A: estimated average requirements (retinol or equivalent)

Age	Daily requirement (µg)
0–3 months	250
1–3 years	300
11–14 years	400
Adult men	500
Adult women	400
Pregnancy (RNI)	Add 100
Lactation (RNI)	Add 350

Vitamin A is essential for growth and development and prolonged depletion is not compatible with life. Vitamin A deficiency is most commonly seen in less developed countries where there is protein-energy malnutrition. The clinical features are impaired adaptation to the dark, followed by night blindness. Dryness of the conjunctiva and cornea (xerophthalmia) can occur, leading to corneal ulceration, superimposed infection and eventually permanent blindness. The initial conditions respond to large doses of vitamin A.

Dietary vitamin A is measured as retinol equivalents (Table 7.6). The most concentrated form of retinol is found in fish liver oil, but it is also present in animal liver, eggs and some dairy products. The precursor, β-carotene, is present in plant sources, particularly dark green and yellow vegetables: the deeper the colour, the greater the β-carotene content. Six micrograms of β-carotene are equivalent to 1 µg retinol. Vitamin A requirements are derived from the amount necessary to maintain a store in the liver of 20 µg/g.

A large body of epidemiological studies suggests that retinol and β-carotene have anti-carcinogenic properties, possibly by modulating the expression of some proto-oncogenes or protein growth factors. Retinoic acid has been shown *in vitro* to promote cellular differentiation and inhibit proliferation of certain tumour cell lines. There is currently considerable interest in assessing the potential of vitamin A and its precursors as agents for prevention of cancer (see below). Furthermore, β-carotene may also act as a protective factor against CHD by virtue of its antioxidant properties.

Excessive intake of vitamin A (retinol) can be dangerous, leading to liver and bone damage. Pregnant women need to be particularly careful because intakes above 3300 µg daily can cause birth defects. Women should avoid eating liver or liver products if they are pregnant or considering becoming so, and should eat green vegetables instead. The precursor, β-carotene, is considered safer because of rate limitations in the conversion to retinol. It has been used for many years at doses up to 180 mg daily and the only documented ill-effect has been yellowing of the skin, which is reversible when the high intake is discontinued.

Vitamin C

The consequence of vitamin C (ascorbic acid) deficiency was one of the first vitamin-related nutritional disorders known – scurvy. This condition is initially characterised by bleeding from small blood vessels, especially in the gums, and slow healing of wounds. The condition is life threatening. The effectiveness of citrus fruits (lemons and limes for example) in preventing scurvy was recognised in the eighteenth century and used by the British Royal Navy: hence the nickname 'limeys'. Vitamin C is also found in vegetables, including potatoes, but not in cereals. The vitamin C content of fruits and vegetables varies widely with the time of harvest, degree of ripeness, variety, storage time and cooking. Small amounts of vitamin C are present in milk.

Unlike most animals, humans cannot synthesise vitamin C. Animal tissues are saturated with the vitamin but very high dietary intakes would be required in humans to reach similar tissue levels. Large doses of vitamin C are poorly tolerated by some people. The DRVs for vitamin C are based on levels that

---

▲ Key points

Biological activity of vitamin A

- ▲ Retinoids regulate proliferation and differentiation of cells
- ▲ Involved in fetal development
- ▲ Functions as chromophore in visual process
- ▲ Carotenoids function as antioxidants

High intakes of vitamin A (retinol) are dangerous, but β-carotene is not toxic in excess

---

Vitamin C deficiency is seen in people who do not eat fruit and vegetables

---

▲ Key points

Effects of vitamin C

- ▲ Deficiency leads to scurvy
- ▲ Required in wound healing
- ▲ May provide protection from cancer and cataracts

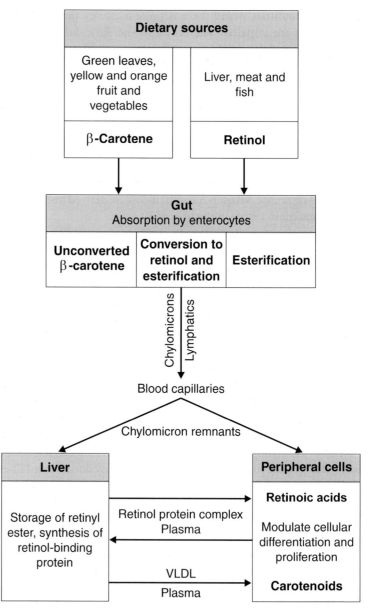

Figure 7.8 Metabolism of vitamin A and its precursors. Most dietary carotenoids are converted to retinol and esterified for transport in chylomicrons and chylomicron remnants. The retinyl esters in chylomicron remnants are taken up by peripheral cells by binding to lipoprotein receptors. Most chylomicron remnants are cleared by the liver. In the liver, retinyl esters are hydrolysed to retinol and coupled to retinol-binding protein. This complex is secreted directly into plasma and is taken up by peripheral cells, probably by binding to specific retinol-binding protein receptors. Within the cell the retinol is uncoupled from the protein and converted to retinoic acid. Some specialised cells, for example in the retina, convert retinol to retinal. Not all dietary β-carotene is converted by the intestinal cells to retinol, and some reaches the peripheral tissues directly in the lymph, in chylomicron remnants, or in VLDL from the liver. For more on lipid metabolism see Chapter 20.

will prevent deficiency disorders such as scurvy and impaired wound healing (Table 7.7).

Table 7.7   Vitamin C: estimated average requirements

Age	Requirements (mg/day)
0–3 months	15
1–3 years	20
Teenagers and adults	25
Pregnancy (RNI)	Add 10
Lactation (RNI)	Add 30

> ▲ **Key points**
>
> **Antioxidant activity of vitamin C**
>
> ▲ Recycles vitamin E in membranes and lipoproteins
>
> ▲ Scavenges free radicals in the aqueous environment, for example ozone and nitrogen oxides in the respiratory tract
>
> ▲ Pro-oxidant effects, for example OH· generation with iron

The DRV (EAR) values for vitamin C are based on the amounts necessary to prevent or cure all clinical signs of scurvy, allowing a generous safety margin. Children require slightly less than adults; pregnant and lactating women require larger amounts. Requirements are significantly increased in smokers. Excessive amounts of vitamin C (1 g or more daily) have been associated with diarrhoea and the development of oxalate kidney stones in susceptible people (the end product of ascorbate metabolism is oxalic acid).

Vitamin C is a water-soluble reducing agent and as such has an antioxidant role, primarily by recycling vitamin E. Plasma vitamin C can react with aqueous free radicals and reactive oxygen species such as might be found as a result of neutrophil activity or as a consequence of smoking. It is notable that mast cells and phagocytes have rich stores of vitamin C in order to neutralise the free radicals that are employed in the breakdown of foreign or unwanted biological substances. Smokers have very low levels of plasma vitamin C, possibly because so much is used in eliminating the excessive free radicals generated.

There are claims that mega-doses (several grams daily) of vitamin C are helpful in preventing or reducing symptoms from the common cold, and that the vitamin might be anti-carcinogenic. Clinical trials have shown that it is of no help for preventing the common cold, and investigations of its possible effects on cancers and CHD are still under way.

Vitamin E

Vitamin E is a fat-soluble antioxidant vitamin and plays an important role in preventing damage to cells by lipid peroxidation. It is believed that sustained damage of this type (mediated by free radicals) increases susceptibility to cancer or CHD. The vitamin acts with selenium in its action against free radical damage. Vitamin E comprises a series of compounds, the most active component being α-tocopherol. It occurs widely in foods, in the lipid phase of meats, fish, vegetables and cereals.

Vitamin E is an essential component in defence against free radical damage

Vitamin E requirements are based on what is needed to prevent the peroxidation of polyunsaturated fats

Haemolytic anaemia: blood disorder characterised by shortened lifespan and excessive destruction of red blood cells.

Thrombocytosis: excess of thrombocytes (platelets) in the blood.

▲ **Key points**

Biological activity of vitamin E

▲ Lipid-soluble antioxidant - contributes to membrane stability

▲ Protects against damage by oxygen free radicals and reactive products of lipid peroxidation

▲ Modulates signal transduction pathways

▲ Regulates cell proliferation by inhibition of protein kinase C activity

▲ Stimulates cell growth and proliferation by inhibition of lipid peroxidation

Clinical signs of vitamin E deficiency are extremely rare. A deficiency syndrome in premature infants (because of their very low fat stores) is characterised by haemolytic anaemia, thrombocytosis and oedema. Children and adults unable to absorb or utilise vitamin E can develop a progressive neurological syndrome.

The amount of vitamin E needed by an individual is related to dietary intake of PUFAs: these have a tendency to become oxidised and potentially atherogenic. As there is wide variation in fat intakes there will be a concomitant variation in the amounts of vitamin E needed – average daily intakes of 7 mg (men) and 5 mg (women) are indicated. Large doses of up to 3200 mg daily may be necessary to achieve protection against the development of cancer or CHD but do not appear to cause significant side-effects. Such high concentrations would be difficult to achieve from normal dietary sources without supplementation.

Antioxidant minerals

Selenium

Selenium is an integral component of the antioxidant enzyme glutathione peroxidase and the availability of selenium can influence the amounts of active enzyme. However, large intakes of selenium do not encourage increased production of this antioxidant enzyme: it is only a deficiency of selenium that might have health consequences. The daily RNI for adult men is 75 µg and for women 60 µg. Lesser amounts are required by children (Table 7.8).

Table 7.8 Reference nutrient intakes for selenium

Age	RNI (µg/day)
0–12 months	10
1–3 years	15
15–18 years (males)	70
15–18 years (females)	60
Over 19 years (males)	75
Over 19 years (females)	60
Pregnant women	No addition
Lactating women	Add 15

Deficiency results in a decrease in production and activity of glutathione peroxidase. In the UK deficiency is very rare, although in some parts of the world (such as Keshan province, China and New Zealand) the soil is deficient in the mineral and consequently so are any crops grown on it. The outcome of severe deficiency is a cardiomyopathy, known as Keshan disease, which is reversible by mineral replenishment.

Zinc

Zinc is an essential trace element present in all tissues. Its principal biological functions are in the regulation or activation of certain enzymes and as a structural component of non-enzyme proteins such as insulin. Zinc-dependent enzymes include those involved in the formation of connective tissues (for wound healing) and the antioxidant superoxide dismutase. Zinc deficiency causes growth retardation. The average dietary intake is 9–12 mg daily. Ingestion of 2 g or more (usually from drinking water that has been stored in galvanised containers) is associated with nausea, vomiting and fever. Chronic ingestion of large amounts of zinc can interfere with metabolism of iron and copper, resulting in microcytic anaemia and neutropenia.

Copper

Copper is a component of cytoplasmic superoxide dismutase. It is also a cofactor in the collagen cross-linking enzyme lysyl oxidase, and hence deficiency of the metal can result in skeletal fragility. Anaemia can develop if deficiency is prolonged and severe but this is very rare. High intakes of copper are toxic but no cases of toxicity have been reported in the UK.

Table 7.9   Copper: reference nutrient intake

Age	RNI (mg/day)
0–12 months	0.3
1–3 years	0.4
11–14 years	0.8
Over 18 years	1.2
Pregnant women	No addition
Lactating women	Add 0.3

Manganese

Manganese is an essential component of many enzyme systems including mitochondrial superoxide dismutase. Manganese deficiency is virtually unknown except in some experimental studies and therefore no DRV has been set. Manganese has a very low toxicity because absorption of the element is low.

Calcium homeostasis

Calcium is required to maintain the strength of bones and teeth, for muscle

Cardiomyopathy: a disorder of heart muscle, often resulting in enlargement of the heart and heart failure.

Microcytic anaemia: an iron-deficiency anaemia characterised by small pale-staining (hypochromic) red blood cells.

Neutropenia: reduction in number of polymorphonuclear neutrophils, associated with increased risk of infection.

Antioxidant vitamins and minerals

Mineral/vitamin	Food source
Zinc	Dairy products, bread and cereals
Manganese	Wholegrain cereals, nuts, tea
Copper	Wholegrain cereals, meat, vegetables
Selenium	Bread and cereals, liver, fish, pork, cheese, eggs, nuts
Vitamin A (retinol)	Liver, whole milk, cheese, butter, eggs, fatty fish
β-Carotene	Yellow and orange fruit and vegetables, spinach, watercress, whole milk and milk products
Vitamin C	Fruit and vegetables, especially kiwi fruit, blackcurrants, citrus fruits
Vitamin E (α-tocopherol)	Oils, almonds and hazelnuts, wholegrain cereals, dark green vegetables, eggs, margarine, cheese and dairy products, fish

contraction, nerve impulses and blood coagulation. Its absorption is controlled by vitamin D.

Vitamin D

Vitamin D deficiency leads to osteomalacia, but could also contribute to osteoporosis

Vitamin D is a fat-soluble vitamin that enhances absorption of dietary calcium from the gut. It also helps to regulate the exchange of calcium and phosphorus between blood and bone. The amount of vitamin D needed is based on how much is necessary to prevent osteomalacia (the failure of bone to calcify). Studies have shown that bone density in middle-aged women is also related to plasma levels of vitamin D.

Most vitamin D is obtained by exposure to sunlight

Vitamin D is produced in the skin by the action of sunlight (ultraviolet radiation) on its 7-dehydrocholesterol precursor. The initial conversion results in cholecalciferol (vitamin D_3), which is then bound to a protein and transported to the liver.

In the liver cholecalciferol is hydroxylated to 25-hydroxycholecalciferol. Measurement of this intermediate in the blood is a good indicator of the bioavailability of vitamin D. The next step in vitamin D metabolism occurs in the kidney, where the 25-hydroxycholecalciferol is further hydroxylated to 1,25-dihydroxycholecalciferol (Figure 7.9). This is the active form of vitamin D.

Normally, adequate amounts of vitamin D are obtained by exposure to sunlight: 15–30 minutes exposure of the forearms, hands and face to the summer sun daily is sufficient. Ultraviolet light intensities in northern climates may be inadequate in winter but, provided that the skin is exposed to sunshine during the summer months, it is possible to build up sufficient stores of the vitamin so that dietary sources are superfluous. Older people, Asian women and children may need dietary supplements.

The relative unimportance of the diet as a source of vitamin D is reflected in the DRV (RNI): for most age groups the value is zero, but it is recognised that children and older adults may be at risk of vitamin D deficiency (Table 7.10). Excessive intakes (above 50 mg daily) have been associated with hypercalcaemia in children. The principal dietary sources are fatty fish, eggs and liver. Limited amounts are also present in butter, and in the UK manufacturers are required to fortify margarine with vitamin D. Several breakfast cereals are also fortified with vitamin D.

Table 7.10 Reference nutrient intakes of vitamin D

Age	RNI (mg/day)
0–12 months	8.5
1–3 years	7
11–18 years (males)	0
11–18 years (females)	0
19–50 years	0
Over 50 years	10
Lactating women	10
Pregnant women	10

Calcium

Calcium requirements are greatest in teenagers and lactating women. The absorption of calcium into the body is less efficient as people get older, and may be related to a decline in the production of vitamin D. Although the EAR for post-menopausal women is only 525 mg daily (Table 7.11), researchers have suggested that larger intakes in women could help to prevent osteoporosis: intakes up to 2 g daily are not usually associated with any detrimental effects. It may be prudent for women who are not on hormone replacement therapy to increase their calcium intake to about 1500 mg/ day.

Extra calcium can be provided by supplements, but the most easily assimilable forms are in foods such as milk and dairy products. Although some people may be worried about the calorie and fat content of dairy foods, low-fat products are good sources of calcium. Calcium supplements, if used, should be taken with increased fluids. Too much calcium can be dangerous: hypercalcaemia or hypercalciuria increases the likelihood of developing renal stones and gallstones.

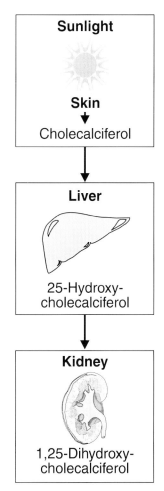

Figure 7.9 Sites of formation of vitamin D.

Table 7.11   Calcium: estimated average requirements

Age	EAR (mg/day)
0–12 months	400
1–3 years	275
11–18 (males)	750
11–18 (females)	625
19–50 years	525
Over 50 years	525
Lactating women (RNI)	Add 550

Dietary iron

Iron is an essential component of the **haem** proteins of haemoglobin and myoglobin. It is also required as a component of cytochromes in the electron transport system, which is vital for cell respiration and generation of energy. Iron, other than that in haemoglobin in red blood cells and myoglobin in muscle, is stored as the protein complexes **ferritin** and, in conditions of excess, as **haemosiderin** in the liver, spleen, bone marrow and muscle. The amount of iron stored is influenced by long-term nutrition and by physiological requirements: more is needed by growing children, adolescents and pregnant women and to make up for losses (menstruating women) or poor absorption (older people).

A variety of dietary factors can enhance or inhibit absorption. Generally the amount of iron absorbed is proportional to its intake. Iron in the haem form (obtained by eating meat) is more readily absorbed than non-haem iron present in vegetables. Absorption is also enhanced by the presence of vitamin C, which reduces ferric iron to the ferrous form. Some amino acids and sugars also enhance absorption, possibly by forming complexes and increasing solubility.

Inhibitors of iron absorption include tannins (in tea for example) and complexing agents such as oxalic and phytic acids in cereals. Some proteins (e.g. those in egg white and yolk) also complex with the metal and inhibit its absorption.

Iron deficiency is the most common nutritional deficiency in children, particularly in those in whom weaning has been delayed. Deficiency causes anaemia, defects in cellular immunity and disturbances in motor function. The EAR values (Table 7.12) are higher for menstruating women. Values for children are lower because of differences in body weight. Iron toxicity is more common in children and very high doses (over 200 mg/kg body weight) can even be lethal. The average iron intake in women aged 18–49 years is 12.1 mg/day.

Ferritin: a ferric iron-protein storage complex.

Haemoglobin: the oxygen-carrying protein of the red blood cells. Red blood cells have a lifespan of only 120 days, and iron from their haemoglobin is broken down and recycled in the liver. It is transported to the bone marrow bound to the glycoprotein transferrin.

Haemosiderin: a storage complex of ferric iron and protein. Deposited in tissues when excessive amounts of iron are stored.

Myoglobin: the oxygen-carrying protein of muscle cells.

Table 7.12 Iron: estimated average requirements

Age	EAR (mg/day)
0–3 months	1.3
1–3 years	5.3
11–18 years (males)	8.7
11–18 years (females)	11.4
19–50 years (males)	6.7
19–50 years (females)	11.4
Over 50 years	6.7

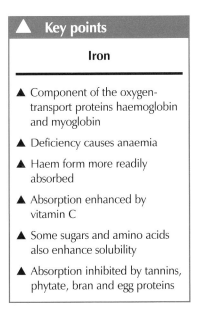

▲ **Key points**

Iron

▲ Component of the oxygen-transport proteins haemoglobin and myoglobin

▲ Deficiency causes anaemia

▲ Haem form more readily absorbed

▲ Absorption enhanced by vitamin C

▲ Some sugars and amino acids also enhance solubility

▲ Absorption inhibited by tannins, phytate, bran and egg proteins

Diet and coronary heart disease

The two main pathological processes leading to CHD are atherosclerosis and thrombosis. Dietary factors are known to influence lipid infiltration into the arterial wall (atherosclerosis) and the tendency of blood to clot (thrombosis).

Dietary fats

Dietary components are important in modulating plasma levels of the cholesterol-containing lipoproteins low-density lipoprotein (LDL) and high-density lipoprotein (HDL). The former is widely regarded as a 'bad' lipoprotein because it can penetrate into the arterial wall and, under certain conditions, initiate atherosclerosis. Conversely, HDL is regarded as a 'good' lipoprotein, because it is involved in 'mopping up' excess cholesterol from the peripheral tissues and transports it back to the liver.

Saturated fatty acids are very effective in raising plasma cholesterol levels; the polyunsaturates tend to have a less marked lowering effect. These observations were behind dietary advice encouraging us to change from the saturated fats in butter to the polyunsaturated fats of margarine and cooking oils (spreading fats and cooking oils comprise about one-third of fat in the British diet).

Saturated fatty acids

The replacement of saturated fats in the diet with monounsaturates or polyunsaturates can lead to reduction in the concentrations of plasma lipids and lipoproteins (see Chapter 20). It is possible to achieve reductions in total cholesterol concentration of up to 20% in normal and hyperlipidaemic men by reducing saturated fat and cholesterol intakes, but the effects in women are not as great. Reductions in cholesterol concentrations of about 20% can be achieved only by a particularly rigorous diet, which many people would find

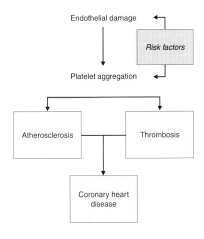

Figure 7.10 The underlying causes of CHD are atherosclerosis and thrombosis. Dietary factors influence events in the atherosclerotic process and the tendency for platelet aggregation.

unacceptable. More modest reductions in cholesterol levels can be achieved by restricting total fat intake to about 30% of total calories – significant changes can be seen in about 6 months.

Trans fatty acids

The molecular structure of *trans* fatty acids bears some similarities to that of the saturated fats. There is therefore some concern that these can influence atherogenesis and thrombosis. In an 8-year prospective study of 85 000 American women (the Nurses' Health Study), of whom 431 went on to develop CHD, *trans* fatty acid intakes were higher in those with CHD than in those without. A case-control study has also revealed higher reported intakes of *trans* fatty acids in British men with myocardial infarction than in matched controls. It is pertinent to note that intakes of *trans* fatty acids have greatly increased over the past 50 years, in parallel with the rise in mortality from CHD.

In early studies, higher contents of *trans* fatty acids were found in adipose tissue from people who died from CHD than in people who died from other causes – however, the large-scale EURAMIC study has failed to confirm this association. The advantage of this particular case-control study concerns the outcome measures used: the fatty acid composition of adipose tissue was determined in people who suffered myocardial infarction and compared it with people who had no history of CHD. This represents an objective biological marker of previous long-term consumption of *trans* fatty acids, since these are not synthesised by the body.

Consumption of *trans* fatty acids increases blood LDL concentrations and lowers HDL levels, although high intakes (about 11% of energy) are necessary to produce these effects. It is estimated that average consumption of *trans* fatty acids in the UK is 2–3%, and perhaps a little higher in the USA. At these more realistic levels the cholesterol-raising effects are not quite as marked as those produced by saturated fats.

There is also some concern about the possible effects of *trans* fatty acids on plasma concentrations of lipoprotein (a). Lipoprotein (a) influences the tendency for both thrombosis and atherogenesis and, when elevated, increases the risk of CHD. This is probably related to similarities in the composition of lipoprotein (a) with both LDL and plasminogen (a component of the fibrinolytic pathway). Plasma levels of lipoprotein (a) were believed to be unconnected with dietary factors, but some studies have shown that consumption of *trans* fatty acids raised lipoprotein (a) levels.

Although it is too soon to draw definitive conclusions, the presence of *trans* fatty acids in margarine may reduce some of the benefits anticipated by changing from saturated fats. Margarine manufacturers have responded to the controversy by reducing the *trans* fatty acid content of some low-fat spreads (Figure 7.11). Paradoxically, the desired hardening is achieved in some products by the addition of butter.

*There is some concern that **trans** fatty acid consumption can increase the risk of CHD*

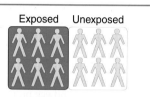

Exposed   Unexposed

Nurses' Health Study

▲ Involved about 85 000 nurses aged 34–59 years

▲ Dietary questionnaire at outset and 2 year intervals

▲ Follow-up for 8 years

▲ Myocardial infarction or death from CHD found in 431 cases

▲ Relative risk 1.5 for high *trans* fatty acid consumption

Data from Willett, W.C., Stampfer, M.J., Manson, J.E. *et al.* (1993) *Lancet*, **341**, 581–5.

Review question 2

How reliable are prospective and case-control studies of dietary intake for proving a causative association between *trans* fatty acid consumption and risk of CHD?

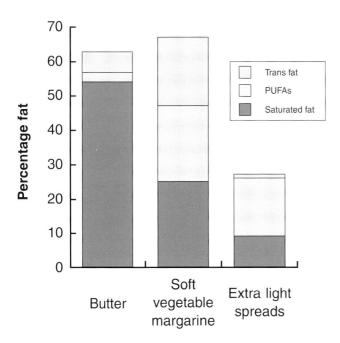

Figure 7.11 The fat composition of butter is predominantly saturated. Margarines, especially the 'light' varieties, contain much more polyunsaturates. *Trans* fatty acids result from the hydrogenation of polyunsaturated fatty acids which is used to produce margarines that are solid at room temperature. (Data from The Flora Project for Heart Disease Prevention, 1994.)

EURAMIC

▲ Involved men aged 70 years and younger from ten centres in nine countries

▲ Compared 742 men with first myocardial infarction in hospital coronary care units with 752 age-matched population controls from hospital catchment areas

▲ Samples of adipose tissue obtained by needle aspiration of buttock

▲ No overall difference between cases and controls in mean proportion of 18:1 *trans* fatty acid

Data from Aro, A., Kardinaal, A.F.M., Salminen *et al.* (1995) *Lancet*, **345**, 273–8.

Are *trans* fatty acids bad for you?

Point	Counterpoint
The increase in consumption of *trans* fatty acids correlates with increases in CHD over the past 50 years	This is simply a secular trend. Other trends were occurring at the same time (cigarette smoking for example). The trends do not show that the people dying from CHD consumed *trans* fatty acids
Case-control and prospective studies show association between *trans* fatty acid consumption and increased risk of CHD	These studies relied on dietary recall as a means of assessing *trans* fatty acid consumption
Early studies showed an increase in the *trans* fatty acid content of adipose tissue of people who had died from CHD	Large multicentre case-control studies have failed to demonstrate any association between adipose *trans* fatty acid concentrations and risk of CHD

Trans fatty acid intakes raise blood levels of LDL and lower HDL	High intakes (11% of energy) are necessary to produce these effects: normal levels of consumption are below 6% and usually in the range 2–3%
Trans fatty acids may increase levels of atherogenic and thrombogenic lipoprotein (a)	Not all studies have shown this effect

Author's view

The structural similarity between *trans* fatty acids and saturated fatty acids makes it difficult to believe that they do not have similar adverse effects. Apart from the possible (but unproved) effects on lipoprotein (a) it is difficult to see how *trans* fatty acids can be worse than saturates, particularly when they will almost invariably be ingested with a high proportion of polyunsaturates (which is not the case with saturated fat consumption). At worst, the switch to polyunsaturated margarines might not be as beneficial as previously thought.

In one sense the controversy is artificial: greater benefits accrue by reducing overall fat consumption to 30–35% of calories. In other words large quantities of spreading fats, biscuits and cakes in the diet are not a good idea, regardless of whether they are made from butter or margarine.

Cis-monounsaturated fatty acids

The advantage of monounsaturated fats is that they do not increase plasma LDL

The only *cis*-MUFA of nutritional significance is oleic acid. Olive oil is particularly rich in this fatty acid. Most studies indicate that *cis*-MUFAs beneficially influence total plasma cholesterol and LDL levels when substituted for saturated fatty acids. Recent meta-analysis of the available studies suggests that the MUFAs are themselves neutral with respect to risk factors for CHD. Their value is in allowing some flexibility in diets aimed at reducing saturated fat consumption: levels of MUFAs can be increased to compensate for the loss of saturates so that the food does not become unpalatable.

Polyunsaturated fatty acids

Polyunsaturates can reduce cholesterol levels and alter the ratio of HDL to LDL

Although the PUFAs have been shown to have generalised cholesterol-lowering effects they can also lower protective HDL levels. It is therefore recommended that overall intake of PUFAs should be limited to 8% of energy. The polyunsaturates are also utilised by the body for synthesis of prostacyclins and thromboxanes, which exert effects on platelet aggregation and vasodilation (Figure 7.12).

n-6 Polyunsaturated fatty acids

These fatty acids are present in cooking oils such as corn oil. A typical n-6 fatty acid is linoleic acid, which in the body is metabolised to arachidonic acid. Arachidonic acid may then be converted to prostacyclin in the endothelium and to thromboxane by platelets (Figure 7.12). These products have opposing effects on haemostasis: the prostacyclin has vasodilatory properties and inhibits platelet aggregation, whereas thromboxane is vasoconstrictive and stimulates platelet aggregation.

The relative amounts of prostacyclin and thromboxane produced depends on the dietary intake of linoleic acid. A high intake decreases the tendency for platelet aggregation and thrombosis, whereas only modest amounts appear to be associated with an increase in the tendency for thrombosis.

n-3 Polyunsaturated fatty acids

An example of an n-3 fatty acid is α-linolenic acid, found in the chloroplasts of green vegetables. This acid can be metabolised to eicosapentaenoic acid and docosahexaenoic acid, both of which can be obtained directly from fatty fish such as sardines, mackerel, herring, trout and salmon. The n-3 fatty acids modulate prostaglandin metabolism and decrease blood triglyceride levels. In high doses they have antithrombotic and anti-inflammatory properties.

> *The n-3 fatty acids, found in fish oils, are believed to inhibit atherogenesis and thrombosis*

Atherosclerosis

The evidence of a beneficial role for dietary n-3 polyunsaturated fatty acids arose from observations that Eskimos living in Greenland who adhered to their traditional fish diet had very low rates of CHD. Their blood lipid profiles revealed lower concentrations of plasma triglycerides, LDL and VLDL, but higher concentrations of HDL, than in Eskimos living in Denmark who had adopted a more 'Western' diet. Intervention studies in Westerners have shown that the intake of extra fish or fish oil can produce changes in blood fatty acid and triglyceride levels, although the effects may not be substantial.

Thrombosis

Eskimos with a relatively high consumption of n-3 fatty acids have been found to have increased bleeding times and a reduced tendency for platelet aggregation probably because thromboxane synthesis is reduced by n-3 acids displacing the n-6 arachidonic acids in the platelet membranes. Consumption of n-3 fatty acids has also been shown to lower lipoprotein (a) levels. It remains to be seen whether reducing lipoprotein (a) by this means also lowers the risk of CHD.

Further advantages of eicosapentaenoic and docosahexaenoic acids are their effects on blood pressure. Hypertension is a significant risk factor for initial endothelial damage and subsequent thrombosis in atherosclerotic lesions. Large intakes of these fatty acids can reduce blood pressure by 3–5 mmHg, particularly in people with high blood pressure. Although the amounts required would be difficult to obtain from the average Western diet, effective amounts might be achieved using fish-oil supplements.

In a prospective study (the Health Professionals Follow-up Study) of middle-aged men who were initially deemed to be free of CHD, increasing fish intake from 1–2 servings to 5–6 servings per week did not substantially reduce risk of

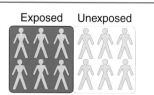

Health Professionals Follow-up Study

▲ Involved 44 895 men aged 40–75 years

▲ Dietary questionnaire at outset and 2 year intervals

▲ Follow-up 6 years

▲ Incidence of myocardial infarction, CHD deaths, bypass or angioplasty procedures in 1543 men

▲ Relative risk of CHD 1.14 for low fish consumption (one serving or less per month) compared with higher intake (six or more servings per week)

Data from Ascherio, A., Rimm, E.B., Stampfer, M.J. *et al.* (1995) *N. Engl. J. Med.*, **332**, 977–82.

Vitamin E may prevent oxidation of LDL in the arterial wall

Laboratory measures show that antioxidant supplementation can delay oxidation of LDL

CHD. There is a potential bias in this kind of study, mainly concerning the accuracy of historical information obtained by questionnaire. However, if the findings are accepted then it would seem necessary to consume more fish, or to supplement with fish oils to obtain significant protection.

▲ Key points	
Effect of dietary fatty acids on CHD risk factors	
Type of fatty acid	**Physiological effect**
Saturated fatty acids	Increase plasma LDL
Cis-monounsaturated fatty acids	Reduce plasma LDL
Cis-polyunsaturated fatty acids: Long-chain n-3	Reduce blood pressure, plasma lipoprotein (a), platelet aggregation and fibrinogen levels
Long-chain n-6	Reduce severity of arrhythmia and plasma LDL
Trans fatty acids	High intake increases plasma LDL and reduces HDL

Antioxidants and coronary heart disease

The prevention of CHD by the antioxidant vitamins is biologically plausible, because the atherosclerotic process involves damage by oxidised LDL. It follows that if LDL oxidation can be prevented or reduced, then so might formation of atherosclerotic plaque.

One cross-sectional epidemiological study (The WHO European Study) has shown an inverse correlation between plasma concentrations of vitamin E and deaths from CHD. In this study, plasma vitamin E concentrations were compared in men living in regions of low, medium and high incidence of CHD. However, this study was population-based and did not measure plasma vitamin E levels in the individuals who actually developed the disease. The study showed that men in southern France have high plasma vitamin E levels, which presents an alternative explanation for the 'French paradox' (see Chapter 20).

The potential of antioxidants to inhibit oxidation of LDL has been investigated by giving daily supplements of 200 mg α-tocopherol (vitamin E), 18 mg β-carotene and 12 mg zinc over a period of 6 months (Abbey et al., 1993). Outcome measures were plasma concentrations of the vitamins and the time taken for serum LDL to be oxidised. Substantial increases in the plasma levels of the vitamins were recorded and LDL oxidation times increased

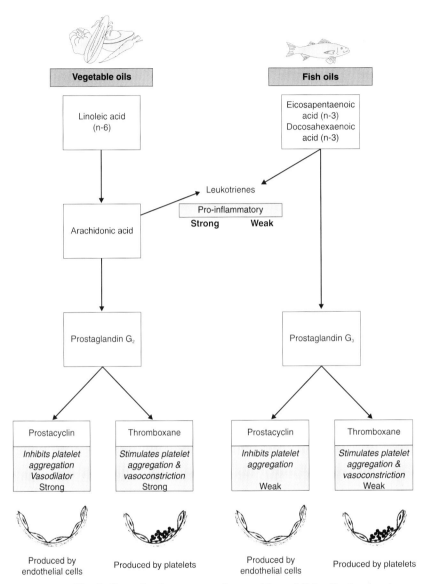

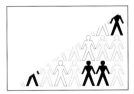

WHO European cross-sectional study

▲ Comparison of plasma vitamin E levels in areas of low, medium and high mortality from CHD (for example southern France, Spain, Denmark, Finland)

▲ Approximately 100 men studied from each centre (16 centres)

▲ Subjects were middle-aged men (40–59 years)

▲ Of the 16 centres 12 had similar blood pressure and cholesterol levels

▲ Inverse correlation found between plasma vitamin E levels and deaths from CHD

▲ Men in southern Europe apparently have higher blood vitamin E levels than those in northern Europe

Data from Gey, K.F., Puska, P., Jordan, P. *et al.* (1991) *Am. J. Clin. Nutr.*, **53**, 326S–34S.

Figure 7.12 Metabolism of polyunsaturated vegetable and fish oils. Leukotrienes, prostacyclins and thromboxanes are synthesised from PUFA precursors in the diet. Products derived from the n-6 PUFAs are usually more potent than their equivalents synthesised from n-3 precursors. The enzymes in the metabolic pathways display enhanced substrate affinity for the n-3 precursors. High intakes of n-3 fatty acids (in fish oils) influence the balance in favour of those prostacyclins that inhibit platelet aggregation.

significantly within 3 months of taking the supplements. The physiological significance of these findings is not clear, but it may be that a delay in LDL oxidation prevents the activation of macrophages, which in turn triggers further oxidation of LDL. The levels of vitamin and mineral given as supplements were far in excess of normal dietary intakes.

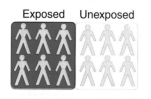

Exposed   Unexposed

Nurses' Health Study, Health Professionals Cohort Study

Women (Nurses' Health Study):

▲ Involved 87 000 nurses aged 34–59 years

▲ Dietary questionnaire at outset and 2 year intervals

▲ Eight-year follow-up

▲ Total of 552 cases of CHD found

▲ Relative risk 0.59 with vitamin E intake above 100 IU/ day

Men (Health Professionals Cohort Study):

▲ Involved 40 000 health professionals aged 40–70 years

▲ CHD found in 667 subjects

▲ Relative risk 0.63 with vitamin E intake above 100 IU/ day

Data from Rimm, E.B. et al. (1993) N. Engl. J. Med., **328**, 1450–6 and Stampfer et al. (1993) N. Engl. J. Med., **328**, 1444–9.

▲   Key points

Vitamin E and coronary heart disease

▲ Antioxidant protector of LDL

▲ Decreased vitamin E concentration is associated with increased platelet aggregation

▲ Vitamin E reduces lipid peroxidation and extent of myocardial infarct

▲ The vitamin also reduces likelihood of reperfusion injury in treated myocardial infarct

Another prospective study of men in Denmark demonstrated a relationship between low serum selenium levels (<1 mmol/l) and increased risk of ischaemic heart disease, after adjusting for other risk factors. It is suggested that selenium supplementation may be beneficial in people with low serum levels, although an intervention trial would be needed to positively demonstrate any benefit.

Recent prospective studies (such as Nurses' Health Study, Health Professionals Study) have provided evidence of an association between higher vitamin E intake and reduced risk of CHD, of the order of 40% for both men and women. However, the benefit was seen only when daily vitamin E intake was above 100 IU, amounts that are not usually obtainable from normal dietary intakes: supplementation would be required.

Two large randomised controlled trials have failed to show any benefit from vitamin E or β-carotene supplementation. In one, the Finnish α-tocopherol [be]-carotene trial (ATBC; see p. 255), all the subjects were smokers, but supplementation with vitamin E or β-carotene did nothing to reduce the risk of CHD. There was even a slight increase in deaths in the group receiving β-carotene. Another trial, the Physician's Health Study, followed more than 22 000 male doctors in the USA for an average of 12 years. This included both smokers and non-smokers (at the beginning of the study in 1982 11% were current smokers and 39% were ex-smokers), randomised to receive β-carotene or placebo on alternate days. There was almost no difference in the overall incidence of CHD, cancer (see p. 253) or in overall mortality between the intervention and placebo groups.

Taken together, these trials show that well nourished men gain no significant benefit from β-carotene supplements. This, seemingly, is in contrast to previous case-control studies which show that fruit and vegetable consumption lowers risks of CHD. The difficulty with case-control studies in any complex relationship between diet and disease is the problem of correct ascertainment: in a lengthy multifactorial disease process such as CHD recent dietary habits probably assume less importance than those earlier in the disease process, and current consumption should not be regarded as an indicator of past consumption. It is also likely that other highly influential risk factors may have changed over the space of 20 years. A similar problem applies to prospective studies: few volunteers are likely to want to complete a comprehensive diet diary over such a prolonged period.

The value of vitamin E supplementation remains unclear, and in large randomised controlled studies appears to have been tested only in men who have a long history of smoking. The disappointing results from the ATBC trial could relate to the short time period of supplementation relative to smoking and, of course, do not convey information relevant to non-smokers.

Diet and cancer

High fat consumption is associated with some of the more common cancers

Dietary fats

It is noteworthy that when people migrate from one country to another they begin to take on the cancer incidence rates of the host country. For example, stomach cancer is very common in Japan, but breast, colorectal and prostate cancers are rare. The incidence of cancer in Japanese immigrants to the USA is lower than in Japan but the rates of breast, colorectal and prostate cancers are higher.

A variety of lifestyle changes accompany migration from one country to another, including changes in living conditions, economic circumstances and social networks. One of the most fundamental changes is likely to be the diet, simply because of differences in local availability and cost of foodstuffs. The most probable dietary change consequent on migration to Western industrialised countries is increased consumption of fat.

Colorectal cancer

A link between dietary fat intake and colonic cancer has been established by epidemiological and laboratory animal studies, although case-control studies have not been consistent in showing the association. A large prospective study (the Nurses' Health Study) has shown that the risk of colonic cancer increases with increase in intake of saturated and monounsaturated fats. It is believed that dietary fat can promote human colonic carcinogenesis by two mechanisms: by promoting cell proliferation and by stimulating the secretion of bile. Bile acids may have a toxic or carcinogenic effect on the epithelium. The increase in risk was associated with high meat intake, but not with consumption of saturated fats as dairy products. It is suggested that the calcium content of dairy products may somehow be protective, possibly by binding and neutralising bile acids.

Other epidemiological studies support an association between calcium consumption and reduced risk of colorectal cancer, but some do not. Randomised controlled trials that will examine the effects of calcium supplementation on the recurrence of colonic adenomas (a precursor for colonic cancer) are currently under way.

Breast cancer

There is a possibility that high intake of dietary fat increases the risk of breast cancer. Although the cause of breast cancer remains unknown certain factors appear to increase the risk. The most important of these is family history, but others (such as early menarche and late menopause) are related to the duration of oestrogen exposure. Some studies indicate that risk of developing breast cancer in post-menopausal women is related to weight and body fat distribution; in turn this may be related to increased production

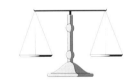

Physician's Health Study

β-Carotene versus placebo
- ▲ Total of 22 071 male doctors aged 40–84 years studied in the USA including smokers, ex-smokers and non-smokers
- ▲ Half (11 036) assigned to receive β-carotene (50 mg) on alternate days, 11 035 assigned to receive placebo
- ▲ Deaths from myocardial infarction in β-carotene group 468, in placebo group 489
- ▲ Deaths from CHD in group receiving β-carotene 338, 313 in group receiving placebo

Data from Hennekens, C.H., Buring, J.E., Manson, J.E. et al (1996) *N. Engl. J. Med.*, **334**, 1145–9.

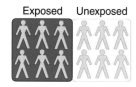

Exposed   Unexposed

Nurses' Health Study

▲ Involved 87 000 nurses aged 34–59 years
▲ Dietary questionnaire at outset and 2 year intervals
▲ Follow-up 6–8 years

Colonic cancer:

▲ Incidence of colonic cancer 150 cases
▲ Animal fat intakes correlate with colon cancer risk
▲ No association with vegetable fat consumption
▲ Relative risk 2.49 for daily consumption of beef, lamb or pork compared with consumption of less than once per month (1.00)

Breast cancer:

▲ Breast cancer seen in 1449 women, of whom 774 were post-menopausal

▲ No association with intake of total or specific types of fat

▲ No protection from dietary fibre

Data from Willett, W.C., Stampfer, M.J., Colditz, G. *et al.* (1990) *N. Engl. J. Med.*, **323**, 1664–72 and Willett, W.C., Hunter, D.J., Stampfer, M.J *et al.* (1992) *JAMA*, **268**, 2037–44.

of oestrogen (a known tumour promoter) from androgen precursors in adipose tissue. There is therefore much interest in the possible role of dietary fats in the development of breast cancer.

Epidemiological studies have shown a correlation between national fat consumption and national figures for incidence of breast cancer and mortality. However, an association has been difficult to prove at the small population or individual level by means of cohort and case-control studies partially because the statistical power of the analyses is limited by small sample sizes. Meta-analysis of the case control studies reveals some relationship between fat intake and breast cancer in post-menopausal women.

The case-control approach is not the most accurate, particularly with respect to determination of aspects such as past consumption of dietary fat, and more reliable results should be obtained from prospective studies. A number of such studies are currently under way – for example, the Women's Health Initiative and the Nurses' Health Study in the USA, and the European Prospective Investigation into Cancer and Nutrition (EPIC). Data for 8 years of follow-up from the Nurses' Health Study have now been published. The results show no relationship between energy, total or specific fat, or dietary fibre intakes.

Prostate cancer

Prostate cancer is the second most common cause of death from cancer in men in the USA, and ranks third in the UK. The cause of the disease is unknown, although the usual genetic and environmental factors have all been suggested. A relationship has been suggested between dietary saturated fat and advanced prostate cancer. In a prospective study of 50 000 men in the USA, there appeared to be an association with the intake of animal fat, particularly α-linolenic acid. The authors of this study suggest that a carcinogen could be formed from α-linolenic acid during the cooking of red meat, but precise mechanisms remain unclear. Another study in Utah suggests that high intakes of dietary fat are associated with more aggressive prostate cancers.

Antioxidants and cancer

It is likely that antioxidants exert a number of biological effects in the transition of cells towards malignancy, probably by neutralising free radicals. There is also evidence that some antioxidants influence the activities of proto-oncogenes and tumour suppressor genes and inhibit mutagenesis. Antioxidants are known to modulate the immune response and increase natural killer cell activity: immune mechanisms are believed to undertake 'surveillance' activities and removal of newly transformed cancer cells. Severely immunocompromised individuals have greatly increased risks of developing cancer.

In support of an association between antioxidants and CHD, epidemiological studies tend to yield promising results in case-control and prospective studies. In contrast, randomised controlled trials of antioxidant supplementation often yield disappointing results, notable examples being the Finland ATBC trial and, in the USA, the CARET and Physicians' Health Study trials. More encouraging results were found in the Linxian trial in China, but this was in a population that could be expected to be relatively poorly nourished.

Colorectal cancer

Epidemiological studies have indicated an inverse relationship between fruit and vegetable intakes and the prevalence of colorectal cancer, probably because of their antioxidant and fibre contents. In a case-control study conducted in the Mediterranean region of France the strongest protective effect was observed with vegetables containing low amounts of fibre. In contrast, meta-analysis of 13 case-control studies indicates that although vitamin C and β-carotene appear to be protective this was a weaker effect than that obtained with fibre intake. Prospective studies are required to examine the relationships between fibre, antioxidant vitamins and colorectal cancer more fully. Intervention studies with vitamin and mineral supplements may go some way to resolving the question of exactly which components of fibre-rich foods have a protective effect.

Breast cancer

The risk of breast cancer has also been examined with respect to the possible influences of dietary fibre and antioxidant vitamins. One prospective study in Canada followed a cohort of 56 837 women, of whom 519 developed breast cancer in a 5-year period. In contrast to the results of the Nurses' Health Study, high dietary fibre intake was associated with a small reduction in risk of developing breast cancer. Smaller reductions in risk were associated with high dietary intakes of the antioxidant vitamins A and C, but not vitamin E.

At best, the estimates attached to the influence of fat, fibre and antioxidant vitamins on the risk of breast cancer point toward only modest changes. This is only to be expected in the face of much stronger influences such as family history and reproductive variables. Any effects of dietary factors would necessarily be subtle, perhaps influencing the time of development of symptoms or diagnosis rather than the overall risk of developing the disease.

Lung cancer

Studies indicate that smokers have an increased turnover of vitamin C. This is possibly related to generation of free radicals by metabolites of the cigarette smoke, and consequent tissue damage. Some of the older epidemiological studies suggest that risks of lung cancer in smokers and non-smokers (a small minority of lung cancers may be attributable to causes other than active smoking) are reduced in populations in whom dietary intake of β-carotene was relatively high. There is therefore some interest in a possible role for antioxidants in preventing cancer or mitigating the effects of smoking.

One of the first randomised clinical trials to report on the effects of deliberate supplemental antioxidant intake was the Finnish ATBC (α-tocopherol, β-carotene) trial, in which male smokers took supplements of α-tocopherol and/or β-carotene for a period of 6 years. No reductions in deaths from lung cancer

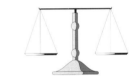

Finland ATBC trial

▲ Involved 29 133 male smokers aged 50–69 years

▲ Average cigarette consumption 20/day for 36 years

▲ Daily α-tocopherol (50 mg) and/ or β-carotene (20 mg) or placebo

▲ Follow-up 5–8 years (median 6.1 years)

▲ Lung cancers newly diagnosed 876 (564 deaths)

▲ No reduction in incidence of lung cancer in group receiving α-tocopherol

▲ Higher incidence of cancer in group receiving β-carotene

Source: The Alpha-Tocopherol, Beta-Carotene Cancer Prevention Study Group (1994) *N. Engl. J. Med.*, **330**, 1029–35.

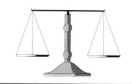

CARET

▲ Involved 18 314 male and female smokers, ex-smokers (aged 50–69 years) and workers exposed to asbestos (men aged 45–74 years)

▲ Subjects randomised to receive 15 or 30 mg β-carotene or 25 000 IU retinol, both, or placebo, daily

▲ Average follow-up 4 years

▲ New cases of cancer: 388

▲ Relative risk of death higher in active treatment groups (1.17 for all-cause, 1.46 for deaths from lung cancer and 1.26 for deaths from CHD)

▲ Supplementation discontinued but follow-up to continue for another 5 years

Source: Omenn, G.S., Goodman, G.E., Thornquist, M.D. *et al.* (1996) *N. Engl. J. Med.*, **334**, 1150–5.

Review question 3

Can dietary antioxidant vitamins and minerals effectively reduce the incidence of cancer?

Dietary factors can act in a similar way to aspirin and reduce inflammation

---

were observed in the groups receiving supplements – in fact there was an excess of cases of lung cancer in the group receiving β-carotene. It may be that the intervention came too late in the multistage process of development of lung cancer as many of the men had smoked for 36 years or more. It is also possible that the vitamin dose was too small, although it was in excess of that achieved by normal (non-supplemental) dietary sources. Perhaps unexpectedly, one positive result of this trial was that men who had received α-tocopherol had a much lower incidence of prostate cancer than those who had not.

Another randomised controlled trial, the β-Carotene and Retinol Prevention Trial (CARET), has been stopped prematurely owing to increased morbidity in the intervention group. The trial, conducted in the USA, was designed to evaluate the combination of retinol and β-carotene in 18 000 people deemed to be at high risk of lung cancer (mainly smokers and asbestos workers). In the people who took the supplement there was a 28% increase in lung cancer and a 17% increase in deaths compared with the control group. Similarly, in the Physicians' Health Study β-carotene trial (see p. 253) no significant differences in the incidence of lung cancer (or indeed in deaths from any type of cancer) between treatment and placebo control groups were found.

Taken together, these results are not encouraging, and it can be concluded that supplementation of antioxidant vitamins in smokers is unlikely to be of significant benefit – and could possibly do harm. Much more can be gained by stopping smoking.

Gastric and oesophageal cancers

Evidence from a number of epidemiological studies suggests that fruit and vegetable consumption reduces the risk of gastric cancer. A recent randomised controlled trial studied vitamin and mineral supplementation in Linxian, China (a rural area in north central China with some of the highest rates of oesophageal and gastric cancers in the world) whose population has a very low intake of vitamins and minerals.

Of the various vitamin and mineral combinations used in the trial, only one (β-carotene plus vitamin E, plus selenium) significantly reduced deaths from cancer, the largest effect being on gastric cancers. As the Linxian population is chronically deficient in micronutrients it is uncertain whether such supplementation will be of any benefit to the relatively well-nourished Western populations. It is notable that the highest prevalence of gastric and oesophageal cancers tends to be in areas of the world that are likely to suffer from nutritional deprivation.

Diet and rheumatoid arthritis

Rheumatoid arthritis is the most common of the autoimmune inflammatory diseases. Although there is little evidence for a role of dietary factors in preventing the disease, there has been interest in the possible benefits of dietary factors such as fish oils, evening primrose oil and olive oil in modulating the inflammatory process and the clinical course of the disease.

▲ Key points

Dietary factors and cancer

Breast cancer:
▲ Relative risks for dietary factors are small compared with age and family history

▲ Early menarche and late menopause relate to duration of oestrogen exposure

▲ Oestrogen exposure influenced by weight and distribution of body fat

▲ Oestrogen is produced in adipose tissue from androgen precursors

▲ Epidemiological studies show a correlation between national fat consumption and rates of breast cancer

▲ An 8-year prospective study (Nurses' Health Study) showed no relationship with energy, fat or fibre intakes

Colorectal cancer:
▲ Epidemiological association with high consumption of red meat and fat, low intakes of fibre, starch and vegetables

▲ Meat intake potential source of carcinogens (for example *N*-nitroso compounds)

▲ One large prospective study shows increased risk with high intakes of monounsaturated and saturated fats (meat, but not dairy saturated fats)

▲ Fats may promote cell proliferation and increase synthesis of bile

▲ Calcium may be protective

▲ Fruit and vegetable consumption protective, including low-fibre types

Lung cancer:
▲ Smokers have an increased turnover of vitamin C

▲ Case-control studies suggest β-carotene intake associated with reduced risk, but this has not been confirmed by randomised controlled trials

Prostate cancer:
▲ Case-control studies show association with increased fat consumption

▲ Vitamin E supplementation may be protective

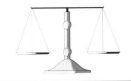

Linxian Trials

Combined daily doses of vitamins and minerals

▲ General Population Trial initiated in 1986, participants aged 40–69

▲ Total of 30 000 people randomised to receive combined retinol and zinc, riboflavin and niacin, vitamin C and molybdenum or β-carotene, vitamin E and selenium, at doses 1–2 times the US recommended daily amounts

▲ After 5 years, reduction in cancer risk found only in the group receiving β-carotene, vitamin E and selenium

▲ Total mortality reduced by 9%

▲ Overall cancer mortality reduced by 13%

▲ Mortality from stomach cancer reduced by 21%

▲ Mortality from oesophageal cancer reduced by 4%

Source: Blot, W.J., Li, J.Y., Taylor, P.R. *et al.* (1993) *J. Natl Cancer. Inst.*, **85**, 1483–92.

Dietary fatty acids and inflammation

The process of inflammation is mediated by a variety of soluble agents, including leukotrienes, prostaglandins and thromboxanes. These substances are produced from fatty acid precursors. Most dietary n-6 fatty acids are converted to arachidonic acid, which is a common precursor for leukotrienes, prostaglandins and thromboxanes. The leukotrienes possess pro-inflammatory properties, while the prostacyclins and thromboxanes influence platelet aggregation and vasoconstriction (see Figure 7.12). In contrast, the n-3 fatty acids (for example, those found in fish oils) are converted not to an arachidonic

Inflammation can be reduced if mediators are derived from n-3 fatty acids

acid precursor but more directly to the leukotriene, prostacyclin and thromboxane end-products. In general these end-products are much less potent than the analogous products derived from arachidonic acid. The n-3 derivatives are preferentially taken up by the cyclo-oxygenase and lipoxygenase pathways at the expense of arachidonic acid, thus favouring the production of the less potent derivatives. It is also postulated that dietary supplementation with the n-3 fatty acids could influence inflammation by reducing the production of IL-1 and tumour necrosis factor by macrophages.

Randomised trials

Randomised trials of fish oil supplementation indicate that the symptoms of rheumatoid arthritis (tender and swollen joints, morning stiffness, loss of grip strength) can be alleviated. There is evidence that the effects are dose-dependent, the best results being obtained with high doses (54 mg/kg body weight eicosapentaenoic acid and 36 mg/kg docosahexaenoic acid) administered daily over 24 weeks. Clinical improvement is accompanied by reduction in production of neutrophil LTB4 and macrophage IL-1. It also seems that the benefits can persist for many months after supplementation is discontinued, and patients become less reliant on NSAIDs such as aspirin.

Evening primrose oil is believed to possess anti-inflammatory activity and has been found to produce clinical improvements in rheumatoid arthritis, particularly reducing reliance on NSAIDs. However, these studies have involved only very small numbers of patients with mild symptoms of rheumatoid arthritis. A larger multicentre study is planned to evaluate the effects of high-dose evening primrose oil. The active component of evening primrose oil is γ-linolenic acid, although its mode of action is not completely understood. It has been suggested that the metabolic products competitively inhibit the synthesis of the strongly inflammatory series 4 leukotrienes and series 2 prostaglandins.

A number of studies have shown that consumption of olive oil can have beneficial effects on symptoms of rheumatoid arthritis. This could be because it reduces the plasma concentration of the pro-inflammatory prostacyclin PGE_2.

In some respects the biochemical changes that are achieved by n-3 fatty acid supplementation are similar to those produced by NSAIDs, which are the mainstay of treatment for patients with rheumatoid arthritis (particularly in the earlier, milder stages) and which work by inhibiting cyclo-oxygenase pathways so that the production of series 2 prostaglandins and thromboxanes is reduced. There are some side-effects associated with aspirin therapy, notably gastrointestinal complications and nausea. In theory these could be avoided by the use of dietary supplements. However, the effects of dietary supplementation are usually much milder than those of NSAIDs and dietary supplementation is very much more expensive. The various supplementation trials have usually been carried out with patients with relatively mild symptoms of the disease that were previously controlled by NSAIDs and the benefits for patients with more severe symptoms are less certain.

Recommendations for a healthy diet

Both the British Committee on Medical Aspects of Food Policy (COMA) and the American National Research Council Committee on Diet and Health have made recommendations to reduce the risk of cardiovascular disease, cancer, and a range of other chronic conditions. These are given below.

- Reduce total fat intake to 35% or less of calories (US recommendation is 30%)
- Reduce saturated fat intake to less than 10% of calories
- No further increases to be made in intake of n-6 PUFAs (UK)
- Intake of cholesterol should not increase beyond current levels
- *Trans* fatty acids should form no more than 2% of dietary intake (UK)
- No specific recommendations have been made for consumption of monounsaturates
- Any energy deficit caused by reduced fat intake should be made up by complex carbohydrates and sugar in fruit and vegetables (UK)
- Five or more servings of a combination of fresh fruit or vegetables should be eaten every day (especially green and yellow vegetables and citrus fruits). Intake of starches and other complex carbohydrates to be increased by eating six or more servings of a combination of breads, cereals and legumes (USA).
- Salt consumption (see Chapters 11 and 20) to be reduced from about 9 g a day to 6 g (UK)

Although the influence of dietary fat on cancers remains largely unproven the influence on CHD and stroke is much clearer. The recommendations to increase intake of fruit and vegetables and complex carbohydrates is designed to increase the availability of fibre, antioxidant vitamins and minerals. There is some evidence that these food types help to prevent CHD and some cancers, but the benefits are not substantial. In the move towards adopting a lower fat diet it will be necessary to replace some high-fat foods: no study has ever shown that there is any harm in increasing the proportion of fruit, vegetables and complex carbohydrates in a mixed diet.

The move towards a low-fat diet often involves reducing the consumption of dairy products. In the British diet these are by far the most important sources of calcium, and there is a danger that intakes of this essential mineral could be reduced to sub-optimal levels. The most obvious consequence would be an increased risk of osteoporosis, although calcium may also have a protective effect in colorectal cancer. The answer is to use lower fat versions of dairy products: skimmed milk actually contains more calcium than whole milk.

Very often the effects of the diet in the development of human disease are very subtle and numerous homeostatic mechanisms are designed to cope with the vagaries of the diet. Although adjustments can be made to the diet, placing less pressure on compensatory homeostasis, these should form part of a wider examination of lifestyle and behaviour.

ANSWERS TO REVIEW QUESTIONS

Question 1

What factors might have influenced the decline in tooth decay?

There are two approaches to the control of tooth decay. One is to reduce consumption of foods that feed the plaque bacteria, the other is to increase defences against acid attack. There has been a decline in the per capita consumption of sugar by people living in the UK, although it is somewhat contentious whether this applies to infants and schoolchildren. Schoolchildren are notorious for snacking on sweets between meals, which is hardly likely to reduce tooth decay (this might explain the merging of the two graphs in Figure 7.2 as the children get older). There is also a disproportionate effect of tooth decay in the lower socioeconomic groups, who tend to consume larger amounts of sugar.

Contributory factors in the decline are likely to be increased surveillance and preventive plaque removal by dentists. Although there remains much to be done, people have become more aware of the importance of oral hygiene. The availability of fluoride toothpaste could also be a factor for people who live in areas where the fluoride content of water is low (the Dudley children for example). Fluoridation of water would have contributed to the overall statistics illustrated in Figure 7.2.

Question 2

How reliable are prospective and case-control studies of dietary intake for proving a causative association between trans *fatty acid consumption and risk of CHD?*

Reliable information about nutritional intake is difficult to obtain. Food frequency analysis is more likely to be representative if undertaken prospectively, while case-control studies will suffer from inadequate recall. Factors that influence the production of chronic diseases such as CHD take years to exert their effects, and no one will remember what they ate, say, 5 years ago. Similarly, very few people will be willing to record everything they eat for some years.

There is also a problem in not knowing what the foodstuff contains, even when evaluated by dieticians, when processed foods are eaten and the respondent is vague about the brand used. This could apply particularly to the assessment of *trans* fatty acids, often present in baked foodstuffs. Alternative brands of biscuits and cakes may have been made from butter or other oils. Accurate estimation of portion size is very difficult. Even when it can be estimated, some respondents may find it difficult to admit that they 'snacked' on half a packet of biscuits! The most reliable information comes from meticulous studies of food intake, ideally in clinical surroundings, where people are isolated or fully supervised. At best, food intake surveys provide only a snapshot of the overall picture – and a rather poor one at that.

Can dietary antioxidant vitamins and minerals effectively reduce the incidence of cancer?

There are strong theoretical arguments that antioxidant vitamins exert some protective influence. However, free radical damage is not the only mechanism involved in carcinogenesis and for many cancer types free radicals and antioxidant availability are secondary considerations. A large body of epidemiological studies shows that dietary antioxidant status has little influence on cancer risk. In particular, smokers cannot completely undo the damage they are doing to themselves simply by increasing their intake of fruit and vegetables.

More convincing epidemiological evidence comes from people who are vitamin-deficient. A marked deficiency of antioxidants appears to be associated with increased incidence of certain cancers such as stomach cancer. The Linxian trial demonstrated that correction of the deficiency is accompanied by significantly reduced cancer incidence. For those who are only marginally deficient (as defined by the current DRVs), the possible benefits of vitamin supplementation are not clear.

Further reading

General

Cheeseman, K.H. and Slater, T.F. (1993) *Free Radicals in Medicine*. Churchill Livingstone, Edinburgh.

Department of Health. (1990) Report of the panel on dietary reference values of the committee on medical aspects of food policy. *Dietary Reference Values for Food Energy and Nutrients for the United Kingdom*, IIMSO, London.

Mera, S.L. (1994) Diet and disease. *Br. J. Biomed. Sci.*, **51**, 189–206.

Rugg-Gunn, A.J. (1993) *Nutrition and Dental Health.*, Oxford University Press, Oxford.

Vitamins

Bates, C.J. (1995) Vitamin A. *Lancet*, **345**, 31–35.

Blomhoff, R. (1994) Transport and metabolism of vitamin A. *Nutr. Rev.*, **52**, S13–S23.

Fraser, D.R. (1995) Vitamin D. *Lancet*, **345**, 104–7.

Gershoff, S.N. (1993) Vitamin C (ascorbic acid): new roles, new requirements? *Nutr. Rev.*, **51**, 313–26

Shearer, M.J. (1995) Vitamin K. *Lancet*, **345**, 229–34.

Dietary fat and CHD

Ascherio, A., Hennekens, C.H., Buring, J.E. et al. (1994) *Trans*-fatty acids intake and risk of myocardial infarction. *Circulation*, **89**, 94–101.

Foley, M., Ball, M., Chisholm, A. *et al.* (1992) Should mono- or polyunsaturated fats replace saturated fats in the diet? *Eur. J. Clin. Nutr.*, **46**, 429–36.

Hegsted, D.M., Ausman, L., Johnson, J.A. *et al.* (1993) Dietary fat and serum lipids: an evaluation of the experimental data. *Am. J. Clin. Nutr.*, **57**, 875–83.

Judd, J.T., Clevidence, B.A., Muesing, R.A. *et al.* (1994) Dietary *trans* fatty acids: effects on plasma lipids and lipoproteins of healthy men and women. *Am. J. Clin. Nutr.*, **59**, 861–8.

Odeyle, O.A. and Watson, R.R. (1991) Health implications of the n-3 fatty acids. *Am. J. Clin. Nutr.*, **53**, 177.

Scott, J. (1991) Lipoprotein (a): thrombotic and atherogenic. *BMJ*, **303**, 663–4.

Simopoulos, A.P. (1991) Omega-3 fatty acids in health and disease and in growth and development. *Am. J. Clin. Nutr.*, **54**, 438–63.

Antioxidants and CHD

Abbey, M., Nestel, P. and Baghurst, P.A. (1993) Antioxidant vitamins and low density lipoprotein oxidation. *Am. J. Clin. Nutr.*, **58**, 523–32.

Riemersma, R.A., Oliver, M., Elton, R.A. *et al.* (1990) Plasma antioxidants and coronary heart disease: vitamins C and E, and selenium. *Eur. J. Clin. Nutr.*, **44**, 143–50.

Fibre and CHD

Ripsin, C.M., Keenan, J.M., Jacobs, D.R. *et al.* (1992) Oat products and lipid lowering – a meta-analysis. *JAMA*, **267**, 3317–25.

Diet and cancer

Dwyer, J. (1993) Dietary fibre and colorectal cancer risk. *Nutr. Rev.*, **51**, 147–8.

Sellers, T.A., Kushi, L.H., Potter, J.D. *et al.* (1992) Effect of family history, body fat distribution and reproductive factors on the risk of postmenopausal breast cancer. *N. Engl. J. Med.*, **326**, 1323–9.

8   The biological basis of ageing

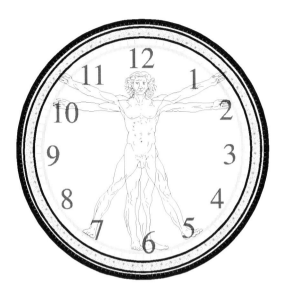

Genetic and environmental factors influence senescence and the rate of ageing. Many of the agents that are implicated in the ageing process also influence the predisposition to disease. An example is oxygen free radicals, which are thought to be partly responsible for the decreased cellular metabolism associated with senescence and the accumulation of waste products like lipofuscin, but which are also involved in the pathogenesis of atherosclerosis and many cancers.

The genetic determinants of senescence have been hard to identify, but these undoubtedly act at the cellular level. There is increasing evidence that the predisposition for certain diseases, and perhaps even the rate of ageing, is laid down in early life. Other than avoiding the obvious risk factors such as poor diet, sedentary lifestyle, smoking and excess of virtually everything that is pleasurable, the best advice is to choose your parents carefully.

Pre-test

- **Why do we grow old?**
- **What are the characteristic biological features of ageing?**
- **What are the signs or symptoms of the menopause? At what age do they arise?**
- **What is hormone (oestrogen) replacement therapy and what is its purpose?**
- **Why is the athletic performance of older people markedly lower than it was in their youth?**

Aims of this chapter

By the end of this chapter you will have increased your knowledge of:
◆   The genetic and environmental contributions to ageing
◆   The age-associated physiological and biochemical alterations that can lead to disabilities and diseases in older people

In addition, this chapter will help you to:
◆   Describe changes due to senescence in cells, tissues and organs and discuss how these may contribute to disabilities or diseases in older people
◆   Identify the biological and environmental factors associated with ageing
◆   Discuss the effect of internal and external factors on ageing of body systems
◆   Distinguish between diseases and disabilities primarily caused by intrinsic senescence changes and those that arise as a function of time (for example, by cumulative exposure to environmental agents)

Introduction

The ageing process occurs throughout the body and at every level of organisation

People now live longer but are more likely to die from the chronic diseases associated with ageing

Ageing is associated with a degeneration of functional capacity in all parts of the body, and at all levels of organisation from molecules to complete organ systems. These functional changes are referred to as senescence. Both genetic and environmental factors govern **senescence**, although the precise mechanisms and the extent of their involvement are largely unknown.

Diseases and disablement may arise because of the ageing process, or simply because wear and tear has caused damage. Senescence changes may be responsible for certain diseases and disabilities associated with old age or they may be a contributory factor in, and increase a person's susceptibility to, particular diseases. This is the case with the most commonly encountered causes of illness and death today, namely atherosclerosis and cancer.

People of the same chronological age show widely different senescence changes and, within an individual, different systems of the body undergo senescence at different rates. Biochemical and physiological senescence is relatively easy to measure and monitor, but the underlying cause of the changes is more difficult to analyse.

Why does ageing take place?

The inevitable consequence of human survival, and indeed that of all other life forms, is the process of ageing. This is accompanied by the capacity to reproduce and a finite capacity for repair. Reproduction is the means by which the species as a whole overcomes senescence, and leads to adaptation. Reproduction ensures the passage of an individual's genes into the next generation, but once this function has been fulfilled and the offspring are safely reared there is no further need for that individual: in short, we pay for sex with our lives.

It can be argued that the forces of natural selection favour the genes that are advantageous during the early stages of life, and any deleterious genes that operate after reproduction are, from a biological point of view, unimportant. What we see as ageing could well represent the operation of these genes after our biological duties have been fulfilled. This concept forms the basis of the **disposable soma theory of ageing**, and is analogous to the manufacture of disposable goods: why invest a lot of money and resources into a product that is expected to have only a short duration of use? It would seem that many organisms are designed on this disposable theory, ensuring sufficient investment, with some reserve, to get past the reproductive stage. Ageing represents the period after that reserve when the body systems can safely (from the biological imperative) be allowed to fall into disrepair.

Species lifespans are to a certain extent correlated with size and basal metabolic rate. Relatively large animals, including humans, live longer than small rodents such as rats and mice which live for only about 4 years (Figure 8.1). There are some exceptions to this generalisation: dogs are larger than cats but have a shorter lifespan. It is also a general rule that the female of the species outlives the male, but again there are exceptions: stallions outlive mares and male hamsters live longer than the females. Women, who on average live 6 years longer than men, have a basal metabolic rate about 6% lower. Similarly, small mammals generally have higher basal metabolic rates than large ones. The insurmountable differences in species lifespan suggests that ageing is at least partly determined genetically.

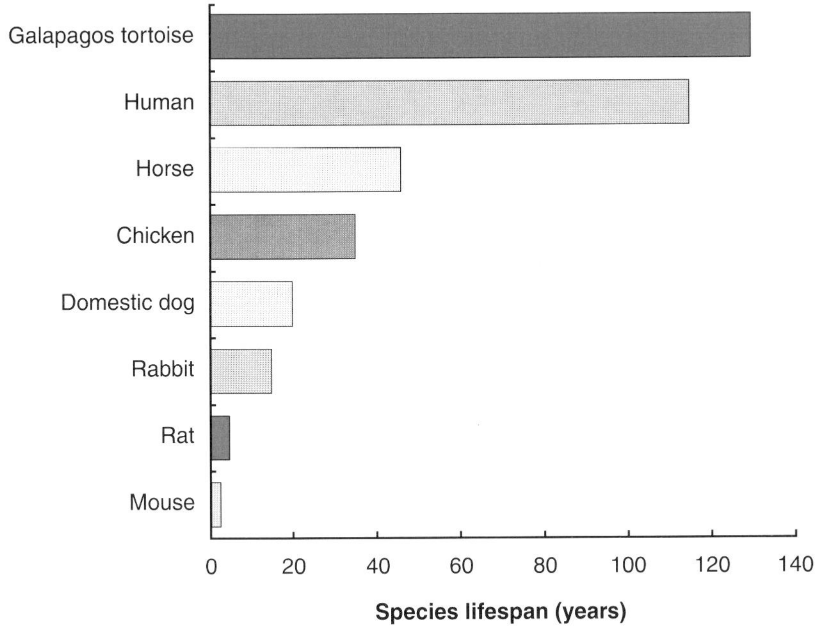

> *Lifespan is species-specific, and may be related to basal metabolic rate and gender*

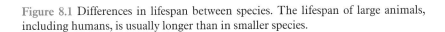

Figure 8.1 Differences in lifespan between species. The lifespan of large animals, including humans, is usually longer than in smaller species.

Theories of ageing

> *Ageing is probably a consequence of genetic susceptibility to damaging intrinsic and extrinsic agents*

The earliest theories on ageing envisaged two possible processes, one based on genetics and the other on generalised wear and tear. The genetic theory sees ageing as a result of a programmed mechanism or 'biological clock' that acts in a similar way to the programmed events which previously occurred during growth and development. The ageing process is simply one more part in the controlled cycle of maturation, synthesis, proliferation and, ultimately, cell senescence and death.

The second possibility is that ageing is the result of wear and tear over a long period of time. It is easy to envisage that 'wear and tear' mechanisms could operate at all levels of the body's organisation. For example, accumulated radiation-induced and chemically induced genetic mutations could lead to errors in transcription and translation. Metabolites and macromolecules, and even cells, can become damaged by free radicals. Larger structures, such as the joints, may suffer from physical damage and erosion of cartilage.

The most probable explanation is that both theories are (at least in part) correct, and that genetic susceptibility is exacerbated by intrinsic and extrinsic 'wear and tear' agents. It would seem reasonable to suppose that genetic characteristics play a fundamental role in maintaining organisms to the reproductive stage and beyond. The disrepair that follows is probably primarily induced by intrinsic and extrinsic agents that cause cell and tissue damage.

There is further evidence for the inheritability of longevity. An old dictum, borne out by some epidemiological studies, is that the best way to achieve a long life is to choose long-lived grandparents. Identical twins (who have exactly the same genes) live to very similar ages whereas non-identical siblings have more diverse life expectancies. It seems likely that no single gene is responsible for initiating the decline of a cell and ultimately the death of an individual: this involves the accumulation and interaction of products from a cascade of genes that are activated or suppressed.

Genetic influences are probably modulated by agents in the environment, causing not only senescence but also some of the diseases of old age. For example, damage by free radicals is implicated in ageing and in a variety of common and life-threatening diseases, including cancer and atherosclerosis.

There is much interest in finding ways to extend the lifespan of the human species. Not surprisingly, a variety of 'quack' elixirs have been promoted ranging from monkey gland extracts to collagen treatments for skin ageing. Recent interest has centred on the administration of melatonin which reportedly extends the life of experimental mice by about 20%. It appears that melatonin modulates the circadian pacemaker system, and for this reason has been used to alleviate the malaise of jet-lag but there is no evidence that this substance has a life-extending effect on humans.

Review question 1

What are the limitations to extending the human lifespan?

Cellular changes due to senescence

Some of the classic studies on cellular ageing were undertaken by Richard Hayflick in the 1960s. Essentially these showed that human diploid cells have a finite life in culture, measured by the number of passages, or doublings, that are produced. The number of doublings is known as the **Hayflick number**, and varies with the chronological age of the person or animal from which the cells were taken.

In human fetal cells in culture the average number of doublings achieved is around 50, but cells from an 80-year-old survive through only 20–30 doublings (Figure 8.2). When the cells are taken out of culture, put into frozen storage and then re-established in culture they appear to retain the 'memory' of the number of doublings completed in the original culture. When cultured again after storage, they go on to complete the 'unused' doublings. These results gave rise to the concept that there is a 'biological clock' within all cells. Such a clock would almost certainly reside within DNA, but no 'senescence genes' have been identified in humans, and the factors that might control their activation are entirely unknown.

Normally cells in culture respond to growth factors, synthesise DNA and divide. When cells undergo senescence in culture cell division slows down because of the production of growth inhibitors. The identity of these inhibitors is not known, but RNA derived from senescent cells will cause the young cells to stop growing. There is evidence that some of the factors controlling cellular senescence in culture are located on chromosome 1. It is also known that a variety of cell types are capable of programmed death (apoptosis), which is undoubtedly mediated by genetic factors (see Chapter 4).

The evidence for a 'biological clock' came from observations that young cells in culture survive longer than cells from older adults

Some genetically controlled factors influence the decline of a cell towards its death

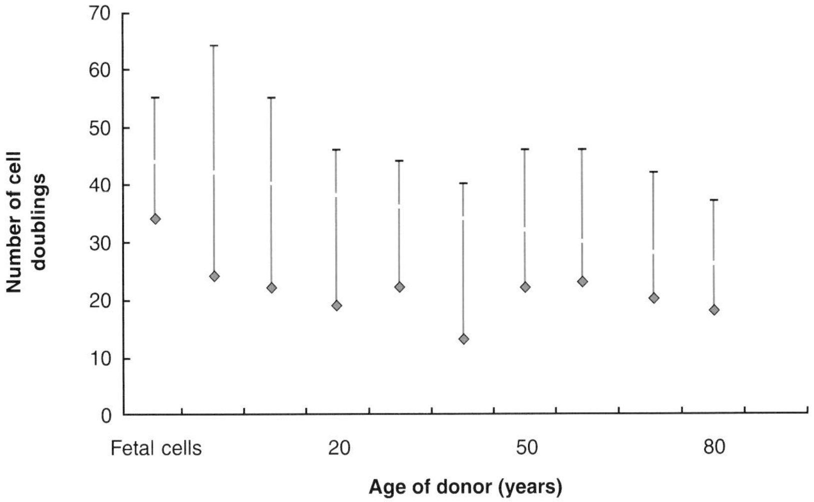

Figure 8.2 Alteration in cell doubling capacity with donor age. It is possible to sustain fetal cells and cells from young people through a greater number of subcultures than cells from older individuals. This variation in cell proliferative capacity with age may be genetically regulated. (Adapted from Kirkwood, T. (1994) *MRC News*, **64**, 14–17.)

> *Certain inherited conditions mimic accelerated ageing, suggesting that senescence is regulated at the genetic level*

▲ **Key points**

Genetic influences on ageing

- ▲ Species differences in lifespan are largely predetermined
- ▲ Cell proliferative capacity appears to be predetermined
- ▲ Apoptosis is a genetically regulated characteristic of all somatic cells
- ▲ Survival is probably influenced by the presence of genes that confer capacity for effective repair and the absence of genes that confer susceptibility to chronic disease
- ▲ 'Long-lived' families and twin concordance studies indicate some inheritability of longevity
- ▲ Progeria syndromes are inherited

> *It is probable that no single gene is directly responsible for normal ageing*

> *Cells are continuously exposed to harmful agents from both inside and outside*

> *There are cellular defences against harmful agents, but in older people these may be impaired and more easily overwhelmed*

Further evidence of a genetic contribution to ageing is demonstrated in the recessively inherited conditions **progeria** and **Werner's syndrome**, which are characterised by an apparently premature ageing process. Progeria sufferers display many of the features of ageing by the time they reach their teenage years, with wrinkling of the skin, osteoporosis and atherosclerosis. Most patients die of heart attack at a median age of 12 years. It is interesting to note that cultured fibroblasts from such patients show severely curtailed doubling capacity. In Werner's syndrome the features of accelerated ageing are not apparent until around 20 years, but individuals have a life expectancy of only 40. Common features of this syndrome are calcification of soft tissues, cataracts, osteoporosis, atherosclerosis, diabetes, premature greying and loss of hair and atrophy of skeletal muscle. Cultured cells from patients with Werner's syndrome also display rapid senescence.

Both of these syndromes are extremely rare, and there is controversy about whether they truly represent acceleration of ageing, because not all the features associated with advanced age, such as senile dementia, are seen. The gene at fault in Werner's syndrome has recently (1996) been located on the short arm of chromosome 8 and, so far, four different mutations have been identified that disrupt the gene and its function. The gene is believed to code for a type of helicase, an enzyme that helps DNA to unwind in preparation for cell replication, DNA repair or gene expression. Disruption of any of these processes has the potential to damage the DNA, which will in turn compromise cell function and, in the case of Werner's syndrome, cause premature ageing.

The extent to which a genetic or cellular 'biological clock' regulates human ageing is unknown. The 'Werner's syndrome' gene may play a part but most human genes probably play some role and are either altered themselves or affect the activity of other genes.

Even though cells appear to have an intrinsic ageing mechanism, transplant studies show that most cells will survive longer than the organism as a whole – in other words there is a substantial inbuilt reserve capacity. It thus seems likely that any intrinsic genetic mechanisms are supplemented or accelerated by other mechanisms, such as the cumulative exposure to toxic agents and general 'wear and tear'.

Cells are continuously exposed to potentially damaging internal and external agents such as UV and γ radiation, heat, free radicals, glucose and exogenous micro-organisms. Many of the external agents can, with prolonged exposure or high doses, kill cells. With intermediate exposure or dosage they may act as initiators or promoters of malignant change. Much lower exposure to the same agents, although not producing immediately apparent effects, may contribute to senescence in the cell by the progressive accumulation of genetic damage.

A number of cellular defence mechanisms have evolved as a response to potentially damaging agents, including enzymes for DNA repair, enzymatic and non-enzymatic antioxidants and the production of heat-shock and other stress proteins. Failure of these mechanisms means that the cell will not be able to maintain homeostasis, and senescence and cell death follow.

In addition to the various 'longevity' genes that control cellular mechanisms and the capacity for repair, survival will be enhanced by not having genes that predispose to the development of chronic life-threatening conditions. For example, the 'oldest-old' (see p. 285) are much less likely to have the apolipoprotein E ε4 gene in their genetic make-up. This gene seems to be associated with an increased risk of early death, probably because of increased susceptibility to Alzheimer's disease.

Molecular changes associated with cell senescence

Cells from aged animals display a reduced capacity for repairing DNA following damage by agents such as UV and γ irradiation or chemical carcinogens. It may be that damaged DNA accumulates in older cells, and that this may cause much of the ageing process by introducing errors in protein synthesis. Indeed, studies on hundreds of proteins have shown age-related changes in concentration, activity, thermal stability and antigenic properties. For the most part the composition of newly secreted proteins produced by young cells differs only slightly from that in senescent cells and it follows that most age-related changes in composition must occur after secretion.

Some cellular defences operate to repair DNA but with age this could be subject to error

The most significant age-associated changes in proteins are probably **racemisation** and **glycation**. Racemisation involves the conversion of the normal laevo stereochemical configuration of amino acids to the alternative dextro form, mostly affecting aspartic acid and serine residues. Glycation involves the addition of sugar molecules to a protein. Other chemical modifications include deamination, carbamylation, oxidation and reactions with other components such as aldehydes and corticosteroids. The precise biological significance of these changes in proteins is uncertain, although they probably contribute to altered properties such as the extent of protein aggregation or cross-linking. These changes are associated with demonstrably deleterious effects. For example, the age-related increases in cross-linking and rigidity of elastin and collagen contribute to lung and cardiovascular pathologies; changes in aggregation of the crystalline proteins in the lens of the eye cause cataracts, which are often a problem in later life.

As well as alterations within cells, changes are seen in most of the important proteins with age

Ageing is also associated with decreased protein synthesis. This affects the production of a wide range of chemicals including enzymes, hormones, receptors, neurotransmitters, antibodies and components of the extracellular matrix. The reduced availability of enzymes may have several consequences for the maintenance of homeostasis, including:

- Repair and normal function of the cell
- Removal of damaged cell components
- Accumulation of abnormal, inactive or damaging macromolecules (such as lipofuscin and amyloid)

Changes in cell function and protein structure can contribute to failure of maintenance and repair and to the functional decline of body organs.

The reduction in function may mean that the body is less able to cope with damaging external agents, so that disease states develop. The failure of maintenance as a consequence of the various age-related changes in the

Lipofuscin: 'wear and tear' pigment composed of undigested lipid-rich cellular material produced by the degeneration of cell membranes and organelles.

Some of the functional alterations of old age can be minimised by following a healthy lifestyle

Even though age-related changes take place throughout the body there is no specific test for age

Ageing changes to the skin are caused by biochemical alterations and the effects of sunlight and general weather exposure

production and modification of macromolecules could contribute to the development and progression of disease. For example, reduced activity of oxidases produced by the liver may impair the detoxification of chemical carcinogens and encourage production of more strongly mutagenic metabolites. Reductions in antioxidant enzymes such as superoxide dismutase will increase susceptibility to damage by free radicals. In turn, free radicals affect carcinogenesis, possibly by activating oncogenes. In addition, alterations in hormone levels and in the number or affinity of hormone receptors may influence a cell's responsiveness to growth regulatory signals. These changes could increase susceptibility to carcinogenesis with age.

Changes in tissues and organs due to senescence

Biochemical and physiological changes

The physiological and biochemical changes that occur with age may influence the presentation of disease, response to treatment and the likelihood of complications. Individuals differ widely, and many of the changes associated with ageing can be modified by lifestyle factors such as diet, exercise and use of tobacco and alcohol. A well-known example is the impaired capacity of older individuals to metabolise glucose: older people have higher blood sugar concentrations in glucose tolerance tests than younger subjects, although many older individuals metabolise glucose just as well as younger people. It seems likely that external and lifestyle factors such as exercise, diet and drugs play a significant part in this variation.

A variety of physiological and biochemical changes that act as markers for senescence can be observed in all organ systems of the body. In some cases the decline in functional efficiency is apparent only when the system is subjected to stress. For example, older people are less able to produce and conserve heat and so may suffer from hypothermia in cold weather.

Skin

The changes induced in the skin as a function of age are probably the most easily recognised, and many people use the appearances of skin and hair to assess the age of an individual. The obvious changes are wrinkling, greying and loss of hair and changes in skin pigmentation. Wrinkling of the skin is to a large extent caused by changes in the proteins of the dermal connective tissue, principally the collagen and elastic fibres. With age these fibres undergo increased cross-linking with consequent reduction in elasticity. To some extent these changes are the result of damage caused by exposure to UV radiation; wrinkling of the skin is usually more severe in sun-exposed skin. Solar damage also contributes to a variety of other skin conditions ranging in seriousness from benign lesions (actinic keratosis) to malignant melanoma.

The follicles producing grey hair lack pigment-forming cells (melanocytes). There is a large variation between individuals concerning loss of hair, caused by genetic and hormonal influences. In some cases new hair growth may occur in older people, in the ears of men, and on the chin in women but, like baldness, these cosmetic changes are not always welcomed.

A common clinical experience is that skin wounds heal more slowly in older individuals, although this has been difficult to show in healthy old experimental animals. A recent study compared the healing of ischaemic and normally vascularised wounds in young and old rats. The normally vascularised wound healed equally well in both populations but ischaemic wounds took much longer to heal in old animals. It may be that the impaired wound healing of older people is caused by disease, such as atherosclerosis, which contributes to ischaemia of the traumatised tissue.

Some wounds can take longer to heal in older people, particularly if they have diabetes or vascular problems

Lungs

The age-related changes to the respiratory system include decreased lung size, decreased elasticity (resulting in enlarged alveolar ducts and alveoli) and reduced mucociliary clearance. The main consequence of these changes is that the vital capacity is reduced and hence gas exchange is reduced. In general the available capacity of the lungs remains adequate for most daily activities of older individuals – but running for the bus may be a little more difficult. Exercise capacity in older people will also be reduced because of reduced cardiovascular function.

Older people are more likely to become short of breath on exertion

Cardiovascular system

A loss of elasticity similar to the connective tissue changes in the skin occurs in connective tissues throughout the body. Most notably, connective tissues form the principal component of arterial walls and loss of elasticity with age makes the blood vessels more rigid. The vessel walls are also prone to calcification in a process called **arteriosclerosis**, often called hardening of the arteries. One consequence of arteriosclerosis is an increase in systolic and diastolic blood pressure, which is progressive with age (Figure 8.3).

In the average older adult most parameters of cardiovascular function are in decline, including work capacity, maximum heart rate, stroke volume and cardiac output. In the heart itself there is a loss of muscle, with replacement by fibrous tissue, and many heart muscle cells contain lipofuscin deposits. These changes may be a consequence of reduced blood supply to the heart, either because of arteriosclerosis, but also because of disease, namely atherosclerosis (see Chapter 20).

Hardening of the arteries impairs cardiovascular function

Actinic keratosis: irregular lesions with a hard keratin surface arising in the sun-exposed skin such as the face, scalp and backs of the hands. It is regarded as a precancerous lesion and can progress to squamous cell carcinoma. The risk is sufficiently great to warrant local excision.

Malignant melanoma: the most serious of the skin cancers, probably caused by excessive exposure to UV light. Usually appears as an irregular pigmented lesion.

Kidneys

The weight and volume of the kidneys decrease 20–30% during adult life. This mainly affects the nephrons, which disappear and are replaced by scar

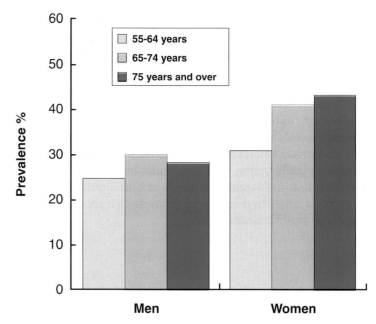

Figure 8.3 Hypertensive disease in the USA, 1980. There is a tendency for systolic and diastolic blood pressure to rise with age. This, however, is not invariably the case in all populations. (Source: 1980 National Medical Care Expenditure Survey (US).)

The kidneys do not function as well in old people and may be more susceptible to infection

tissue, decreasing filtration rate, impairing elimination of nitrogenous waste and increasing the glucose threshold.

As a result of these functional changes older people are at risk of developing renal disease. Early renal disease is commonly asymptomatic and the usual tests may not reveal disease – up to half of renal functional capacity can be lost before it is revealed by measurable changes in blood urea, nitrogen or serum creatinine concentrations.

Liver

The liver may not work as well as people get older, which means that drugs and alcohol are not as easily tolerated

Between the ages of 60 and 90 years the liver shrinks in size and contains fewer cells. Standard liver function tests are within normal ranges in disease-free older people, but changes in some enzymes, particularly the microsomal enzymes concerned with oxidation and detoxification, are seen. Thus there is a decline in some liver functions and diminished capacity for metabolism of drugs and hormones. This is of clinical importance, and drug prescriptions and dosages should take account of the fact that many medications are metabolised and cleared from the body much more slowly. Tolerance for alcohol also decreases markedly with age.

Gastrointestinal tract

The absorption of vital elements such as calcium can be impaired in older people

Motor function and muscle tone of the large intestine decrease with age, leading to decreased motility, frequent constipation and diverticular disease. Atrophy of the mucosal lining of the stomach can result in chronic gastritis. There may also be impairment of the digestive and absorption capacity of the small intestine.

The mucosa of the aged gut is susceptible to anoxic damage due to reductions in blood supply in the splanchnic circulation as a consequence of atherosclerosis. Loss of tensile strength of the connective tissues in the gut wall can lead to diverticulosis of the small and large intestines.

Most gastrointestinal disorders that occur in older people are also commonly seen in the young and are not attributable only to the ageing process. Exceptions include atrophic gastritis and pernicious anaemia, which are more common in people over 50. The most important gastrointestinal problems for the older person are dysphagia, constipation, diarrhoea and faecal incontinence, often complications of disease or side-effects of drugs.

Many older people suffer from constipation, diarrhoea and incontinence

Bone

Bone loss starts in the third or fourth decades of life (see Chapter 22). The pattern of loss differs in trabecular and cortical bone, initial losses occurring in trabecular bone. The amount of bone lost is more severe in women, particularly in the menopausal and early post-menopausal years. The maintenance of bone depends on the reproductive hormones oestrogen and testosterone, but their production declines with age. In men the decline in testosterone levels is much more gradual than the decline in oestrogen during the menopause, and so men experience smaller losses of bone mass.

Bone loss with age increases the risk of fractures

Cartilage

Changes occur in the cartilages of both weight-bearing and non-weight-bearing joints, starting at 20–30 years of age. These alterations principally concern the activity of cartilage-forming cells so that there is reduced turnover. The 'old' cartilage has a yellowed appearance, compared with the bluish cartilage of youth.

The function of cartilage is to protect bone by providing an intervening 'springy' layer in the joints. Cartilage contains a high proportion of glycosaminoglycans, large macromolecules that are able to hold a large amount of water as a gel and give cartilage its 'springiness'. With age the amount and type of these glycosaminoglycans reduce, causing a decline in physical resilience. The result is that the cartilage splits, becomes fragmented and is worn away. General wear and tear of the weakened cartilage leads ultimately to osteoarthritis.

'Wear and tear' of joint cartilages causes damage and pain

Osteoarthritis: a common degenerative disease involving the cartilage, bone, synovium and joint capsule. In late stages the bone surfaces are exposed because of erosion of the cartilage. Bone and cartilage debris causes thickening of the synovial membrane and inflammation.

Muscle

The age-related changes in striated muscle are similar to those produced by

Reduced muscle strength in older people may be the result of ageing or under-use

inactivity: muscles atrophy (Figure 8.4). Atrophy leads to reductions in the size of muscle groups and to loss of individual muscle fibres. As a result there is a decrease in work capacity. A simple confirmation of this is in the performance of athletes: very few Olympic gold medal winners are over the age of 40.

Other factors, such as cardiovascular, respiratory and joint functions, can influence muscle strength. The older person disabled by arthritis is not able to move about easily, and muscles will atrophy unless specific exercises are taken. Very often changes due to ageing, when considered separately, appear to be minor, but they can assume major significance when organ systems interact.

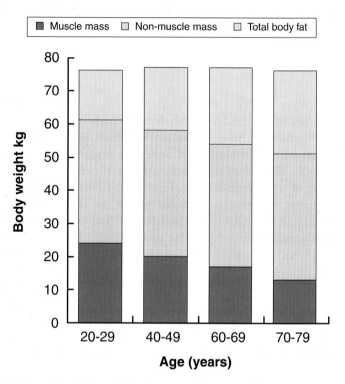

Figure 8.4 Age-related change in body composition. The proportion of lean muscle mass declines progressively with age. This is accompanied by an increase in the proportion of body fat (otherwise known as 'middle-age spread'), so that there is little overall change in body weight. (Data from Young, V.R (1990), in Nutrition and ageing (eds D.M. Prinsley and H.H. Sanstead), *Progr. Clin. Biol. Res.*, **326**, 279–300.)

Sense organs

Older people often do not realise that their eyesight has become impaired

It is common to see older people wearing spectacles. According to General Household Survey statistics, more than 95% of people over the age of 65 wear corrective lenses at some time. With age, the ability of the lens to change shape decreases, making it more difficult to focus on near objects: hence the need for reading spectacles. Older people also show a decreased sensitivity to light. Changes in the protein composition of the lens produce light scattering and absorption, and less light reaches the light-sensitive surface of the retina. This does not present much of a problem in daylight but artificial illumination needs to be bright, particularly in homes for older people. The change in protein composition of the lens also means that it becomes more yellow with age, so that colour perception is no longer 'true'.

It is estimated that about 30% of those over 65 have hearing difficulties, and that one in ten has a hearing aid. Sounds need to be louder before they are audible, and high-frequency sounds can be lost altogether. Usually both ears are affected because of a general physiological deterioration of the auditory system.

Hearing losses make communication with older people more difficult

Other changes in the sense organs include loss of smell and taste, decreased sensitivity to touch and an increased pain threshold.

Brain

There is a loss in the weight of the brain with age, from a typical 1.4 kg at age 20 years to about 1.3 kg at 60. This weight loss is the result of changes in brain composition, which include an enlargement of the fluid-filled ventricles and a widening of the sulci (surface channels). In some areas nerve cells are lost, and those that remain display a reduction in their branching dendritic network. Amyloid deposits are associated with blood vessels and as extracellular plaques in the aged brain. There is also evidence of neuronal degeneration in the form of intracellular neurofibrillary tangles (Chapter 26). The 'wear and tear' pigment lipofuscin accumulates within certain neurons in the ageing brain.

Changes in the brain with age means that older people find it more difficult to learn and memorise things and are more easily confused and forgetful

The consequences of these changes are seen as alterations in reaction times, problem-solving and learning capability, impaired memory and altered sleep patterns. Many of these age-related changes described are seen to excess in dementia, and particularly in Alzheimer's disease. There is thus some controversy over whether the changes to the brain are the result of true ageing processes or are manifestations of disease. Fortunately for most individuals, age-related changes in the brain do not result in catastrophic loss of function.

Severe degeneration and loss of neurons can cause dementia

Immune system

Age-related alterations occur in both the cell-mediated and humoral immune responses of humans. The most obvious change is a reduction of about 15% in the number of circulating lymphocytes, mostly T cells. This is accompanied by reductions in the functional capacity of immune system cells.

Changes in the immune system with age increase vulnerability to viral pneumonia

Reduced immune function is caused by a number of changes affecting the surface membrane, cytoplasm and nucleus of T and B cells, monocytes or macrophages. The decline in T-cell function is probably related to the involution of the thymus which occurs in adults. Impairment of humoral immunity is similarly related to loss of T-cell function: there is evidence that B-cell functions that do not depend on T cells are only modestly curtailed in older people. This may explain why older people are more susceptible to viral infection, while their resistance to bacterial infections remains relatively unaltered. The relative loss of T-cell function may also contribute to a breakdown of tolerance, leading to autoimmunity. Generally, prevalence of autoimmune diseases increases with age, although the incidence of many autoimmune diseases (rheumatoid arthritis, for example) peaks before old age.

Endocrine system

The endocrine system is complex and interwoven with the nervous system and other systems to control the overall body metabolic functions. The effects of ageing are just as diverse as the effects of hormones on different target tissues and it would not be surprising if some of the senescence changes in the body were secondary to age-related alterations in components of the endocrine system. Endocrine function declines because of decreases in hormone production and in the numbers of hormone receptors in target tissues. Examples are the age-related functional decline in the reproductive organs, altered thyroid hormone status, altered immunity and the development of diabetes.

The menopause

The menopause has very unpleasant physical and psychological effects on some women

One inescapable endocrine change in women is the menopause. This is usually defined by the cessation of menstruation, and is most likely to occur between the ages of 45 and 55. Women who smoke and have a poor nutritional status are more likely to commence the menopause at an earlier age. Premature menopause may also be produced by chemotherapy, pelvic radiotherapy and surgical removal of the ovaries. Some women are born with an unusually small number of primary ovarian follicles and menopause commences when most of these are lost. In some women an autoimmune reaction is responsible for follicular destruction; their menopause begins in their twenties or thirties.

▲ **Key points**

Causes of early menopause

- ▲ Smoking
- ▲ Chemotherapy
- ▲ Pelvic radiotherapy
- ▲ Surgical removal of both ovaries
- ▲ Autoimmune reaction
- ▲ Small number of primary follicles at birth

Some effects of the menopause are not immediately obvious

Menstruation gradually decreases or becomes irregular in some women; in others it suddenly ceases. The cessation of menstruation results from a decline in production of sex hormones by the ovaries, which become insensitive to stimulation by the pituitary hormones follicle-stimulating hormone (FSH) and luteinising hormone (LH). After the menopause the ovaries produce only androstenedione, which is converted in peripheral fat to the less active oestrogenic hormone oestrone.

The cause of ovarian failure is the progressive loss of primary ovarian follicles. The blood levels of oestrogen fall, but concentrations of FSH and LH increase as the ovaries become less responsive to their effects (Figure 8.5). When only a few thousand follicles are left cyclical activity cannot be sustained. A number of other signs may accompany the menopause: hot flushes, atrophy of glandular breast tissue, atrophy of the vaginal mucosa, changes in libido and decreased elasticity of the skin. These physical symptoms are often accompanied by psychological effects such as sudden changes in mood, anxiety, depression and irritability.

After the menopause blood cholesterol levels rise significantly, contributing to the risk of CHD. Oestrogen also affects the activity of cells responsible for bone formation and resorption; osteoporosis is a problem in post-menopausal women.

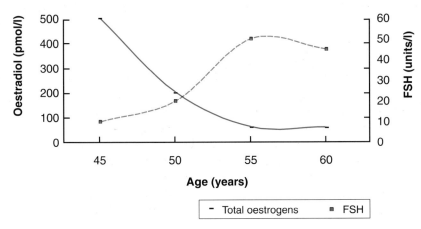

Figure 8.5 Changes in serum levels of FSH and total oestrogens during the menopause. In most women blood concentrations of FSH and LH begin to rise during their late forties. This is part of the feedback mechanism, in response to the reduced oestrogen produced by fewer ovarian follicles, and disrupts the menstrual cycle. Eventually the menopausal pattern of low oestradiol and elevated FSH and LH concentrations is established.

Hormone replacement therapy

Hormone replacement therapy (HRT) aims to prevent or minimise some of the distressing symptoms of the menopause by compensating for the fall in ovarian oestrogen production (Figure 8.6). It has the added advantage that other long-term protective benefits of oestrogen, such as slowing bone loss and modulating blood lipids, are also restored. Three natural oestrogens are commonly used for HRT: conjugated equine oestrogens, oestrogen valerate and 17β-oestradiol.

The treatment may be employed in several ways, most commonly as an oral preparation, oestrogen skin patches, subcutaneous implants or vaginal creams or pessaries. The oral oestrogen preparation is usually cycled with progesterone because oestrogen alone increases the risk of endometrial cancer. Women who have had a hysterectomy will not be at risk.

Many of the symptoms of the menopause begin before the cessation of menstruation and there is no reason why HRT cannot be initiated at this stage. However, menstrual bleeding can become a problem particularly if the imposed cycle becomes out of step with the natural ovarian cycle. The doses used in HRT are insufficient to have a contraceptive effect.

▲ **Key points**

Effects of the menopause

Immediate physical effects:
▲ Hot flushes
▲ Sweats and palpitations
▲ Panic attacks
▲ Insomnia

Psychological symptoms:
▲ Mood changes
▲ Anxiety
▲ Depression
▲ Irritability
▲ Poor memory and concentration
▲ Decreased libido

Changes to the genitourinary tract:
▲ Breast atrophy
▲ Genital tract atrophy

Late-onset effects:
▲ Osteoporosis
▲ Crush fractures of vertebrae
▲ Hip fractures
▲ Cardiovascular disease

Most menopausal changes (except for fertility!) can be corrected by hormone replacement therapy

Some women find HRT difficult to tolerate, but different preparations are available which may be better tolerated

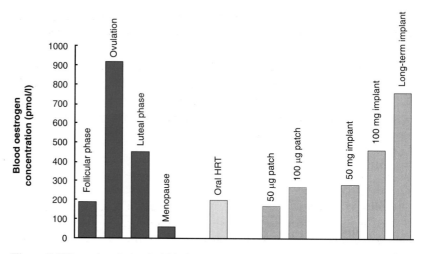

Figure 8.6 Natural variation in blood oestrogen levels and influence of HRT. None of the hormone replacement regimens replicate the pattern of oestrogen production found in premenopausal women. High levels of blood oestrogen after the menopause are only attainable with hormone implants. (Adapted from Studd, J.W.W. and Smith, R.N.J. (1993) Oestradiol and testosterone implants. *Bailliere's Clinical Endocrinology and Metabolism*, 7, 203–23.)

Oral HRT

Oestrogen: produced by the ripening ovarian follicle. Stimulates the proliferation of endometrium and is responsible for the development of secondary sexual characteristics.

Progesterone: produced by the ovarian follicle in the luteal phase. Stimulates secretory changes in the endometrium. Progesterone production is essential for the maintenance of pregnancy; it also influences breast structure and function.

Virtually all the epidemiological data concerning the risks and benefits of HRT have been obtained from the use of oral preparations. The oral route is most frequently used and a wide choice of preparations and doses is available. The hormones are absorbed from the gastrointestinal tract and pass through the liver before reaching the systemic circulation. Most of the oestradiol is converted to the weaker-acting oestrone in the gut and liver. A consequence of oestradiol processing by the liver is an increase in the production of blood clotting factors. Because of this, a history of deep-vein thrombosis or pulmonary thrombo-embolism during pregnancy or previous oral contraceptive use are contraindications for oral HRT.

The conversion of oestradiol into oestrone also means that the normal premenopausal balance between 17β-oestradiol and oestrone (a 2:1 ratio in favour of 17β-oestradiol) cannot be achieved. In addition, oral oestrogens cause a surge of plasma hormones that would not be encountered during premenopausal physiological production. It is not possible to achieve the usual premenopausal oestrogen levels by oral administration because the high doses that would be necessary induce severe nausea.

Oestradiol patches

Oestradiol patches and implants offer the advantage that the hormone is absorbed directly into the systemic circulation. Liver induction is avoided and there are no measurable changes in the production of clotting factors. The resulting blood oestrogen levels are much more consistent than those produced by oral administration, and the normal ratio between oestradiol and oestrone is maintained.

One disadvantage of oestradiol patches is that the premenopausal hormone levels cannot be attained. Practical problems include the adhesiveness of the patches in hot weather, skin irritation and their cosmetic appearance. Endometrial protection can be achieved with oral progestogen or in a combined oestrogen and progestogen patch.

Oestradiol implants

A minor surgical procedure is required for the placement of oestradiol implants. Many women prefer this method of administration because once it is in place they do not have to concern themselves with the practicalities of repeated doses. The implants are renewed every six months and testosterone implants can be placed simultaneously to counter low libido. Implants offer the only means of restoring plasma oestrogens to premenopausal levels. In some women higher than normal physiological levels, which appear to be associated with an increased incidence of psychiatric disorders, are produced. This situation is easily avoided by adherence to the correct starting doses and interval between maintenance doses.

Vaginal preparations

Vaginal oestrogen preparations can be used to relieve vaginitis and vaginal dryness. Low-dose preparations have no systemic effects and do not induce uterine bleeding. They may be given in women for whom systemic HRT is contraindicated.

HRT and risk of cardiovascular disease

Oral HRT has a positive effect on some of the strongest determinants of cardiovascular disease risk – plasma lipid and lipoprotein concentrations. It may also have beneficial effects on blood pressure and on the coagulation and fibrinolysis systems. Unopposed oral oestrogen raises the plasma level of HDL-cholesterol, especially the beneficial HDL_2 fraction (see Chapter 20), while lowering LDL levels. Oral oestrogen also elevates triglyceride concentrations, but this is unlikely to cause problems unless the woman is diabetic. Administration of oestrogen by patches or implants has a less marked effect on both HDL and LDL levels. The addition of progestogen to the therapy also reduces the favourable impact of oestrogen on the blood lipid profile.

HRT and osteoporosis

The most important influence on osteoporosis in women is the availability of

> ▲ **Key points**
>
> **Advantages of HRT**
>
> ▲ Amelioration of acute physical and psychological effects of menopause
>
> ▲ Increases in bone density
>
> ▲ Reduced risk of coronary heart disease and stroke due to positive effect on blood lipid profile
>
> ▲ Treatment for premature menopause

oestrogen and HRT protects against osteoporosis whether or not the oestrogen is opposed by a progestogen. For any worthwhile protection against osteoporosis HRT must be continued for at least 5 years, usually until the woman is 55–60 years of age. Not only can bone loss be stopped, but some studies show that there can be a modest increase in bone density, usually in the first few years of therapy. These gains in bone density translate into reductions in the incidence of vertebral and femoral fractures. Discontinuation of HRT is associated with resumption of bone loss at a rate similar to that seen in untreated women of similar age.

The gains in bone density are related to the oestrogen dose and duration of use (Figure 8.7); the greatest benefits are associated with oestradiol implants. Long-term use of oestradiol patches also leads to increased bone density, but oral HRT is the least potent (low dose vaginal preparations have no systemic effect).

HRT and endometrial cancer

Unopposed oestrogen therapy stimulates the endometrium and increases the risks of endometrial hyperplasia and cancer. The risk of cancer is related to the dose and duration of oestrogen use. Growth of endometrial cells is stimulated by oestrogen, but these cells are shed under the influence of progesterone. Adding progesterone to the therapy eliminates the opportunity for prolonged oestrogenic stimulation and hence the risk of hyperplasia or cancer.

The usual progestogens used in HRT are norethisterone, medroxyprogesterone and dydrogesterone. Side-effects include headache, depression, loss of libido and a bloated feeling, not unlike the premenstrual syndrome. Because of the side-effects, progestogen therapy is usually limited to 7 days per month.

Breast cancer

The use of HRT appears to be associated with an additional risk of breast cancer; this cannot be modified by the addition of a progestogen to the therapy. Risk estimates vary, some epidemiological reports showing virtually no change in risk, others showing a very small decrease in risk. The more recent larger studies support an increased risk (see Chapter 15), particularly when the recipients of HRT are compared with women who have never used the therapy. The risk appears to fall if the therapy is discontinued.

It is known that oestrogen stimulates the growth of tumour cells and that treatment with the anti-oestrogen drug tamoxifen improves survival rates of women with breast cancer – even if epidemiological studies do not always show it, an adverse effect of oestrogen on breast cancer is biologically plausible. It would therefore seem prudent to advise any woman who has had breast cancer or who has a strong family history of the disease against using HRT.

▲ **Key points**

Risks of HRT

▲ Fluid retention

▲ Unwanted uterine bleeding

▲ Premenstrual syndrome

▲ Not advised in women with previous or strong family history of breast cancer

▲ Oral HRT not suitable for women who had deep vein thrombosis or pulmonary thrombo-embolism during pregnancy or previous oral contraceptive use

▲ Unopposed oestrogen therapy increases risk of endometrial cancer

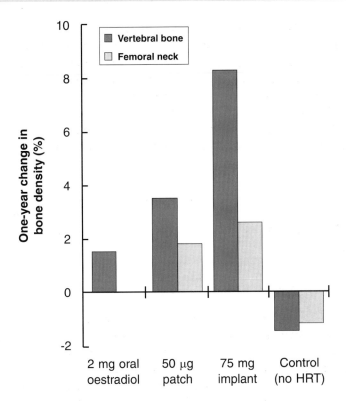

Figure 8.7 Changes in bone density in the vertebrae and femoral neck with HRT. Bone density increases with HRT in a dose-dependent manner. Gains of 8% a year are possible in vertebral bone although it is currently uncertain how long this can be sustained. The increase in bone density translates into reduced risk of fracture. (Adapted from Studd, J.W.W. and Smith, R.N.J. (1993) Oestradiol and testosterone implants. *Bailliere's Clinical Endocrinology and Metabolism*, **7**, 203–23.)

Withdrawal bleeding

The main reason that women who have not had a hysterectomy discontinue HRT is the return of bleeding which can be heavy, prolonged and painful. There are several ways in which bleeding can be controlled. One of these is to give the progestogen in a combined low-dose therapy, rather than cyclically. However, some women will still experience irregular breakthrough bleeding and discontinue the treatment. The main concern surrounding combined low-dose progestogen therapy is endometrial pathology, and any bleeding that occurs after prolonged amenorrhoea should be investigated. There are new synthetic derivatives of oestrogenic hormones on the horizon which are only weakly oestrogenic and offer the prospect of bleed-free therapy. However, these may not be as effective in modifying blood lipid profiles or in preventing osteoporotic fractures. Currently the only approach that guarantees amenorrhoea and avoids the need for progestogen is hysterectomy.

The protective benefits of HRT increase with duration of use, but few women

Review question 2

What are the main changes that happen to a woman as she reaches the ages of 20, 50 and 70 years? Think not only about the biological and developmental changes that take place but also about the changes in lifestyle that are likely to occur.

want to put up with monthly bleeds in old age. Although some of the overt symptoms of the menopause remain difficult to treat, other strategies can be employed to reduce the risks of bone loss and coronary heart disease – such as cessation of smoking and excessive alcohol consumption, proper diet and adequate exercise.

ANSWERS TO REVIEW QUESTIONS

Question 1

What are the limitations to extending the lifespan of humans?

Improvements in lifespan will be difficult to achieve because they will entail interference with the fundamental processes of ageing which are undoubtedly to a large extent determined genetically, although the genes involved have not been identified. It seems likely that these genetic mechanisms would be exerted in most cells of the body, rather than in a single 'controlling' organ. The problems are thus to identify the genes and find ways to alter their activity – in virtually every cell of the body.

It is likely that cells are somehow sensitive to the passage of time and in particular to the number of cell divisions that have taken place. A simpler approach might be to find some way of fooling the cells into 'thinking' that time had not passed or that previous cell divisions had not taken place. This would probably involve artificial modification of the body's biorhythms, although it is difficult to see how this might be achieved without modifying, for example, natural sleep/wake patterns which could produce undesirable psychological effects.

Question 2

What are the main changes that happen to a woman as she reaches the ages of 20, 50 and 70 years?

At age 20 a woman is at the peak of her physical abilities; her muscle strength and athletic prowess (depending on the particular sport) will be at a maximum, her hair will be at its thickest and her skin will be unwrinkled. She will be sexually mature, although in many women the desire for sexual activity is not at its strongest until their thirties. For many women this age is marked by fundamental changes in lifestyle. She may be involved in a serious relationship, contemplating marriage or setting up home for herself. She may also be taking advantage of educational opportunities or taking the first steps in her career. Without the constraining influences of children she may have a large variety of interests and activities outside the home. Alternatively, she could already have had children and will be closely involved in caring for their needs.

At the age of 50 a woman could be experiencing symptoms of the menopause (the average age of onset in Western women is 50 years, but is often earlier in women who smoke). She will probably be 5–10 kg heavier than she was at 20 due to metabolic changes and decreased activity. She will be slightly shorter and her hair may be thinning and going grey. Her skin will be wrinkled due to loss of elasticity. Muscle strength and lung function will become reduced.

By the age of 70 the woman may experience minor memory losses, although for the most part the intellect remains sharp. There will also be a decline in muscle mass and overall weight. Height decreases due to the changes in bone volume and there is a decrease in lung capacity. Her skin sags as the amount of facial fat decreases. There may also be impairment of hearing and eyesight. A decline in the efficiency of a variety of organs may mean that a number of medical conditions arise. Loss of function of the immune system can increase susceptibility to infection and cancer. A build-up of fatty deposits in the arteries can clog the circulation and lead to heart problems and the disruption of other vital organs such as the brain and the lungs.

References

Behnke, J.A., Finch, C.E. and Moment, G.B. (1978) *The Biology of Ageing*, Plenum Press, New York.

Brookbank, J.W. (1990) *The Biology of Ageing*, Harper & Row, New York.

Finch, C.E. and Hayflick, L. (eds) (1977) *Handbook of the Biology of Ageing*, Van Nostrand Reinhold, New York.

Finch, C.E. (1990) *Longevity, Senescence and the Genome*, University of Chicago Press, Chicago.

Hayflick, L. (1965) The limited *in vitro* lifetime of human diploid cell strains. *Exp. Cell. Res.*, **37**, 614–36.

Hulka, B.S. (1990) Hormone replacement therapy and the risk of breast cancer. *CA Cancer J. Clin.*, **40**, 289–96.

Kanungo, M.S. (1994) *Genes and Ageing*, Cambridge University Press, Cambridge.

Makinodan, T. (1990) Immunologic aspects of ageing, in The Ageing Process (ed. M.C. Geokas) *Ann. Intern. Med.*, **113**, 455–66.

Mera, S.L. (1992) Senescence and pathology in ageing. *Med. Lab. Sci.*, **49**, 271–82.

9   The impact of ageing

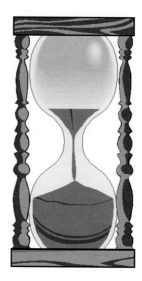

In the developed world people are living longer than was previously the case. This can be ascribed to general improvements in social and economic conditions as well as technological and medical advances. In many countries the proportion of the population aged 65 years and over is 15% or more. A more recent demographic phenomenon has been the increase in the proportion of the 'oldest-old' (people aged 85 years and over) in the older population.

As they get older many people are affected by disabling conditions such as arthritis, coronary heart disease, stroke and Alzheimer's disease. The continued expansion of the oldest-old population poses the question of how best to provide social and medical support. Fears that society will have to provide for larger and larger numbers of infirm people appear to be unfounded, because the oldest-old represent the survivors in our society, who are less likely to suffer chronic morbidity.

The combination of physiological, social and economic changes that accompany ageing is often reflected in poor nutritional status. Malnutrition becomes a real possibility, especially in those with chronic disabling conditions. Activity levels are often very low so that there is little desire for food. This leads to inadequate energy intake and accompanying depletion of essential vitamins and minerals. Although overt nutritional deficiencies are rare in older people, susceptibility to disease can be increased because of inadequate nutrition. A further problem for older people is that, because of a variety of concomitant symptoms and pathologies, many are on multiple drug regimens that can interact and produce untoward effects.

Pre-test

- **Describe how you think being old affects a person's life**
- **Estimate the proportion of older people (over 65 years) in your country**
- **What special requirements do older people have?**
- **What diseases are older people susceptible to?**

Aims of this chapter

By the end of this chapter you will have increased your knowledge of:
◆   The reasons why life expectancy has increased in the UK
◆   The social, demographic and health consequences of increased life expectancy
In addition, this chapter will help you to:
◆   Recognise the difficulties in maintaining proper nutritional status in older people
◆   Describe the disabilities and diseases that older people are most likely to suffer from and discuss how these affect their lives

Introduction

Life expectancy of people living in the developed countries has markedly increased over the last century because of changes in the principal causes of death. People are more likely to die of diseases related to the ageing process rather than infectious diseases.

Definition of terms

Definitions vary as to what constitutes 'older people' or 'the elderly'. In this book these terms are taken to mean men and women over the age of 65 years. Another expression, the 'oldest-old', refers to people aged 85 and over. However, different people age at different rates and functionally an 80-year-old person can be just as physically and mentally fit and agile as someone aged 65 who has led a sedentary life. In essence, you are as young as you feel.

Life expectancy refers to that period for which 50% of a cohort of people born in a certain year are expected to live. There will, of course, be much variation in the survival of individuals, some surviving only for hours and others passing 100. The maximal attainable age for members of a particular species is known as their **lifespan**. Hence the reductions in the mortality rates of infants and young children that have been achieved over the past century have concerned life expectancy, but nothing has yet appreciably altered the known human lifespan of about 120 years.

Ageing is accompanied by fundamental changes in social and economic circumstances

Life expectancy has increased markedly over the past 100 years, but lifespan remains unaltered

Demographic changes in the UK

The life expectancy of people living in the UK has increased markedly in the last 100 years (Figure 9.1). At the turn of the century the average life expectancy was less than 50 years, whereas today most people can expect to live into their seventies or eighties, and beyond that is not uncommon. This improvement is mainly because of reductions in perinatal mortality and deaths from infectious diseases such as influenza, pneumonia and tuberculosis. The principal factors

Average life expectancy in the UK is now about 73 years of age for men and 79 years for women

Review question 1

Comment on the differences in male and female survival in 1855 and 1981

Review question 2

Why has life expectancy in the UK improved so markedly over the past century? What further strategies will be necessary to further increase life expectancy?

involved are improved nutrition, housing and health care. Nowadays most people die of chronic degenerative diseases such as coronary heart disease and cancers, which are in some respects related to the processes of ageing.

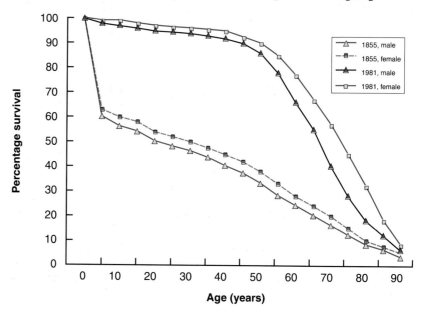

Figure 9.1 Survival rates in 1855 and 1981, Scotland. (Source: Registrar General, Scotland.)

The proportion of people living in the UK aged 65 years and over was about 15% in 1981 (Figure 9.2). This is not expected to alter substantially in the first part of the next century, although within this group it is anticipated that there will be an increase in the proportion of the 'oldest old'. This subgroup is expected to increase by about two-thirds over the next 20 years (Table 9.1). Similar trends are predicted in the USA.

Table 9.1   Percentage of people of 65 years of age and over in the UK

Year	Age 65–74 years	Age 75+	Total
1901	3.4	1.4	4.8
1941	8.9	3.4	12.3
1981	9.3	5.9	15.2
2001 (predicted)	8.1	7.2	15.3

Source: Central Statistical Office, 1984.

Generally, life expectancy for men is shorter than that for women. In the UK, more boys are born than girls. By middle age the gender distribution is equal, but there is a progressive imbalance in favour of women (Table 9.2). The consequence is that the older woman is much more likely to live alone,

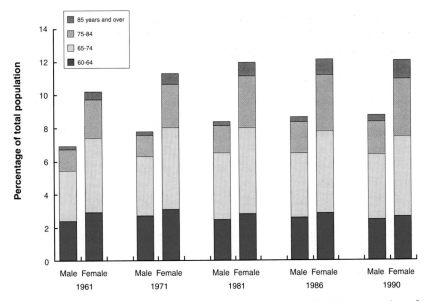

Figure 9.2 Variation in age structure of the population of the UK. The proportion of people over 60 in the population has increased since 1961, with some stabilisation after 1986. The 85-year and above subgroup continues to increase. The ratio of women to men is greater in all age categories over 60 years. (Source: OPCS, 1991.)

having lost her male partner (Table 9.3). The proportion of people living alone increases with age, and is usually because of loss of a partner. This affects women more than men, because of their longer life expectancy. It is also traditional for a woman to choose a partner older than herself.

Table 9.2   Ratio of men to women living in the UK

Year	Age 65–74	Age 75+
1901	1:1.2	1:1.5
1941	1:1.2	1:1.6
1981	1:1.3	1:2.2
2001 (predicted)	1:1.2	1:1.8

Source: Central Statistical Office, 1984.

Table 9.3   Percentage of people living alone in the UK

Age	Men	Women
45–64	9	13
65–74	16	37
75+	31	58

Source: General Household Survey, 1989.

Growing old

Ageing can affect a person's lifestyle, causing illness, disability and changes in social and economic circumstances

The physiological and biochemical changes that are associated with ageing suggest that this phase of life is characterised by a progressive and irreversible decline. Such changes reduce the ability of the older person to adapt to the challenges and stresses of everyday life, which may be exacerbated by the social conditions of older people. Factors such as social class, occupational status, and loneliness contribute significantly to the health of older people. Loneliness and social isolation may contribute to both psychological and physical illness, leading to depression, which may itself suppress the immune system and predispose to disease.

> *For far too many, old age is a wretched time characterised by a sense of uselessness, by physical and social neglect, and by increasingly severe physical and mental deterioration. The urgency of this problem is evident in countless personal tragedies, in the loss to society of the potential for self-reliance and productiveness of millions of our citizens...*
>
> **Moment (1978)**

Not all the features of ageing are negative: increased free time may mean that we can do more things

There are, however, opportunities for developmental growth in older people. Increased leisure time may mean that new or old interests can be pursued; friendships can be enhanced and educational courses pursued. Things can be done to minimise the effects of ageing but these need to be acted on by society at large, not just the individual. Many of the disabilities of older people can be lessened by lifestyle changes such as diet, exercise and cessation of smoking. Health promotion for older people can be targeted to emphasise the physical, mental and social facets of positive health and to counteract traditional 'ageism' attitudes. Feelings of well-being, independence and self-esteem have as much to do with being healthy as physical capacity.

Attitudes towards older people

It is easy to stereotype older people as slow, set in their ways and dependent on others

Many younger people have strong attitudes towards older people which may be expressed as shunning and discriminatory behaviours. These prejudices may be based on stereotypes in which older people may be perceived as childlike, isolated, inactive, non-productive and unhappy. Many of the diseases that afflict older people may themselves elicit negative attitudes, for example the degenerative diseases such as Parkinson's disease and Alzheimer's disease are associated with overt mental or physical disabilities. Similarly, there is some prejudice against people who require some form of prosthesis: spectacles, hearing aid, walking frame or wheelchair.

We should concentrate on adding life to the years, not just years to life

Communicating with older people who are confused, depressed or even demented can present enormous problems, particularly if additional barriers of poor sight and hearing are to be overcome. The older person may hold low opinions and expectations of himself, which can act as a 'vicious circle' and exacerbate functional impairments such as incontinence, depression, fatigue, pain and poor balance. The end result is that the person can become depressed, confused and difficult to communicate with.

Efforts should be made to counteract these negative stereotypes. A positive attitude by both older people and those around them can minimise many of the difficulties faced in old age by increasing general awareness of the problems and by health promotion. In particular, the professionals with whom older people frequently come into contact – community nurses, general practitioners and social care workers – can do much to promote positive coping behaviours.

Helping the older person to understand that dependency is a normal part of human relationships can bring a new perspective to events that might otherwise increase despondency. In this way the older person can be given a sense of control and from this may come improvement in the management of health problems. It is a mistake to characterise all older people with the attitudes and disabilities seen in a minority.

Reflect on your own attitudes towards older people. Think of the older people you know personally and consider how their lifestyles differ from your own.

- Describe your positive feelings about older people
- Describe your negative feelings about older people
- List the things you can easily do now, but may find more difficult as you get older
- Describe in general terms how the social and economic circumstances of older people differ from your own

Activity 1

Nutrition and older people

A variety of dietary habits can potentially affect the nutritional status and health of older people.

- Altered meal frequencies
- Lack of motivation to prepare food, particularly hot cooked meals
- Social isolation and loneliness – many older people are forced to eat alone
- Lack of money
- Lack of dietary awareness

Nutritional problems can also arise because of the underlying health status of the individual.

- Impaired appetite
- Poor dentition
- Mental disturbance
- Reduced gastrointestinal absorption
- Physical disability
- Chronic disease
- Alcohol intake
- Drug therapy

The institutionalisation of older persons will inevitably cause a change in dietary habits as new meal types and frequencies are imposed. It is to be hoped that the diets devised by institutions are well founded and professionally informed rather than based on purely economic considerations. Other factors

Older people may find it difficult to cook for themselves and their diets may not be nutritionally adequate

A loss of appetite, reduced taste sensation and depression may contribute to poor diet in older people

that may contribute to poor diet include the emotional state of the person; someone depressed by recent bereavement is unlikely to devote much consideration to preparing balanced meals, particularly if that person is also socially isolated.

The limited economic circumstances of many older people often preclude the purchase of fresh foods – and this can become more difficult if the person has mobility problems and cannot easily get to the shops. Lifting heavy or bulky containers of foodstuffs out of cupboards can cause difficulties for older people with disabilities.

Both obesity and underweight may present as problems in older people, although obesity is by far the most common. In the later years of adult life the proportion of lean body mass usually declines relative to fat. In women this occurs most dramatically after the menopause. Consequently the basal energy requirement decreases, and this may be exacerbated by reduced physical activity. Thus it is not only the nutritional balance that needs to be addressed but also the increased sedentary behaviour of older people.

> *Nutritional problems in older people are more likely to be caused by obesity than malnutrition*

Obesity

Obesity is associated with a number of health risks, including diabetes, stroke, cardiovascular disease, osteoarthritis, digestive disorders, kidney failure, and a variety of cancers. Reduction in fat intake and increasing physical activity are the most effective ways of reducing weight. Reductions in food items such as sugar and alcohol are also appropriate because they provide energy but no other nutrients.

Excess body fat adversely affects plasma lipoprotein concentrations, particularly the atherogenic LDL and VLDL. Blood concentrations of these lipoproteins can be altered by a low-calorie diet. Successful long-term weight loss improves the adverse lipoprotein profiles of obese subjects.

> *Obesity is associated with a number of health risks that reduce life expectancy*

Underweight

Underweight is most commonly associated with young adults and children, but after middle age the prevalence of this condition increases (Figure 9.3). The problems of underweight include depression of the immune system, which leads to increased susceptibility to infection or even the development of cancer.

Underweight and eventual malnutrition can arise from:

- Dietary inadequacy
- Underlying disease
- Behavioural problems
- Dependency on drugs or alcohol

Dietary inadequacy may be due to a variety of social, economic or educational reasons and may be secondary to a medical condition that causes loss of appetite (for example, in cancer). Many of the treatments for underlying medical conditions (for example, chemotherapy and radiotherapy treatments for cancer) can cause loss of appetite or other gastrointestinal symptoms such as nausea,

> *It is easy for underweight people to become deficient in essential vitamins and minerals*

vomiting and diarrhoea. Even relatively mild infections and antibiotic treatment can cause dietary disturbances for some months.

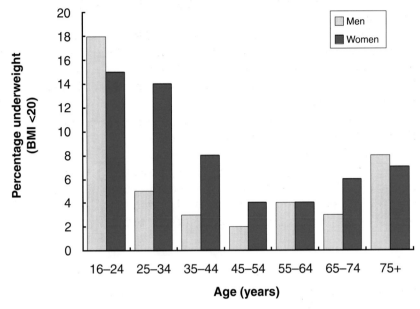

Figure 9.3 Percentage of underweight adults in the UK. (Source: OPCS, 1993.)

A number of behavioural problems afflicting older people can lead to general neglect, including inadequate attention to the diet. These may be consequent on depressive illness as well as more serious functional disorders such as Alzheimer's disease. Another possible reason, although not restricted to older people, is alcohol consumption: in heavy drinkers the dependence on alcohol takes precedence over other body requirements, most notably the need for proper and regular meals. Malnutrition inevitably occurs when most calories are obtained from alcohol.

Some causes of underweight and even malnutrition are relatively simple, and once recognised can be easy to correct. A common reason for inadequate food intake is poor dentition: at present the proportion of older people with no natural teeth remains high since conservative dentistry is a relatively recent practice (Figure 9.4). The pain induced by chewing with ill-fitting dentures can discourage many older people from eating a balanced diet.

Malnutrition

It becomes extremely difficult to meet the requirements for vitamins and minerals when food intake is low (energy intake below 1500 kcal). Although frank vitamin and mineral deficiencies such as scurvy are rare in older people, suboptimal intakes can still affect health adversely. For example, vitamins and minerals are essential in wound healing and for maintaining the immune system and bone mass. Mild deficiencies can increase susceptibility to infection,

▲ **Key points**

Common nutritional deficiencies in older people

▲ Energy

▲ Vitamins, mainly because consumption of fruit, vegetables and meat is low

▲ Fluid

▲ Fibre

▲ Minerals, particularly calcium, also magnesium, zinc, iron, phosphorus, potassium

pressure sores, leg ulcers or bone fracture. Adequate intake of antioxidant vitamins and minerals is important in reducing the risks of cancers and cardiovascular disease.

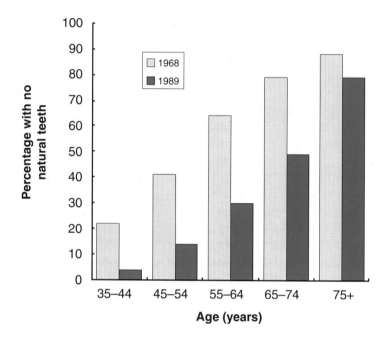

Figure 9.4 The proportion of people with no natural teeth increases with age. There are also historical differences reflecting the move to more conservative dental practice. Currently, more than 70% of people over 75 have no teeth of their own. It can be expected that the older people of the future will have had the benefit of conservative dental treatments, so that the proportion with no natural teeth will decrease further. (Source: General Household Survey, 1989.)

Only 1–2% of older people in the UK show clinical evidence of serious malnutrition, which mainly occurs in people with other physical or mental disabilities and in those with acute and chronic illnesses. However, low body weight is common in old people with chronic or disabling conditions and hence low activity levels, particularly those in institutional care. The main problem of inadequate energy intake may be accompanied by low vitamin and mineral status because of a lack of fresh fruit and vegetables in the diet.

In the chronically sick older person malnutrition can arise through a combination of poor appetite and a diet low in nutritional density. In these circumstances it is sensible to relax restrictions on fatty foods in the diet. Fat enhances the palatability of food as well as providing a vehicle for fat-soluble vitamins.

Attention should also be paid to the fluid needs of older people who tend to become dehydrated, mainly because of diminished thirst sensation. Dehydration is a significant cause of confusion, headaches and irritability in older people.

Special dietary needs

Older people may have particular dietary needs as a consequence of disease or disability. For example digestive disorders, particularly constipation and diverticular disease but also ulcers and colitis, are common. Many of these conditions can be improved by dietary means, such as by the inclusion of fibre. Up to 50% of the older population regularly take laxatives, and reliance on these could be reduced by incorporation of wheat bran, soy polysaccharide and other fibre sources into the diet. However, large amounts of bran should not be taken, because it interferes with the absorption of essential vitamins and minerals – more is not necessarily better.

It is estimated that 17% of Americans over 65 years of age have some form of diabetes. Glucose tolerance can be improved by the incorporation of fibre-rich foods or by supplementing the diet with extracted fibre such as wheat bran, guar gum, apple fibre or cellulose.

Because of concerns that absorption of vitamins and minerals can be inhibited by the inclusion of very high amounts of fibre it is sensible to adjust the amount of fibre in the diet to the total calorie intake (10–13 g of fibre per 1000 kcal per day is recommended).

> *Diet should contain adequate fibre, but too much can be detrimental*

Dietary trends and longevity

Paradoxically, one of the largest improvements in diet which influenced life expectancy came in the UK about the time of World War II. The government decided to enforce changes in the diet, presumably with the intention of benefiting the fighting man. Synthetic vitamin B_1 was added to flour, vitamins A and D to margarine, milk and potato production was encouraged, as was the production of green vegetables in a 'dig for victory' campaign. It is, of course, this population who are old today and it remains to be seen whether older people of the future, brought up on highly processed 'convenience' foods rich in sugar and fat but low in fibre, will be as fit.

There is evidence to suggest that a diet that is nutritionally balanced but low in calories may be conducive to longevity in a variety of mammals and possibly even in humans. For example, rats on a very low-calorie diet can live for up to 4 years, compared with the usual maximum of 3 years in a captive environment. Examination of organs such as the brain in these animals indicates that some of the changes due to senescence may be delayed, although various age-related alterations of the neurons and their supporting neuroglia do ultimately occur. The mechanism by which calorie restriction works in extending the longevity of laboratory animals is unknown, and its relevance to humans uncertain. If a low-calorie dietary regime does work, it seems likely that it would have to operate throughout the lifetime. It is interesting to note that in parts of the world (such as parts of Russia and China) where some people reportedly live to a very old age (if accurate), the way of life is simple, rural, subsistence. However, it is easy for a low-calorie diet to become nutrient

▲ Key points

Lifestyle recommendations for older people

- ▲ Eating and lifestyle patterns should be similar to those recommended for younger people
- ▲ Avoid obesity: reduce intakes of fat and simple sugars
- ▲ Increase intake of starchy and non-starch polysaccharides
- ▲ Ensure adequate intake of fruit and vegetables
- ▲ Chronic or recurrent illness in some older people may mean that they become underweight: ensure dietary intake is generous and food is nutrient-rich
- ▲ Ensure some exposure to sunlight, or consider vitamin D supplementation
- ▲ Maintain an active lifestyle, and resume activities as quickly as possible after illness
- ▲ Do not smoke
- ▲ Avoid excessive alcohol consumption

deficient, which in the long term would lead to greater susceptibility to illness and slower recovery.

Exercise

In older people regular exercise can mean the difference between independence and institutionalisation. Lack of exercise may be responsible for up to three-quarters of the risk of stroke and probably doubles the risk of CHD, mainly because of its influences on obesity and hypertension. It also helps to avoid osteoporosis and consequent hip fracture, which is one of the main causes of disability in older people.

All surveys indicate that levels of physical activity are markedly reduced in most older people (Figure 9.5). Some decline in physical fitness is inevitable, mainly because senescence changes in the connective tissue affect lung and respiratory functions and joint flexibility. However, there is good evidence that much of the decline in exercise capacity in older people is caused by disuse and, with care, this lost capacity can be regained. Part of the problem is a 'chicken and egg' situation: once an older person suffers from a disabling illness (fracture, for example) it becomes difficult to re-establish activity. Conversely, a lack of activity can make disabling conditions (such as osteoporosis) worse.

The psychological gains of exercise particularly benefit older people: exercise can make people feel good by reducing depression and anxiety and increasing confidence and self-esteem. It can provide a reason for the lonely person to get out of the domestic environment.

A *Health of the Nation* survey published in 1995 showed that activity levels are so low that sustaining a reasonable walking pace for several minutes on level ground constitutes severe exertion for 50% of women over the age of 55. About 30% of men and 50% of women aged between 65 and 74 years have insufficient strength in their thigh muscles to rise from a chair without using their arms.

The main recommendation of the report is that people who take no regular exercise should aim to complete 30 minutes of moderate activity every week. This should be gradually increased to 30 minutes moderate activity each day. Moderate activity is classed as energy expenditure of at least 5 kcal/min, which leaves an individual warm and slightly out of breath (brisk walking, cycling, dancing and swimming are suitable activities).

Frequency of disease and disability in older people

There is an expectation among many that life for older people becomes marred by disability and disease. Unfortunately this can be true, and there are many examples of people crippled by arthritis, debilitated by stroke and experiencing loss of memory and mind that characterises Alzheimer's disease. These conditions are not amenable to cure and affected individuals require long-term care and management.

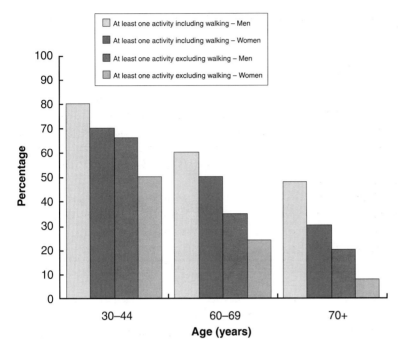

Figure 9.5 Physical activity by age and gender (UK, 1990). Self-reported activity in 4 weeks before interview. Physical activity levels decline markedly as people get older. Many people below 70 years of age claimed to have undertaken a walk of at least 2 miles in the 4 weeks before interview. The other most popular activities include swimming, cycling, keep fit, weight training and yoga. At all ages participation in men is more common than in women, but after 70 years of age only 20% of men and 8% of women participate in some activity other than walking. (Source: OPCS, General Household Survey, 1992.)

A substantial majority of older people suffer from long-standing illness. By the age of 75, 50% of people report that their illness is severe enough to interfere with their activities (Figure 9.6). Illness in older people is reflected by an increased number of consultations with their general practitioner (Figure 9.7).

Inspection of almost any of the statistics for chronic diseases (Figure 9.8) confirms an inexorable increase with age. However, there is evidence that many of the oldest-old lead relatively healthy lives. This is because people in this age group represent life's survivors: they are more robust and more resistant to the diseases that disable and kill most people before they enter the oldest-old category. Moreover, many of the oldest-old lead lives that are relatively free of disabilities and death, when it comes, is preceded by a much shorter period of illness.

Exactly what gives the oldest-old their survival advantage is uncertain. Undoubtedly there is a genetic advantage, if only by freedom from those genes that predispose to certain categories of illness, rather than the possession of 'longevity' genes. The other factors are in the environment, and it is probably no coincidence that centenarians are more likely to ascribe their longevity to exercise, keeping busy and life-long avoidance of 'rich' foods, smoking and excessive alcohol consumption. What is clear is that the oldest-old do not

People in their nineties suffer less chronic disease and disability than many in their seventies and early eighties

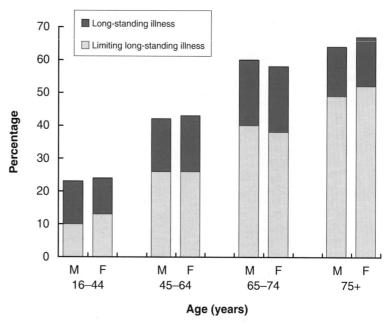

Figure 9.6 Self-reported illness in the UK, 1992. The prevalence of self-reported long-standing illness increases with age. This trend is mainly because of increased prevalence of limiting long-standing disease: with age the illness is more likely to interfere with daily activities. The increase in prevalence with age is related to age-specific functional decline and altered socioeconomic circumstances. Individuals with low income and social standing are much more susceptible to disease. It should be noted that the chart shows *self-reported* illness, which will include both perceived and diagnosed illnesses. (Source: OPCS General Household Survey, 1992.)

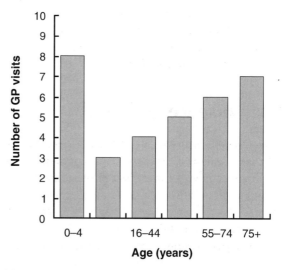

Figure 9.7 Problems with disability and disease in older people are reflected by increases in the number of consultations each year. (Source: General Household Survey, 1989.)

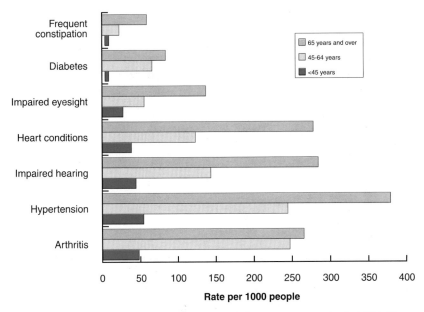

Figure 9.8 Frequency of chronic conditions in different age groups in the USA. Heart disease and hypertension are the most common causes of morbidity and mortality in older people in the USA. (Source: National Center for Health Statistics.)

have the burden of poor health that might be expected by simply extrapolating morbidity data for older people in general.

In actuarial tables the chances of survival are recalculated with increasing age. This takes into account a 'survival of the fittest' phenomenon in which the length of time already survived indicates an individual who is fit and more likely to survive into old age. The life expectancy for men being born in the UK is 73.4 years, and for females 79 years. At 70 years of age men are expected to live another 11.2, and women 14.5, years (Figure 9.9) – longer than the original life expectancy estimates at birth.

Age-related disease and disability

The diseases most commonly associated with old age are atherosclerosis, arthritis, osteoporosis, cataract, chronic renal failure, diabetes, senile dementia and most types of cancer. Contributory factors in causing these diseases may include:

- The physiological and biochemical changes of normal ageing
- Cumulative exposure to harmful agents
- Increased sensitivity to agents or environments with increasing age

Older people are susceptible to a large array of chronic diseases including coronary heart disease, cancer and arthritis

Cancer

Cancer is a common cause of illness and death in older people, with over 50%

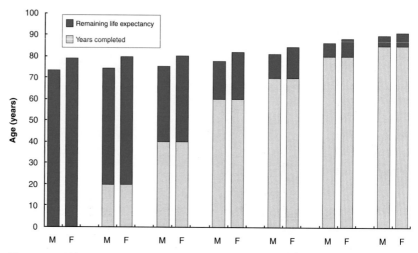

Figure 9.9 Life expectancy in England and Wales, 1990–1992. Actuarial tables take account of the fact that people who have already lived to a certain age have shown themselves to be survivors, and so life expectancy is continuously upgraded according to the length of time a person has already lived. (Source: OPCS, 1992.)

Most cancers occur in older people and are responsible for one-third of all deaths in people over 65

of all cancers occurring in those over the age of 65 years. In general the incidence of cancer increases with age (Figure 9.10). The precise role of ageing in this is uncertain; it may be that many of the cancers are caused by a continuous and prolonged exposure to a carcinogenic agent and are nothing to do with the ageing process itself.

The types of cancer seen at different ages also differ (see Chapter 13). Leukaemias and sarcomas are more common in children and young adults; in older adults, carcinomas and lymphomas are more common. A contributory factor in childhood cancer may be that cells throughout the body are in a phase of rapid proliferation, increasing their susceptibility to carcinogenic agents.

The combination of cumulative exposures and increased sensitivity to damaging agents may contribute to increased cancer rates in older people

Several hypotheses have been proposed to explain the greater frequency of cancers in the older population. They may arise from an age-related accumulation of carcinogens, the total dose received being a function of age in susceptible individuals. This process is independent of the senescence changes that take place in the body.

A second hypothesis takes account of senescence changes which are thought to make cells more vulnerable. Changes in physiological function (for example, immune, nutritional, metabolic and endocrine status) concomitant with age create a more favourable environment for the induction of cancer. These altered responses may affect a variety of internal cell processes, such as those involving the detoxification of mutagenic agents, repair of damaged DNA and responses to oncogene activation. In addition, some cells and tissues may enter an altered state of growth regulation, resembling that of tumour promotion, as part of the process of senescence. Entry into this state could precipitate cancer in previously initiated or mutated cells.

An interesting facet of the age–incidence pattern of cancer is that the increase

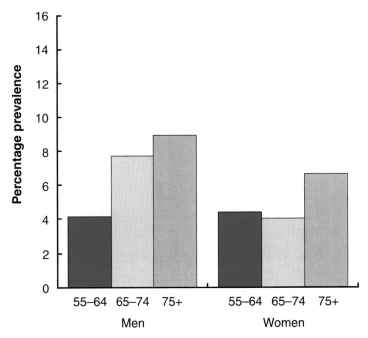

Figure 9.10 Cancer prevalence in the USA, 1980, with age. (Source: 1980 National Medical Care Expenditure Survey (US).)

is not exponential: cancer risk does increase with advancing age, but at a rate that is constantly decreasing. This could arise from two opposing processes in the ageing individual.
- Genetic mutations accumulate with time, predisposing to neoplastic transformation
- Cells tend to lose proliferative potential with age – loss of proliferative potential tends to reduce the risk of neoplastic transformation

Diseases of the cardiovascular system

Many of the altered cardiovascular functions in the older adult, such as reduced maximal heart rate, stroke volume and cardiac output, may be caused by disease rather than old age.

Plasma cholesterol concentrations tend to increase with age, and cumulative exposure over many years is thought to be responsible for increased mortality from coronary heart disease, first in middle-aged men and later in older women (Figure 9.11). The current consensus is that risk can be reduced by controlling the factors that influence the tendency for formation of atherosclerotic plaque and thrombosis. This can be achieved by lifestyle changes involving diet, smoking habits and amount of physical activity.

Lifestyle and behavioural risk factors primarily operate in adult life, but there is evidence that susceptibility to cardiovascular disease could be laid down much earlier in life. It is believed that growth characteristics of fetal and infant life influence later measurements of blood pressure, glucose tolerance,

Age-related changes in blood lipid profiles increase the likelihood of coronary heart disease in later life

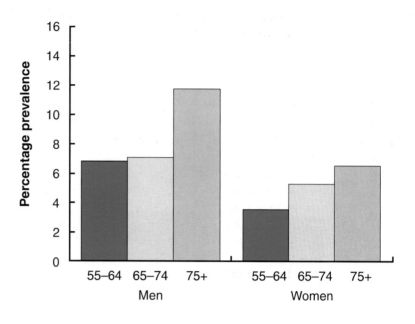

Figure 9.11 Prevalence of CHD in the USA. (Source: 1980 National Medical Care Expenditure Survey (US).)

The strongest risk factors for disease are determined by what we do as adults, but some risks are laid down very early on in life

and concentrations of cholesterol and fibrinogen, all of which are risk factors in cardiovascular disease. Indeed, our early lifetime experiences appear to affect a wide range of later disease outcomes and physiological changes, including stroke, chronic bronchitis and late-onset diabetes.

It has been suggested that susceptibility to CHD could be influenced by whether the person was breast fed or bottle fed as a baby and by the age of weaning (see Chapter 20). Breast milk is rich in saturated fat and cholesterol and strongly influences plasma cholesterol concentrations in the infant. Higher plasma cholesterol concentrations in infancy appear to track through to later life, affecting the predisposition for atherosclerosis and its complications. This is one of the few instances when breast-fed babies may be at a disadvantage.

Respiratory disease

Older people are more likely to have bronchitis and emphysema, particularly if they are smokers

A common problem in older people is chronic obstructive airways disease, which often causes reduced pulmonary capacity and functional disability. It is a range of conditions including chronic bronchitis and emphysema, which are generally caused by the interplay of physiological ageing and environmental factors such as cigarette smoking. The classic and progressing symptom of this complex of diseases is dyspnoea, often accompanied by cough and sputum production and secondary symptoms such as fatigue and weight loss.

Chronic obstructive airways disease is a leading cause of death in the UK and is also a factor in deaths from pneumonia and influenza. Death usually occurs within 10 years of the onset of dyspnoea. The most effective treatment is cessation of smoking, but bronchodilators, corticosteroids and inhaled anticholinergic therapies can also be employed.

Late-onset diabetes

Most older people exhibit some degree of glucose intolerance. This can be severe enough to be classified as non-insulin-dependent diabetes mellitus. The main reason for the raised blood sugar levels appears to be an increased resistance to the effects of insulin in peripheral tissues with age, and is associated with increased post-prandial insulin levels. In turn, a high insulin profile is thought to be a significant contributor to mortality from coronary heart disease.

Diabetes in older people is strongly influenced by exercise and diet

There is evidence to suggest that the correlation between age and post-prandial blood glucose and insulin levels is modulated by exercise, diet and drugs (see Chapter 23). In particular the effects of exercise are so favourable that carbohydrate intolerance and insulin resistance may no longer be demonstrable in non-obese healthy older men.

Cataract

A cataract causes the lens of the eye to become partially or completely opaque, affecting the passage of light through the lens and causing blindness. There are many different types and causes of cataracts, but one of the most common is senile cataract. This affects about one in 1000 people of 60 years in the UK and the prevalence rate doubles with each 6–7-year increment in age thereafter. People who are short-sighted are more likely to develop senile cataract. Another risk factor for cataract is diabetes, which can also develop in later life. The treatment is to remove part or all of the opacified lens tissue and to implant a substitute plastic lens into the eye.

Changes in the connective tissues of the eye lens mean that older people are more likely to develop cataracts

Osteoporosis

Osteoporosis is a common disorder among older people, and is characterised by a reduction in bone mass which can lead to fractures and collapse of the vertebrae (kyphosis). The fractures most frequently occur in the distal radius (wrist), femoral neck and vertebral bodies. The combined prevalence of fractures in these sites is about 40% in women over 65 years.

Osteoporosis is a very common problem in older women and can lead to fractures and curvature of the spine

Osteoporosis represents an imbalance between bone formation and osteoclastic resorption (see Chapter 22). Bone resorption is influenced by the reproductive hormones, particularly oestrogen in women and testosterone in men. The condition is most commonly seen in women after the menopause; because loss of testosterone production is not as marked osteoporosis usually occurs at a later age in men. In women, the rate of bone loss can approach 10% per decade from the menopause and as much as 40% of original bone mass can be lost by the time a woman is in her eighties. The rate of loss is slower in men. Probably the most common manifestation of the disease is lower back pain.

The most common joint disease in older people is osteoarthritis

Collagen: protein component of fibrous and non-fibrous connective tissues. Imparts tensile strength to the connective tissue.

Glycosaminoglycans: conjugates of sugar and protein. Components of the non-fibrous extracellular matrix.

Rheumatoid arthritis is common in older people, but onset occurs at any age, even in children

A number of treatments are available for osteoporosis, perhaps the best known of which is hormone replacement therapy in women. This is best initiated around the menopause, but can still benefit the older woman. Various risk factors influence the development of the condition, most notably exercise, smoking and intakes of alcohol, calcium and vitamin D. It would be prudent to adjust these factors rather than rely exclusively on hormone replacement therapy.

Many older people are not very mobile and do not go out enough to synthesise adequate amounts of vitamin D from sunlight. They also generally have low dietary vitamin D intakes, together with a decreased capacity to synthesise the vitamin D metabolites in the skin and kidney. In addition, the aged intestine is less responsive to the calcium-absorbing effects of vitamin D metabolites. The net result is that many older people may have a negative calcium balance, and supplementation with vitamin D should be considered. Exercise can do much to attenuate the age-related reduction in bone mass.

Disorders of the joints

Joint disorders are a major cause of disability in the older population. In particular, the arthropathies increase with age, although spinal conditions have a peak incidence in middle age. In a recent survey conducted in Yorkshire, 5% of people between 16 and 24 years old reported having some problems with their joints, and over half of those over 85 reported joint problems. The most commonly affected sites were the knee and the back.

Osteoarthritis is essentially a non-inflammatory disorder of movable joints, characterised by deterioration and abrasion of the articular cartilages. The injury to cartilage may be followed by proliferation of new bone at the joint surfaces. Occasionally small pieces of bone and cartilage may slough off to form loose bodies in the joint, causing pain and transient inflammation.

The disease can be caused by injury to the joints. Advancing age is also a factor, which may reflect cumulative damage to the articular tissues, together with senescence changes of cartilage (altered amounts of glycosaminoglycans and changes in collagen). Other prime causes are excessive use of the joints arising from occupation, obesity or physical abnormality. The course of osteoarthritis is usually progressive, with no exacerbations or remissions. The disease is not life-threatening and does not usually cause severe disability.

In contrast, the other common disease of the joints, rheumatoid arthritis, often causes severe disability and pain. This is not only a disease of ageing, although the prevalence increases with age, affecting about 2% of individuals over the age of 50. The disease is characterised by chronic inflammation, arising from an autoimmune reaction in an immunogenetically susceptible individual.

The exact initiating factors are unknown, although a variety of bacteria have been implicated, most notably mycobacteria. Treatment of the disease initially involves NSAIDs, but more aggressive treatment with steroids, immunosuppressant drugs or even low-dose methotrexate (a cytotoxic drug used in cancer chemotherapy) may be needed later on. There is now some evidence that early intervention with steroids can minimise the severity of the disease. Surgical replacement of hip or knee joints may be the only option for patients who become severely disabled.

Dementia

Dementia is a deterioration of intellectual and cognitive functions affecting orientation, memory and judgement. These functions can become so impaired that a patient no longer recognises his or her spouse or children (or even remember that they have a spouse or children) and forgets what they were doing even a few moments ago. Of all the disabilities and diseases associated with old age, the loss of mental capacity probably invokes more distress than any other.

About 1% of those between 65 and 74 suffer from dementia. Of those over 75 years of age the proportion rises to 10%, and more than 20% of people over 85 years of age may suffer. The principal causes of dementia are Alzheimer's disease and multiple infarcts in the brain.

Dementia is age-related and is becoming more common as people live longer

Alzheimer's disease

Alzheimer's disease is a degenerative condition of the brain in which some nerve cells gradually lose function and die. The clinical course of Alzheimer's disease averages about 8 years. Death is usually caused by pneumonia, accidents and, occasionally, respiratory arrest. The onset may be insidious, starting with periods of forgetfulness, proceeding to a confusional state and, ultimately, frank dementia. Life expectancy is about 2–3 years once severe dementia develops (see Chapter 26).

The pathological hallmarks of Alzheimer's disease are large numbers of neurofibrillary tangles and plaques in cortical areas of the brain. These reflect neuronal degeneration and death. There is also a loss of brain mass, with widening of the sulci and ventricles. These changes are also found, but to a lesser extent, in the brains of functionally normal older people. There is some speculation that the changes of Alzheimer's disease merely represent an acceleration of ageing processes that would take place anyway in people if they lived long enough. However, there is mounting evidence that genetic factors underlie the pathological process in Alzheimer's disease, particularly involving genes controlling the metabolism of amyloid proteins. It seems most likely that Alzheimer's disease is a condition associated with age, rather than intrinsic to the ageing process itself.

Most cases of dementia are caused by Alzheimer's disease

 Key points

Features of rheumatoid arthritis

Prevalence:
▲ 0.5% overall prevalence
▲ 1.5% in people over 30 years of age
▲ 2–3% in those over 50

Signs and symptoms:
▲ Insidious onset: joint aches and stiffness, followed by swelling, warmth, redness and tenderness
▲ Sudden onset in about 20% of patients, with multiple joint inflammation

Pathology:
▲ Polyarticular in most patients
▲ Involves small joints in hands and feet
▲ Joints usually involved symmetrically

Parkinson's disease

The prevalence of Parkinson's disease in those over 70 is 1–2%. Symptoms usually develop after the age of 50 years, with an average survival time of 8–10 years following diagnosis. Parkinson's disease is very distinct from Alzheimer's disease: different nerve cells are affected and there is a loss of motor co-ordination, which is usually unimpaired in Alzheimer's disease.

The brain changes in Parkinson's disease comprise degeneration of dopamine-producing nerve cells

Histological and biochemical studies of the brain in Parkinson's disease show loss and degeneration of dopaminergic neurons. This causes a reduction in the concentration of dopamine in the substantia nigra and locus ceruleus. Some degeneration of non-dopaminergic neurons and depletion of other neurotransmitters also occurs. It is believed by some researchers that the degeneration of neurons is caused by an excess of free radicals.

The pathological hallmarks of the disease are the loss of dopaminergic neurons and the appearance of eosinophilic cytoplasmic inclusions, known as Lewy bodies, in some of the surviving neurons. Lewy bodies have also been reported in some older patients with psychiatric syndromes, particularly dementia, but are considered to be very rare in people without Parkinson's disease or dementia (see Chapter 27). Thus, Lewy body formation cannot be regarded as a general age-associated neurodegenerative change. However, losses in the numbers of dopaminergic neurons and in the concentrations in dopamine also occur in non-symptomatic older people. These changes may be exacerbated in Parkinson's disease by an unknown causative agent.

Drug metabolism in older people

Ageing affects the absorption, distribution, metabolism and elimination of drugs

Older people often respond to drugs differently than younger adults. Ageing changes in the gastrointestinal tract, liver and kidneys affect the ability to metabolise and eliminate drugs and the absorption and distribution of the drug to the peripheral tissues are altered. The general pattern is that drug doses need to be lower, and adverse reactions are more frequent than in younger people.

Absorption

Reduced intestinal motility can affect the amount of drug absorbed by increasing its contact time. This will be exacerbated if antispasmodic drugs are taken as part of a multiple drug regimen. In contrast, some ageing changes militate against the purposes of drug therapy. For example, delayed gastric emptying and breakdown by enzyme or acid may mean that the activity of some short-acting drugs is diminished. Enteric-coated drugs can lose their protection and cause gastric irritation. A decrease in gastric acidity in the older person will reduce the action of acid-dependent drugs.

Distribution

The distribution of drugs to their target tissues depends on the adequacy of the blood circulation, which may be impaired in the older person because of arteriosclerosis or atherosclerosis. Reduced circulation could also delay drug metabolism and excretion from the body. Many drugs are transported in the plasma bound to albumin. Albumin concentrations may be very low in older people with chronic illnesses or poor nutrition, so that the drugs may be transported in their more toxic free form.

Age-related changes in lean body mass, body water and body fat may mean that drug concentrations in blood and tissue fluids become too high. Storage of lipid-soluble drugs in adipose tissue can ensure that the agent persists in the body for an unduly long time.

Metabolism

Drugs are primarily metabolised by microsomal enzymes in the liver. With age, liver function and enzyme induction are reduced so that drug clearance is slower. This may be exacerbated by reduced blood supply to the liver. Slower metabolism will cause the drug to remain in the body longer, increasing the possibility of side-effects.

Excretion

Most drugs are excreted through the urinary system. The clearance of drugs slows in older people because renal blood flow and glomerular filtration rate are slower.

Drug interactions

A further problem in older people is **polypharmacy**: many older people take a number of different drugs aimed at alleviating a variety of symptoms and pathologies, increasing the possibilities for adverse drug interactions. Reactions may interfere with drug potency or increase toxicity and create a new range of side-effects.

Another possible problem is related to drug interactions with nutrients in people who may already have poor nutritional status. The influence of drugs on the metabolism of nutrients is of two types. (1) The drug may inhibit an enzyme essential for intermediary metabolism, so that the nutrient cannot be used. For example, isoniazid treatment (for tuberculosis) reduces the availability of vitamin B_6. (2) Drugs can stimulate enzyme activity, causing increased breakdown and elimination of important micronutrients – this occurs with the anticonvulsant drug phenytoin, resulting in loss of vitamin D and folic acid. Diuretics and laxatives will also affect the absorption or elimination of important nutrients, for example, the diuretic thiazide increases the excretion of potassium, magnesium and zinc.

Talk to an older relative or friend. Try to establish the main changes that person feels has taken place in their life since they were young. Concentrate on:
- Diet
- Activities and amount of exercise
- Illness and disability
- Use of medications

▲ Key points

Factors influencing responsiveness to drugs with age

Absorption:
- ▲ Reduced intestinal motility
- ▲ Delayed gastric emptying
- ▲ Reduced gastric acidity

Distribution:
- ▲ Decrease in uptake by peripheral tissues
- ▲ Reduced blood flow to peripheral tissues
  Changes in body composition

Metabolism:
- ▲ Reduced metabolic capacity of liver
- ▲ Decrease in blood flow to liver
  Decreased plasma albumin

Excretion:
- ▲ Decrease in renal blood flow
- ▲ Reduction in glomerular filtration rate and urine output

Review question 3

What actions can be taken to maximise the chances of enjoying a healthy old age? What are their limitations?

Activity 2

Devise a checklist for the topics listed, designed to ensure all the relevant issues are raised during the conversation.

ANSWERS TO REVIEW QUESTIONS

Question 1

Comment on the differences in male and female survival in 1855 and 1981

Your list could include the following points:
- Female life expectancy is generally higher than that for males
- There was a substantial improvement in life expectancy between 1855 and 1981. In 1855 life expectancy was only about 30 years; this had increased to over 70 years by 1981
- The improvement in survival is mostly due to a reduction in perinatal mortality: in 1855 only about 65% of infants survived beyond 3 years of age

Question 2

Why has life expectancy in the UK improved so markedly over the past century? What further strategies will be necessary today to further increase life expectancy?

Your list would probably include:
- Improved sanitation, housing and social conditions
- Improved diet
- Prevention of disease by immunisation
- Advances in medical care

Improved social conditions apply to both the work and home environments. Working hours have been reduced, and changes in work practices arising from various Factories Acts and Health and Safety legislation designed to regulate and improve working conditions. Improved housing conditions have arisen because of a combination of legislative and technological improvements such as more efficient and effective central heating in houses, indoor toilets and bathrooms, and the control of building standards through building regulations. Together with less overcrowding in homes these have helped to reduce the incidence of infectious diseases such as tuberculosis. Water purification and sewage treatment standards and regulation have dramatically reduced the risk of acquiring a wide range of infectious diseases.

Medical advances cover all aspects of primary, secondary and tertiary prevention. Improved maternal care, immunisation and the availability of antibiotics have done much to reduce both perinatal mortality and deaths from pneumonia and other infectious diseases in older people.

Improvements in diet include the increased availability and variety of foods, increased purity of ingredients, and reduced spoilage from the use of processing and preservation methods such as canning and freezing.

Further improvement in life expectancy will be difficult. The medical improvements so far have largely been due to success in treating acute infectious diseases but the chronic diseases such as heart disease, dementia and cancer are much more intractable, difficult and costly to treat. However, technological improvements continue to be made, for example chemotherapy and radiotherapy for cancer, the introduction of screening for asymptomatic disease, angioplasty and coronary bypass treatments for CHD.

Much more can be done to prevent disease. The largest single cause of ill-health and premature death is smoking. Alcohol consumption is another leading cause of chronic disease, as well as causing accidental deaths.

There is a case for saying that some improvements have gone too far and can be detrimental to health and life expectancy. For example, highly processed convenience foods are often reduced in vitamin and fibre content, but are high in sugars and fats. These may contribute to heart disease as well as some cancers (see Chapter 7).

What actions can be taken to maximise the chance of enjoying a healthy old age? What are their limitations?

Question 3

We lack understanding of the basic processes underlying ageing and associated disabilities and diseases. For example, the basic genetics and molecular biology of dementia are only just beginning to be elucidated and at this stage the risk factors and the ways they can be modified are unknown.

The general strategy is to avoid risk factors, which are for the most part present within our general lifestyles as diet, exercise levels, alcohol consumption and tobacco use. These are not always easy to address because of the many psychological, social and economic reasons which underlie these behaviours. Further improvements in social support and employment conditions need to be made.

Most of the chronic diseases of older people are multifactorial in their causation, and the modification of only one risk factor may do little to arrest initiation or progress of the disease. Furthermore, most of these diseases are, to a greater or lesser extent, influenced by genetic traits that cannot be altered. There is also evidence to suggest that many of our predispositions to disease are determined very early in life, perhaps even during fetal development. It is obviously not possible to modify risks to which we have already been exposed.

Positive feelings towards older people could focus on their useful roles in the community:

Activity 1

- Through the years people accumulate a wealth of experience which can be passed on as 'wisdom' to the younger generation – in many societies older people are accorded great respect as 'elders' of the community

- Many older people remain active in the economic sense. For example, they take on part-time jobs to supplement their income, or voluntary and charitable work
- In the extended family grandparents assume many responsibilities for the welfare and development of children
- Old age can still be a time for personal development. In retirement there is more time to develop and participate in social networks; educational opportunities and exercise classes are still available.

Negative feelings about older people probably centre on associated disabilities and diseases:

- Older people can appear physically and mentally slow. For example, some cannot walk quickly and get in the way. Slight deafness may impede understanding of conversations. Some people become 'set in their ways' and are reluctant to accept new ideas and concepts: they appear unwilling or unable to adapt to the changes in attitudes and structures of contemporary society
- Some older people are perceived as doing nothing useful and as a drain on resources. They may require care either in the home or within an institution

Differences in activities centre around the changes in physical, social and economic circumstances, for example:

- The death of a spouse may severely restrict both the desire and opportunity for social activities
- People of an athletic disposition will find it more difficult to achieve the same results. This is not to say that exercise does not remain an enjoyable, and indeed desirable pastime for older people
- The loss of income on retirement may mean that social activities have to be curtailed. A person may not be able to afford to run a car, further limiting mobility and social opportunity. Physical disability in old age may mean that driving a car is no longer possible
- Many older people have difficulty with the simple daily activities that most younger people take for granted, such as getting out of bed, dressing, washing, cooking a meal and shopping

Activity 2

The checklist of questions might include the following (bear in mind that you may not be able to ask all the questions of a friend or relative because of their personal nature or for reasons of confidentiality).

Diet:

- Are there foods you would like to buy but feel you cannot afford?
- Is your appetite as good as it used to be?

Activities and exercise levels:

- Do you have trouble with strenuous activities, such as carrying a heavy bag or suitcase?
- Are you able to get out to the shops?
- Do you go for walks? Do you have difficulty taking a long walk?
- Do you have to stay in a chair or bed for most of the day?

- Do you need help with eating, dressing, washing yourself or using the toilet?
- Are you limited in the household jobs that you can do?
- Do you take any exercise such as playing golf, swimming?

Illness and disabilities:
- Do you easily get short of breath?
- Do you need to rest often?
- Do you have trouble reading?
- Do you have difficulty hearing?
- Do you have difficulty remembering things?
- Do you think you easily become confused? depressed?
- Do you have trouble sleeping?
- Do you need a stick or other aid for walking? Have you had any falls?
- Do you have problems with your feet?

Drug use:
- Do you take any tablets?
- If so, how many different types, how many times a day?
- Do you always remember to take your drugs? Do they make you feel unwell?
- Do you need to take something to help you sleep?
- Do you take tablets to help with depression?

Further reading

Brookbank, J.W. (1990) *The Biology of Ageing*, Harper & Row, New York.

Dix, D. (1989) The role of ageing in cancer incidence: an epidemiological study. *J. Gerontol.*, **44**, 10–18.

Ebersole, P. and Hess, B. (1994) *Toward Healthy Aging*, Mosby, St Louis.

Fall, C.H.D., Barker, D.J.P., Ostiond, C. *et al.* (1992) Relation of infant feeding to adult serum cholesterol concentration and death from ischaemic heart disease. *BMJ*, **304**, 801–5.

Finch, C.E. and Hayflick, L. (eds) (1977) *Handbook of the Biology of Ageing*, Van Nostrand Reinhold, New York.

MacLennan, W.J. (1988) The ageing society. *Br. J. Hosp. Med.*, 112–20.

Moment, G.B. (1978) in *The Biology of Aging* (eds J.A. Behnke, C.E. Finch and G.B. Moment), Plenum Press, New York.

Suzman, R.M., Willis, D.P. and Manton, K.G. (eds) (1992) *The Oldest Old*, Oxford University Press, New York.

Timiras, P.S. (1990) Alzheimer disease compared with normal ageing of the brain, in The Ageing Process (ed. M.C. Geokas), *Ann. Intern. Med.*, **113**, 455–66.

Zimmerman, J.A. and Carter, T.H. (1989) Altered cellular responses to chemical carcinogens in aged animals. *J. Gerontol.*, **44**, 19–24.

10   Principles of screening

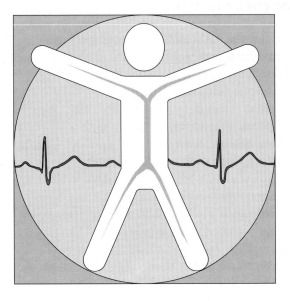

The detection and elimination of a life-threatening disease before an individual has even become aware of symptoms is an alluring prospect. By definition, screening requires the investigation of people without symptoms for latent disease or for risk factors that will probably result in disease. Most people who do not have any symptoms of disease are actually healthy, and screening for even common diseases necessitates the examination of many people for each person who is ultimately identified as having the disease. Hence there are substantial cost implications in performing tests that are 'wasted' on healthy people. In addition, people who believe themselves to be healthy may be very reluctant to be screened.

Screening tests therefore need to be non-invasive and cheap to apply and because of this screening tests often lack sensitivity and specificity; any suspicious results need to be investigated further. More seriously, lack of sensitivity means there will be false negatives and people may be falsely reassured. As most diseases can occur at any age, screening tests need to be repeated at regular intervals – a 'negative' screening result does not represent a lifelong clean bill of health.

When disease is detected in an asymptomatic individual treatments must be available that would give a better outcome than the normal treatment applied at the symptomatic stage of the disease. For some diseases treatment at an early stage not only improves the outcome by enabling a complete cure, but also ensures that the treatment itself is less extensive and has fewer associated complications. However, in some conditions the treatment at the asymptomatic stage is little different from that as the symptomatic disease, and the outcomes are much the same.

Pre-test

- **What is the purpose of screening?**
- **What disease conditions do you know about for which screening is carried out?**
- **Have you at any stage been screened for a disease or risk factor?**
- **Do you think it likely that you will be offered screening in the future?**

Aims of this chapter

By the end of this chapter you will have increased your knowledge of:
◆ The reasons for health care screening
◆ Principles governing the establishment of effective screening and
  surveillance programmes

In addition, this chapter will help you to:
◆ Discuss the rationale for screening and surveillance programmes
◆ Describe the ways in which screening programmes can be evaluated
◆ Assess the merits and disadvantages of screening programmes

Introduction

A variety of checks and screening tests are available in the UK that are designed
to monitor either the health status of the population as a whole or that of
individuals at various times. These include:
- Ultrasound monitoring of fetal growth
- Surveillance of growth and development in neonates and infants
- Health checks in schoolchildren
- Detection of specific diseases and risk factors in adults
- Assessment of functional ability in older people

These tests fall under two main categories, referred to as **surveillance** and
screening.

Surveillance measures usually comprise a number of health checks aimed
at anticipating future problems and preventing disease. Another aspect of
surveillance concerns the gathering of data on disease or risk factors in
populations rather than individuals. The information obtained may not directly
benefit the individuals concerned. Examples of this are studies to determine
the prevalence of a condition, such as HIV infection. Occasionally the spread
of HIV has been monitored by testing blood taken for other purposes, without
the individuals being identified and without their knowledge.

In a variant of this investigations are carried out to identify individuals
who pose a threat to the health of others, for example, the identification of
hepatitis B carriers. This should more properly be described as **testing**.

By contrast, screening is aimed more directly at benefiting the individual,
tests being designed to detect the presence of disease or a predisposition to
disease in individuals without specific symptoms. The screening process can
expose a need for treatment or other intervention in people who were probably
unaware of any problem.

Screening has been defined by Cuckle and Wald (1984) as:
the identification, among apparently healthy individuals, of those who are
sufficiently at risk of a specific disorder to justify a subsequent diagnostic test or
procedure, or in certain circumstances direct preventive action.

One advantage of screening asymptomatic people is that if disease is detected

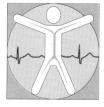

*Screening is designed to detect
the presence of disease or risk
factors in people without
symptoms*

> *Screening is intended to advance the time of diagnosis*

it will probably be at an earlier stage than would be the case if symptoms were produced (Figure 10.1). This should mean that any treatment is more efficient and effective. Some screening tests are designed to assess vulnerability to a particular disease (cholesterol testing as a predictor for heart disease for example). The screened person has the option to alter various lifestyle factors such as smoking, exercise and diet in order to reduce the risk of developing the disease.

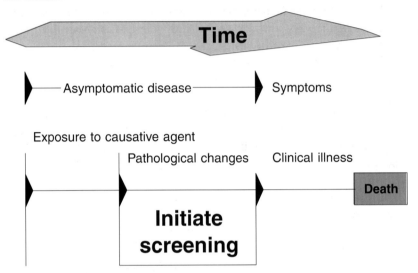

Figure 10.1 The progression of disease. In many diseases, pathological processes are under way in the cells and tissues for some years before symptoms develop. The aim of screening is to detect these changes and therefore advance the time of diagnosis. This should be accompanied by earlier and more effective treatment, thereby avoiding premature death.

Screening programmes will usually be divided into three distinct phases:

1. The **screen** itself: this involves the application of a test procedure which should be rapid and simple to apply, low cost, accurate, reliable and non-invasive
2. A **diagnostic** phase: any positive results or suspicious findings will usually need to be confirmed by more accurate diagnostic investigations. For example, the diagnosis of cancer or precancer usually involves obtaining a cell or tissue sample for cytological or histological evaluation. The diagnostic stage may also involve assessment of the degree of spread of the cancer (tumour staging) and determination of other prognostic factors.
3. A **treatment** phase: for curable cancers this usually involves some degree of surgical intervention, which may be supplemented by radiotherapy, chemotherapy or hormonal therapy.

Criteria for screening

Screening programmes are aimed at those diseases which are common and life-threatening, such as CHD and various types of cancer, or at those rarer diseases where the target population can be tightly controlled, as occurs in some genetic disorders. Successful screening programmes must satisfy a number of criteria, proposed by Wilson in 1965:

- It must be possible to detect the disease in asymptomatic people
- Once detected, treatments and resources must be available to do something about the disease
- It should be possible to initiate treatment at an earlier stage of the disease process and this should influence the outcome in terms of morbidity and mortality
- Ideally, treatment in an earlier stage of the disease should be much less damaging to the patient but at the same time have a far greater chance of cure
- The disease should be common and serious enough to warrant resources being spent on screening procedures – there is no point in having a screening programme for ingrowing toenails where there would be little impact on morbidity and none on mortality; this condition is adequately treated when symptoms arise. There would also be little economic point in screening large numbers of people for very rare diseases

In many instances it can be difficult to fulfil these criteria. Very often the only methods available for screening are exactly the same as the methods used for the diagnosis of disease in symptomatic patients. Sometimes these methods are highly invasive and can be associated with discomfort, pain or even more serious side-effects. For a symptomatic patient with a possibly life-threatening disease the advantages of arriving at the correct diagnosis, and hence the appropriate treatment, usually outweigh any possible hazards of the test.

Some screening programmes are let down by the detection methods available and reluctance of people to attend

As far as the person who attends screening is concerned, there are no symptoms and therefore every reason to believe that nothing is wrong: indeed, in the large majority of people who attend screening there is nothing wrong. Understandably, people are less willing to submit to invasive procedures unless clear and substantial benefits can be demonstrated. The problem is that non-invasive tests often have a poor information yield (Figure 10.2) and lack sensitivity and specificity. The general screening principle is to use the least invasive test possible without producing too many false-positive or false-negative results, and then to refer the positive cases on to a diagnostic phase in which more reliable, but probably more invasive, tests are used.

Screening tests

The requirements of a screening test are that it should be non-invasive, quick to perform and inexpensive compared with a 'gold standard' diagnostic test. At the same time, there are circumstances in which the inferior screening test is expected to give better performance than the diagnostic test – for example in the detection of cancers where an asymptomatic tumour will commonly be smaller than those usually diagnosed in people with symptoms. Clearly, this is asking too much, and inevitably sensitivity and specificity are lost.

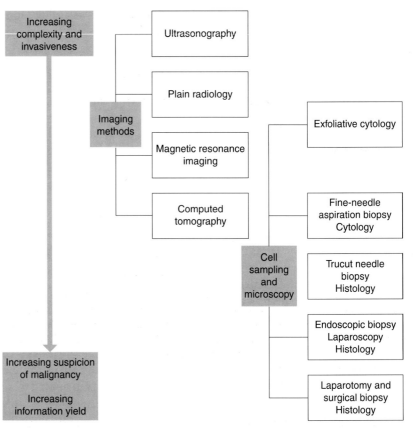

Figure 10.2 Investigations for cancer. Investigative procedures differ in their degree of invasiveness and information yield. The 'gold standard' test for the identification of cancer is based on the microscopic examination of cells. Unless the cells are on the surface, or are exfoliated into accessible body cavities, cell sampling is an invasive procedure unsuitable for screening purposes. Imaging methods are not usually physically invasive (there may be radiation risks) but the information yield is relatively poor. The exceptions are computed tomography and magnetic resonance imaging but these are specialist and expensive procedures more suited to cancer staging.

Test sensitivity and specificity

The sensitivity of a test is its ability to pick out all the people with the disease

Tests for cancers usually depend on visualisation of the tumour mass by some means, or estimation of proteins produced by the tumour which find their way into blood or other body fluids (tumour markers). Naturally, the smaller the tumour the more difficult it will be to visualise and the less likely it is to produce any marker in measurable quantities. In other words, the tests may not be sufficiently sensitive to detect tumours in their early stages. As a consequence, a test with poor sensitivity will produce **false-negative** results (Figure 10.3). Some of these undetected tumours, if slow-growing, will be picked up in the next screening round but a proportion of undetected tumours will be more aggressive and will cause symptoms before the next screening round. These cases, arising in the interval between screening, are known as **interval** cases.

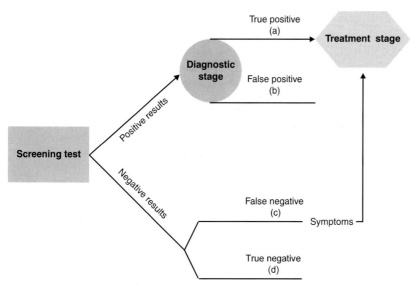

Figure 10.3 Outcomes of screening. A non-invasive test used for screening purposes may lack sensitivity and specificity compared with the more invasive 'gold standard' diagnostic tests. All positive results will be referred to a diagnostic stage in which a proportion is inevitably revealed as falsely positive (b) because of a lack of specificity. Conversely, a screening test with poor sensitivity will place some positive cases in the negative category (c). These false negatives will ultimately be revealed at the next screening round or when symptomatic disease develops.

Specificity refers to the ability of the test to identify all the people without disease, thereby avoiding their misclassification – a test with poor specificity produces **false-positive** results. The sensitivity and specificity of a particular test may be adjustable, but these are inextricably linked; an increase in one parameter will be offset by a decrease in the other. As an analogy, anyone who has ever bought a cheap radio will know that as the volume is turned up (to increase sensitivity) the sound becomes fuzzier (decreased specificity).

The sensitivity and specificity of a particular test can be calculated when the numbers of true positives and negatives become known:

A specific test does not misclassify people without disease as sufferers

	Disease truly present	Disease truly absent	
Test positive	a	b	a + b
Test negative	c	d	c + d
	a + c	b + d	

a = True positives; b = false positives; c = false negatives; d = true negatives

$$\text{Sensitivity} = \frac{a}{a + c} \qquad \text{Specificity} = \frac{d}{b + d}$$

▲ **Key points**

Sensitivity and specificity

▲ Sensitivity: ability of a test to correctly identify people with disease

▲ A test with 100% sensitivity yields no false-negative results

▲ Specificity: ability of a test to correctly identify non-diseased people in the population

▲ A test with 100% specificity yields no false-positive results

Sometimes tests are quoted in terms of their **predictive value**. The predictive value of a positive result (called the **positive predictive value**) reflects the probability that the result corresponds to someone who actually has the disease. It is influenced by test sensitivity and specificity and the frequency of the disease: given reasonable sensitivity and specificity the chances of getting it right increase if there are more positive cases in the test population anyway. The positive predictive value is calculated by dividing the number of true positives by the sum of true and false positives:

$$\text{Positive predictive value} = \frac{a}{a + b}$$

The predictive value of a negative test result (the **negative predictive value**) reflects the probability that the result corresponds to someone who does not have the disease. It is calculated by dividing the true negative figure by the sum of true and false negatives:

$$\text{Negative predictive value} = \frac{d}{c + d}$$

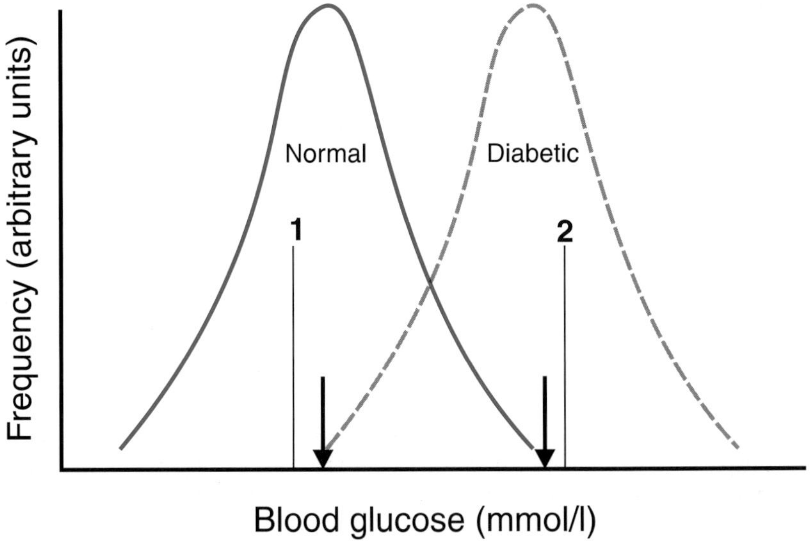

Figure 10.4 Effect of cut-off values on test sensitivity and specificity. In this example there is a cross-over in blood glucose values for normal and diabetic subjects so that anyone with a value between the arrows could be either normal or diabetic. A low cut-off value (1) will guarantee that all subjects who have glucose values below this value (to the left of line 1) are normal. However, there will also be normals to the right who will be misclassified as false positives – the test lacks specificity. A high cut-off value (2) will ensure that all those subjects above that value are classed as diabetic but some diabetics (on the left of line 2) will be misclassified as negatives – the test lacks sensitivity.

Some tests are either positive or negative – for example the cytological examination of a cervical smear can show either precancerous changes or normal cells. In contrast many other tests produce a continuum of values into which 'normal' and 'abnormal' fall. This is a characteristic of many biochemical and haematological tests, for which there is a **normal range**. Very often there will be an overlap between the normal and abnormal ranges, and hence the definition of a positive or negative test result depends on the cut-off value chosen. The cut-off value chosen will therefore affect the sensitivity and specificity of the test (Figures 10.4 and 10.5).

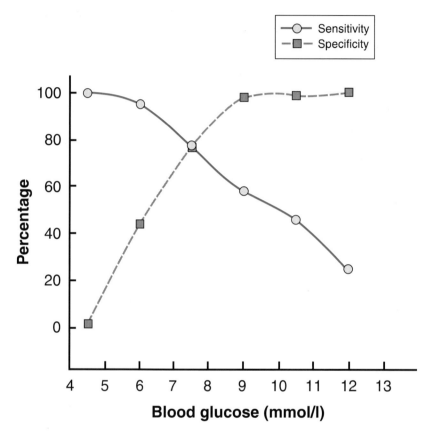

Figure 10.5 Sensitivity and specificity of a blood glucose test for diabetes. In this example, a cut-off value of 9.0 mmol/l in a blood glucose test for diabetes would be almost 100% specific, but only 58% sensitive (some people with diabetes would not be recognised).

Blood glucose (mmol/l)	Sensitivity (%)	Specificity (%)
4.5	100	1
6.0	95	44
7.5	77	77
9.0	58	99
10.5	46	100
12.0	24	100

Treatment of screen-detected disease

Treatments that would markedly improve the outlook for the patient must be available

It is also necessary to consider the treatment aspects of the disease. For screening to be effective, the programme must offer treatment in the asymptomatic stage of the disease which is better than the treatment necessary for symptomatic disease. With some diseases (cervical cancer, for example) the treatments available for the early phases of the disease are far less severe than those necessary to treat the later symptomatic stages, and result in very much higher cure rates. The patient will therefore avoid morbidity from the side-effects of treatment as well as morbidity (and mortality) related to the disease itself (Figure 10.6).

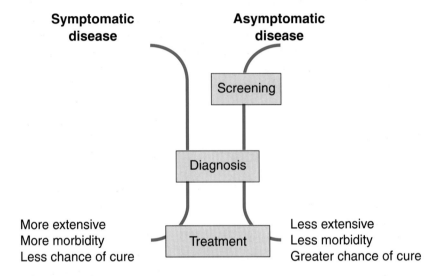

Figure 10.6 Outcomes of screening. The treatment of screen-detected disease should be less extensive than that required for symptomatic disease and have fewer side-effects. The chances of treatment success should be greater for diseases detected at an earlier stage.

With other diseases (prostate cancer, for example) the treatments available are very similar for both the asymptomatic and the symptomatic stages of the disease. These treatments can be debilitating and, although this would clearly represent a worthwhile trade-off in someone with invasive cancer, it might be more difficult to convince someone with asymptomatic disease of the necessity for extensive treatment. The picture is further complicated because the biology of some early-detected lesions in prostate cancer is uncertain: in some men prostate cancer grows so slowly that it is never life-threatening and therefore any treatment given would be unnecessary. It is therefore essential to understand the natural history of the disease and the stages at which interventions would be of most benefit.

Goals of screening

Screening is aimed at the earlier detection of life-threatening disease in asymptomatic people. The logical outcome measure for evaluating such a screening programme would be death from the disease. In practice, screening programmes differ in their ability to reduce mortality. For example, in cervical screening a clearly defined precancerous stage can be identified, and intervention at this stage is very effective in preventing progression to malignancy. The outcome of the screening programme, if it reaches the target population and the results are acted on, would be a substantial reduction in the disease-specific death rate. In contrast, with other types of cancers a clearly defined precancerous stage may not be identifiable and thus the screening test will detect only active cancer. Although the screen-detected cancer is much more likely to be at an earlier stage in its natural history, with more favourable treatment options and prognosis, such a screening programme cannot be expected to be as effective as detection and treatment of a precancerous condition.

> *The main goal of screening should be to reduce deaths from the disease*

The natural time-course of some life-threatening diseases can be very long, and it may take many years before a positive effect is seen in terms of reducing the number of deaths from the disease. As a consequence, alternative or **surrogate** measures are often used to check if the programme is working. These include:

- Assessment of the average survival time after detection and treatment
- Assessment of the severity of the disease at the time of detection
- Measurement of interval disease rates

These secondary measures can be misleading. In cancer screening the average survival times of the screened population will be influenced by **lead-time** and **length-time** bias, with the effect that the screening programme appears to be working much more effectively than it actually is. Similarly, although it is possible to compare the severity of the disease in screened and unscreened groups, this may not always translate into differences in survival. For example, detection of smaller breast lumps by mammographic screening does not necessarily mean that a woman will live longer. However, a screening programme does have some impact on the incidence of symptomatic disease, and this can be measured as interval disease fairly soon after its inception.

Lead-time bias

Screening should bring forward the time at which a diagnosis is made (lead time). The presence of disease will therefore be known for a longer period of time and survival rates (measured from the time of diagnosis) will inevitably be improved. There is therefore an inherent bias in evaluating the treatment of screen-detected disease – some of the apparent benefit may well result from earlier treatment, but some will be a result of prolonged awareness of the disease. This bias is referred to as lead-time bias.

> *Survival rates measured from the time of diagnosis will automatically be better in screened patients*

Length-time bias

Length-time bias is a common problem in cancer screening. The screen-detected cancers, because they are found in people without symptoms, are more likely to be slower-growing tumours of longer duration. Many of the more aggressive tumours will rapidly produce symptoms and cause the patient to seek immediate medical attention, outside the screening programme. The effect, therefore, will be that screening appears to increase survival rates, even though many of these slower-growing tumours might never do the patient any harm and, without screening, would have remained undetected.

Monitoring screening programmes

It is desirable that new screening programmes should be evaluated by randomised trials before they are implemented: a population cohort should be identified and randomised into a screening group, while a control group of similar size and characteristics is left unscreened. In the case of cervical screening the benefits were believed to be so substantial that programmes were introduced, albeit haphazardly, on a wide scale before proper randomised trials were evaluated. The benefits of breast cancer screening are not so obvious and several randomised controlled trials were set up although the political and social climate in the UK favoured the introduction of breast screening on a national scale before the trial results were fully known.

Established health screening programmes must be monitored to ensure that the benefits achieved are consistent with those obtained in previous randomised trials or demonstration projects. The factors that influence the effectiveness of a screening programme include proper targeting of the population, compliance (attendance) rates and the sensitivity and specificity of the test. The ultimate outcome measure is death from the disease, but in the short term other (less accurate) outcome measures can be applied.

Opportunistic and formal screening

There are two main processes in which individuals are recruited into screening programmes: first, a subgroup of the population at risk from the disease under study is identified, and individuals from that population are invited to attend a screening session by letter; secondly, the screening process can be undertaken opportunistically. In practice this means that when a patient attends a surgery or clinic for some other reason he or she is informed of the availability of the screening test and invited to participate. Opportunistic screening has the advantage of being cheap to administer and may reach a section of the population who would not attend a clinic for preventive advice alone. However, its main disadvantage is that it cannot offer 100% coverage of the target population.

With formal call–recall screening a comprehensive coverage of the target population can be planned. Usually letters are sent out with explanatory leaflets about the screening programme. This gives the participants more time to understand and act on the advice given. However, these screening programmes need to be highly organised, and problems occur when eligible people cannot be contacted, particularly in the large cities where the population is more mobile, and when people do not respond to the invitations.

Call–recall screening is more effective in reaching the target population

Costs of screening

Costs to the provider

Some screening programmes involve millions of people – for example in the UK nearly 5 million women are eligible for breast screening. The financial costs and human resources are tied up at all levels of the screening programme, from provision of computerised call–recall systems to employment and training of health professionals to carry out and analyse the tests and provide explanations or counselling when the results are known. It will also be necessary to monitor the effect of the programme on the quality and quantity of life of its participants. Sometimes the costs can be partly offset by savings made in initiating more conservative treatments but overall costs will be increased owing to the lengthier observation time of the disease and of any follow-up procedures. The imbalance of the far greater numbers of people who are screened and those that need treatment usually ensures that screening programmes are fairly costly ventures.

Mass screening programmes have extremely high cost implications

Review question 1

Give reasons why screening could be expected to reduce morbidity and mortality from a disease

Costs to the individual

By their very nature screening programmes are aimed at detecting life-threatening diseases. Unless proper measures are taken to explain the purposes of the programme an invitee may believe that something ominous is already known about his or her health status, which is the reason for the invitation. Anxiety can be induced by inadequate explanation of what the test is designed to do, and what it will and will not detect.

Once a person submits to screening his or her status changes from that of an asymptomatic 'healthy' individual to that of a patient. This may be reinforced by the attitudes of the health care professionals involved in the test and in informing the 'patient' of the result. The outcomes of some screening tests can have profound effects on an individual's way of life. For example, someone found to be HIV positive may find that they can no longer obtain life assurance and mortgage loans, and the attitudes of friends and colleagues at work may change so that he or she can no longer sustain normal social relationships or even remain in employment.

It is also possible that people may be falsely reassured by a negative screening test. With breast cancers the incidence of interval cancers can be quite high and a woman who is 'cleared' by a mammographic test could none the less

Attending a screening session is an anxious time in a person's life

Review question 2

How can the treatment of screen-detected disease actually represent over-treatment?

have breast cancer in its early and undetectable stages. In such a situation the cancer is likely to become symptomatic before the next screening appointment is due. It is also not unknown for a person to be informed of a positive test result and subsequently to be found not to have the disease. In this situation reassurance may not be enough and the anxieties produced on first hearing the positive test result can persist for many years.

Practical problems of mass screening

Some screening may not work because the criteria have not been fulfilled: for example, the technology available is not good enough to detect disease at an earlier stage, or earlier treatments may make no impact on survival. One example of this was the British mass screening programme for tuberculosis and lung cancer, which relied on chest radiography. There was initially much optimism about the chances of improving survival from lung cancer by earlier surgery in the screened population. However, it took 10 years for sufficient data to become available to demonstrate that the cumulative mortality from lung cancer was the same in both the control and screened populations.

Even when screening has been shown to work in demonstration projects, a programme can fail when applied on a large scale. The impact of formal mass screening programmes depends on achieving maximum compliance, which depends on precise identification of the target population for screening and follow-up. A programme will be undermined if the population registers are poorly maintained and updated. This is often the situation in inner-city areas where the population tends to be relatively mobile.

Even when invitations for screening reach the right people at the right time, individuals may choose not to attend. There is often a predominance of the better-educated or the 'worried well' in attenders, which can bias the results and effectiveness of the screening programme because those most in need of a screening service are often from the lower socioeconomic groups who tend to have more lifestyle risk factors.

Rigorous quality control is needed in performing and validating the test. For example, cervical screening can fail because of inadequate training of the smear-takers, the smears may have inadequate numbers of cells for analysis, may have been taken from the wrong site or may be poorly preserved. The staff in the laboratory where the smear analysis is to be performed must be highly trained and must follow established internal and external quality control protocols so that the results may be monitored.

All aspects of the screening programme, from the call–recall systems to the testing, intervention and follow-up procedures, must be closely audited. Performance comparisons must be made with other equivalent programmes. Morbidity and mortality data for the disease must be collected and compared with data obtained before the programme was implemented, in the non-attenders, and with comparable unscreened populations elsewhere. This will allow strategic planning for the future of the screening programme.

ANSWERS TO REVIEW QUESTIONS

Question 1

Give reasons why screening could be expected to reduce morbidity and mortality from a disease

Screening is meant to advance the time of diagnosis by the detection of asymptomatic disease, so that treatment can be given earlier. One problem concerns the sensitivity of the methods available for detection: by the time a disease can be shown to be present it may be too late for early treatment to make any significant difference to the outcome.

A further aim of screening is to prevent a disease arising. Most notably this can be achieved by screening for risk factors, on which the development of the disease depends. A problem is that few common diseases are directly caused by a single, or even a few, risk factors. Cholesterol screening is used to assess the risk of CHD but, because the disease has multiple risk factors, screening for cholesterol alone has a poor predictive value.

Question 2

How can the treatment of screen-detected disease actually represent over-treatment?

This question is related to what we know about the biology of disease. In some people a disease (for example prostate cancer) can behave very aggressively, producing symptoms and ultimately cause death. In other individuals the same kind of disease does no harm and may not even cause symptoms. There may be no reliable methods for differentiating between these two states, which means that people with the harmless form of disease will also be treated by a possibly radical treatment that will markedly affect quality of life.

References

Cuckle, H.S. and Wald, N.J. (1984) Principles of screening, in *Antenatal and Neonatal Screening* (ed. N.J. Wald), Oxford University Press, Oxford.

Further reading

Mant, D. and Fowler, G. (1990) Mass screening: theory and ethics. *BMJ*, **300**, 916–18.

Marteau, T.M. (1990) Screening in practice: reducing the psychological costs. *BMJ*, **301**, 26–28.

Miller, A., Chamberlain, J. and Day, N. (eds) (1991) *Cancer Screening*, Cambridge University Press, Cambridge.

Wilkinson, C., Jones, J.M. and McBride (1990) Anxiety caused by abnormal result of cervical smear test. *BMJ*, **300**, 440

Wilson, J.M.G. (1966) Some principles of early diagnosis and detection, in *Proceedings of a Colloquium*, Magdalen College, Oxford, July 1965 (ed. G. Teeling-Smith), Office of Health Economics, London.

11   Cohort screening and surveillance

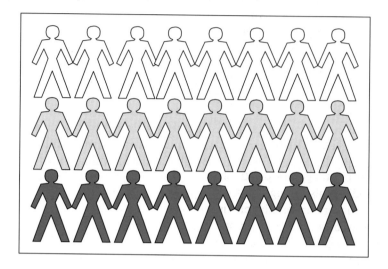

Screening and surveillance can begin before a person is born and continue to old age. The intention throughout is to prevent disease or minimise its effects.

Screening involves the application of investigative procedures, designed to detect disease before symptoms develop, to selected cohorts of the population thought to be at particular risk, such as pregnant mothers, older people, those with a family history of a disorder or certain racial subgroups.

Surveillance is more about careful observation with a view to implementing preventive measures or detecting symptoms of disease as soon as they appear. In this way treatment or support can be given early to lessen the impact of disease.

A further role of screening and surveillance is in health promotion, by ascertaining who is at risk and encouraging appropriate lifestyle changes.

Aims of this chapter

By the end of this chapter you will have increased your knowledge of:
◆ The application of screening and surveillance programmes in various population cohorts such as expectant mothers, neonates and older people

In addition, this chapter will help you to:
◆ Describe the technologies available for the screening and surveillance of defined population groups
◆ Evaluate the usefulness of screening and surveillance programmes in defined population groups

Introduction

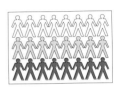

In the UK the general practitioners' contract provides for regular health checks of individuals throughout their lives. This extends the role of the general practitioner from reactive provision of general medical services towards disease prevention and health promotion – the family doctor has a **surveillance** role. In this context 'surveillance' refers to an ongoing process which includes preventive and anticipatory measures that go beyond identifying and treating disease.

> *Health checks aimed at reducing disease morbidity and mortality can be carried out throughout a person's life*

Surveillance and screening measures are generally carried out in selected population cohorts considered vulnerable, such as preschool children or older people. Surveillance usually involves a home visit by the practice nurse or an invitation to attend for a consultation if the person has not visited the surgery for some time. In addition, 'well-man' and 'well-woman' clinics are often set up for the remaining population. Pregnant women are subject to a range of interviews, physical examinations and tests in the practice or hospital clinic situations.

> *Surveillance is a monitoring process that anticipates the need for intervention*

Screening, particularly genetic screening, raises a number of ethical issues. In pregnancy, screening for untreatable fetal abnormalities implies that an abortion will be offered when positive results are found. Occasionally the inherent lack of specificity of some screening and diagnostic tests means that some false-positive and false-negative results will be obtained.

Health promotion: a process of enabling people to improve their health by increasing their awareness and control.

It is now becoming possible to screen for genetic abnormalities that become evident only in later life. The symptoms of Huntington's disease (see Chapter 3) usually become evident at 40–50 years of age. Should a fetus with the condition be aborted? Will a young adult wish to know that he or she has the condition and may pass it on their own offspring? It is likely that this conundrum will soon be extended for a range of more common conditions, such as Alzheimer's disease and familial hypercholesterolaemia.

Screening itself is often a traumatic event, if not physically then certainly emotionally. Considerable anxiety and depression may be experienced while waiting for the results of screening and diagnostic tests. A 'positive' result, particularly after fetal screening and diagnosis, may then mean that a 'life or death' decision will have to be made. Consequently, no screening should be contemplated unless properly trained counsellors are available to give advice.

The counsellor should have a good understanding of the clinical outcomes of the various disorders and the investigative procedures necessary to confirm the diagnosis. Information should be provided about the prognosis and the options available and should include an evaluation of the risks inherent in the diagnostic and treatment procedures and the possibilities for misdiagnosis.

Screening before conception and birth

The main purpose of screening before and during pregnancy is to reduce the incidence of congenital malformations, either by preventive measures (if they are available) or by the termination of an affected pregnancy. The priorities are to establish

- Family history of the prospective parents
- Presence of current or previous infections with organisms that can cause congenital abnormalities
- Presence of any other maternal medical condition which could influence the outcome of the pregnancy

Ideally, all of the above should be established before the woman becomes pregnant. However, many women do not present themselves for medical attention and advice until after they become pregnant.

The family history is of prime importance in establishing the risk of inherited genetic abnormalities. However, not all genetic disorders are inherited and other risk factors need to be considered. For example, maternal age is an important risk factor for Down's syndrome (Table 11.1) and other disorders involving alterations in the number of chromosomes (aneuploidy). If there is a history of genetic abnormalities genetic counselling can be arranged so that the parents can make an informed decision about prevention or termination of pregnancy. Pregnant women who are over the age of 35 may be offered amniocentesis or chorionic villus sampling to identify fetal genetic abnormalities. All women should receive nutritional supplementation with folic acid if they intend to become pregnant, especially those who have a previous history of neural tube defects.

Some infective agents (rubella, for example) affect fetal development. If the woman has had a previous infection and has detectable antibodies against the agent then the risk of reinfection and transfer to the fetus is much reduced: alternatively, appropriate immunisation can be offered. The diagnosis of infection during pregnancy can influence the choice of how the baby is to be delivered. Caesarean section may be preferred if there is a possibility that infection can be acquired by the baby in the birth canal (for example in a mother with herpes simplex virus).

The most common maternal medical condition that could adversely affect the outcome of pregnancy is diabetes mellitus. Without proper management the risk of pregnancy loss is increased, as is the likelihood of congenital malformations such as heart defects, central nervous system defects (anencephaly, spina bifida and hydrocephalus), and defects of the renal system.

The risk of congenital malformations is often determined by conditions which existed before the woman became pregnant

Congenital malformation: a condition present at birth. Abnormalities most often involve the heart and circulatory system, central nervous system and renal system.

Anencephaly: most of the brain and skull are absent, causing stillbirth or neonatal death.

Hydrocephalus: excess fluid in the brain causing raised intracranial pressure. Maintenance of cerebral function depends on the degree and duration of the hydrocephalus and can be compatible with normal development and intelligence. In some cases the build-up of pressure stops spontaneously but if it does not the pressure can be relieved by surgical implantation of a bypass valve.

Table 11.1 Risk of live birth aneuploidy with maternal age

Maternal age (years)	Risk at live birth	
	Down's syndrome	**Any aneuploidy**
30	1 in 950	1 in 385
32	1 in 770	1 in 315
34	1 in 500	1 in 205
36	1 in 300	1 in 130
38	1 in 175	1 in 80
40	1 in 105	1 in 50

Adapted from Hook, EB (1981) *Obstet Gynecol*, **58**, 282; and Hook EB *et al.* (1983) *JAMA*, **249**, 2043.

Genetic screening

Screening for genetic and congenital disorders has several purposes (see Chapter 3). If carried out before pregnancy it may allow a decision to be made to avoid a high-risk pregnancy. In contrast couples who, because of their family history, had been reluctant to start a family might be reassured by a negative screening result. Screening in early pregnancy gives advance warning that the child will be handicapped, providing the option of termination or allowing advance preparation and optimal management of delivery and postnatal care.

With improved medical care, women who have an autosomal recessive genetic disorder (for example, cystic fibrosis, sickle-cell anaemia, phenylketonuria) often reach reproductive age and may wish to start their own families. Provided that the male partner is not a carrier of the recessive disorder, all the offspring will be carriers and completely unaffected by the disease. However, if the man is a carrier there is a 50% chance that the child will be affected (see Chapter 21) and therefore his genetic status should also be ascertained if possible.

Genetic screening can be carried out in many ways:

- Screening of the entire population at risk, for example all newborn babies for phenylketonuria
- Carrier screening of high-risk subgroups within the population, such as particular ethnic groups (Table 11.2)
- Screening for carriers or asymptomatic disease in high-risk families (for example cystic fibrosis or Huntington's disease)

These screening strategies can be used to detect people who have a genetic disorder but which has not yet become apparent, and people who are carriers of a disorder and are themselves disease-free but who could have an affected child if their partner is also a carrier.

Screening for genetic disorders can be carried out on the prospective parents, the fetus and the newborn baby. The potential for effective intervention is greater the earlier that screening is carried out. Ideally, a woman should be screened before conception but this is not likely to happen unless she has a family history of an inherited disorder. For the information to be useful, her partner should also be screened for carrier status.

Table 11.2 Carrier screening of high-risk population subgroups

Genetic disorder	Population at risk	Screening method
Sickle-cell anaemia	African Americans	Haemoglobin electrophoresis, DNA analysis for haemoglobin S gene
Tay-Sachs disease	Ashkenazi Jews	DNA analysis
β-Thalassaemia	Italians, Greeks, Mediterranean French	Haemoglobin electrophoresis
Cystic fibrosis	Northern European	Direct gene analysis of most common mutations (not routine in the UK); direct gene analysis of previously identified mutations in other family members

The metabolic changes inherent in some genetic disorders can be detected by biochemical tests

The types of test used in screening vary according to the condition sought. **Biochemical tests** evaluate the phenotypic expression of the genetic disorder (for example the absence of a particular protein or excessive production of precursor metabolites). As such, biochemical tests are not capable of distinguishing the phenotypically normal carriers of a genetic disorder. They are usually rapid and cheap to administer but can give misleading results because the phenotypic marker may not be produced in sufficient quantities to measure accurately, or production of the marker may be altered in a range of other conditions. Consequently, biochemical tests are often used as a primary screening method, positive results being followed by more definitive diagnostic tests.

Genetic tests can detect gene abnormalities in both affected people and carriers

Cytogenetic screening is used to detect chromosomal abnormalities such as changes in chromosome number (aneuploidy) or the inappropriate transfer of genetic information from one chromosome to another (translocations). **Genetic** methods probe for the gene abnormality itself (or related genetic sequences, see Chapter 3). In recessive disorders a gene abnormality can be detected in carriers who are not themselves affected by the disorder. Once an abnormality is detected there is no need for any further testing by other methods. Some genetic disorders are the result of a number of possible mutations and it is not possible to test for them all. Because of this, there is a slight risk (in cystic fibrosis, for example) that a negative test result could conceal a true positive.

Maternal screening and surveillance

Correction of metabolic imbalance (diabetes, for example) and prompt recognition and treatment of some infections (Table 11.3) can markedly affect the outcome of pregnancy and the frequency of congenital malformations. Unfortunately, in some circumstances maternal screening allows only the early detection of congenital malformations, for which the possible outcomes are a handicapped child, stillbirth or elective termination. Sometimes it is only possible to provide an estimate of the risk that the fetus is affected, rather than a definitive diagnosis. Attendance at an antenatal clinic also provides an opportunity to 'catch-up' on cervical screening if the woman has not had a recent smear taken.

> *The aim of maternal screening and surveillance is to ensure the health of the mother and fetus*

Surveillance measures include assessment of the mother's nutrition, alcohol consumption and smoking habits. Well-nourished mothers are most likely to produce healthy well-grown babies, and most mothers will need to increase their consumption of protein and other nutrients (see Chapter 7). Smoking has a major impact on pregnancy because it reduces placental blood flow and thus retards fetal growth. Babies who are small for their gestational age are at increased risk of perinatal death.

Alcohol consumption during pregnancy is also associated with fetal growth retardation and a small increase in congenital heart malformations. Virtually all addictive drugs (drugs of abuse), whether legally prescribed or not, have adverse effects on the fetus. The effects range from growth retardation, congenital malformations, addiction of the newborn baby to fetal or neonatal death.

On confirmation of the pregnancy a variety of screening tests will usually be performed on blood and urine samples. A full blood count should be made to exclude anaemia. The most common reason for anaemia in pregnancy is iron or folate deficiency because of the increased burden of the growing fetus. Urine is tested for the presence of protein, blood, and glucose, to exclude diabetes or nephropathy (see Chapter 23), and to detect any urinary tract infections which are common but often asymptomatic in pregnant women.

Diabetes mellitus

With proper recognition and management the risks of a poor pregnancy outcome in diabetic women are not substantially different from women who do not have diabetes. In many cases the diabetes is already known, but screening of blood and urine is designed to detect undiagnosed cases. In addition, glucose intolerance may develop during pregnancy. This condition, known as **gestational diabetes**, improves after delivery but predisposes for non-insulin-dependent diabetes in later life. It carries pregnancy-associated problems

> *Poorly managed diabetes is associated with an increased risk of stillbirth or congenital abnormalities*

Table 11.3 Maternal infections affecting the fetus and neonate

Infection	Effect on fetus or neonate	Intervention
Toxoplasmosis	Spontaneous abortion, CNS developmental abnormalities: mental retardation, epilepsy, spasticity. Organism does not always pass across placenta and less than 50% of fetuses become infected. Complications are most severe when infection occurs in first trimester	Termination
Rubella	Heart malformations, eye lesions, mental retardation and deafness. Chance of fetal infection 90% in first trimester, risk diminishes thereafter	Termination
Cytomegalovirus	Spontaneous abortion, CNS abnormalities, mental retardation, hepatitis. Affects fetus in about 40% of infections during pregnancy, but 90% of infected infants develop normally	Termination
Herpes simplex	Intrauterine infection can cause CNS defects. Infections acquired during vaginal delivery may be localised to skin or mucous membranes but can be fatal after general spread	Congenital malformation is rare. Avoid vaginal delivery; specific antiviral therapy of infected baby should start immediately, but brain damage is still likely
Human immunodeficiency virus	AIDS (although this is not inevitable)	AZT taken in pregnancy can prevent vertical transmission
Hepatitis B virus	Acute or chronic hepatitis, liver cirrhosis	Risk of complications reduced by immunisation soon after birth
Group B *Streptococcus*	Septicaemia, pneumonia	Antibiotic therapy Avoid vaginal delivery
Gonorrhoea	Severe conjunctivitis	Antibiotic therapy
Syphilis	Stillbirth, skin lesions. Late disease similar to that in adults	Antibiotic therapy
Candida albicans (thrush)	Infections of mouth and gastrointestinal tract acquired during vaginal delivery	Antibiotic therapy

similar to those of pre-existing diabetes. The condition can be controlled by diet but most women require insulin during their pregnancy. Oral hypoglycaemic agents are inappropriate because they cross the placenta. Ultrasound is used to detect any fetal anomalies during the pregnancy.

Pre-eclampsia (pregnancy-induced hypertension)

Protein in the urine may also signify pregnancy-induced hypertension in the second and third trimesters. The condition is defined as the onset of sustained diastolic blood pressure above 90 mmHg, and its severity correlates with the amount of protein in the urine. Pre-eclampsia occurs in about 10% of all pregnant women in the UK. Baseline blood pressure levels are measured on the initial visit to the antenatal clinic and at every visit thereafter.

There are risks to both the mother and fetus. In most cases little or no serious harm is done, but the condition can cause growth failure or even death of the fetus. The condition is managed by bed rest in hospital and careful monitoring for signs of maternal renal or liver function impairment, together with ultrasound monitoring of the fetal heart and circulation.

Left untreated, pre-eclampsia can develop into eclampsia, a condition characterised by severe headache, a rapid rise in blood pressure, shock and fits. This is accompanied by disseminated intravascular coagulation (Chapter 6) leading to infarcts in vital organs and can be fatal. Surveillance and management of pre-eclampsia have ensured that eclampsia is now a very rare complication of pregnancy in the UK.

Pre-eclampsia: a syndrome of increased blood pressure, protein in the urine and peripheral oedema. A reduction in placental blood flow predisposes to fetal hypoxia in late pregnancy, especially during labour, increasing the risk of perinatal mortality. Fetal growth may be retarded, and the baby has a low birthweight. The condition is more likely in women who are over the age of 35 at a first pregnancy, have diabetes, a multiple pregnancy, or rhesus isoimmunisation.

Infections in pregnancy

Many infections that can cause serious malformations in the fetus or illness in the newborn are asymptomatic in the mother but are detectable by screening. Although screening for rubella and syphilis is routine in the UK, screening for other maternal infections is usually carried out only if the woman is at risk or is suspected of having an infection.

Maternal infections can affect the fetus or may be acquired by the baby during or after delivery

Vaginal infections

Vaginal swabs are taken towards the end of the pregnancy if there is reason to suspect infection (usually if the woman complains of vaginal discharge). Treatment will then be given before the onset of labour in order to reduce the risk of infection to the baby in the birth canal. Vaginal swabs may also be taken if a group B *Streptococcus* has previously been cultured from the vagina. If these organisms are present the baby could develop streptococcal septicaemia and so should be screened for bacteria and given prompt antibiotic therapy if the cultures are positive or if fever develops. Primary genital herpes may also be detected by taking vaginal swabs; the management of this condition in pregnancy is contentious because the chances of intrauterine infection or infection during delivery are low, although the consequences of infection can be serious.

Other maternal infections that can cause problems for the neonate include HIV, hepatitis B virus and gonorrhoea. Screening of pregnant women for HIV is currently carried out anonymously and the results are not made known to the mother or her carers. In women known to be HIV-positive, therapy with zidovudine (AZT) during pregnancy reduces the risk of viral transmission to the fetus. Although gonorrhoea is often asymptomatic in women the condition is not routinely screened for in the UK. Infection in the baby causes a severe conjunctivitis which if left untreated leads to blindness. This condition is easily recognised and treated with local and systemic antibiotics. Hepatitis B infection can cause acute hepatitis or may be completely asymptomatic. Infection is more common in intravenous drug users and in women who have had multiple sexual partners. The virus can be transmitted to the baby at birth or later on through infected blood and body secretions. A chronic asymptomatic carrier state develops in most infants but development of acute hepatitis can be fatal, although this is rare. Babies of known carriers should be immunised soon after birth. Without immunisation there is a risk that they could develop chronic hepatitis or liver cirrhosis in later childhood. In the UK, screening for hepatitis B infection is carried out in high-risk women.

Infections causing congenital malformation

Some maternal infections cross the placenta and cause developmental abnormalities in the fetus. Their impact is generally most severe when the infection occurs in the first trimester of pregnancy, although later infections can still be damaging. A combined screen, known as the TORCH (**t**oxoplasmosis, **r**ubella, **c**ytomegalovirus and **h**erpes simplex virus) test, was once routinely used in the UK to detect infections in the mother and newborn baby. During pregnancy TORCH infections can cross the placenta, causing mild or severe congenital malformation, abortion or stillbirth. The consequences are usually more severe if infection occurs in the first trimester.

There is a move away from routine TORCH testing as a screen for all mothers and towards specific testing based on clinical indications in the mother or suspicion of congenital infection in the neonate. The organisms are detected indirectly by the specific IgG antibodies that are produced in response to infection. In the UK, screening for rubella and syphilis (not included in the original TORCH test) remains routine, while tests for other infections are carried out if the need arises.

Toxoplasmosis

In the mother toxoplasmosis is most often asymptomatic, although it can cause a febrile illness with neck stiffness, headache, sore throat and rash. The organism does not always cross the placenta but when it does it can cause spontaneous abortion or developmental abnormalities of the central nervous system (CNS). Survivors of congenital infection usually have mental retardation, epilepsy or spasticity. The risk is greater in the first trimester of

Cytomegalovirus: in most individuals infection is asymptomatic and harmless but it can cause encephalitis, retinitis, pneumonia and gastrointestinal involvement in the immunocompromised.

Herpes simplex virus (HSV): HSV-2 causes genital herpes and systemic infections in immunocompromised patients, leading to severe hepatitis or encephalitis.

Rubella, 'German measles': caused by viral infection with peak incidence at about 15 years. Symptoms include general malaise and fever, mild conjunctivitis and swollen lymph nodes, followed by macular rash of face, trunk and limbs. Complications in adults are rare but intrauterine infection can cause congenital abnormalities.

Toxoplasmosis: caused by the protozoan *Toxoplasma gondii*. Infection is from eating lamb or pork or ingesting infected animal faeces (for example, from hand contamination in children after playing outdoors).

pregnancy and later infections are associated with fewer complications or no effect at all.

In the UK screening is offered to women who demand it and to those who may be at higher risk by regular contact with cats (a common host for the organism).

Rubella

Screening is still carried out for rubella (German measles) antibodies. Vaccination is not recommended once a women becomes pregnant but should be given after the birth. Intrauterine infection is almost certain if infection occurs in the first trimester, causing fetal abnormalities in 15–30% of cases. The onset of infection in later stages of pregnancy is associated with a smaller risk. The main fetal abnormalities comprise heart malformations, eye lesions, mental retardation and deafness. These abnormalities may not be detectable by ultrasound and therefore the pregnant mother with rubella must face the difficult decision of terminating what could be a perfectly normal pregnancy.

There is a high risk of congenital malformation when rubella infection occurs early in pregnancy

Cytomegalovirus

Cytomegalovirus infection is often asymptomatic in the mother but intrauterine infection can cause jaundice, motor disorders and CNS abnormalities in the fetus. The infection affects the fetus in about 40% of cases regardless of the stage of pregnancy. Only about 10% of babies show clinical evidence of infection and 90% of these develop normally. There is therefore little point in screening for cytomegalovirus because nothing can be done to eradicate the infection, and the termination of infected pregnancies would result in the loss of many normal babies.

The risk of congenital malformations arising from maternal cytomegalovirus infection is small

Herpes simplex

Herpes simplex infections can cross the placenta and cause congenital malformations but this is rare. It is much more likely to be acquired during vaginal delivery if the mother has active genital lesions. This can be prevented by Caesarean delivery.

Herpes simplex infection is more likely to be acquired during delivery

Syphilis

The early stage of syphilis starts as a small papule at the site of contact. This may go unnoticed if it is inside the cervix or rectum. Routine blood screening tests for syphilis are carried out in pregnant women in the UK and as a result of this policy the congenital form of the disease is extremely rare, affecting no more than about a dozen babies a year. The infection is not acquired by the fetus before the fourth month of pregnancy. This means that there is opportunity to identify maternal infection by screening and treat the condition before it affects the fetus.

Treatment of syphilis early in pregnancy can prevent infection of the fetus

Meningocele: protrusion of the meninges through a defect in the vertebral column, without spinal cord elements, into a skin-covered sac.

Meningomyelocele: protrusion of the spinal cord and meninges through a defect in the vertebral column. Usually covered by only a thin membrane which oozes moisture.

Neural tube defects: developmental defects of the brain, spinal cord, skull and spinal column, such as anencephaly and spina bifida.

Spina bifida: failure of the spinal canal to close, thereby exposing and damaging the spinal cord and nerves. Excess fluid in the brain (hydrocephalus) is a frequent complication. The physical disabilities are of varying severity but can include paralysis of the spine and bladder. Largely preventable by adequate dietary folic acid before and during pregnancy.

Screening for neural tube defects and Down's syndrome

Most infants with congenital abnormalities are born to couples who have no obvious identifiable risk factors. It is therefore necessary to apply screening tests to the general maternal population (Table 11.4).

A number of markers, present in maternal blood, can now be used to predict pregnancies affected by Down's syndrome and neural tube defects. These markers are α-fetoprotein, unconjugated oestriol (uE₃) and human chorionic gonadotrophin (hCG). Although suitable for general screening these markers lack sensitivity and specificity, and any positive results need to be investigated further. Women who have identifiable risk factors should in any case be investigated further.

Neural tube defects

Neural tube defects can cause spontaneous abortion or severe physical and mental disabilities in the child. The frequency of known neural tube defects in the UK, detected in pregnancy or at term, is about 5–7 per 1000 pregnancies. The number of affected live births is much lower (about 0.3 per 1000), because of spontaneous abortion, stillbirths and the impact of antenatal screening. Neural tube defects include anencephaly and spina bifida. Spina bifida usually occurs with meningomyelocele or, less commonly, with meningocele only.

Risk can be identified by screening maternal blood for α-fetoprotein, and the presence of a meningomyelocele can be confirmed or excluded by ultrasound examination. The outlook for survival and quality of life for spina bifida with meningomyelocele is poor, and only about 25% of affected babies are considered for surgical treatment. Spina bifida with meningocele has a much better prognosis and, after surgery, there are usually no neurological complications or mobility problems.

α-Fetoprotein

High α-fetoprotein levels are associated with neural tube defects

α-Fetoprotein: the fetal precursor of albumin, produced in the yolk sac and the fetal liver. Fetal blood levels of α-fetoprotein increase until around 30 weeks' gestation and then gradually decline as it is replaced with albumin.

Some fetal α-fetoprotein normally finds its way into the amniotic fluid through fetal renal excretion. An open defect of the fetal spine or cranium, with exposure of fetal blood vessels, leads to leakage of α-fetoprotein into the amniotic fluid. Hence, α-fetoprotein concentrations become markedly raised in both the amniotic fluid and the maternal blood circulation as it is cleared.

Screening of maternal blood for α-fetoprotein is capable of identifying nearly all fetuses with anencephaly and about 80% of those with open spina bifida. The optimum time for screening is 16–18 weeks' gestation. Because of normal changes in the concentration of α-fetoprotein with gestational age, it is vital that gestational age is determined accurately, usually by ultrasonography. Levels of α-fetoprotein are affected by the weight and race of the mother and by insulin-dependent diabetes. In about half of pregnancies in which the α-fetoprotein concentration is raised no abnormality can be detected during or after the pregnancy and because of this all instances of raised α-fetoprotein in maternal blood require further diagnostic investigation.

The initial investigative step comprises ultrasound examination of the fetus and placenta. Abnormal or equivocal results from this examination are then investigated by amniocentesis. Raised α-fetoprotein levels in the amniotic fluid, together with detection of acetylcholinesterase (derived from neural tissues) confirms diagnosis.

Down's syndrome

Although Down's syndrome is a genetic disorder it is not usually inherited through genetic defects already present in the parents. The practice in the UK used to be to offer cytogenetic screening to pregnant women at high risk of having a child with Down's syndrome (older mothers, usually over the age of 35). The availability of a simpler blood test now means that screening can be offered to all pregnant women, regardless of age. Positive results are confirmed by amniocentesis and cytogenetic analysis.

Unfortunately, the blood screening test is associated with high rates of false-positive and false-negative results. The most accurate screening protocol is a combination of assays for uE_3, hCG and α-fetoprotein. The detection rate is about 60%, with a false-positive rate of about 5%.

Current indications for amniocenteses or chorionic villus sampling and cytogenetic investigation are

- Maternal age alone
- Maternal age in conjunction with a positive blood test
- Family history of Down's syndrome (the less common chromosomal translocations are inherited)
- Abnormalities detected on ultrasonographic examination

Screening for haemolytic disease of the newborn

Haemolytic disease of the newborn is caused by production of maternal antibodies to fetal red blood cell antigens. The most common type of haemolytic disease is ABO incompatibility, in which the mother is usually of blood group O and the fetus is group A. **Rhesus haemolytic disease** can occur if the mother's blood group is rhesus-negative and the father is rhesus-positive because the baby might also be rhesus-positive. In both types of haemolytic disease sensitisation of the mother's immune system occurs by passage of fetal red blood cells into the maternal circulation. This usually occurs at the time of delivery so that first pregnancies are rarely affected by maternal antibodies. However, amniocentesis, chorionic villus sampling and threatened miscarriage can also result in exposure to fetal red blood cells.

In a subsequent pregnancy red cells of the blood group- or Rhesus-incompatible fetus will be subjected to attack by maternal antibodies, causing anaemia, jaundice, stillbirth or neonatal death. Severe jaundice in the neonatal period can result in the deposition of bilirubin in the basal ganglia of the brain, causing mental retardation, deafness, epilepsy and spasticity. Haemolytic

ABO blood groups: a blood grouping system based on red blood cell surface antigens. Type A blood contains type A antigens, type B blood contains B antigens, AB blood has both and type O blood neither. Antibodies to the absent antigens develop soon after birth. A person with type A blood has anti-B antibodies, someone with type B blood has anti-A antibodies. No AB antibodies are produced in people with type AB blood. Both anti-A and anti-B are found in people with type O blood.

Antibody-mediated red cell destruction in haemolytic disease leads to anaemia and jaundice

Bilirubin: a yellow pigment that is released into the blood following destruction of red blood cells. Normally, bilirubin is taken up by the liver, incorporated into bile and excreted. Excessive amounts lead to the characteristic yellow colour of jaundice. Bilirubin has an affinity for lipids, particularly in brain tissue, where it causes damage in babies. Adults with jaundice are protected from brain damage because bilirubin does not pass across the fully developed blood–brain barrier.

Exchange transfusion: exchange transfusion is used to reduce circulating bilirubin and maternal rhesus antibodies, and to correct anaemia. The technique involves insertion of catheters into the umbilical artery and vein and running cross-matched blood into the venous catheter while removing a similar amount of blood from the artery.

Rhesus factor: based on red blood cell antigens originally identified in rhesus monkeys. There are about 25 rhesus antigens but the D (RhD) antigen is the most common cause of incompatibility. About 85% of whites are RhD-positive. Unlike the ABO group antigens, antibodies to the Rh antigens do not develop spontaneously and exposure to incompatible transfused or fetal blood is required before antibodies are produced.

disease associated with ABO incompatibility is usually mild. There are three main forms of rhesus haemolytic disease:

- **Hydrops fetalis**, in which the baby is often stillborn with gross oedema and anaemia
- Jaundice, which usually arises within the first few hours after birth. This is not immediately evident because the baby had previously been able to excrete bilirubin through the placenta
- Anaemia, which occurs gradually over several weeks, with only slight jaundice

All pregnant women in the UK are routinely tested for their rhesus blood group. If anti-D antibodies are detected the test should be repeated to check for a raised titre. If the titre is raised an amniocentesis may be performed to confirm haemolytic disease in the fetus. This will also influence decisions regarding the timing of the eventual delivery. Intrauterine blood transfusion may be necessary to provide the fetus with sufficient red blood cells for oxygen transport.

The treatment of rhesus haemolytic disease depends on its severity. The aim is to restore normal haemoglobin concentration and eliminate biliverdin before it builds up and causes damage. Exchange transfusions, in which the baby's rhesus-negative blood is removed and replaced with rhesus-positive blood, may be needed after birth. Phototherapy is used for babies with mild haemolytic jaundice to convert bilirubin to water-soluble biliverdin which is excreted by the kidneys. About 95% of babies born with rhesus haemolytic disease can be expected to survive although neonatal deaths are more likely in the more severely affected babies with hydrops fetalis.

Rhesus haemolytic disease can be prevented in future pregnancies by injection of anti-D antibody within a few hours of delivery (or miscarriage) of the first child (which eliminates the fetal cells before the mother has time to develop her own, more permanent, antibodies). The extent of maternal exposure to fetal red blood cells can be estimated by the **Kleihauer test** and used to determine how much anti-D should be given.

Antenatal screening methods

Perhaps the most common perception of screening during pregnancy is the use of ultrasound. This is used as a general screening method to check dates and confirm that the fetus is viable and as an adjunct to other screening tests, particularly to check for fetal abnormalities. The results of this examination may indicate the need for more invasive procedures aimed at sampling amniotic fluid and fetal cells or blood such as amniocentesis, chorionic villus sampling or cordocentesis. There are no risks to the mother or fetus consequent on ultrasound examination. Both amniocentesis and chorionic villus sampling carry risks of spontaneous abortion and placental bleeding, resulting in maternal exposure to fetal red blood cells (the rhesus-negative mother should routinely be given anti-D antibodies after the procedure). Some studies suggest that additional risk of fetal limb abnormalities is associated with chorionic villus sampling, particularly if the procedure is carried out before 9 weeks' gestation.

Ultrasound screening

Ultrasound examination can be used in the first trimester to confirm pregnancy, and to determine the gestational age and viability of the fetus. Second-trimester (usually at 16–20 weeks) ultrasound examination is valuable for the detection of fetal anomalies such as cardiac, CNS or renal tract abnormalities or limb reduction.

Ultrasound can be used to detect structural malformations in the second trimester of pregnancy

Most of the structural abnormalities that are responsible for an increase in maternal α-fetoprotein are observable by ultrasound examination, although proper identification requires a high degree of skill and experience. Many of the appearances are extremely subtle and are easily missed.

Amniocentesis

All pregnant women over the age of 35 may be offered amniocentesis to exclude the possibility that the fetus is affected by Down's syndrome or other chromosomal abnormality. A triple test result suggestive of Down's syndrome or neural tube abnormalities will be further investigated by amniocentesis. Down's syndrome and other chromosomal abnormalities are detectable by cytogenetic analysis of fetal cells shed into the amniotic fluid.

Amniocentesis has become a routine diagnostic procedure for confirmation of suspected genetic or neural tube abnormalities

Detection of neural tube defects relies on the estimation of α-fetoprotein in the amniotic fluid. This is a far more accurate indicator of fetal abnormality than testing of maternal blood. Amniocentesis is also useful for assessing the severity of rhesus haemolytic disease, by estimating antibody concentration and the degree of contamination by bile salts.

Another application of amniocentesis is for determining the maturity of the lungs in a fetus which may need to be delivered early. A threat to premature babies is **respiratory distress syndrome**, caused by the inability of the lungs to secrete sufficient surfactant. Normally, surfactant coats the alveoli, reducing surface tension and decreasing the pressure required to keep the alveoli open. Without it, breathing becomes much more difficult because the alveoli tend to collapse. The test is based on the estimation of the **lecithin:sphingomyelin ratio** in amniotic fluid. If the ratio is low (<1.5) at birth the risk of respiratory distress syndrome is high. It is now possible to treat the condition with natural or synthetic surfactant in aerosol form, which can be extremely effective provided it is administered before the condition becomes severe.

Respiratory distress syndrome: primarily a condition of premature infants, caused by immaturity of the lungs at birth which cannot synthesise adequate amounts of surfactant. Without surfactant the alveoli collapse and the infant becomes hypoxic. This damages the epithelium and blood vessels so that the airways become filled with plasma exudate. Death is usually from brain damage (because of hypoxia) or heart failure.

Amniocentesis is usually carried out at 15–18 weeks of gestation but can be performed as early as 12 weeks. Most procedures are carried out with continuous ultrasound to monitor the needle location (Figure 11.1). Potential complications of amniocentesis are bleeding, rupture of the membranes and spontaneous miscarriage and fetal abnormalities can be caused by accidental insertion of the needle into the fetus. Fortunately, this is extremely rare when ultrasound monitoring is used and is usually confined to minor skin injury, although more serious damage has been reported. The risk of pregnancy loss from an amniocentesis performed at 15–20 weeks' gestation is about 1%.

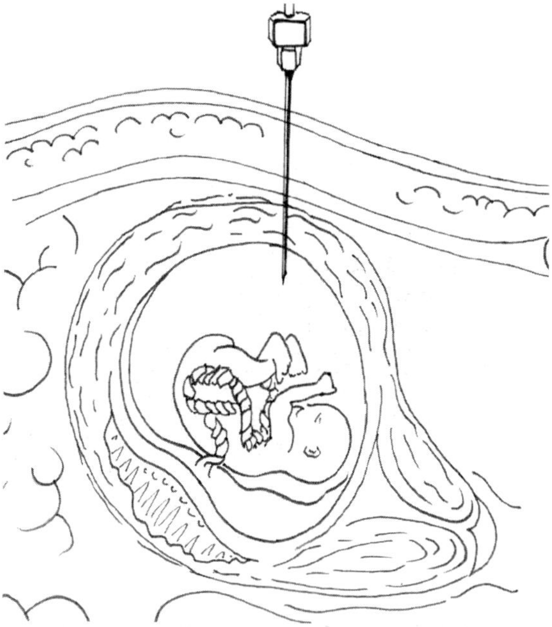

Figure 11.1 Amniocentesis. Amniotic fluid is sampled transabdominally under ultrasound guidance.

Chorionic villus sampling

Chorionic villus sampling may be contemplated as a diagnostic procedure when standard biochemical or ultrasonographic screening have yielded positive or equivocal results. The procedure is usually performed at 10 weeks of pregnancy and offers earlier detection of genetic defects than is possible by amniocentesis. Inadequate sampling is more of a problem in chorionic villus sampling than in amniocentesis. In experienced hands, with ultrasound guidance, the risks of spontaneous abortion are only slightly higher than those of amniocentesis.

The procedure can be carried out by transabdominal or transcervical routes (Figure 11.2). Not all women are suitable for transcervical sampling because of vaginal infections or the position of the uterus. The safety and complication rates of the two procedures appear to be comparable. The transabdominal route is associated with more discomfort but is more familiar to practitioners used to performing amniocentesis.

The main advantage of chorionic villus sampling is that it brings forward the time in which genetic abnormalities can be diagnosed. However, because the sample is principally composed of cells, biochemical markers in the amniotic fluid cannot be evaluated.

▲ Key points

Routine screening tests in pregnancy

- ▲ Full blood count: detection of anaemia and other blood disorders
- ▲ Rhesus and ABO blood grouping: assess risk of haemolytic disease
- ▲ Rubella antibodies: assess risk of congenital rubella
- ▲ Syphilis antibodies: assess risk of congenital syphilis
- ▲ Urine testing: diabetes, nephropathy
- ▲ Random blood test for diabetes
- ▲ Triple test: assess risk of Down's syndrome and neural tube defects
- ▲ Genetic screening: sickle-cell disease or thalassaemia in selected populations
- ▲ Cystic fibrosis carrier screening in some areas of the UK
- ▲ Ultrasound: check dates, fetal growth and viability, malformations

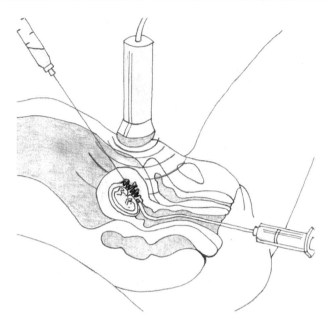

Figure 11.2 Chorionic villus sampling. A catheter can be passed through the cervix or abdomen under direct ultrasound guidance and placed within the chorionic villi for sampling.

Fetal blood sampling

Fetal blood can be obtained in the second trimester by **cordocentesis**. This involves insertion of a needle into the umbilical cord under ultrasound guidance, preferably at the site of its insertion into the placenta but blood can also be obtained from a free loop of the cord, at the insertion of the cord into the fetal abdomen, or directly through the fetal abdominal wall into the umbilical vein. The choice of insertion site is usually governed by accessibility and clarity of the ultrasound image. The technique is performed without anaesthesia or sedation. The risk of fetal loss depends on the gestational age at sampling, the site of the puncture, the number of attempts and the presence of fetal anomalies. The average loss is 1–2% of fetuses with normal ultrasound appearances.

Cordocentesis is less frequently used than either amniocentesis or chorionic villus sampling, for the diagnosis of haemoglobin and bleeding disorders.

Screening the newborn

At birth a brief physical examination is made and if all is well the baby is returned to its mother. Some babies may require resuscitation following a difficult delivery. The need for resuscitation is based on a quantitative clinical evaluation known as the **Apgar score**, which is derived from assessment of

> ### ▲ Key points
>
> #### Techniques in antenatal diagnosis
>
> ▲ Ultrasound: safe, no risks to mother or fetus, mainly performed in second trimester to assess fetal abnormality
>
> ▲ Amniocentesis: performed in second trimester to assess genetic abnormalities, neural tube defects, rhesus haemolytic disease and fetal lung maturity
>
> ▲ Chorionic villus sampling: performed in first trimester, to assess genetic abnormalities
>
> ▲ Cordocentesis: performed in second trimester to assess haemoglobin and bleeding disorders

the baby's physical condition including heart rate, respiratory effort, muscle tone, and reflex response.

In the UK all newborn babies are given an injection of vitamin K at birth to prevent **haemorrhagic disease of the newborn**. This is a bleeding disorder caused by a deficiency of vitamin K, needed for the synthesis of clotting factors. The condition usually develops within a week of birth and is more likely to occur in breast-fed babies because there is very little vitamin K in breast milk. Further doses of vitamin K may be given to susceptible breast-fed babies.

Biochemical and genetic screening

Biochemical and genetic screening tests are routinely carried out on small samples of dried blood

In the UK all newborn babies are screened for phenylketonuria and congenital hypothyroidism. Screening for phenylketonuria was initiated in the early 1970s and the screen for congenital hypothyroidism was added in 1981. It is now possible to detect a wider range of genetic disorders from a small blood sample, and some centres also screen for sickle-cell disease, cystic fibrosis and amino acid disorders. Pilot schemes are also being followed to evaluate the effectiveness of screening for Duchenne muscular dystrophy and familial hyperlipidaemia. Anonymous surveillance of neonatal HIV infection is performed in some areas.

Phenylketonuria

Normal development is possible if phenylketonuria or congenital hypothyroidism is recognised and treated early

Screening for phenylketonuria and congenital hypothyroidism fulfil the classical requirements of a screening programme: the conditions are serious but can be ameliorated by prompt identification and treatment. Phenylketonuria may be diagnosed from a sample of heelprick blood placed in a capillary tube or spotted on to filter paper. The commonly used **Guthrie test** relies on the measurement of phenylalanine in the blood by a bacterial inhibition assay. The filter paper blood spots have become known as Guthrie spots and usually a strip of four spots is assessed. Some laboratories use chromatographic methods which can also identify other amino acid disorders.

Treatment of the disorder is to restrict dietary phenylalanine. This is highly effective when initiated before 4 weeks of age, but must be continued throughout childhood and beyond (see Chapter 3). Untreated, the disorder causes mental deficiency. It affects about one in 10 000 neonates in the UK.

Congenital hypothyroidism

Congenital hypothyroidism is the inadequate production of thyroxine, either because the thyroid tissue is absent or because it does not function properly. By a feedback mechanism, the pituitary attempts to correct the deficiency by secretion of thyroid stimulating hormone (TSH). The blood therefore contains very low levels of thyroxine, but high levels of TSH. The screening test is an assay for thyroxine or TSH in blood (the methods can be adapted for use with Guthrie spots). Affected neonates usually appear normal at birth because they have been able to use thyroxine from the mother. Affected babies who are not identified and treated promptly suffer mental retardation and growth failure.

Treatment is by oral thyroxine. The frequency in the UK is about one in 4000 live births.

Other genetic disorders

Pilot studies have been set up in Wales and some other countries to evaluate screening for Duchenne muscular dystrophy. The test relies on determination of creatine kinase in dried Guthrie spots. However, early diagnosis does not affect outcome and the advantage of routine screening is that possible further cases could be avoided through genetic counselling. The disadvantage is that it entails informing parents that their son has a fatal illness well before he has any symptoms. The incidence of the disease in the UK is one in 4000 boys.

Similarly, early identification and treatment of cystic fibrosis do not currently do much to improve prognosis (see Chapter 21), although early identification allows the option of antenatal diagnosis in subsequent pregnancies. The screening test in the neonatal period relies on the detection of raised levels of immunoreactive trypsin in dried blood spots.

Haematological and genetic tests are available for neonatal screening of haemoglobin disorders. Some 5% of the UK population consists of ethnic minorities at risk from these diseases and 10% of births occur in these groups. The thalassaemias can be diagnosed by red cell indices and abnormal haemoglobins identified by electrophoresis. Sickle-cell anaemia can be detected by a sickle solubility test – this disease can affect up to 2% of some ethnic groups.

Child health surveillance

A large number of health checks are carried out at intervals in infants and schoolchildren. In preschool children these are carried out in medical general practice. The medical conditions to be excluded include congenital dislocation of the hip, congenital heart disease and undescended testicles in boys. A programme of immunisation may also be initiated.

The following checks are recommended at 6–8 weeks or earlier:

- Assessment of mother–baby bonding
- Identification of any feeding problems
- Exclusion of congenital dislocation of the hip
- Assessment of physical and neurological development
- Exclusion of congenital heart disease

Vaccination

In the UK, childhood vaccination programmes are aimed at immunisation against diphtheria, tetanus and whooping cough (DTP triple vaccine), polio and measles, mumps and rubella (MMR). In addition BCG (for protection against tuberculosis) may be given to babies who are at high risk. Immunisation

Review question 1

What are the main causes of congenital malformation?

Table 11.4   Antenatal and neonatal screening for non-infectious disorders

Time of screen	Disorder	Population at risk	Screening method
Antenatal period	Rhesus haemolytic disease	All mothers	Blood group serology; amniocentesis
	ABO haemolytic disease	All mothers	Blood group serology
	Diabetes mellitus	All mothers	Blood glucose
	Pre-eclampsia	All mothers	Urine protein
	Congenital malformations	All mothers	Ultrasound
	Down's syndrome	All mothers over 35 years	Triple test; amniocentesis or chorionic villus sampling (also detects other chromosomal abnormalities
	Neural tube defects	All mothers	Triple test: not routine in all areas of UK; amniocentesis
	Haemoglobinopathies (sickle-cell disease, thalassaemia)	All mothers not of northern European descent	Determine if parents are carriers; cordocentesis
	Cystic fibrosis	All mothers of northern European descent	Carrier detection by direct gene analysis; not routine in the UK
Neonatal period	Phenylketonuria	All neonates	Biochemical test
	Hypothyroidism	All neonates	Biochemical test
	Cystic fibrosis	All neonates of northern European descent	Immunoreactive trypsin; not routine in the UK
	Sickle-cell disease	Selected ethnic groups	Biochemical test
	Duchenne muscular dystrophy	All neonates	Biochemical test; not routine in the UK

against hepatitis B is given to babies whose mothers were positive for hepatitis B surface antigen during pregnancy.

The Department of Health recommendations for vaccination are:

- At 8 weeks: DTP triple vaccine and oral polio vaccine
- At 12–18 months: MMR
- Preschool (4–5 years): boosters of diphtheria, tetanus and polio vaccines
- Girls of 10–14 years: rubella vaccine if they have not already received MMR.

The incidence of measles, mumps, rubella and whooping cough in the UK fell in the early 1990s (Figure 11.3, and see Figure 6.5), which correlates with uptake in vaccination. There has been a small but steady rise in the incidence of tuberculosis, possibly because of a previous fall in BCG coverage, but other factors affecting the adult population have also influenced this change (see Chapter 6). Compared with MMR and poliomyelitis vaccines BCG is not the most effective form of immunisation.

At 8–10 months of age assessments of vision, hearing and manipulation skills are undertaken. Deafness can go unnoticed because the child uses other clues from its surroundings. Sensorineural loss (nerve deafness) occurs in about one in 1000 children; conductive hearing loss caused by otitis media with effusion ('glue ear') is more common. Early language delay can be detected at 18–24 months.

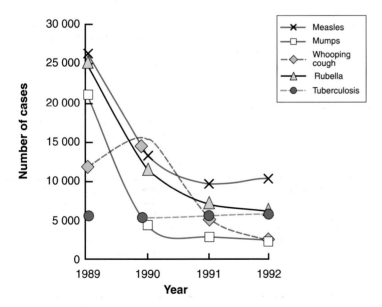

Figure 11.3 Incidence of infectious diseases in England and Wales. Measles, mumps, rubella and whooping cough are all common infectious diseases for which vaccines are available. Tuberculosis is steadily increasing in incidence, while incidence of the other infectious disease is falling, presumably because of the impact of effective immunisation. Occasional 'scares' about the safety of vaccination are followed by more cases of the disease (whooping cough in 1990). Diphtheria and tetanus are currently rare (about 10 cases a year).

Diphtheria: caused by *Corynebacterium diphtheriae*, producing systemic symptoms (by an exotoxin) and a localised inflammatory reaction, or membrane, on the surface of the tonsils, pharynx or larynx. Complications include myocarditis which can lead to acute circulatory failure and death.

Measles: a common childhood infection, particularly in less developed countries. Viral infection causes general malaise and fever, characteristic spots in the mouth (Koplik's spots), followed by a maculopapular rash, initially on the face, and then on the rest of the body. Usually a mild disease in the healthy child, but mortality is high in malnourished children.

Mumps: primarily a disease of school-age children and young adults, caused by infection with paramyxovirus. Symptoms include severe pain and swelling of the parotid glands. Meningitis occurs in about 5% of infected patients, often without evidence of salivary gland involvement. After puberty, mumps in boys can cause inflammation of testis and epididymis, but causes sterility in only a minority of these patients.

Otitis media with effusion (OME), 'glue ear': commonly associated with upper respiratory tract infections. Mucus secretions accumulate in the middle ear cavity because they cannot drain through the eustachian tube, which is very narrow in the child or becomes blocked by inflammation of the adenoids. The thick fluid or 'glue' can be drained by insertion of a grommet.

Poliomyelitis: caused by infection with a poliovirus, which has a propensity for the nervous system. Spread is by the faecal–oral route. Incidence has fallen dramatically because of improved hygiene and sanitation and the widespread use of vaccination. Infection can be asymptomatic or self-limiting, but causes paralysis in about 0.1% of children and 1% of adults.

Serious defects in vision are very rare in children but require prompt investigation and treatment. Causes include retinoblastoma, cataract and glaucoma. Many are of genetic origin and hence genetic counselling may be offered to advise on the likelihood of further affected pregnancies. It is more common to find moderate visual impairment, early recognition and treatment of which can prevent worsening. For example, untreated squint can result in permanent damage as well as causing reading difficulty.

Further checks of vision, language and hearing are made at about 36 months. Finally, a preschool check of gross motor performance, vision, fine manipulation, hearing and language is included at 4–5 years.

These health checks ensure that children with special teaching requirements can be identified and that treatments can be started without delay for children with congenital diseases such as deafness, cataracts, hip dislocation, and acyanotic heart disease. Children with cerebral palsy may receive therapy at an earlier age. Undescended testicles in boys are usually corrected by orchidopexy before the age of six.

School-age children

Children over the age of 5 years are especially vulnerable to physical, emotional, social and intellectual problems. Screening for occult defects generally involves tests for vision and hearing only.

Almost one in five children at some stage have disorders of communication and learning. These problems can be minimised if identified at an early stage and may require referral to health care professionals or specialist teachers. There is also potential for health promotion in the 'captive' audience at school. Particular issues covered are those of solvent abuse, drug taking, drinking, smoking and teenage sexual activity.

Health checks in adults

In recent years 'well-man' and 'well-woman' clinics held by general practitioners have proliferated. In the UK it is a condition of the general practice contract that all patients of 16–74 years who have not consulted their doctor for 3 years must be offered a 'health check'. This might include physical checks and assessments of hypertension, smoking habits, alcohol consumption, obesity and hyperlipidaemia (see Chapter 12).

More formal mass screening programmes are aimed at specific sectors of the adult population, most notable of which are cervical screening (see Chapter 16) and breast cancer screening (see Chapter 15). There is also interest in extending screening to the detection of other cancers such as colorectal and prostate cancers, but this is more problematic because of limitations of the screening tests and treatments available (Chapters 17 and 18).

At present the methods used for cancer screening are based on detection of the cancer itself or a precursor lesion. It is likely that genetic methods will become more commonly employed. This might be useful for identifying the small group of women at risk of inherited breast and ovarian cancers. It is also possible to test for the gene responsible for familial adenomatous polyposis, an inherited condition that leads to colorectal cancer (Chapter 17); this is already being undertaken in families known to be at risk.

A current issue surrounding genetic screening is the detection of carrier status for cystic fibrosis. A precedent for carrier screening of adults has already been set with the tests for carriers of thalassaemia, sickle-cell disease and Tay–Sachs disease in Asian, Afro-Caribbean and Jewish people, and there is no technical reason why screening for cystic fibrosis carriers could not be carried out, particularly in people who are contemplating having a family.

Screening implies that something will be done with the knowledge obtained, that is, to terminate an affected pregnancy. The commonly perceived picture of cystic fibrosis is one of chronic ill health, yet there are many patients who are fit and active and their prospects are improving all the time with the help of new treatments. The advantage of carrier screening is that it allows an unhurried decision to be taken on whether to become pregnant or continue with a pregnancy and it is possible to avoid having a first child with the disease (fetal testing requires amniocentesis or chorionic villus sampling and is usually undertaken only when the condition is suspected because there is already an affected child in the family).

However, the knowledge about a condition (or possible condition) brings about anxiety and pressure. A further complication of general carrier screening is that the knowledge of carrier status in one individual is useless unless the partner or prospective partner is also screened. Knowledge about carrier status may therefore have to be given to other people, with possibilities for stigmatisation.

Another issue in genetic screening is the application of tests for Huntington's disease. Not only is it possible to determine who has inherited the condition but it is becoming possible to predict the age of onset based on the number of CAG repeats (see Chapter 3), although not reliably. This leaves people who have a family history of the disease with the agonising choice of whether to be tested, with implications for both themselves and their families.

Surveillance of older people

In the UK general practitioners are required to offer an annual home visit to patients who are over 75 years of age. One purpose is to assess the need and availability of helpers and carers. A variety of assessments of the individual are made, including:
- Mobility (walking, sitting, use of aids)
- Mental state
- Hearing and vision
- Continence
- General function

- Social (lifestyle, relationships)
- Review of medication

There is something of a misconception that the disabilities seen in older people are an inevitable part of the ageing process, and that there is little that can be done to overcome them. In a minority of cases this may be true, but the older person may have this attitude and not seek help even though it is likely that some improvements to the quality of life can be made. One purpose of surveillance in older people is to identify these problems and remedy them. Unlike screening for asymptomatic disease, surveillance in older people is more about searching for symptomatic disease already affecting the patient. Older people often consider that it is not worth presenting symptoms which they believe to be an inevitable consequence of ageing for medical attention, and their perceptions of any possible benefit are low.

Sensory impairment

Loss of vision

A loss of visual acuity and hearing range is universal as people get older

Loss of visual acuity tends to be accepted by both patients and their carers. However, other causes may be superimposed on age-related sight loss and people with failing vision should not be regarded as a homogeneous group. Some problems (cataracts, for example) can be treated: it is estimated that 50% of the population over 75 years have some form of cataract. In addition, many older people may not realise that their eyesight has changed since their last prescription for glasses and that they would benefit from a change.

Loss of hearing

The view that hearing loss is to be expected in old age leads many people to ignore the problem until it is a severe handicap. About one-third of people over the age of 65 suffer from hearing loss that inhibits social interaction but only a minority of older people become deaf. Screening for hearing impairment has the advantage that recognition of the problem alone can ease the situation for both the patient and their relatives: communication can be improved by speaking clearly and from the direction in which the patient hears best. In some cases hearing can be improved by the simple expedient of removal of ear wax; others may benefit from a hearing aid.

Mobility

A variety of conditions contribute to mobility problems in older people. Each condition in itself may not be serious, but the combination of minor pathologies in the muscles, nerves, joints and arteries commonly disables the older person. A simple grading system can be used to assess mobility, based on the distance the person is able to walk unaided and the degree of reliance on mobility aids or assistance by another person. It is also important to assess the person's mobility in a familiar environment rather than rely on the analysis of gait in a strange setting. Improvements can be made for some people by the proper evaluation and treatment of any medical condition which may contribute to impaired mobility; the quality of life of others can still be improved by ensuring the correct mobility aids are used, giving information about mobility allowances and by improvements in the home.

Bladder and urinary tract disorders

The most common urological disorder that affects older people is urinary incontinence. People with stroke are particularly susceptible. Urinary incontinence can be reversible, partially reversible, or irreversible. The reversible causes include:

- Urinary tract infection, often associated with prostate disease in men
- Use of diuretics, sedatives or anticholinergic drugs
- Mechanical effects caused by faecal impaction, prostatic hypertrophy, urethral prolapse or bladder neck obstruction

The irreversible causes are usually dementia, complications of radical prostatectomy or radiotherapy, and neuropathic bladder.

Surveillance of older people means that the reversible causes of urinary incontinence can be identified and treated appropriately. Even when irreversible incontinence is diagnosed, much can be done to improve matters by regular use of the toilet and appropriate absorption pads, collection devices or catheters. A home visit is essential to check the availability of toilets or commodes.

Faecal incontinence

Faecal incontinence is common in older people, particularly in the infirm or those with dementia. Overflow incontinence is usually secondary to faecal impaction arising from constipation. Other causative factors include rectal prolapse, colorectal cancer, infection, inflammatory bowel disease and diabetic neuropathy. Surveillance allows proper identification of the cause, which may be improved by treatment, or provision of incontinence aids.

> ### ▲ Key points
>
> **Surveillance of older people**
>
> ▲ Based on an annual home visit by doctor or practice nurse
> ▲ Social assessment: lifestyle, relationships
> ▲ Mobility assessment: walking, climbing stairs, balance, use of aids
> ▲ Sensory function: hearing and vision
> ▲ Continence assessment: changes caused by urinary tract infections, prostate disease, constipation, colorectal cancer
> ▲ General functional assessment: activities of daily living (cooking, shopping, washing, dressing)
> ▲ Mental assessment: depression, mental tests for dementia
> ▲ Review of medication

Neuropathic bladder: interruption of sensory nerve pathways between sacral spine and cortical centres can result in loss of sensation of bladder fullness. Associated with multiple sclerosis and diabetes.

ANSWERS TO REVIEW QUESTIONS

What are the main causes of congenital malformations?

Question 1

Congenital malformations are caused by disturbances in metabolism such as maternal diabetes, lack of essential nutrients (folic acid for example), chromosome aneuploidy or translocation, intrauterine infections and maternal exposure to teratogens (see Chapter 5).

Most malformations are anomalies of the heart and circulatory system.

Abnormalities of the CNS comprise less than 10% of malformations, a figure that has decreased over the years because of the impact of screening.

Further reading

Best, J.M. and Sutherland, S. (1990) Diagnosis and prevention of congenital and perinatal infections. *BMJ*, **301**, 888–9.

Brown, A.D. (1985) Newborn screening for inborn errors of metabolism and related disorders. *Clin. Biochem. Rev.*, **6**, 3–13.

Bull, M.J.V. (1990) Maternal and fetal screening for antenatal care. *BMJ*, **300**, 1118–20.

Freer, C.B. (1990) Screening older people. *BMJ*, **300**, 1447–8.

Hall, D., Hill, P. and Elliman, D. (1995) *The Child Surveillance Handbook*, 2nd edn, Radcliffe Medical Press, Oxford.

Hart, C.R. and Burke, P. (1992) *Screening and Surveillance in General Practice*, Churchill Livingstone, Edinburgh.

Johnston, P.G.B. (1994) *Villiamy's The Newborn Child*, 7th edn, Churchill Livingstone, Edinburgh.

King's Fund Report. (1987) King's Fund forum consensus statement: screening for fetal and genetic abnormality. *BMJ*, **295**, 1551–3.

Modell, B. (1990) Biochemical neonatal screening. *BMJ*, **300**, 1667–8.

Tuke, J.W. (1990) Screening and surveillance of school age children. *BMJ*, **300**, 1180–2.

Wilson, D., McGillivray, B., Kalousek, D. *et al.* (1989) Multicentre randomised clinical trial of chorion villus sampling and amniocentesis. *Lancet*, **i**, 1–6.

12 Screening for coronary heart disease and stroke risk factors

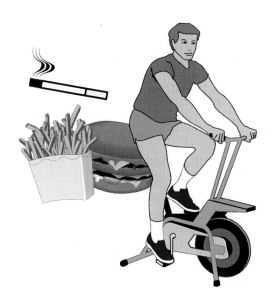

The prevention of coronary heart disease (CHD) and stroke has become a priority in the UK and other developed countries. These conditions are difficult to identify in their early asymptomatic stages, and secondary prevention by screening for disease is inappropriate. Instead, the aim of screening is to identify susceptible individuals by the presence of risk factors. This would seem to have far greater potential than secondary prevention. However, risk factors are generally poor predictors of subsequent disease.

Primary prevention also requires greater compliance because active intervention may be required for many years, changing a lifetime's habits and exposure to factors deemed to represent risk. Furthermore, a large number of risk factors must be considered for the primary prevention of CHD and stroke, many of which act in concert and multiply the risk. Most attention has focused on cholesterol screening as a preventive measure but attention should also be paid to other lifestyle and behavioural factors.

Some high-risk conditions, including hypertension and raised blood cholesterol levels, may require intensive drug intervention. A variety of drugs is available which effectively reduce blood pressure or cholesterol concentration, but their use does not always translate into substantial survival benefits. It may be that treatment often comes too late in the disease process although some patients do benefit, even when treatment is initiated in older people.

Pre-test

- **What are the principal lifestyle risk factors involved in the development of CHD?**
- **What risk factors are involved in stroke?**
- **Is cholesterol testing alone of any value?**
- **What is the best means of reducing hypertension?**

Aims of this chapter

By the end of this chapter you will have increased your knowledge of:

◆ The risk factors that influence the development of atherosclerosis and stroke

◆ Ways in which risk factors can be identified and modified

In addition, this chapter will help you to:

◆ Understand the difficulties in measuring and modifying disease risk factors

◆ Select the most appropriate medical and non-medical interventions for people identified as having excessive risk of coronary heart disease and stroke

◆ Evaluate the potential of risk factor modification for reducing morbidity and mortality from coronary heart disease and stroke

Introduction

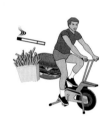

> *It is never too late to alter lifestyle risk factors for CHD and stroke*

Unlike established screening programmes such as those used for the early discovery of breast and cervical lesions, risk factor screening is aimed at preventing the development of detectable disease. Screening for risk factors is also applicable in people who have already experienced symptoms or have been treated for disease. In the latter situation, the aim is to identify and remove the risk factors, to slow down further progression of disease or prevent its recurrence.

In common with other types of screening, identification of risk must come early enough in the disease process to allow appropriate interventions to have a significant impact on morbidity and mortality. Unlike secondary prevention, modification of risk factors places a far greater responsibility on individuals to look after themselves and compliance can be difficult.

Most risk factor screening is aimed at controlling lifestyle and behavioural factors which influence the development of vascular diseases such as CHD and stroke. These conditions are major causes of illness and death in the developed countries. Evidence from population-based epidemiological studies suggests that there is much potential for avoiding premature death from these diseases.

The risk factor whose modification is likely to bring the greatest benefit is smoking – by stopping smoking men reduce their risk of death from CHD by 20%. Taking aspirin after a myocardial infarction is nearly as effective. Cholesterol-lowering and anti-hypertensive treatment are estimated to have a smaller, but worthwhile, impact on CHD and will also reduce the risk of stroke.

Coronary heart disease

> *Positive changes to risk factors can slow the progress of atherosclerosis*

A number of clinical trials have been conducted which show that reductions in death rate from CHD can be achieved by attention to risk factors. The main benefit is in preventing *premature* deaths: risk factor modification is more likely to slow down the progression of the disease than prevent it completely.

Cohort studies in which people were regularly monitored by serial ECG measurements indicate that up to 50% of all myocardial infarcts are clinically silent. It is believed that a silent myocardial infarction carries the same prognosis as a clinically evident infarct, yet these patients remain untreated. As a consequence, in many patients the first intimation of coronary artery disease is also the last – sudden death. Treatment of myocardial infarction and angina has contributed greatly to improving survival, and probably accounts for a substantial proportion of the decrease in deaths from CHD in the USA and the UK. Substantially more can be done by identifying people at risk, and then modifying lifestyle risk factors or correcting increased blood pressure and markedly high cholesterol concentrations by drug therapy.

Assess your own risk of heart disease

This table has been adapted from The Arizona Heart Institute Cardiovascular Risk Analysis devised by C.D. Cataldo, L.K. De Bruyne and E.N. Whitney in *Nutrition and Diet Therapy*, 3rd edn, published by West Publishing, Saint Paul, 1992.

Activity

	Points	Your score
Age (years):		
56 or over	1	
55 or under	0	
Gender:		
Male	1	
Female	0	
Family history -		
do you have a blood relative who has had:		
A heart attack before age 60	12	
A stroke before age 60	12	
A history of heart disease	10	
A heart attack after age 60	6	
A stroke after age 60	6	
No history of heart disease	0	
Personal history - are you:		
50 or under and have had a heart attack, stroke or cardiovascular surgery	20	
51 or over and have had a heart attack, stroke or cardiovascular surgery	10	
If you have diabetes:		
It occurred before the age of 40 and you take insulin	10	
It occurred after the age of 40 and you take insulin	5	
It occurred after the age of 50 and is controlled by diet	3	
No diabetes	0	

Do you smoke?	
40 or more cigarettes a day	10
20–40 cigarettes a day	6
Six or more cigars a day	6
Smoke a pipe regularly	6
Fewer than 20 cigarettes a day	3
Stopped smoking over a year ago	3
Never smoked	0

Select the group of foods closest to your normal diet:	
Red meat daily, more than seven eggs a week, butter, whole milk and cheese daily	8
Red meat 4–6 times a week, margarine, low-fat dairy produce and some cheese	4
Poultry, fish and little or no red meat, no more than three eggs a week, some margarine, non-fat milk and milk products	0

Weight:	
Using the formulae	
110 lb + 6 lb per inch over 5 ft for men	
100 lb + 5 lbs per inch over 5 ft for women	
Are you:	
25 lb overweight	4
10-24 lb overweight	2
Less than 10 lb overweight	0

Do you engage in aerobic exercise for 20 min or more:	
Less than once a week	4
Once or twice a week	2
Three or more times a week	0

When waiting in a queue are you:	
Frustrated and easily angered	4
Impatient and occasionally moody	2
Comfortable and easy going	0

Score:	
High risk:	40 or above
Medium risk:	20–39
Low risk:	19 and below

Stroke

Stroke is a leading cause of death, accounting for 10–12% of all deaths in developed countries, most of which are in people over the age of 65. About 80% of strokes are caused by cerebral infarction (usually as a consequence of atherosclerosis), the remainder being caused by intracerebral haemorrhage. The distinction between the various types of stroke is not always made, since this would require computed tomographic (CT) scanning or post-mortem examination.

Stroke, or **cerebrovascular accident** (CVA), is a term for sudden loss of brain function, lasting longer than a day. There are two main types: **ischaemic** stroke and **haemorrhagic** stroke. Some strokes are preceded by a 'small' stroke that causes a temporary episode of neurological dysfunction, usually lasting between 5 minutes and an hour, and never longer than 24 hours. This is the most common form of cerebral ischaemia and is known as **transient ischaemic attack** (TIA). The cause is usually a small thrombus that has formed around an atheromatous plaque.

Larger deficits in the blood supply to the brain cause **cerebral infarction**. This is usually the result of complete occlusion of an artery by thrombus (very often at the bifurcation of the internal carotid or middle cerebral artery), leading to **thrombotic** stroke. Less commonly, the artery may become occluded by embolus, usually a fragment of thrombus from the heart, causing **embolitic** stroke.

Haemorrhagic strokes are caused by rupture of a blood vessel in the brain, interrupting blood supply. Further damage can be caused to cerebral tissue by the pressure of blood escaping from the artery.

Epidemiology of stroke

Each year about 100 000 people in the UK suffer their first stroke. Strokes are more common in older people because of the cumulative effects of atherosclerosis and hypertension, but are not confined to this age group. As well as being a prime cause of death, stroke is a significant cause of long-term disability. Post-menopausal women have a higher incidence of stroke than men of similar age, but incidence rates are lower in younger women. Mortality from stroke in most developed countries has fallen over the last 20–30 years (Figure 12.1), accompanied by population-wide changes in the main risk factors.

Although death rates from both stroke and CHD have started to fall, the population distribution of the two conditions is different: in Japan, for example, there are high rates of stroke but low rates of CHD. The importance of environmental factors in the aetiology of stroke is illustrated by migrant studies; Japanese men living in the USA have comparatively lower rates of stroke but higher rates of CHD. These patterns may well be influenced by changes in diet.

Risk factors in CHD and stroke

As atherosclerosis and thrombosis are common to both ischaemic stroke and CHD (see Chapters 7 and 20) it would seem reasonable to expect that the risk factors would be similar for both diseases. In many respects this is the case and the various physiological (blood pressure, cholesterol and fibrinogen concentrations, for example) and lifestyle factors (diet, smoking, alcohol

Cerebral infarction: caused by thrombus formation or embolus, occluding one of the cerebral arteries, the internal carotid artery or the basilar artery.

Embolitic stroke: emboli originating from pathological changes in the left side of the heart, such as in endocarditis, rheumatic heart disease and myocardial infarction, can become logged in the smaller branches of the cerebral arterial tree. Insertion of artificial heart valves, pacemaker failure and arterial fibrillation are all associated with this type of stroke.

Thrombotic stroke: the most common type of stroke, associated with atherosclerosis, hypertension, diabetes and coronary or peripheral vascular disease. Often preceded by TIA.

Transient ischaemic attack (TIA): caused by a temporary impairment of blood flow to the brain (cerebral ischaemia) by atherosclerosis or a small embolus. This leads to an episode of neurological dysfunction which lasts no longer than 24 hours. Symptoms appear very suddenly and can last for minutes or hours. The most common symptoms are slight paralysis of one side of the body, vertigo and difficulty with speech. The patient usually remains conscious. Complete recovery usually occurs between attacks, but a TIA can be a warning sign of impending stroke.

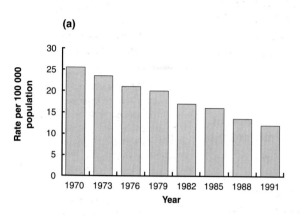

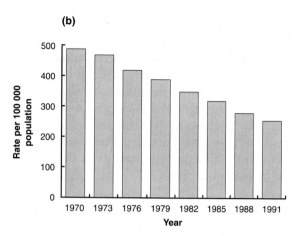

Figure 12. 1 Mortality rates for stroke, England 1970–1991 in (a) people under 65 years and (b) people between 65 and 74 years. In common with most other developed countries, the mortality rates for stroke in England have progressively declined in all age groups. (Source: OPCS.)

consumption) are all implicated in both ischaemic stroke and CHD.

Haemorrhagic stroke is quite different, and factors that inhibit ischaemic stroke (for example, n-3 fatty acids in fish oils) by decreasing platelet aggregation, blood viscosity and fibrinolytic activity could adversely affect the risk of haemorrhagic stroke. Unfortunately, most epidemiological studies fail to distinguish between the two main types of strokes, and the overall findings are likely to reflect the larger contribution by the more common ischaemic stroke.

Diet and alcohol consumption

The contribution of dietary risk factors (such as antioxidant vitamins and minerals, fibre and lipid composition) and alcohol consumption to CHD are discussed in Chapters 7 and 20. Fewer studies have evaluated the effect of dietary factors on the risk of stroke. The strength of association between blood cholesterol levels and all types of stroke is similar to that for CHD, probably because of their impact on ischaemic stroke. Obesity is a risk factor mainly because of its association with hypertension.

The association between alcohol consumption and the risk of ischaemic stroke is also expected to be similar to that for CHD but there appears to be a dose–response relationship between moderate alcohol consumption and the risk of haemorrhagic stroke.

Smoking

Cigarette smoking is associated with both ischaemic and haemorrhagic stroke. The risk increases with the number of cigarettes smoked and decreases with smoking cessation. Smoking probably contributes to the risk of ischaemic stroke in much the same way as it does to CHD – by affecting blood fibrinogen, clotting factors, platelet aggregation, plasma cholesterol levels and by directly damaging the endothelium (Chapter 20). Smoking can bring about an acute rise in blood pressure, which may contribute to arterial rupture and haemorrhagic stroke.

Diabetes mellitus

Epidemiological studies have shown the risk of CHD is higher than normal in people with diabetes (Chapters 20 and 23) and the same holds true for stroke. The risk is greater for ischaemic stroke (relative risk 3.0), the risk for haemorrhagic stroke being little different from those in people without diabetes. The pathology is probably related to the increased likelihood of atherosclerosis, increased plasma levels of fibrinogen and clotting factors, increasing the propensity for platelet aggregation.

Hypertension

Hypertension is associated with the most common causes of death in older people in the UK. The 30-year follow-up data from the Framingham Study (Slovick and Bulpitt, 1992) demonstrate that the risk of coronary heart disease increases with age and both systolic and diastolic blood pressure in men and women (Figure 12.2). Increased pressure in the blood circulation imposes stresses on the heart and the blood vessels (Figure 12.3). Workload on the heart is increased because it is pumping against increased peripheral resistance, and hypertrophy of the left ventricle can occur as an adaptive response, particularly if heart muscle has been compromised by an infarction. Left ventricular hypertrophy has a very poor prognosis and is a good predictor of impending death. Some regression of the condition can be achieved by antihypertensive therapy.

The risk of stroke also rises with systolic and diastolic blood pressure (Figure 12.4). Hypertension contributes to the development of atherosclerosis, which further elevates blood pressure. The combination of high blood pressure and atherosclerosis weakens the blood vessel walls, and they are liable to rupture.

Other complications of hypertension include kidney disease and aortic aneurysm. Despite its seriousness, hypertension is often asymptomatic and is detected only by measuring blood pressure although occasionally it may be detected by the damage that has been done to target organs – changes in heart sounds arising from hypertensive heart disease, protein in urine caused by kidney damage, abnormal peripheral pulses caused by atherosclerosis or changes in the appearance of the retinal blood vessels.

Hypertension may be defined as primary or secondary. **Primary (essential)** hypertension is hypertension in which no specific cause can be identified and is responsible for more than 90% of cases. **Secondary** hypertension is associated with a specific disease. The most common cause is reduced blood flow in the kidney which stimulates the release of renin and activates the angiotensin

Hypertension increases the risks of CHD, stroke and peripheral vascular disease

The most reliable predictor of stroke is hypertension

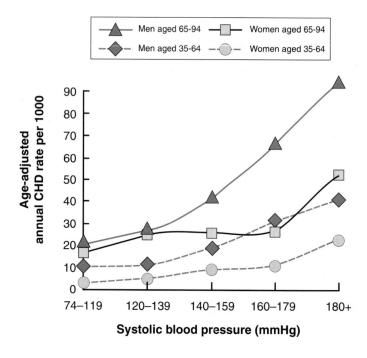

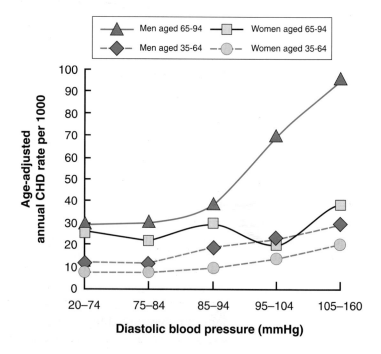

Diastolic pressure: blood pressure at the moment the heart relaxes between contractions.

Hypertension: consistent elevation of blood pressure. Defined as a systolic blood pressure ≥160 mmHg, and/or diastolic blood pressure ≥95 mmHg.

Systolic pressure: peak pressure at the moment the heart ventricles contract.

Figure 12.2 Correlation between risk of CHD with age and (a) systolic and (b) diastolic blood pressure. The incidence of CHD increases with age and is associated with increased systolic and diastolic blood pressure in both men and women. (Data from Slovick and Bulpitt, 1992.)

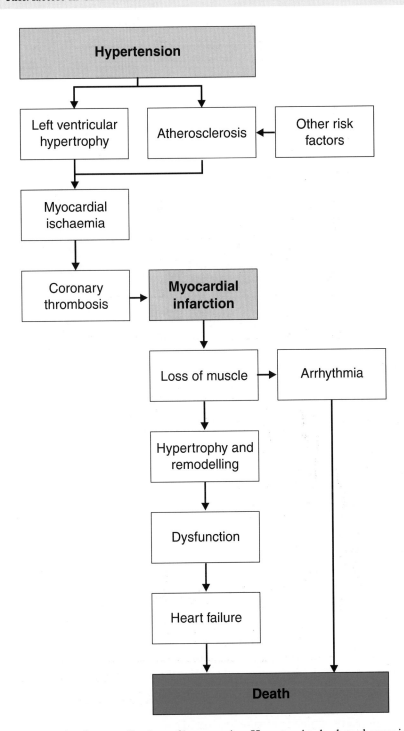

Figure 12.3 Cardiac complications of hypertension. Hypertension leads to changes in the heart and blood vessels. These influence progression to myocardial ischaemia, thrombosis and myocardial infarct. Several processes then lead to myocardial remodelling, left ventricular dilatation and dysfunction. Heart failure progresses either as a slow decline in function or causes sudden death.

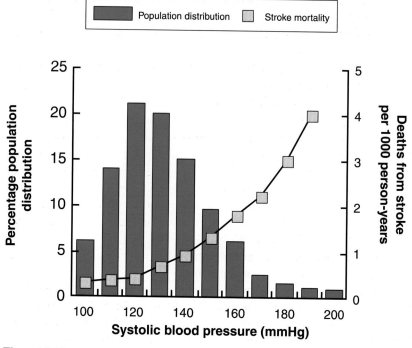

Figure 12.4 Systolic blood pressure and age-adjusted deaths from stroke. The risk of death from stroke increases with systolic and diastolic blood pressure. (Adapted from Marmot, M.G. and Poulter, N.R., in *Stroke Octet* published by *The Lancet*, London, 1992.)

system (see Chapter 20).

Regardless of cause, most hypertension is ultimately fatal unless treated. In most cases the progression is very slow (**benign** hypertension) but in up to 5% of hypertensive people the progression is extremely rapid – this condition is referred to as **malignant** hypertension and is usually triggered by kidney damage arising from benign hypertension or other causes. The rapid increase in blood pressure causes endothelial damage, which in turn promotes the formation of small thrombi, causing restriction of blood flow and destruction of red blood cells.

Risk factor intervention in hypertension

The main uncertainties that surround the treatment of hypertension are the threshold at which interventions should be given and the type of drugs to be used in the initial treatment. There may also be difficulties in accurately measuring hypertension, which is best achieved by taking several measurements of blood pressure in a seated patient, on several occasions. It is generally accepted that interventions are indicated if the diastolic pressure regularly exceeds 100 mmHg.

Non-pharmacological intervention may be adequate for controlling mild hypertension. In patients who have high blood pressure requiring drug therapy,

▲ **Key points**

Non-pharmacological management of hypertension

▲ Stop smoking
▲ Lose weight if you are obese
▲ Avoid high intakes of saturated fat
▲ Avoid excessive alcohol consumption
▲ Reduce salt intake
▲ Take regular exercise

concomitant non-pharmacological measures can produce better control at lower drug doses.

Alterations in lifestyle factors appropriate for lowering blood pressure comprise:

- Achieving ideal body weight by reducing total energy intake and taking regular physical exercise
- Avoiding excessive alcohol intake
- Reducing salt intake

Blood pressure rises with increasing obesity and hypertensive people may lower their blood pressure by losing weight. Exercise can be an effective means of obtaining and sustaining weight reduction. The exercise needs to be vigorous enough to produce a training effect on the cardiac and respiratory systems. After a gradual build-up, the activity should be intense enough to double the resting pulse rate, and should be carried out at least three times a week. The benefits of exercise are discussed further in Chapters 2 and 9.

> *Blood pressure can be reduced by 1.5 mmHg for each 1 kg of weight lost*

Alcohol consumption causes a rapid rise in blood pressure. Case-control studies show that alcohol intakes tend to be higher in people with hypertension. Acute withdrawal of alcohol may cause temporary elevation of blood pressure, but in the long term blood pressure is reduced by lowering alcohol intake.

> *Reduction in or cessation of alcohol consumption can decrease blood pressure by 5–10 mmHg*

The association between salt consumption and hypertension is controversial. Undoubtedly, salt consumption is much higher in the developed countries, where the prevalence of hypertension and its complications is higher. In the few populations in which blood pressure does not rise with age, and where there are few cases of primary hypertension, salt consumption is very low. Individual responses vary, but reduction in dietary salt intake can lead to reduction in average blood pressure.

Drug treatment for hypertension

The principal drugs used for the treatment of hypertension are diuretics and β-blockers. Other, newer agents include angiotensin-converting enzyme (ACE) inhibitors, calcium-channel blockers and α-blockers (Table 12.1).

Diuretics

Diuretics act on the kidney to increase urinary output and are used to reduce oedema in congestive heart failure, some kidney diseases and liver cirrhosis. Some diuretics are used to treat hypertension, and work by reducing oedema (if present) and peripheral resistance by dilating the peripheral arterioles. Diuretics are relatively inexpensive and effective treatments in older people.

> *Diuretics are usually the first-line drug to treat hypertension*

The benefits of reducing hypertension are partly negated by some adverse effects on risk of CHD, including increased likelihood of arrhythmia and increased plasma LDL-cholesterol concentrations. Nevertheless, the advantages gained by lowering blood pressure appear to outweigh these adverse effects in most patients. Diuretics are preferred in patients who have heart failure or peripheral vascular disease but are contraindicated if the patient has diabetes because they increase blood glucose levels. The main side-effect in men is impotence.

Table 12.1   Antihypertensive agents and their uses

Drug class	Example	Mechanisms	Recommended use	Contraindications
Diuretics	Thiazides (bendrofluazide, cyclopenthiazide)	Dilation of arterioles, mild diuretic effect, absorption of sodium ions from distal convoluted tubule	Uncomplicated hypertension with normal lipid profile	May precipitate gout, worsen glucose intolerance
	Loop diuretics (frusemide, bumetanide)	Dilation of arterioles, additional diuretic effect by absorption of sodium ions from the loop of Henle	Patients with cardiac or renal impairment	
β-Blockers	Oxprenolol, propranolol	Reduce force of cardiac contraction and production of renin	Patients with angina	Asthma, heart failure, peripheral vascular disease, diabetes
ACE inhibitors	Captopril, lisinopril, enalapril	Block conversion of angiotensin I to the more powerful vasoconstrictor angiotensin II	Patients with left ventricular hypertrophy	Renal artery stenosis
Calcium-channel blockers	Amlodipine, long-acting nifedipine	Arteriolar dilation, reduce force of cardiac contraction	Appropriate for most hypertensive patients, especially if diuretics or β-blockers are inappropriate	Bradycardia, headaches, flushing, oedema and constipation limit use in some patients
α-Blockers	Prazosin, doxazosin, terazosin	Vasodilatation	Appropriate for most hypertensive patients, especially if diuretics or β-blockers are inappropriate	Initial dose causes hypotension

Two main classes of diuretics are available, the **thiazide** diuretics and the **loop** diuretics. Thiazide diuretics block sodium absorption in the distal convoluted tubules of the kidney but the loop diuretics block the absorption of sodium ions from the loop of Henle portion of the nephrons. In addition to their transient effect on reduction in blood pressure by altering sodium and water excretion, diuretics act by dilating arterioles. The thiazide drugs have a longer duration of action and are not as strongly diuretic as the loop diuretics.

β-Blockers

> *β-Blockers are recommended for patients with angina*

The β-blockers lower blood pressure and reduce the heart rate and peripheral vascular response to stress. Experimental studies have shown that most β-blockers reduce atheroma formation in animals, despite their tendency to raise plasma triglyceride and decrease HDL-cholesterol levels. They also help to reduce anxiety levels.

The β-blockers are preferred drugs for patients with angina. They are not suitable for people with asthma, and are contraindicated for patients with heart failure or peripheral vascular disease.

Calcium-channel blockers

Calcium-channel blockers (antagonists) are used extensively in the treatment of angina and hypertension. They reduce blood pressure mainly by arteriolar dilation but also by reducing the force of cardiac contraction. The drugs affect the activity of the heart muscle cells by blocking the entry of calcium.

Calcium-channel blockers are suitable for most patients with hypertension, except those with heart failure

There has been some concern about the safety of calcium-channel blockers, but not all drugs in this class are alike. The long-acting dihydropyridine drugs (amlodipine, modified-release nifedipine) are generally safe and effective. They do not adversely affect blood lipid profiles and they have a weak diuretic effect. The main side-effects are flushing, headaches, constipation and oedema.

Although calcium-channel blockers are effective in controlling blood pressure in most hypertensive patients there are no clinical trial data to support the contention that therapy could prevent a first myocardial infarction. This question is being addressed in several ongoing clinical trials.

The ACE inhibitors

The ACE inhibitors are used in the treatment of hypertension and heart failure. They regulate blood pressure by reducing angiotensin II (a component of the renin–angiotensin system). They also appear to improve sensitivity to insulin and inhibit early processes in atheroma formation.

Renal artery stenosis: usually caused by atheroma in the aorta, occluding one of the renal arteries. This causes the affected kidney to become hypoxic, and the kidney shrinks in size. The response to reduced blood flow in the kidney is over-production of renin which, through the renin–angiotensin system, causes hypertension. The hypertension may be cured in the early stages by removal of the kidney. The unaffected kidney undergoes compensatory hypertrophy so that overall function is largely unaffected.

There is some uncertainty about the value of ACE inhibitors in patients who do not have abnormal left ventricular function. In the Survival and Ventricular Enlargement (SAVE) trial (1992) an ACE inhibitor (captopril) given to patients with left ventricular dysfunction after myocardial infarction led to a 19% reduction in mortality during 3.5 years of follow-up. Another post-infarction trial (CONSENSUS II, 1992) showed no benefit after 6 months, but not all the patient groups had left ventricular dysfunction. To date there is little information on the value of ACE inhibitors for the prevention of coronary events in people with hypertension. The question is being examined by the Captopril Prevention Project (CAPPP, 1990), but the results had not been reported at the time of writing.

The ACE inhibitors are generally safe and effective and are particularly appropriate for diabetic patients who have secondary nephropathy (therapy can reduce the degree of proteinuria). Side-effects include hypotension and cough. The drugs are contraindicated in patients with renal artery stenosis because their effect is to reduce renal blood flow further and to stimulate production of renin.

α-Blockers

The α-blockers (adrenergic antagonists) reduce hypertension by vasodilatation. Their advantages are that they do not adversely affect blood lipid profiles, improve insulin resistance and, unlike β-blockers, do not cause impotence. Side-effects include palpitations and marked hypotension, particularly after the first dose.

Management of hypertension

Antihypertensive treatment is beneficial at any age

There is now ample evidence that drug treatment of hypertension can reduce the frequency of complications such as myocardial infarction or stroke. Most clinical trials have evaluated treatment with diuretics and β-blockers and demonstrate that benefits are applicable to both younger (below 60 years) and older people (including those in their eighties). In general, reduction in blood pressure by anti-hypertensive therapy appears to have a greater effect on the incidence of stroke than on CHD. Diuretics seem to offer greater benefit, but β-blockers are probably more effective in preventing CHD.

The benefits are not always substantial. There is a problem in measuring just how great the benefit is, as it would be unethical to give placebo to people with moderate or severe hypertension. Consequently most of the trials compare one kind of treatment with another, or placebo is given only to people with mild hypertension.

One such trial, completed in the UK, was the MRC trial of hypertension (MRC, 1985; Figure 12.5). In this study 17 354 men and women aged 35–64 with mild hypertension (diastolic blood pressure 90–109 mmHg) were randomised to receive placebo, thiazide diuretic (bendrofluazide) or β-blocker (propranolol). Over 85 572 patient-years there were 60 strokes in the treated groups, compared with 109 in those receiving placebo, but there were no significant differences in CHD events. Using these data, it is estimated that if 850 mildly hypertensive patients are given antihypertensive drugs for 1 year, one stroke will be prevented.

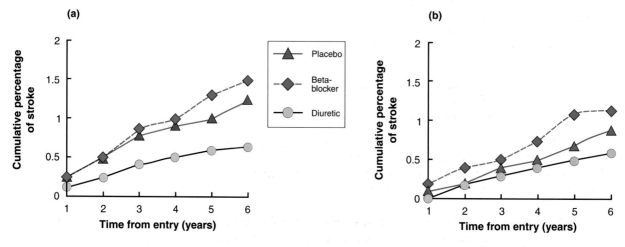

Figure 12.5 MRC mild hypertension trial: cumulative incidence of stroke in (a) men and (b) women aged 35–64 with mild hypertension. The incidence of stroke is reduced by administration of the thiazide diuretic bendrofluazide. The β-blocker propranolol had a less substantial effect. (Data from MRC, 1985.)

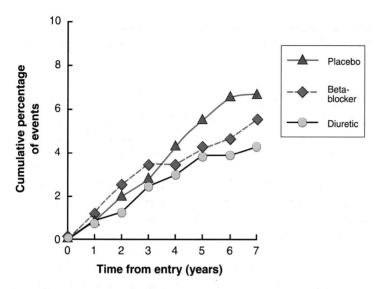

Figure 12.6 MRC older adult hypertension trial: cumulative percentage of patients who developed stroke. After 7 years of treatment the group receiving diuretics showed a significant reduction in risk of stroke. (Data from MRC, 1992.)

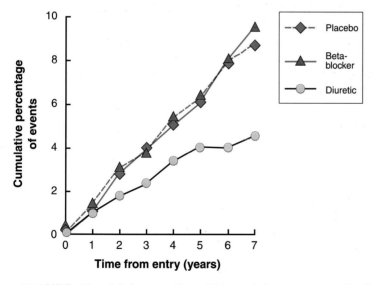

Figure 12.7 MRC older adult hypertension trial: cumulative percentage of patients who developed CHD. After 7 years of treatment the group receiving diuretics showed a significant reduction in risk of CHD events, compared with placebo. There was no advantage for β-blocker treatment. (Data from MRC, 1992.)

A later MRC study (MRC, 1992) was confined to 4396 older adults aged 65–74, who had diastolic blood pressure below 115 mmHg. They were randomised to receive placebo, thiazide diuretic and β-blocker (atenolol). Active treatment reduced the risk of stroke, particularly in non-smokers taking diuretics (Figure 12.6): the β-blocker had little impact on the incidence of CHD (Figure 12.7).

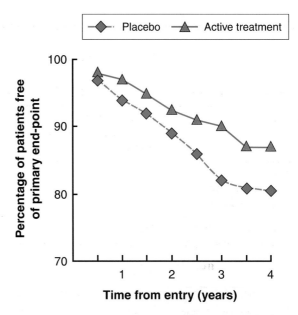

Figure 12.8 Primary end-points in the STOP-hypertension trial. In this Swedish trial of older patients (aged 70–84) with hypertension the proportion reaching a primary end-point (morbidity or mortality from stroke or CHD) was less in the active treatment group than in those receiving placebo. (Data from Dahlof *et al.*, 1991.)

In contrast, a Swedish trial of older patients with hypertension (STOP-hypertension; Dahlof *et al.*, 1991) showed reductions in all-cause and coronary deaths in those given diuretic or β-blocker treatment for mild hypertension (Figure 12.8).

Although all the studies indicate that there is some benefit to be gained by treating hypertension whatever the age of the patient, the largest gains will probably be seen in middle-aged people.

The British Hypertension Society has made recommendations about the appropriate blood pressure thresholds for pharmacological intervention (Table 12.2), assuming that all patients are advised on how to reduce hypertension by non-pharmacological means.

Traditionally, antihypertensive agents were given in a stepwise fashion, starting with a diuretic or β-blocker. If these agents fail to reduce hypertension substantially then further agents are added, such as diuretic and β-blocker and, failing this, by adding another vasodilator. A more logical approach is to tailor therapy to the individual patient profile, taking into account the patient's age, desire to remain sexually active (if male), presence or absence of angina, left ventricular hypertrophy, diabetes, asthma, gout or raised blood cholesterol concentration.

Table 12.2 Blood pressure thresholds for pharmacological intervention

Category	Treatment (in addition to non-drug intervention)
Malignant hypertension at any age	Treat with drugs
Severe hypertension	(diastolic blood pressure ≥110 mmHg) Repeat measurements and treat with drugs
Sustained diastolic blood pressure 100–109 mmHg, with evidence of target organ damage	Treat with drugs
Diastolic blood pressure 100–109 mmHg, no evidence of target organ damage	Observe weekly and treat with drugs if sustained. A downward trend obtained by non-drug treatment can be monitored monthly
Diastolic blood pressure 90–99 mmHg, with evidence of target organ damage	Treat with drugs
Diastolic blood pressure 90–99 mmHg, no evidence of target organ damage or diabetes	Treat with drugs if there are other risk factors (male, advanced age, smoker, raised blood cholesterol levels, strong family history of CHD)
Sustained systolic hypertension (>160 mmHg), irrespective of diastolic blood pressure in middle-aged and older people	Treat with drugs

Plasma cholesterol

Risk of stroke

The relationship between plasma cholesterol and stroke is complicated by the fact that cholesterol influences ischaemic stroke and haemorrhagic stroke in different ways. High plasma cholesterol levels could lead to atherosclerosis of the internal carotid artery and the larger cerebral arteries, increasing the likelihood of ischaemic stroke. Conversely, low plasma cholesterol levels are associated with haemorrhagic stroke. The mechanism of action is uncertain. It has been suggested that low cholesterol may contribute to the increased fragility of endothelial cell membranes, rendering them more susceptible to damage, although this hypothesis is by no means proven.

Risk of CHD

High blood cholesterol levels are associated with increased risk of cardiovascular disease. The relationship between plasma cholesterol concentration and mortality is curvilinear, with no clear cut-off point (Figure

12.9) and it is difficult to decide what levels of plasma cholesterol represent a risk. There are also concerns about the validity and application of cholesterol measurement because the lipoprotein system is very complex and cholesterol is just one of the many components that can influence atherogenesis. Estimation of relative HDL and LDL concentrations is much more informative (Table 12.3) but total cholesterol concentration is the lipid marker of greatest predictive value for eventual CHD outcome, and triglyceride concentration the poorest predictor (Pocock *et al*, 1989).

Table 12.3 Plasma lipoproteins and risk of CHD

	Concentration (mmol/l)		
	Desirable	**Borderline**	**Increased risk**
Total cholesterol	<5.2	5.2–6.4	>6.4
LDL-cholesterol	<4.0	4.0–5.0	>5.0
HDL-cholesterol	>1.0	0.9–1.0	<0.9
Triglyceride	<2.0	2.02.5	>2.5

LDL-cholesterol is not usually measured directly but calculated from total cholesterol, HDL-cholesterol and triglyceride concentrations.

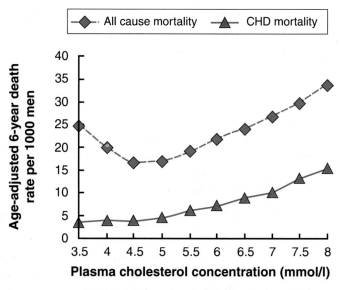

Figure 12.9 Correlation between plasma cholesterol and mortality from CHD compared with all-cause deaths. The risk of death from CHD and other causes increases with total plasma cholesterol concentration. The risk of all-cause mortality is a J-shaped curve, with increased risks at low and high cholesterol concentrations. At low levels excess deaths tend to be from haemorrhagic stroke, cancers, accidents, suicides and respiratory and benign liver disease. (Data from Martin, M. *et al*. (1986) *Lancet*, **ii**, 933–6.)

About 50% of deaths due to CHD occur in individuals with blood cholesterol concentrations greater than 6.5 mmol/l and it may be appropriate to target people above this cut-off point for intervention. If such a cut-off is chosen, the intervention necessary for most individuals will be alteration of lifestyle risk factors. Drug intervention is usually reserved for higher cut-offs (7.5 mmol/l, for example), and their use at lower entry levels is likely to be less beneficial in terms of efficacy, cost and prevalence of side-effects.

In the USA, the National Cholesterol Education Program has set a slightly lower cut-off point at 6.2 mmol/l. It is intended to screen all adults over the age of 20, and those with cholesterol levels above 6.2 mmol/l will be referred for further lipoprotein analysis, individual risk assessment and intervention. Extension of such a programme to the UK will have considerable cost and organisational implications. The mean blood cholesterol concentration in the UK population is higher than in the USA (about 6.3 mmol/l) and setting the same values for intervention would mean that most of those screened will require further investigation and follow-up.

Individuals who have very high blood cholesterol concentrations (in familial hypercholesterolaemia, for example) would undoubtedly benefit from cholesterol screening. However, screening of the whole population is probably not the most appropriate way of identifying this relatively small group of people. An alternative is to use more selective screening of a high-risk population ('high-risk' in this context means anyone with known symptoms of CHD or peripheral vascular disease, family history of coronary disease at a young age, obesity or diabetes). Although smokers are also at high risk, their inclusion would considerably increase the number of people who would be eligible for cholesterol measurement (Figure 12.10).

Outcomes of cholesterol screening

In theory, each 1% reduction in total plasma cholesterol should lead to a 2% reduction in the risk of death from CHD. In practice, this is not always the case, and some clinical trials of diet restriction and drug treatments have failed to show reductions in either CHD or all-cause mortality. There is evidence that obstructive fibrous plaques can be formed without obvious lipid infiltration and lowering the blood lipoprotein levels in these cases could not be expected to resolve this type of plaque.

The initial intervention in anyone found to have persistently raised blood cholesterol levels is dietary control: normally a patient will be re-assessed 3 months after diagnosis to see how well dietary control is working. Unfortunately, it is not always successful even with good compliance, and anyone who achieves a 20% reduction in cholesterol concentrations by non-drug interventions alone is doing extremely well. In most people (without familial hyperlipidaemia) a rigorous diet can reduce blood cholesterol by about 10%. With a more reasonable dietary regime (total fat less than 30% of energy) the fall in total plasma cholesterol may be only 2–3%.

Raised blood cholesterol is always initially managed by diet

Therefore, for many patients a decision has to be made whether to offer drug therapy. The decision to give lipid-lowering drugs is based on individual

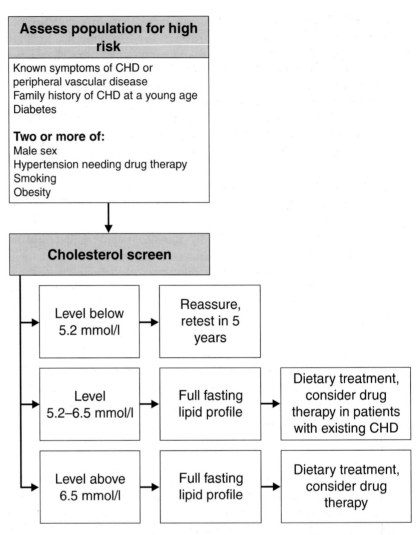

Figure 12.10 Strategy for cholesterol screening. A high-risk population for cholesterol screening can be identified on the basis of symptoms of CHD, a strong family history, diabetes or the presence of two or more risk factors such as male sex and obesity. Values below 5.5 mmol/l are below the 'safe' limit (it is still possible to develop CHD even with a low plasma cholesterol concentration, but reducing cholesterol further by diet or drugs is unlikely to be helpful). People who have cholesterol concentrations in the range 5.5–6.5 mmol/l should be recalled for a full lipid profile and, if confirmed, need to restrict their diet. People who have cholesterol concentrations above 6.5 mmol/l should be placed on a cholesterol-lowering diet and drug therapy considered if the elevation persists at re-assessment in 3 months. (Based on European Atherosclerosis Society guidelines.)

Lipid-lowering drugs are more likely to be given if cholesterol is persistently raised and other risk factors are present

merits, with intervention at different levels of cholesterol concentration, depending on any other risk factors or conditions present. The following guidelines are consistent with recommendations made by the American Heart Association and the European Atherosclerosis Society.

One priority group is people who already have coronary or peripheral vascular disease. The aim is to maintain total blood cholesterol below 5.2 mmol/l (with fasting triglycerides below 2.3 mmol/l and HDL-cholesterol above 1.0 mmol/l). A further priority are those with higher than average cholesterol concentrations (above 6.5 mmol/l) and multiple risk factors such as hypertension, diabetes, and smoking.

Patients with familial hypercholesterolaemia, diagnosed by the clinical signs of arcus xanthelasma or tendon xanthoma (see Chapter 20) will almost invariably require lipid-lowering drug therapy at some stage. Without treatment, men with the condition have a 50% risk, and women a 15% risk, of myocardial infarction by the age of 60. Systemic drug therapy is usually given to young men in late adolescence or their early twenties. Treatment can be delayed for a decade or so beyond this in women, but should be avoided in pregnancy and when breast-feeding.

Men with a high cholesterol concentration (>7.8 mmol/l) are likely to need drug therapy if dietary control has proved unsuccessful. Concentrations in this range are common in menopausal women and are often accompanied by high HDL-cholesterol levels but as HDL-cholesterol is protective simple dietary restriction may be adequate. An alternative for the menopausal woman who does not have a high HDL-cholesterol level is HRT.

Adoption of these guidelines in the UK would mean that 2–3% of the population would be taking lipid-lowering drugs. At present, the use of lipid-lowering drugs in the UK is much lower than France, Italy and the USA, which historically have experienced lower CHD mortality, or more dramatic reductions in mortality, than the UK.

Lipid-lowering drugs
Several categories of drugs will reduce blood cholesterol and triglyceride levels: ion-exchange resins, fibric acid derivatives, nicotinic acid, statins (HMG-CoA reductase inhibitors) and probucol. These drugs should always be used as an adjunct to dietary control. The choice of drug depends on the patient's lipid profile and tolerance of side-effects.

Ion-exchange resins
The ion-exchange resins (cholestyramine, colestipol) are recommended as first-line drug therapy for hypercholesterolaemia. They work by binding bile acids in the intestinal lumen so that they are excreted rather than returned to the liver for reprocessing. This drains the bile acid pool and stimulates new synthesis of bile acids from cholesterol in the liver. However, large doses are usually required and the side-effects of constipation, dyspepsia, and flatulence, as well as interference with the absorption of other drugs and nutrients are common. Although LDL-cholesterol levels can be reduced by about 15% the ion-exchange resins do not reduce plasma triglycerides.

▲ **Key points**

Target population for cholesterol screening

Symptomatic screening:
▲ All patients with known coronary artery or peripheral vascular disease

▲ All patients with diabetes

Asymptomatic screening (men and women aged 30–60 years):
▲ Patients with a family history of hyperlipidaemia or premature (<65 years) coronary artery or peripheral vascular disease

▲ Patients with clinical signs of hyperlipidaemia (arcus xanthelasma, tendon xanthoma)

▲ Patients with two or more risk factors: male gender, hypertension requiring drug treatment, smoking, obesity

Review question 1

Explain the limitations of dietary control alone in lowering plasma cholesterol levels in normal and hyperlipidaemic subjects

The statins block the endogenous synthesis of cholesterol

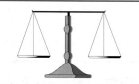

4S

Simvastatin vs. placebo

▲ 4444 patients on lipid-lowering diet with angina or previous myocardial infarction, and serum cholesterol 5.5–8.0 mmol/l

▲ Randomised to simvastatin or placebo

▲ Median follow-up 5.4 years

▲ Mean 25% reduction in total cholesterol, 35% reduction in LDL-cholesterol, and 8% rise in HDL in simvastatin group

▲ 12% of patients in placebo group died compared with 8% in group receiving simvastatin

Fibric acid derivatives

Fibric acid derivatives (bezafibrate, gemfibrozil, ciprofibrate, fenofibrate) are effective in lowering plasma triglycerides and are recommended as first-line drug treatment for hypertriglyceridaemia (familial, or associated with diabetes). Generally, they interfere with lipoprotein production and promote lipoprotein catabolism by activation of lipoprotein lipase. Some agents in this group (fenofibrate, for example) are also effective at reducing total plasma cholesterol concentrations.

Nicotinic acid

Nicotinic acid (niacin) and its derivatives (such as acipomox) lower plasma VLDL and LDL concentrations, but the precise mechanism of action is unknown. Complications include liver damage, which can occur at low doses, gastrointestinal symptoms and flushing.

Statins

The statins (lovastatin, pravastatin, simvastatin) inhibit hydroxymethylglutaryl coenzyme A reductase (HMG-CoA reductase) which is a rate-limiting enzyme in the cellular synthesis of cholesterol. These agents can produce very marked dose-dependent reductions in blood LDL-cholesterol levels of up to 30%, without adversely affecting HDL-cholesterol. Triglyceride levels are also reduced by up to 25%. Reductions of this order are not available with any other class of drugs or dietary intervention. The drugs appear to be well tolerated by patients and it is likely that their use will become much more widespread once their long-term safety has been confirmed.

Clinical trial data for these new drugs are only now becoming known. The first study to be completed was the Scandinavian Simvastatin Survival Study (4S; 1994) in which men and women who already had angina or a previous myocardial infarction were randomised to receive simvastatin or placebo. After 5 years of follow-up the drug was proven effective in producing beneficial changes in blood lipid profiles and reducing the risk of a non-fatal myocardial infarction or death from coronary heart disease. There was no difference in deaths from other causes, attesting to the safety of this class of drugs.

A further trial, conducted in the West of Scotland (Shepherd *et al.*, 1995), showed that the benefits of statin therapy are applicable to people who do not have overt CHD. The trial demonstrated that substantial reductions were obtainable in total and LDL-cholesterol levels, and that these were translated into reductions in the incidence of CHD (by about one-third) and the need for coronary angioplasty or bypass graft. The benefits became apparent after only 1 year of therapy, and were independent of baseline plasma cholesterol levels. This has led some observers to suggest that the current advice to consider using drugs when the total cholesterol concentration exceeds 6.5 mmol/l is too restrictive. It is possible that most healthy people with cholesterol concentrations above 5.5 mmol/l could benefit, particularly if they are male or have other CHD risk factors.

Although statins appear to have few significant side-effects they are expensive and, despite therapy, many subjects in the trials still suffered coronary events. Although a truly effective cholesterol-lowering drug is a welcome advance, too much reliance should not be placed on drug therapy in the absence of risk factor modification. Intuitively, drug therapy seems an odd way of going about the primary prevention of multifactorial diseases and taking cholesterol-lowering drugs does not make smoking or a high-fat diet acceptable.

Aspirin and primary prevention

Aspirin is an established therapy for the tertiary prevention of myocardial infarction in people who have already experienced angina or a heart attack. Meta-analysis of 31 clinical trials by the Antiplatelet Trialists' Collaboration (reported in 1994) indicated that the incidence of serious vascular complications could be reduced by up to 25%.

Relatively few studies have examined the effects of aspirin therapy for the *primary* prevention of coronary heart disease and stroke. In the Physician's Health Study conducted in the USA (1989), 22 071 men were randomised to receive 325 mg aspirin (11 037 men) or placebo (11 034) every other day for 5 years. There was a marked decrease in the incidence of first myocardial infarction (44% relative risk reduction) in the aspirin group but this was accompanied by increased risks of stroke, especially haemorrhagic stroke. The total number of deaths in the aspirin and control groups was very similar.

In the UK, a randomised clinical trial of 500 mg aspirin given daily to male British doctors showed no significant difference in the incidence of either CHD events or stroke compared with a group receiving placebo (Peto *et al.*, 1988).

Hormone therapy

Oral contraceptives

The original studies which examined the possible detrimental effects of the use of oral contraceptives showed that risks of stroke increased in some women, particularly those who had other risk factors such as smoking and hypertension. Following concerns about increased thrombosis and high blood pressure the amounts of oestrogen and progestogen in the formulations were substantially reduced. More recent epidemiological studies have examined the effects of the newer formulations and suggest that there is no association between use of oral contraceptives and risk of stroke.

HRT

Oestrogens exert their effect on the cardiovascular system primarily by influencing lipoprotein metabolism. As this is mainly regulated by the liver, oral HRT is likely to be more effective than the other routes of administration, which avoid first-pass liver metabolism.

Primary prevention with aspirin can prevent death from CHD, but this may be offset by increased risk of stroke

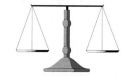

West of Scotland Study

Pravastatin vs. placebo

▲ Studied 5695 men aged 45–64 and mean plasma cholesterol 7.0 mmol/l

▲ None had previous infarction, 5% had stable angina at start of trial

▲ Randomised to receive pravastatin or placebo

▲ Mean follow-up 4.9 years

▲ Mean 20% reduction in total cholesterol, 26% reduction in LDL-cholesterol, 5% increase in HDL in treatment group

▲ Risk of death or non-fatal myocardial infarction reduced by 31%

▲ Need for coronary angioplasty reduced by 31% or coronary bypass graft by 37%

Oral HRT should reduce the risk of CHD

Oestrogen receptors are found in the blood vessel walls and unopposed HRT (without progestogens) can improve vascular tone and blood flow. Various mediators of vascular tone and platelet adhesiveness such as the thromboxanes and prostacyclins (see Figure 7.5) are also favourably influenced by oestrogen.

The actual value of HRT in reducing the risks of CHD and stroke is uncertain, mainly because there has been no major randomised control clinical trial of the currently available oral and parenteral preparations. Nevertheless, the less reliable case-control prospective studies largely favour a benefit of HRT on CHD risk although the effect on stroke is less marked. For example, in a prospective Nurses Health Study trial of 48 470 post-menopausal women (Stampfer *et al.*, 1991) the risk of CHD in those taking oestrogen was about half that of those who had never taken HRT, after adjusting for age and other risk factors. There was no change in the risk of stroke.

Strategies for screening

Targets for CHD

A multifactorial approach is needed to deal with a multifactorial disease

Many intervention studies have focused on reducing blood cholesterol levels. Unfortunately, estimation of blood cholesterol concentration alone is poorly predictive of CHD because of an overlap in the values of affected and unaffected people – those with relatively high blood cholesterol are often unaffected while it is possible to have low blood cholesterol levels and still develop CHD. In practice, most deaths from CHD occur in people who do not have strongly elevated blood cholesterol (Figure 12.11). Cholesterol screening is therefore an inexact tool, having high predictive value only when very high levels are detected (such as in familial hypercholesterolaemia).

Because CHD is multifactorial in nature (Figure 12.12), any intervention strategy must take into account other risk factors. It also should be directed at the whole population. This is an aim of the *Health of the Nation* strategy for reducing the number of deaths from CHD.

Targets for stroke

The *Health of the Nation* targets for stroke are, like those for CHD, set against a background of reducing mortality over the past two or three decades. This has probably been achieved by general improvements to lifestyles (diet, smoking and exercise), and increasing use of antihypertensive treatment. Further reductions could be expected to accrue by reinforcing the health education message about risk factors and by screening for hypertension.

Blood pressure can be lowered in some individuals by reducing salt consumption. It is calculated that the effect of lowering the mean blood pressure of the whole UK population by 5 mmHg would produce a 10% reduction in deaths from stroke. This should be easily achievable through attention to salt intake, body weight and alcohol consumption. The control of hypertension

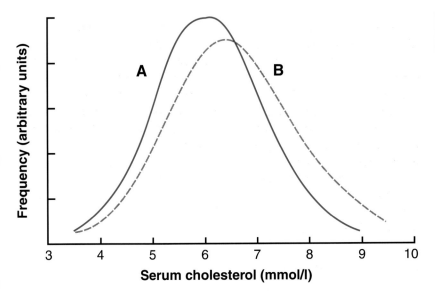

Figure 12. 11 The distribution of serum cholesterol concentrations in men who have had a major coronary event (B) overlaps the distribution in unaffected men (A). The mean cholesterol concentration in men who experienced a major coronary event was 6.5 mmol/l (SD 1.32), compared with a mean of 6.0 (SD 1.2) in unaffected men. Data from the British Regional Heart Study (Pocock *et al.*, 1989) are similar, but with slightly higher mean values for both groups. (Data from US Pooling Project (1978) *J. Chron. Dis.*, **31**, 201–306.)

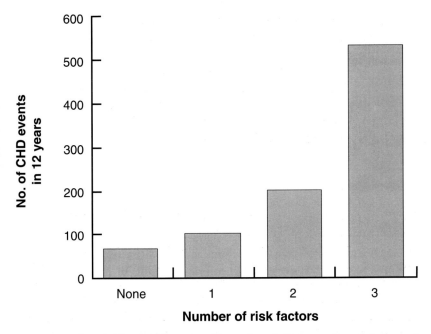

Figure 12.12 Correlation of CHD events with number of risk factors (serum cholesterol >6.5 mmol/l, hypertension, cigarette smoking). The risk of CHD events (myocardial infarction for example) increases with the number of risk factors present. (Data from Kennel, W.B. (1988) *Am. J. Cardiol.*, **62**.)

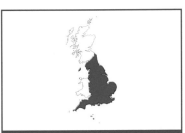

HEALTH OF THE NATION

Coronary heart disease

▲ Reduce CHD deaths in people under 65 years by at least 40% by year 2000 (from 58/100 000 in 1990)

▲ Reduce CHD deaths in people aged 65–74 by at least 30% by the year 2000 (from 899/100 000)

Smoking:

▲ Reduce smoking prevalence to 20% or less, by year 2000 (1990 prevalence 31% in men and 28% in women)

Diet and nutrition:

▲ Reduce energy derived from fat by at least 12% by the year 2005 (from 40% in 1990 to less than 35%)

▲ Reduce energy derived from saturated fats by at least 35% by 2005 (from 17% in 1990 to less than 11%)

Obesity:

▲ Reduce the proportion of obese people by at least 25% (men) and 33% (women) by year 2005 (from 8% of men and 12% of women in 1986/7)

Blood pressure:

▲ Reduce mean systolic blood pressure in adults by at least 5 mmHg, by year 2005

Alcohol:

▲ Reduce proportion of men drinking more than 21 units of alcohol a week from 28% (in 1990) to 18% by year 2005

▲ Reduce proportion of women drinking more than 14 units a week from 11% to 7% by 2005

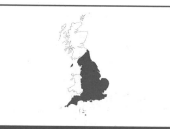

HEALTH OF THE NATION

Stroke

▲ Reduce the death rate for stroke in people under the age of 65 by at least 40% by the year 2000 (from 12.5 per 100 000 in 1990)

▲ Reduce the death rate for stroke in people aged 64–75 years by at least 40% by the year 2000 (from 259 per 100 000 population in 1990)

would be beneficial in preventing both haemorrhagic and non-haemorrhagic strokes.

The BMA has proposed a strategy for screening for CHD and stroke risk factors, in which health promotion programmes can be offered by general medical practices at different levels of intervention (bands 1–3), depending on the resources available.

Band 1

At the very least general practices should discourage smoking, by offering advice to people aged 15–74 years. Information about smoking habits should be collected opportunistically when the patient presents for other reasons.

Band 2

A second stage is aimed at reducing illness and deaths from hypertension, CHD and stroke. This entails regular measurement of blood pressure, carried out opportunistically on the target population (aged 15–74 years) who are not known to have raised blood pressure. A register should be maintained of patients with hypertension, CHD and stroke. Where appropriate, patients are managed by lifestyle intervention.

Band 3

The most intensive intervention involves primary prevention aimed at reducing the incidence of CHD and stroke. It requires the collection of information concerning smoking, family history, alcohol consumption and measurement of body mass index. Dietary habits and physical activity levels are also monitored so that lifestyle advice and other interventions can be offered as appropriate.

Evaluation of risk factor intervention in CHD and stroke

Health promotion activities are effective in modifying risk, but have little impact on morbidity and mortality

One of the first randomised control trials designed to evaluate the effectiveness of risk factor modification for the prevention of CHD deaths was the Multiple Risk Factor Intervention Trial (MRFIT, 1982). In this American study men deemed to be at high risk of CHD on the basis of smoking, hypertension and cholesterol risk factors (for example combination of 30 cigarettes a day, diastolic blood pressure above 95 mmHg, serum cholesterol above 7.6 mmol/l) were randomised to receive special intervention or usual care. Participants in the special intervention group were seen every four months by a team of nutritionists, nurses, physicians and general health counsellors. The initial aim was to reduce hypertension by means of weight reduction and, if necessary, medication. Subjects were encouraged to restrict their diet to less than 10% of calories from saturated fats, to reduce calorie intake if overweight, and to stop smoking.

The interventions were effective in reducing risk factors. About 50% of the intervention group gave up smoking, compared with 29% in the control group. Diastolic blood pressure was reduced by an average of 10.5 mmHg (7.3 mmHg in controls) and serum cholesterol levels were reduced by about 5% in the intervention group (3% in the control group). Despite this, there were no significant differences in deaths from CHD or other causes.

A problem with modification of risk factors is that the pathological process of atherosclerosis occurs early in life, and then takes many years to develop fully. A substantial time delay could be expected before any benefits accrue: in other words, modification probably should be initiated at an early age or should be maintained for a long period. It could be that the lack of impact on mortality shown in the MRFIT trial is simply because the intervention had not been carried out early or long enough. Delayed impact of risk factor modification has been reported in other trials. Some trials of cholesterol-lowering have shown an effect on CHD within 4 years but, universally, the effect is much greater when the treatment is given for a longer period of time. Similarly, some studies have shown early benefits from stopping smoking, but the full effect is not seen until many years later.

A second report of the MRFIT trial, after 10.5 years of follow-up, supports this view (MRFIT, 1990). In this, analysis of a subgroup of 8012 hypertensive men showed that death rate was markedly lower in the intervention group (15% lower for CHD and 11% for all causes). The effect was even greater for men who started in the trial with diastolic blood pressure of 100 mmHg or more – a 26% improvement in CHD mortality and 50% fewer deaths from all causes. The picture is complicated by an amendment that was made to the antihypertensive treatment protocol 5 years after randomisation in which hydrochlorothiazide was replaced by chlorthalidone, which may be more effective. Whatever the interpretation, long-term multifactor intervention, with the inclusion of specific drug treatment for hypertension, is undoubtedly beneficial.

One of the largest evaluations of general practice risk factor interventions conducted in the UK was the OXCHECK study (Imperial Cancer Research Fund, 1991, 1994, 1995). In this, patients on general practitioner registers were randomised into intervention and control groups. The intervention groups received regular health checks and advice from practice nurses. The intervention was effective in encouraging people to eat a better diet and take more exercise. Cholesterol concentrations fell by about 3% in the intervention group, and were sustained over 3 years. It is too soon to say what impact these results have on mortality.

Disappointingly, the study produced no reduction in smoking prevalence or alcohol consumption – the very factors likely to produce most benefit. The study consumed substantial resources and non-attendance was high, particularly by men. Women were much better attenders at the clinics and were more likely to comply with the interventions suggested (in the OXCHECK study the mean serum cholesterol concentration in the intervention group was 3.1% lower in men, and 4.5% lower in women). Paradoxically, in terms of

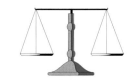

MRFIT

Special intervention vs. usual care

▲ Involved 12 866 men with high CHD risk (smokers, high blood pressure, high cholesterol levels), aged 35–57 years
▲ Randomised to receive dietary advice and risk factor counselling or usual community care
▲ Average follow-up 7 years
▲ Risk factor reduction greater in intervention group
▲ No significant differences in deaths from CHD or total mortality

potential years of life to be gained, it is men who stand to benefit most from risk factor intervention.

A cost analysis of the OXCHECK data indicates that universal screening and intervention strategies is an inefficient approach for reducing the burden of CHD and stroke. Probably the best approach would be to target patients who have raised blood pressure or a history of CHD.

ANSWERS TO REVIEW QUESTIONS

Question 1

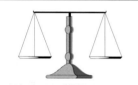

OXCHECK

Regular health checks and advice vs. single health check

▲ After randomisation, 2205 men and women aged 35–64 in intervention group and 1916 in control group

▲ Intervention group allocated to an initial health check and further checks annually or after 3 years

▲ Control group received initial health check only

▲ Outcome measures serum total cholesterol, blood pressure, BMI, smoking prevalence, self-reported dietary, exercise and alcohol habits

▲ Mean cholesterol concentration, dietary fat consumption, BMI, systolic and diastolic blood pressure lower in intervention group

▲ No significant differences in smoking or excessive alcohol use

▲ Conclusion: regular health checks promote dietary change and reduce cholesterol concentrations

Explain the limitations of dietary control alone in lowering plasma cholesterol levels in normal and hyperlipidaemic subjects

The main determinant of plasma cholesterol levels is genetic (see Chapter 20). It is possible to reduce plasma cholesterol levels by up to 20% in men with very high initial plasma concentrations, but this requires a severe dietary regime. A less strict diet, in which fat intake is confined to 30% or less of total calories, is probably more appropriate for people who are not markedly hyperlipidaemic: this can reduce cholesterol levels by up to 10% although reductions of up to 5% are more usual. High intakes of soluble fibre (in cereals, for example) can also reduce plasma cholesterol concentrations.

It is just as important to pay attention to the ratio of HDL-cholesterol and LDL-cholesterol. This can be favourably influenced by reducing saturated fats and switching (if they still have to be included) to polyunsaturates and monounsaturates.

High plasma cholesterol levels are not the only factor influencing atherosclerosis. There is also the contribution to endothelial injury by factors such as smoking and hypertension. Attention should therefore be given to other lifestyle risk factors in conjunction with dietary control.

References

Antiplatelet Trialists' Collaboration (1994) Collaborative overview of randomised trials of antiplatelet therapy. I. Prevention of death, myocardial infarction and stroke by prolonged antiplatelet therapy in various categories of patients. *BMJ*, **308**, 81–106.

The CAPPP Group (1990) The captopril prevention project: a prospective intervention trial of angiotensin-converting enzyme inhibitor in the treatment of hypertension. *J. Hypertens.*, **8**, 985–90.

The CONSENSUS II Study Group (1992) Effects of the early administration of enalapril on mortality of patients with acute myocardial infarction. *N. Engl. J. Med.*, **327**, 678–84.

Dahlof, B., Lindholm, L.H., Hansson, L. *et al.* (1991) Morbidity and mortality in the Swedish trial in old patients with hypertension (STOP-hypertension). *Lancet*, **338**, 1281–5.

Imperial Cancer Research Fund OXCHECK Study Group (1991) Prevalence of risk factors for heart disease in OXCHECK trial: implications for screening in primary care. *BMJ*, **302**, 1057–60.

Imperial Cancer Research Fund OXCHECK Study Group (1994) Effectiveness of health checks conducted by nurses in primary care: results of the OXCHECK study after one year. *BMJ*, **308**, 308–12.

Imperial Cancer Research Fund Study Group (1995) Effectiveness of health checks conducted by nurses in primary care: final results of the OXCHECK study. *BMJ*, **310**, 1099–1104.

MRC Working Party (1985). MRC trial of treatment of mild hypertension. *BMJ*, **291**, 97–104.

MRC Working Party (1992). Medical Research Council trial of treatment of hypertension in older adults: principal results. *BMJ*, **304**, 405–12.

Multiple Risk Factor Intervention Trial Research Group (1982) Multiple risk factor intervention trial. Risk factor changes and mortality results. *JAMA*, **248**, 1465–77.

Multiple Risk Factor Intervention Trial Research Group (1990) Mortality after 10.5 years for hypertensive participants in the multiple risk factor intervention trial. *Circulation*, **82**, 1617–28.

Peto, R., Gray, R. and Collins, R. (1988) Randomised trial of prophylactic daily aspirin in British male doctors. *BMJ*, **296**, 313–16.

Pocock, S.J. *et al*. (1989) Concentrations of high density lipoprotein cholesterol triglycerides, and total cholesterol in ischaemic heart disease. *BMJ*, **298**, 998–1002.

The SAVE Investigators (1992) Effects of captopril on mortality and morbidity in patients with left ventricular dysfunction after myocardial infarction. *N. Engl. J. Med.*, **327**, 669–77.

Scandinavian Simvastatin Survival Study Group (1994) Randomised trial of cholesterol lowering in 4444 patients with coronary heart disease: the Scandinavian Simvastatin Survival Study (45). *Lancet*, **344**, 1383–9.

Shepherd, J., Cobbe, S.M., Ford, I. *et al*. (1995) Prevention of coronary heart disease with pravastatin in men with hypercholesterolaemia. *N. Engl. J. Med.*, **333**, 1301–7.

Slovick, D.I. and Bulpitt, C.J. (1992) Hypertension: a guide to successful management. *Geriatric Med.*, **22**, (March), 59–63.

Stampfer, M.J., Colditz, G.A., Willett, W.C. *et al*. (1991) Post-menopausal estrogen therapy and cardiovascular disease: ten-year follow-up from the Nurses Health Study. *N. Engl. J. Med.*, **325**, 756–62.

Steering Committee of the Physicians Health Study Research Group (1989) Final report on the aspirin component of the ongoing Physicians Health Study. *N. Engl. J. Med.*, **321**, 129–35.

Further reading

Bronner, L.L., Kanter, D.S. and Manson, J.E. (1995) Primary prevention of stroke. *N. Engl. J. Med.*, **333**, 1392–1400.

Family Heart Study Group (1994) Randomised controlled trial evaluating cardiovascular screening and intervention in general practice: principal results of British family heart study. *BMJ*, **308**, 313–20.

General Medical Services Committee (1993) *The New Health Promotion Package*. BMA, London.

Kendall, M.J. and Horton, R.C. (1994) *Preventing Coronary Artery Disease*. Martin Dunitz, London.

McCormick, J.S. and Skrabanek, P. (1988) Coronary heart disease is not preventable by population interventions. *Lancet*, **ii**, 839–41.

Sever, P., Beevers, G., Bulpitt, C. *et al.* (1993) Management guidelines in essential hypertension: report of the second working party of the British Hypertension Society. *BMJ*, **306**, 983–7.

Smith, W.C.S., Kenicer, M.B., Davis, A.M., Evans, A.E. and Yarnell, J. (1989) Blood cholesterol: is population screening warranted in the UK? *Lancet*, **i**, 372–3.

Strandberg, T.E., Salomaa, V.V., Naukkarinen, V.A. *et al.* (1991) Long-term mortality after 5-year multifactorial primary prevention of cardiovascular disease in middle-aged men. *JAMA*, **266**, 1225–9.

Working Group of the Coronary Prevention Group and the British Heart Foundation (1991) An action plan for preventing coronary heart disease in primary care. *BMJ*, **303**, 748–50.

13 Understanding cancer

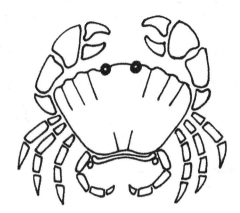

Cancer is the second most common cause of death in developed countries: particularly lung, colorectal and prostate cancers in men and breast, lung, colorectal, ovarian and cervical cancers in women.

The most frequently encountered cancer in either sex is skin cancer. Fortunately, most types are slow growing, do not spread to other parts of the body and can be successfully managed by local treatment, usually surgical excision or radiotherapy. Local control forms an important part of treatment of other cancers but eventual death is usually due to tumour spread to the lungs, liver, bones or brain. These metastatic deposits are often much more difficult to control and treatment must be instituted on a systemic basis.

The diagnosis of cancer is usually made from the clinical history together with imaging techniques such as radiography and ultrasonography and laboratory investigation (particularly cytology and histology). The prognosis depends on the size of the tumour and the degree of spread at presentation. This is ascertained by a staging system in which tumour size, degree of local spread and involvement of lymph nodes and other organs are evaluated. Tumour staging may require CT scanning or MRI, sometimes with guided needle biopsy of lymph nodes or secondary deposits. Occasionally accurate tumour staging is determined only after laparotomy.

Unfortunately, with many cancers symptoms do not develop until significant tumour spread has already taken place. The prognosis for these people is poor.

Pre-test

- **What is cancer?** Can you describe the fundamental changes which have taken place in cancer cells?
- **Who is likely to develop cancer?** Are there any genetic, geographical, socioeconomic, lifestyle or behavioural determinants of cancer?
- **When does cancer arise?** Does the incidence of cancer change with age? Do different types of cancer predominate in specific age groups?
- **How is cancer diagnosed?** Can you list some of the laboratory investigations and imaging methods commonly employed?
- **Can cancers be cured?** What methods are used in treatment?

Aims of this chapter

By the end of this chapter you will have increased your knowledge of:
◆ The known causes of cancer
◆ The pathological processes leading to cancer
◆ General approaches to diagnosis and treatment of cancer
In addition, this chapter will help you to:
◆ Describe the causative factors involved in the development of precancer and cancer and discuss the role of risk factors
◆ Describe the processes leading to cancer at the cellular level
◆ Describe the various kinds of cancer and discuss their distribution in different populations
◆ Describe the strategies available for diagnosing cancer and how prognosis can be determined
◆ Discuss the application and relative merits of the different approaches to treating cancer
◆ Understand the reasoning behind the *Health of the Nation* strategy for reducing deaths from cancer and discuss how targets can be met

Introduction

> *Cancer is the second most common cause of deaths in developed countries*

'Cancer' is a Latin word meaning 'crab'. The disease may be likened to a crab because of its tendency to spread out, just as a crab does with its four pairs of legs. A cancer is a new growth (**neoplasm** or **tumour**) which results from a continuous proliferation of abnormal cells. These have the capacity to invade and destroy other tissues and to spread to other parts of the body. Tumours with these characteristics are described as **malignant**, as distinct from **benign** (non-cancerous) tumours that grow only so far and then stop. **Oncology** describes the study of tumours.

Cancer is, after heart disease, responsible for most adult deaths. In Western countries the most common cancer is skin cancer, but fortunately this is rarely a cause of death (with the exception of malignant melanoma). In contrast, lung cancer is associated with very high mortality rates: in most European countries and in the USA lung cancer is the largest single cause of deaths in men due to cancer.

There are many causes of cancer, and these exert their effects on the cells in many different ways to produce a variety of changes. Cancer can arise from any type of cell and in any body tissue: it is not a single disease entity. Although there are common approaches to the treatment of cancer, not all types of cancer, or indeed patients, respond in exactly the same way.

> *Prevention of cancer is better than cure*

The most common cancers are caused by a combination of genetic, environmental and behavioural factors, although not all of these factors will be of the same relative importance in the development of cancer. For example, smoking is of fundamental importance in most cases of lung cancer, but not all smokers develop lung cancer, presumably because some have genetic protection. A genetic predisposition for cancer cannot be altered but many of the environmental or behavioural factors can. Perhaps two-thirds of all cancers are preventable: tobacco smoking alone is probably responsible for more than 30% of all deaths from cancer. For the foreseeable future, a preventive approach is likely to save more premature deaths than any treatment.

Concerted efforts are currently under way to reduce the deaths from cancer, most notably promulgated by the *Health of the Nation* strategy for health in the UK. Similar objectives have been set out by the American government in their pathfinder document *Healthy People 2000*. The number of deaths from cancer can be reduced only by the adoption of a range of approaches, with particular focus on preventing cancer and, when the disease does arise, by earlier diagnosis.

Some progress is being made: lung cancer is declining in the USA and the UK, although deaths from the disease are still rising in many other countries. Avoidance of excessive exposure to natural and artificial forms of UV radiation would have considerable impact on the frequency of skin cancers. Some dietary constituents are thought to promote a wide range of common cancers, including those of the stomach, breast, colon, rectum and prostate. Some of these cancers could possibly be avoided by limiting saturated fat intakes and increasing the consumption of fruit and vegetables, although the evidence for the effectiveness of such measures is presently inconclusive (see Chapter 7).

Unfortunately, not all the risk factors are known for some cancer types, or the risks we do know about cannot be modified. Therefore a secondary preventive measure is to try and identify the disease at an earlier stage, by the use of **screening**. In both the UK and USA asymptomatic women have been screened for cervical abnormalities for many years, and there is no doubt that this measure can reduce the number of deaths from invasive cervical cancer. More recently, screening for breast cancer has been introduced on a wide scale, and there is considerable interest in developing screening methods to cover many more cancers.

At present the treatments available for many kinds of cancer are imperfect and the goal of eradicating all the cancer cells is not always reached. Usually sufficient cancerous cells are removed to slow down substantially the progress of the disease, so that the expectation of survival is increased. Very often the survival gains are so great that the person dies of something else: in other words, a personal cancer cure has been achieved. However, with many cancers the patient will eventually succumb to the disease, even after treatment.

Anyone can develop cancer, regardless of age, place or occupation. However, there are factors that can influence the likelihood of developing some cancers. First, there is that unalterable factor, genetic constitution. Some cancers can be directly inherited (such as retinoblastoma and the precancerous condition familial adenomatous polyposis coli), but these are relatively rare. More commonly, a clustering of some cancers may be seen in families: the cancers are not inherited in a predictable way but more cases occur in the family than the law of averages would suggest. A notable example is breast cancer, which is more likely to occur in a woman if her mother, aunt or daughter is affected.

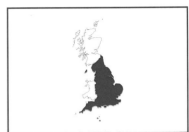

HEALTH OF THE NATION

Targets for cancer

▲ Reduce the death rate for lung cancer in people under the age of 75 by at least 30% in men and 15% in women by the year 2010 (from 60 per 100 000 men and 24.1 per 100 000 women in 1990)

▲ Reduce the death rate for breast cancer in the population invited for screening by at least 25% by the year 2000 (baseline 1990)

▲ Reduce the incidence of invasive cervical cancer by at least 20% by the year 2000

▲ Halt the year-on-year increase in the incidence of skin cancer by 2005

Genetic predisposition and damage by environmental factors are the causes of most cancers

Familial adenomatous polyposis coli: a rare condition of the colon which contains hundreds of polyps. Progression to colorectal cancer is inevitable.

Prognosis: prediction of the course of disease and likelihood of recovery.

Retinoblastoma: a rare cancer of the retina, usually in children below two years of age. Treatable by radiotherapy or in more advanced cases by removal of the eye.

Undoubtedly, most cancers appear as sporadic events, probably arising from the combination of genetic predisposition and exposure to factors in the environment.

In general the risk of cancer increases with age, although some types of cancer are more common in young people (see Chapter 9). There is also widespread geographical variation in the frequency of certain types of cancer, often reflecting differences in diet, smoking prevalence, alcohol consumption and other behavioural and lifestyle risk factors rather than geography itself (see Figure 1.6).

A small minority of cancers are caused by occupational exposure to precipitating agents. Examples are mesothelioma of the pleura and peritoneum and some lung cancers (see Chapter 14), which are caused by exposure to asbestos dust, particularly in combination with smoking. Workers in the aniline dye and rubber industries are at increased risk of bladder cancer because of exposure to benzidine and 2-naphthylamine. Other cancers can arise from exposure to vinyl chloride (in the plastics industry), arsenic, nickel and chromium (miners, chemical workers) and radioactive ores (miners).

In recent years the mortality rates from cancer have changed. A marked increase in deaths from lung cancer has been observed in men since about 1940 (somewhat later in women) but deaths from all the other types of cancer taken together have fallen slightly, mainly because of declines in the rates for cervical (recorded within the figures for uterine cancer), stomach and liver cancers. Slight increases in death rates continue to be recorded for prostate and, until very recently, breast cancers (see Figures 13.1 and 13.2 for American data: broadly similar trends have been observed in the UK).

Many cancers have low cure rates and therefore it is usual to express prognosis in terms of 5-year survival. The most common type of cancer is skin cancer, but this hardly figures in mortality statistics because skin cancers are generally very slow growing and very rarely spread to other parts of the body (malignant melanoma is a notorious exception). In addition, they are easily visible and readily accessible, so that treatment is sought early on. In contrast, cancers of the lung and pancreas are associated with very poor survival rates (Figure 13.3) because they are usually well advanced before any symptoms develop and their relative inaccessibility can make surgical intervention difficult.

Environmental factors in cancer

A variety of environmental agents can act in concert with a genetic predisposition to cause cancer. These agents include physical agents such as ionising and UV radiation, chemical agents and biological agents such as viruses.

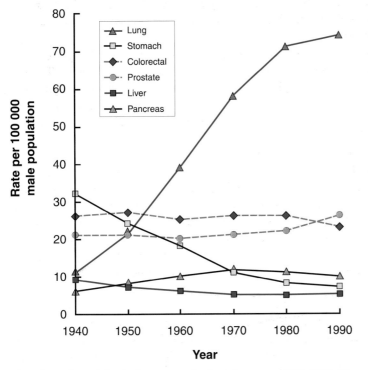

Figure 13.1 Age-adjusted deaths from cancer in American men, 1940–1990. The most striking trend is the increase in deaths from lung cancer. There has also been a moderate increase in deaths from prostate cancer; deaths from liver and stomach cancer have fallen in most developed countries but incidence of colorectal cancers has remained fairly constant. (Source: US National Center for Health Statistics.)

> ▲ **Key points**
>
> **Strategies for reducing deaths from cancer**
>
> ▲ Prevent the development of cancer by alterations to risk factors (primary prevention)
>
> ▲ Diagnose and treat the disease at an earlier stage in its development by the application of screening (secondary prevention)
>
> ▲ Improve treatments for cancer

Ankylosing spondylitis: a chronic inflammatory condition affecting fibrous tissue and ligaments of sacroiliac joints, spine and large joints.

Radon: a gas released from the breakdown of uranium in granite.

Radiation

A causative association between radiation and cancer has long been suspected and became evident when survivors of the Hiroshima and Nagasaki atomic bombs developed leukaemia. Excessive exposure to X-rays (a form of ionising radiation) can cause cancer: at one time a treatment for ankylosing spondylitis was intensive X-ray therapy, but many patients subsequently developed leukaemia.

Radiation can damage germ cells, causing a variety of birth defects. In the UK, an increased incidence of leukaemia was found in children whose fathers had worked at the Sellafield nuclear reprocessing plant, although there remains considerable controversy over whether radiation or other factors were responsible for causing the leukaemias (Chapter 5). Naturally occurring radiation is also harmful: high levels of radon are believed to cause some lung cancers. Ultraviolet radiation is responsible for a number of benign and malignant tumours of the skin, the most serious of which is malignant melanoma. Excessive exposure should be avoided and sunscreens used wherever possible.

> *Radiation causes genetic damage to both germ cells and mature body cells*

> *Radiation damage can be transmitted as a genetic mutation to the next generation*

Review question 1

Why have deaths from cervical cancer fallen? (see Figure 13.2: cervical cancer is included within the statistics for uterine cancer)

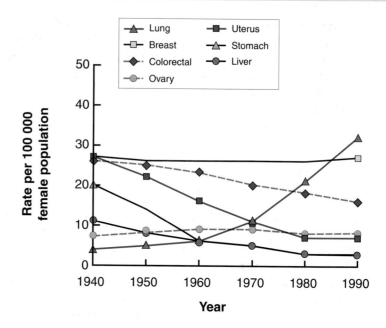

Figure 13.2 Age-adjusted deaths from cancer in American women, 1940–1988. The most common cause in the USA has been breast cancer. In some countries (including the USA) death rates from lung cancer are now higher. (Source: US National Center for Health Statistics.)

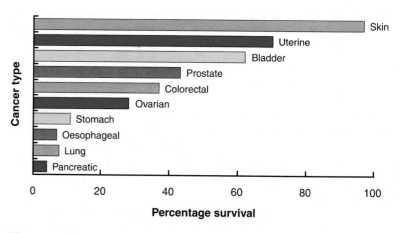

Figure 13.3 Five-year survival from cancers, England and Wales, 1981. Many cancers are well advanced by the time symptoms develop and survival is poor. Note: the skin cancer figure does not include malignant melanoma. (Data from Austoker, J. (1994) *BMJ*, **308**, 1415–20.)

Chemicals

Chemical agents can act as initiators and promoters of cancer

Environmental chemicals can behave as initiators or promoters of malignant change. The chemicals most strongly implicated are the polycyclic aromatic hydrocarbons, aromatic amines, aromatic nitro and *N*-nitroso compounds.

These may be encountered in a number of forms, as components of the air and our diet, and as occupational hazards. The classic example is the polycyclic aromatic hydrocarbon 3,4 benzpyrene, a product of incomplete combustion and present in cigarette smoke, soot, tar, oil, water and food. Well documented examples of occupational cancers include bladder cancers in workers in the aniline dye industries, skin cancers caused by arsenic used in sheep dip and mesothelioma, which is related to asbestos exposure.

Diet and cancer

There are a variety of components in the diet that are either carcinogens or tumour promoters, or act as protective agents against the development of cancer (see Chapter 7). N-nitroso compounds (for example dimethylnitrosamine) are highly potent animal carcinogens although their ability to induce cancer in humans has not been substantiated. They are present in the salty fish and pickled vegetables which are frequently consumed in the Chinese diet. Chinese populations have a particularly high incidence of oesophageal cancer, and a recent case-control study (Cheng *et al.*, 1992) suggests that consumption of pickled vegetables increases the risk for this type of cancer.

There is some concern about the safety of nitrates used in food preservation because they can be reduced by bacteria in the gut to nitrites, which can then react with secondary amines (found in a variety of foods) to produce N-nitroso compounds. The higher incidence of stomach cancer in Japan is believed to be linked to the diet, which includes a higher proportion of raw food and uncooked preserved foods – these often contain high amounts of nitrates.

The typical Western diet has fallen under suspicion because of the high frequency of some cancers, such as colorectal and breast cancer, in Europe and the USA. Western diets usually contain a high proportion of high-density foods rich in calories and often with a high saturated fat content. These diets are usually low in fibre compared with those generally consumed by people in parts of Asia, Africa and South America where the frequency of colorectal and breast cancers is lower. It is believed that the incidence of cancer could be reduced by limiting saturated fat and overall fat intake to about 30% of calories and avoiding obesity.

Some of the cellular damage leading to cancer is believed to be mediated by free radicals. Much of this damage could be prevented through the scavenging of free radicals by antioxidants in the diet. Foods rich in antioxidants (notably vitamins A, C and E) include whole grains, fruit and vegetables. Epidemiological studies have indicated that people who have low intakes of these antioxidant vitamins, have increased risks of some cancers (Chapter 7).

Alcohol is a significant factor in causing cancers of the mouth, throat, oesophagus and stomach, and can lead to the development of liver cancer in people who have alcoholic cirrhosis.

▲ **Key points**

Chemical carcinogens

▲ Polycyclic hydrocarbons (e.g. 3,4 benzpyrene): present in soot, tar, cooked foods, cigarette smoke

▲ N-nitroso compounds (e.g. dimethylnitrosamine): may be produced from nitrates used as food preservatives and amines in food

▲ Aromatic amines and azo dyes: can cause bladder cancer

▲ Plant products (aflatoxin): toxin produced in mouldy food contaminated with *Aspergillus flavus*

▲ Alkylating agents: developed for chemical warfare, now used as cytotoxic agents in cancer therapy

▲ Inorganic chemicals, e.g. arsenic, asbestos, nickel, cadmium

---

Mesothelioma: a cancer of the surface lining (pleura) of the lungs.

Smoking

The most common exposure to carcinogenic chemicals is by inhaling cigarette smoke

There is strong epidemiological and experimental evidence for a causative association between smoking and lung cancer. Smoking is also a contributory cause in cancers of the mouth, throat, bladder, cervix and pancreas. Agents in cigarette smoke act as tumour promoters which, in concert with other agents such as asbestos and alcohol, are capable of completing the cell transformation to malignancy. The most important measure anyone can take to avoid cancer is not to smoke.

More than 90% of lung cancers, causing 26 000 deaths a year in England alone, are directly attributable to smoking. The risk is related to the number of cigarettes smoked and benefits can be gained by cutting down or, better still, by ceasing altogether: after 5 years the risk of lung cancer in ex-smokers is much reduced and after 15 years the risk is similar to that of people who have never smoked.

Although there are encouraging signs that the prevalence of smoking is in decline it will be some time before these trends become evident as changes in deaths from lung (and other) cancer because of the long time lag (sometimes 20–40 years) between exposure to the aetiological agent and production of the disease.

Geographical variation in incidence of cancer

Cancer rates vary around the world, mostly reflecting differences in exposure to risk factors

The incidence of many cancers varies dramatically in different parts of the world. In Africa there is a high incidence of liver cancer, in China of nasopharyngeal cancer, in Australia there are more cases of malignant melanoma, and the UK and USA are notable for high rates of lung, breast and colorectal cancer. These variations could arise from differences in lifestyle and exposure to environmental risk factors or could reflect differences in genetic make-up; probably a combination of both. Migration studies (see Chapter 1) demonstrate that environmental factors play a very strong role in many cancers. The trend in migrant populations is towards the incidence rates of the host country, and children of migrants display an even closer correlation with the incidence rates of the host country.

Viruses and cancer

Viruses can cause cancer, but most common types of cancer show no evidence of viral infection

At one time viruses were believed to be a prime cause of human cancers. This is now known not to be true, but still a number of human cancers are associated with viruses. In some cases it is uncertain whether the virus is directly involved in the causation of the cancer, or whether the malignancy alters the host response, which allows infection by the virus; it may be that viruses act as tumour initiators or promoters, and cofactors are required to complete the transformation to malignancy.

DNA viruses

Among the DNA viruses, human papillomavirus (HPV), Epstein–Barr virus (EBV) and hepatitis B virus are most strongly implicated in certain human cancers.

Human papillomavirus

Infection with HPV is associated with a variety of benign and malignant tumours, usually of the skin or the genital tract. About 70 types of HPV have been identified, and some tumours are particularly associated with certain HPV types. Benign wart-like lesions of the female genital tract (condylomata acuminata) are associated with infection by HPV types 6 and 11. Cervical cancer, including the morphologically identifiable precancerous stages, is principally associated with HPV types 16 and 18 (see Chapter 16). These viruses may also be present in the normal female genital tract, and it is likely that other factors (such as cigarette smoking) are required to complete the transformation to cancer.

Epstein–Barr virus

This virus is implicated in Burkitt's lymphoma and nasopharyngeal carcinoma. Burkitt's lymphoma is most commonly seen in children in central Africa and in New Guinea. Antibodies to EBV are present in almost all cases of Burkitt's lymphoma. However, many cases of infection with EBV do not result in malignancy – it is believed that almost all adults have at some time been infected, without symptoms.

In some individuals infection with EBV results in infectious mononucleosis (a self-limiting disease affecting B lymphocytes). It is possible that in the regions of Africa where Burkitt's lymphoma is endemic, host immunity is compromised by concomitant malaria and that, rather than causing the benign B lymphocyte proliferation of infectious mononucleosis, uncontrolled replication of the virus in the host cells eventually causes them to mutate. With time further genetic abnormalities may develop, such as the chromosome 8:14 translocation that appears to be a consistent feature of the tumour (see p.397).

Nasopharyngeal carcinoma is common in some parts of China, Africa and the Arctic. There is a 100% correlation between this type of cancer and infection with EBV, strongly implicating the virus as a causative factor in the disease. However, the geographical distribution of nasopharyngeal carcinoma is much more restricted than that of the virus, suggesting that other genetic or environmental cofactors are involved.

Hepatitis B virus

Infection with HBV is associated with primary liver cancer (hepatocellular carcinoma). This cancer is more common in countries of the Far East and Africa. However, many individuals suffer only acute hepatitis as a result of infection, and many people are asymptomatic carriers of the virus. It is therefore likely that other environmental or dietary factors are needed for neoplastic transformation and that their influence is probably dependent on the immune system response to the original infection.

▲ Key points

Most frequent cancers world-wide

Males (% all types):

Lung	15.8
Stomach	12.6
Colorectal	8.8
Mouth/pharynx	7.9
Prostate	7.3
Oesophagus	6.2

Females (% all types):

Breast	18.4
Cervix	15.0
Colorectal	9.2
Stomach	8.4
Corpus uteri	4.8
Lung	4.7

Data from Muir, 1990.

Burkitt's lymphoma: A tumour of B lymphocytes, typically involving the jaw, orbit and abdominal organs.

DNA virus: a virus containing double-stranded DNA that (with the exception of poxviruses) replicates in the nucleus of the host cell.

Infectious mononucleosis, 'glandular fever': infection with Epstein–Barr virus causes lymph node enlargement, sore throat, fever, enlargement and proliferation of blood lymphocytes. Benign but follows an irregular course.

Nasopharyngeal carcinoma: cancer arising in the region behind the nose, above the level of the soft palate and in close proximity to the base of the skull. Treatment is by radiotherapy.

RNA viruses cause cancers in many species

Oncogenic: tumour-forming, especially malignant tumours.

RNA viruses

All the RNA viruses that are capable of causing cancer are retroviruses, so named because they contain reverse transcriptase, which allows the virus to convert its RNA into DNA (the normal sequence of events in the cell is transcription from DNA to RNA). The viral DNA can then become incorporated into the DNA of the host cell (see Figure 13.6). When this occurs the normal genes of the cell become disrupted. If the disrupted genes are involved in control of cell growth, this can cause the cell to become malignant. Only a few RNA viruses are implicated in human cancers but many are oncogenic in other species.

Human oncogenic retroviruses include the human T-cell leukaemia/lymphoma virus (HTLV) and human immunodeficiency virus (HIV): HTLV-I is associated with adult T-cell leukaemia/lymphoma, HTLV-II with hairy cell leukaemia, and HIV with AIDS-associated lymphoma.

Other infectious agents

Other infectious agents (such as bacteria and fungi) are not implicated in cancer. One exception is *Helicobacter pylori*, which is associated with stomach cancer and probably plays a role in the initial pathological stages (Chapter 19).

Review question 2

Assess the potential of reducing deaths from cancer or improving survival by the three main strategies of risk factor modification (primary prevention), screening (secondary prevention) and improved treatment. In the table opposite, use a scoring system for each type of cancer and strategy based on a scale of 1 (very little potential for improvement) to 5 (likely to produce a large improvement)

1. Give the historical picture, over the past 20 years

Cancer site	Primary prevention	Screening	Improved treatment
Lung			
Breast			
Colon/rectum			
Cervix			
Prostate			
Stomach			
Skin			

2. Assess the potential for improvement over the next decade

Cancer site	Primary prevention	Screening	Improved treatment
Lung			
Breast			
Colon/rectum			
Cervix			
Prostate			
Stomach			
Skin			

Review question 3

Why were the *Health of the Nation* objectives for cancer (see page 381) chosen and how might they be achieved?

▲ **Key points**

Cancer risk factors

Principal risk factors	Potential for prevention
Lung:	
Tobacco smoking	Do not smoke or give up smoking
Exposure to asbestos	Substitute with other materials
Exposure to radiation	Ventilation of buildings prevents build-up of radon
Stomach:	
Exposure to chemical carcinogens	Avoid foods preserved with nitrates
Infection with *H. pylori*	Antibiotic eradication of *H. pylori*
Breast:	
Hormonal influences	Attend screening
Cervical:	
Related to HPV infection and sexual transmission	Attend screening: use condoms with new partners
Increased incidence in smokers	Do not smoke
Colorectal:	
High-fat, low-fibre diet	Increase consumption of fruit and vegetables, decrease consumption of red meat and saturated fats
Mouth (including pharynx):	
Tobacco smoking and chewing, alcohol consumption	Do not smoke and avoid excessive alcohol consumption
Skin:	
Skin cancers and malignant melanoma: exposure to UV radiation	Avoid sunburn and use of sunbeds
Liver:	
Infection with HBV	Extend vaccination
Nasopharyngeal cancer and Burkitt's lymphoma:	
Infection with EBV	None
Kaposi's sarcoma:	
Infection with HIV	Avoid risk behaviours

Lymphoid tissue: organised as nodes along the course of lymphatic vessels, source of lymphocytes in the peripheral blood, eliminates toxic agents or foreign matter in the lymph fluid.

Reticuloendothelium: network of cells involved in blood cell formation and destruction, they also play a role in inflammation and immunity.

The pathology of cancer

Cancer can occur at any age. Generally, cancers become more frequent with increasing age. The cancers of childhood are likely to be leukaemias or sarcomas, whereas cancers in adults are more commonly carcinomas or lymphomas.

Terminology

The suffix **-oma** designates a benign or a malignant tumour. A prefix specifies the type of tissue or cell from which a tumour is derived. Nomenclature of malignant tumours also incorporates a designation of the cell type.

For example, the prefix adeno- refers to gland tissue, and fibro- to fibrous connective tissue. The terms **adenoma** and **fibroma** would describe benign tumours of glandular and fibrous tissues respectively. A mixed tumour containing the two components would be described as a **fibroadenoma**: a common benign tumour of the female breast.

A **carcinoma** is a malignant tumour of epithelial cells (any cell that lines an organ, body surface or passageway). This could be further elaborated as an **adenocarcinoma**, which would describe a malignant tumour of glandular epithelium (for example in the breast, uterus, prostate), or **squamous** cell carcinoma, which denotes a tumour derived from stratified epithelium (for example, skin).

Malignant tumours of connective and supportive tissues (for example bone, cartilage, nerves, blood vessels, muscle and fat) are described as **sarcomas**, with a prefix to describe the tissue site. **Osteosarcoma** would represent a malignant tumour of bone and **osteoma** its benign counterpart.

Lymphomas describe tumours which arise in the lymphoid tissues. Leukaemias are usually characterised by an over-production of immature blood cells. This type of malignancy usually involves the bone marrow, lymphatic and reticuloendothelial systems.

A further type of tumour is known as a **teratoma**. In contrast to the preceding tumours, teratomas contain more than one type of cell or tissue. Teratomas are usually derived from primitive germ cells in the gonads which have the potential to differentiate into any tissue type.

Malignant tumours contain genetically altered cells

'Cancer' refers to proliferation of malignant cells to form a tumour which invades adjacent tissues. In most cases the cells are attached to each other or surrounding tissues only loosely and so can easily spread to distant sites in the body via the blood and lymphatic circulations. The fundamental feature of malignant cells is that they are unresponsive to normal growth control mechanisms, and compared with normal cells, exhibit preferential and rapid growth. Cancer cells often perpetuate as a clone of cells because they fail to die by apoptosis (see Chapter 4). In all cases the transformation of cells to malignancy is caused by alterations to the DNA.

Cancer cells are invasive

Malignant tumours exhibit a number of characteristics that are not present in either normal cells or benign tumours, including their uncontrolled growth and propensity to invade surrounding tissues. Cancer cells produce proteolytic enzymes which facilitate their spread through the connective tissue by dissolving it. It is hoped that this property can be exploited by the use of drugs that will specifically inhibit these enzymes. One such drug, a metalloproteinase inhibitor called marimastat, has been found in preliminary trials to be effective against pancreatic and ovarian cancer. It will be some years yet before this class of drugs will become routinely available.

A tumour can develop its own blood supply by producing growth factors which stimulate the production of new blood vessels (this process is called **angiogenesis**). Occasionally a malignant tumour will grow so fast that it outstrips this blood supply and as a result becomes necrotic in the middle.

> *Cancer cells display uncontrolled growth and invade surrounding tissues*

Most cancers metastasise

Invasive cancers will eventually find their way into the blood or lymphatic circulation and are carried to other parts of the body where, after a dormant period, they resume their growth. This process is known as **metastasis**, and the new growths in other tissues are referred to as **secondary** deposits. The original site of the tumour is the **primary** site.

Another mode of spread is **seeding** of body cavities and surfaces: some cancers can penetrate the surface of an organ from within and extend into a cavity. The cells may then break away from the surface and become implanted on the surface of adjacent organs. The peritoneal cavity is most commonly involved by this process. Ovarian cancers spread in this way.

Some cancers appear to spread preferentially to particular organs. For example, breast cancers are most likely to metastasise to the lung, liver, bone and brain. Very often the first evidence that a cancer has begun to spread elsewhere is by enlargement of the adjacent lymph nodes. This is a very important prognostic indicator, and its assessment forms part of the examination of a patient who has cancer.

For reasons which are not understood some metastatic cancer cells may divide only a few times, forming a small nest of cells called a **micrometastasis**. These can remain dormant for many years but unfortunately will eventually grow again. An example is breast cancer; the primary tumour may be completely eradicated by surgery and the woman apparently be free of all disease, but overt metastases may become evident 20 years later.

> *Invading cancer cells may reach lymphatics and blood vessels and spread to other organs*

> **▲ Key points**
>
> **Properties of malignant cells**
>
> ▲ Altered genetic constitution, conversion of proto-oncogenes into oncogenes and loss or inactivation of tumour suppressor genes
>
> ▲ Loss of growth control
>
> ▲ Invasiveness
>
> ▲ Metastasis
>
> ▲ Poor differentiation
>
> ▲ Fatal if left untreated

Cancer cells grow uncontrollably

Cancer cells lose their specific functions (their **differentiation**) for the tissues from which they are derived and instead concentrate their activities into growth. Generally, the less differentiated the cells become the more aggressive the tumour and the worse the prognosis. The rate of growth also depends on the cell type and host factors such as the immune and nutritional state. The change

> *Cancer cells lose their specific functions, instead concentrating their activities into growth*

in cell function is accompanied by a change in appearance and staining properties, which can be assessed histologically (tumour **grading**).

With time many cancers become more aggressive

Poorly differentiated cancers are said to be **anaplastic**. One characteristic of malignant tumours is their heterogeneity. As the cells proliferate they become more susceptible to mutation and because the mutations are chance occurrences the tumour often contains a mixture of cells in various altered states.

Further genetic change usually gives rise to more aggressive growth patterns so that there is growth selection in favour of the more aberrant cell subpopulations.

The cancer process: neoplastic transformation

There are numerous staged events in the progress of a cell towards cancer

A cancer is the result of a cascade of alterations affecting DNA and the growth of cells. The cells have gone through the process of **neoplastic transformation** to produce a limited benign growth or an unlimited malignant growth. Neoplastic transformation is a multistage process (Figure 13.4), in which internal and external agents act sequentially to produce cellular changes of increasing severity. The multistage process towards malignancy has been demonstrated in animals and cultured normal cells lines by exposure to **carcinogens** (agents that can initiate cancer). The processes involved can occur over many years, and may be reversible until the stage in which the cancer cells become invasive.

The initial stage involves mutations to DNA on exposure to a carcinogen

The first part of the sequence is **initiation**, exposure to a chemical carcinogen or other agent such as a virus or radiation causes irreversible changes to the DNA. Only a single exposure to the initiating agent may be necessary. With time the initiated cells may die and be removed – or can persist in the tissues. This is much more likely if the cells become stimulated into repeated division, as would happen in tissues subjected to cyclical hormonal stimulation or in sites of tissue damage or inflammation. The result will be a larger clone of proliferated cells. At this stage no morphological changes can be detected in the cells.

The initiated cells may be exposed to and altered by another agent, such as a chemical or by exposure to radiation. This is known as the **promotion** stage. Promoters do not change the DNA but stimulate genes controlling growth and other functions (for example the proto-oncogenes) into abnormal expression. Exposure to the promoter must be repeated, perhaps over many years, for a permanent effect to occur. This has important health consequences. For example, cigarette smoke contains a variety of promoters but because the exposure needs to be repeated the damage may not be irreversible: the risk of lung cancer is dramatically lower in ex-smokers than in smokers.

The initiated cells proliferate and are further transformed by a promoting agent

The promoted cells may then proliferate into focal benign lesions such as polyps, papillomas or nodules. These lesions can regress and regain a normal appearance or may persist and exhibit further changes such as continued proliferation accompanied by changes in the size and shape of the cells and

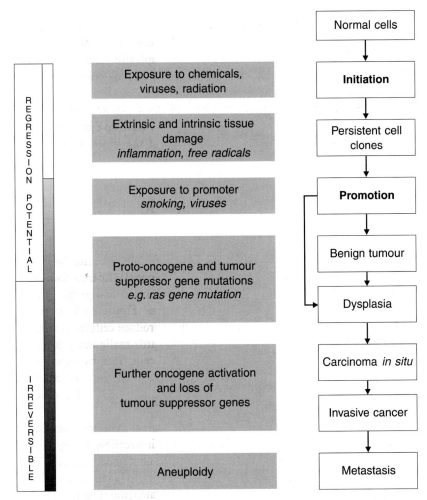

Figure 13.4 The multistage development of cancer. Cells undergo a series of changes before the final manifestation as invasive cancer. In the primary event (initiation) DNA mutations are caused by exposure to chemicals, viruses or radiation. Initiated cells are usually eliminated by apoptosis, but persist in some circumstances to be damaged by tumour promoters. At this stage the genetic damage probably involves activation of oncogenes or loss of tumour suppressor gene activity. The condition is still precancerous and some potential for regression to normal remains. Further genetic damage, by other agents, or persistence of the original agents is likely to result in progression, first to cancer *in situ* and then to invasive cancer. Metastatic tumour cells often show marked absence of differentiation and gross genetic changes (aneuploidy). Most benign tumours do not exhibit further change, and many cancers proceed from the cell promotion stage without entering a stable, morphologically identifiable benign stage.

their nuclei, known as **dysplasia**. Dysplastic changes are still potentially reversible but these lesions in certain sites will progress to malignancy, first as a preinvasive lesion (carcinoma *in situ*) and then to invasive cancer which has the potential for metastasis. Because of the possibility of its progression to

Mutation: a change in genetic structure. Can cause catastrophic alteration to cell function or have no effect at all, depending on where in the DNA the mutation takes place.

Promoted cells can form benign tumours or progress through further stages to invasive cancer

▲   Key points

Initiation of normal cells

▲ Requires single exposure to chemical carcinogen, virus or radiation

▲ Results in irreversible changes to DNA

▲ Initiated cells may persist or be removed

Clones of initiated cells are much more likely to become established in:

▲ Tissues in which normal cell turnover rates are high – gastrointestinal tract, skin

▲ Tissues subjected to cyclical hormonal influence

▲ Cells subjected to repeated trauma – those associated with inflammation

The most important genes in cancer development are oncogenes and tumour suppressor genes

cancer, dysplasia is regarded as a precancerous condition.

The progression of promoted cells through dysplastic change and ultimately into an invasive malignant tumour is poorly understood compared with the stages of initiation and promotion. Endogenous alterations to DNA probably occur, causing mutations to proto-oncogenes and tumour suppressor genes (growth-controlling genes: see p. 395). The alterations affect gene activity, and there is a failure to correct the defects during DNA repair. Eventually gross changes to the DNA take place, manifest as chromosomal deletions or even multiple copies of some chromosomes (referred to as aneuploidy). Aneuploidy is associated with a poor prognosis.

The neoplastic process can stop at any stage before invasive cancer is reached, and the tissue can regress to normal. Regression most probably occurs by the immune system eliminating the abnormal cells – this function is often referred to as **immune surveillance**. At various stages in neoplastic transformation the changes in DNA not only alter the way the cell behaves but also cause changes to the structure and composition of the cell. These changes may be recognised by cells of the immune system as 'foreign' and an immune response can be activated to eliminate them.

The integrity of the immune system is therefore an important factor in the development of cancer. If it becomes compromised in any way the neoplastic process may continue unchecked. Known states of immuno-deficiency are associated with increased risk of cancer, for example people on long-term immunosuppressive therapy are at risk of developing lymphoma and patients with AIDS develop an otherwise rare cancer known as Kaposi's sarcoma (see Chapter 25).

Another possible end-point of the neoplastic process is the production of benign tumours. These tumours grow slowly and then stop, without invading local tissues and metastasising. In most sites benign tumours stay that way, but occasionally become malignant. An example is adenoma of the large intestine, which may remain unaltered or may progress to colorectal cancer.

Benign tumours, even if they do not progress to malignancy, are not totally innocuous and can cause problems because of their size: for example, they can press against other tissue components and organs, perhaps blocking the blood supply or compressing nerves. The cells in benign tumours remain fully differentiated and are capable of performing the usual functions of the tissue in which they are in. If this happens to involve a cell which normally produces a hormone, excess hormone will be produced, often with profound physiological consequences.

The genetics of cancer

Most malignant tumours represent the clonal expansion of a cell type that has undergone genetic change in response to chemical, physical or biological agents. The changes involve the genes that normally regulate cell growth and development. Two major classes of genes are involved in the transformation of cells and progression of malignancy: cellular proto-oncogenes can become activated abnormally, causing over-expression of the gene product; tumour suppressor genes can lead to malignancy if they become inactivated for any reason. Proto-oncogenes act to accelerate cell proliferation, tumour suppressor genes act as a brake, slowing down the cycle of cell division.

Oncogenes and proto-oncogenes

Oncogenes were first discovered through work with retroviruses which cause cancer in animals. In some species (chickens, rodents, cats) cancer develops within weeks of exposure to the retrovirus. One of these viruses, the Rous sarcoma virus, was found to carry a specific gene which transforms normal cells into malignancy.

Proto-oncogenes have functions concerned with normal cell division and maturation

Similar genes are present in the normal cells of many species, including humans. The normal version of the gene is a **proto-oncogene**. Proto-oncogenes are expressed only at certain stages of the growth cycle, coding for growth factors, growth factor receptors and various nuclear proteins (Table 13.1). About 50 of these genes are known. They are also referred to as cellular proto-oncogenes (*c-onc*).

Oncogenes, or tumour-causing genes, result from aberrant expression of normal proto-oncogenes. In humans this can occur by mutation or by the translocation of other active genes to a site near the proto-oncogene. Both these processes can change the activity of the proto-oncogene so that the cell is stimulated into accelerated growth. In other species extra copies of proto-oncogenes or oncogenes can be introduced into the DNA of the host by retroviral infection.

Oncogenes stimulate the growth of cells along a pathway to malignancy

Table 13.1 Oncogenes: their products and association with human tumours

Oncogene	Product	Retrovirus	Human tumour (type of alteration)
src	Protein kinases	Rous sarcoma virus	None known
abl	Protein kinases	Abelson murine leukaemia virus	Chronic myeloid leukaemia (translocation and activation of undamaged proto-oncogene)
fes	Protein kinases	Feline sarcoma virus	Acute myeloid leukaemia (translocation)
erb-B	Protein kinases	Avian erythroblastosis virus	Squamous cell carcinoma cell lines (amplification)

GTP, guanosine triphosphate: an energy source used in the synthesis of DNA purine and pyrimidine bases.

Protein kinases: intracellular enzymes that add phosphate groups to other enzymes, activating or deactivating them. These alter the activity of genes in DNA.

neu (erb-B2)	Protein kinases		Breast cancer (amplification)
H-ras	GTP-binding proteins	Harvey murine sarcoma virus	Bladder, lung, colon carcinomas (point mutation)
K-ras	GTP-binding proteins	Kirsten murine sarcoma virus	Leukaemias, neuroblastoma (point mutation)
sis	Growth factors	Simian sarcoma? virus?	Breast cancer
myc	Nuclear proteins		Burkitt's lymphoma (translocation); anaplastic carcinomas (amplification)

Mechanisms of proto-oncogene activation

Human proto-oncogenes can be converted into active oncogenes by point mutation, chromosomal translocation or deletion of a regulatory gene.

Point mutation

Alteration to the genome, resulting in malignant transformation, can occur by point mutation. This involves alteration of a single base pair in a proto-oncogene, resulting in its aberrant activation as an oncogene. Point mutation of c-ras can result in human leukaemia.

Chromosomal translocation

Chromosomal translocation is a well known anomaly associated with a variety of myeloid and lymphoid tumours such as Burkitt's lymphoma and chronic myeloid leukaemia.

In Burkitt's lymphoma a balanced translocation occurs between chromosomes 8 and 14. Chromosome 8 contains the myc gene on its long arm; but this can become transferred to the long arm of chromosome 14 close to the gene for immunoglobulin heavy chain. The gain of genetic information on the long arm of chromosome 14 is balanced by the transfer of genetic material from chromosome 14 to chromosome 8. Normally the myc gene is active only at certain stages of the cell growth cycle, although the immunoglobulin genes are usually very active. When translocated, its new site imposes a high activity state on the myc gene. The result is aberrant expression of the myc gene product, a nuclear protein causing gene transcription. In the new site the myc gene behaves as an oncogene (Figure 13.5).

A balanced translocation also occurs in chronic myeloid leukaemia, between

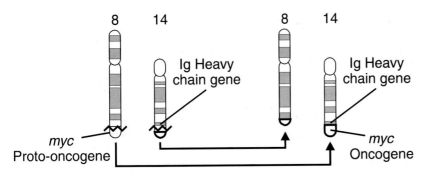

Figure 13.5 Chromosome 8:14 translocation in Burkitt's lymphoma. In Burkitt's lymphoma genetic material containing the *myc* gene is translocated from chromosome 8 to chromosome 14. The new site is close to the highly active gene for production of immunoglobulin heavy chain.

the long arms of chromosomes 9 and 22. The *abl* gene, coding for a tyrosine kinase, is translocated from chromosome 9 to chromosome 22, giving rise to the **Philadelphia chromosome**.

Trisomy

Some cancer cells have an extra copy of a chromosome. For example in chronic lymphocytic leukaemia an extra copy of chromosome 12 is present. This contains the *ras* gene, and the extra copy means excessive production of the *ras* gene product (GTP-binding protein). This stimulates cell proliferation: the extra *ras* gene has oncogenic potential.

Oncogenic retroviruses

Retroviruses have three of their own genes – ***gag, pol*** and ***env***. The *gag* gene codes for viral core protein, the *env* gene for envelope protein and the middle *pol* gene codes for reverse transcriptase, the enzyme used by the virus to make a DNA copy of its RNA. Some retroviruses, the **acute transforming retroviruses**, contain an additional gene that is similar to proto-oncogenes normally present in the DNA of birds and mammals. This additional gene was probably acquired in a previous incorporation of the virus into host DNA. During the process of incorporation the original proto-oncogene becomes mutated to an oncogene (Figure 13.6).

When the virus infects a new host cell it (and its oncogene) will be incorporated into the host DNA: the host cell now has an extra copy or copies of genes that cause uncontrolled growth (Figure 13.7). As these cancer-causing genes are carried within the viral genome they are called **viral oncogenes** or **v-oncs**.

Retroviruses can induce the neoplastic transformation of a host cell, even if they do not carry oncogenes, if the viral DNA is inserted near a normal host cell proto-oncogene. Because viral genes are usually highly active they can change the activity of adjacent genes in the host cell DNA (Figure 13.8). The

Balanced translocation: an exchange of genetic material from one chromosome to another, without loss of genetic material.

Philadelphia chromosome: a distinctive chromosome abnormality associated with chronic myeloid leukaemia, detectable in granulocyte, red cell and platelet precursors by standard cytogenetic methods.

Retroviruses have genes coding for core and envelope proteins and reverse transcriptase: gag, pol, env

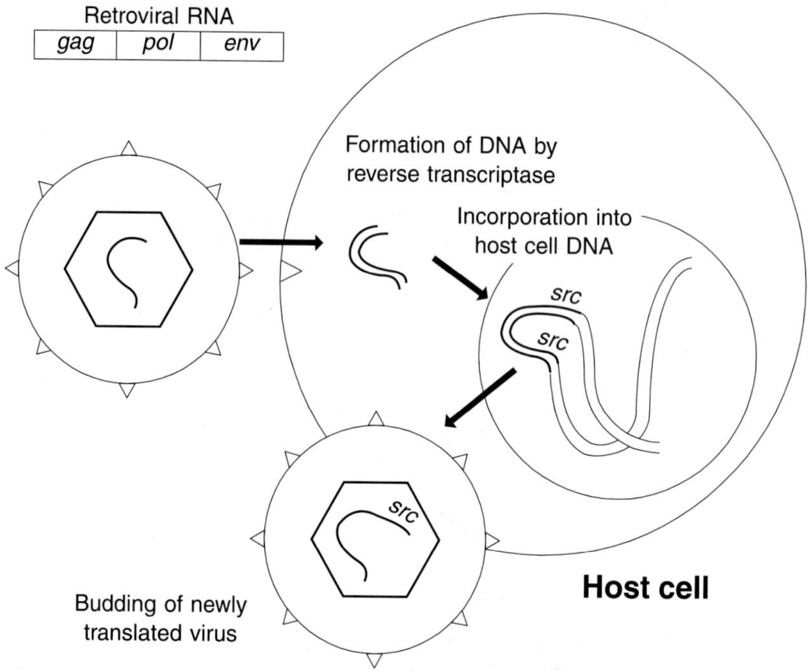

Figure 13.6 Acquisition of mammalian oncogene by retrovirus. Once inside the host cell a retrovirus makes a DNA copy of its RNA, using the enzyme reverse transcriptase. The viral DNA is then incorporated into the host cell's DNA. The virus uses host cell DNA and replicative machinery to produce new viral RNA. Viral core and envelope proteins are assembled and the completed viral particles are shed from the cell, available to infect more host cells. Occasionally, retroviral DNA becomes inserted into the host DNA adjacent to a proto-oncogene sequence (for example *c-src*). This will be replicated along with the viral sequences, and can become incorporated within the virus. By this means new virus particles consist of viral RNA and sequences 'stolen' from the host cell. During this process the 'stolen' sequences often become mutated.

sustained and abundant expression of normal proto-oncogenes can cause uncontrolled cell growth. This is believed to be the mechanism of action of the **slow transforming retroviruses**. Some of the viruses in this category cause leukaemia in rodents, and are also referred to as **chronic leukaemia viruses**.

Insertion of viral DNA into the host genome inevitably causes some structural damage to the host's DNA. Damage in the vicinity of proto-oncogenes can cause them to mutate to oncogenes.

Tumour suppressor genes

The loss or inactivation of tumour suppressor genes can lead to malignancy

Tumour suppressers have opposing effects to proto-oncogenes: proto-oncogenes act as cell accelerators, tumour suppressor genes apply the brakes on cell growth. Suppressor genes normally operate to inhibit tumour formation, so their loss or inactivation can cause uncontrolled growth and malignant change. Many tumours are associated with the loss of genetic material and many of these

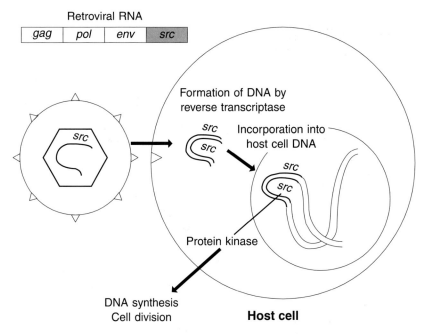

Figure 13.7 Incorporation of retroviral oncogene into host DNA. Some retroviruses can carry oncogenes into the cell. The mutated gene initiates production of a protein involved in control of cell growth. For example, incorporation of *src* will result in abnormal production of protein kinase, which can influence the rate of DNA synthesis and hence cell division.

deletions are consistent, the lost genetic material probably corresponding to tumour suppressor genes. Non-random allele losses have been reported in breast cancer (11p, 13q, 17p), colonic cancer (5q, 17p, 18q), osteosarcoma (18q) and a variety of other malignancies.

Tumour suppressor genes and retinoblastoma

Tumour suppressor genes were first identified in retinoblastoma. This tumour can be inherited or may arise sporadically. In both instances a gene on the long arm of chromosome 13 (the **Rb gene**) is mutated.

Like all genes there are two copies of the *Rb* gene, one on each chromosome. For the disease to occur both copies of the gene must be affected: the gene behaves as a recessive cancer gene. In the inherited form of the disease one copy of the gene is defective in the zygote. At this stage the retinal cells are functionally normal but there is a very high chance that the remaining normal gene will be damaged. Retinoblastoma usually develops by the time a child is 6 or 7 years old because the second gene copy in any one of the somatic retinal cells is lost or damaged. This has been described as the 'two-hit' mechanism of tumorigenesis: one 'hit' is inherited, the other is a chance occurrence. Only one cell needs to be damaged for it to develop into a cancer clone. Sporadic cases of the cancer are caused by both 'hits' occurring within a single somatic

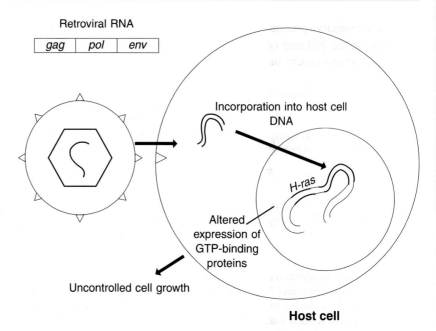

Figure 13.8 Retroviral activation of host cell proto-oncogenes. Integration of viral DNA sequences into host cell DNA can affect the activity of host proto-oncogenes. For example, excessive expression of *H-ras* could result in production of excessive GTP-binding protein, causing uncontrolled cell growth. Incorporation of viral sequences could cause structural alterations in adjacent host proto-oncogenes, resulting in their aberrant expression.

retinal cell.

Abnormalities of the *Rb* gene have been detected in other tumours, notably sarcomas, breast cancer, small-cell lung cancer and bladder cancer. Patients with familial retinoblastoma are at increased risk of developing osteosarcoma and other soft-tissue sarcomas.

Short arm deletion of chromosome 17: the *p53* gene

One of the most common deletions of genetic material in cancer cells is the loss of part of the short arm of chromosome 17, which corresponds to the position of the so-called *p53* gene. Loss of *p53* is associated with progression of a wide variety of tumours, including those found in the adrenal glands, bladder, brain, breast, cervix, gastrointestinal tract, liver, kidney, lungs, testes and bones. The *p53* gene codes for a phosphoprotein, normally present in the nucleus, with functions that include control of the cell cycle, DNA repair and synthesis, cell differentiation and programmed cell death (apoptosis; see Chapter 4).

Normally when cells sustain significant but non-lethal damage (for example by DNA-damaging chemicals or ionising radiation) they become committed to degeneration and death through the activities of *p53* and related genes. Inactivation of *p53* could lead to a proliferation of mutated cells, and a *p53*

> *Programmed cell death is a protective response that avoids the continuation of DNA mutations*

mutation is usually a precancerous event. For example, in colonic cancer point mutations in the *p53* gene typically arise during the transition from the benign precursor tumour (adenoma) to malignancy (Figure 13.9).

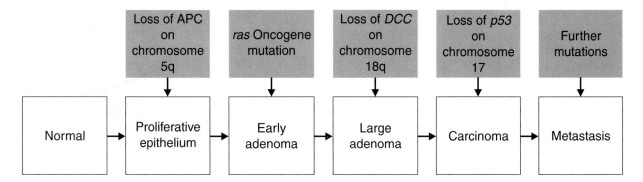

Figure 13.9 Genetic alterations in the development of colonic cancer. Most colonic cancers arise from adenomas. The initial change is a cellular proliferation caused by deletion of the *APC* tumour suppressor gene on chromosome 5q. Activation of the *ras* oncogene gives rise to adenoma. Further mutations to tumour suppressor genes follow, eventually resulting in invasive cancer with metastases.

The *bcl-2* 'survival' gene

Experimental evidence suggests that cells can escape from apoptosis and persist in the tissues, even when the *p53* gene remains intact. One of the genes that mediates this phenomenon is the *bcl-2* gene (or 'survival' gene). Expression of this gene has been observed in some human lymphomas, presumably enabling the tumour cells to adopt a 'death suppression' strategy.

Genetic alterations as a prognostic indicator

The amplification of cellular oncogenes and loss of tumour suppressor gene activity are predictors of the eventual outcome in several human cancers. Usually oncogene amplification is associated with the more aggressively growing cancers and hence holds a poorer prognosis. For example, up to 25% of primary breast cancers show amplification of the *c-myc* gene; these patients are more likely to have invasive cancer with metastases. Loss of *p53* activity correlates with shorter survival in patients with breast and lung cancer. This information can be of importance in treatment decisions: women with node-negative breast cancers but with *p53* mutations have a poorer prognosis and should be treated more aggressively (usually by adjuvant chemotherapy).

Symptoms of cancer

The early stages of cancer may have no symptoms whatsoever, although

Review question 4

Why are changes in proto-oncogenes and tumour suppressor genes of fundamental importance to the development of cancer?

metastases may have already occurred. In some cases the symptoms are so vague that the patient does not seek medical attention until the condition has reached an advanced stage. Fear of what might be found causes some patients to delay seeking attention. It is imperative that attention is sought at the earliest opportunity because the prognosis depends on how far the cancer has spread: the earlier a cancer is diagnosed and treated the greater the chance of cure.

If the cancer is on or near the surface of the body one of the most obvious signs of the disease is the appearance of a lump. Not all lumps are caused by cancer, for example only about one in ten lumps in the breast that are investigated turn out to be malignant.

General symptoms include weakness, breathlessness, loss of weight, bleeding or pain. Very often cancers come to attention because they obstruct a tract – colonic or rectal cancers cause disturbances in bowel function, prostate cancer causes urinary retention, lung cancer can cause persistent cough and bronchial infections. Some cancers can cause anaemia by chronic blood loss (lung and stomach for example) or profuse bleeding.

Pain is not the most common presenting feature of cancer but usually occurs later because the tumour presses on nerves, distends internal organs, or erodes bone.

Weight loss is associated with most cancers, particularly if the tumour has caused gastrointestinal obstruction. This may be reversed once the tumour is removed. Rapid weight loss is usually an ominous sign of advanced malignancy and almost always occurs in the later stages of disease. The terminal phase of the disease may be accompanied by pain and **cachexia** (the patient becomes wasted, weak and lethargic), which can be marked even when there is only a small tumour mass.

Diagnosis and staging of cancer

The diagnosis of cancer is based on a series of approaches which together lead to definitive identification of the disease. The methods include:

- Clinical examination
- Imaging methods
- Laboratory investigation

Clinical examination and imaging methods are primarily used to find a tumour and any metastases. Laboratory investigations are usually needed to determine the type of tumour.

Once a diagnosis of cancer has been made, the extent, or **stage**, of the disease must be determined. This is the means by which the best treatment and the likely prognosis for the patient are determined. Most cancers are staged according to the **TNM** classification (**t**umour, lymph **n**odes, **m**etastasis), which takes account of the degree of invasion into surrounding tissues, whether the lymph nodes are involved and whether metastatic spread to other organs has taken place. The stage categories have progressively more severe prognostic implications:

- Stage I – small local tumour
- Stage II – more extensive local tumour (locally invasive)
- Stage III – regional lymph node involvement
- Stage IV – with distant metastases

Very often staging procedures are carried out at the same time as, or form part of, the initial diagnostic investigation. The aim is to determine whether there is any metastatic spread to lymph nodes and organs such as the liver, lungs and bone.

Clinical examination

The diagnosis of cancer usually begins with a thorough clinical examination, which usually includes history taking, inspection and palpation. All accessible sites should be examined, especially the skin, neck, breasts, abdomen, testes and lymph nodes. Some cancers of the rectum and prostate can be felt with a finger (digital rectal examination), and a pelvic examination should be performed for suspected cancers of the cervix or body of the uterus.

Endoscopy

Tumours inside the body can be viewed with an endoscope provided they are on the inside surface of a hollow tract or on the external surface of an organ that is accessible through a small abdominal incision. The latter technique, known as **laparoscopy,** is useful for examination of the abdominal organs and pelvic structures (uterus, tubes and ovaries).

Rigid instruments are most commonly employed to examine accessible areas such as the bladder (cystoscopy), rectum (proctoscopy) and pharynx (pharyngoscopy). For more distant sites flexible fibreoptic instruments are employed. In the gastrointestinal tract, endoscopes can reach as far as the duodenum and (from the other direction) a colonoscope permits examination of the entire colon. The airways can be examined as far as the bronchial branches within the lungs. The vagina and cervix are easily accessible for examination. It is now possible to examine the kidney, ureter and bile duct with flexible instruments.

These instruments allow biopsy or therapeutic procedures to be directed through them. For example, snare diathermy of a gastrointestinal polyp can be completed through the endoscope, providing material for microscopic examination and (usually) providing adequate treatment for benign polyps.

> *Flexible fibreoptic instruments can be used to visualise the surfaces of hollow organs*

Endoscopy: a rigid or flexible fibreoptic instrument allows visualisation of the surfaces of a hollow organ. Instruments contain a central biopsy channel for removal of tissue and a lens at the tip that can be manipulated by remote control for forwards or sideways viewing. Video endoscopes replace the lens and fibreoptic bundle with an electronic sensor at the tip. The image is transmitted electronically to a video processor and displayed on a television monitor.

Imaging methods

Imaging methods are used in the diagnosis and staging of cancer, to monitor the effects of treatment and to guide biopsy and treatment procedures. The cheapest and simplest procedures are plain film radiography, contrast radiography (using barium for example) and ultrasonography. In most cases these are sufficient to arrive at the diagnosis, but more sophisticated methods may be needed for tumour staging. The common imaging methods used in diagnosis, staging and follow-up are:

- Chest and abdominal radiography
- Ultrasonography
- Radioisotope scanning
- Computed tomography (CT) scanning
- Magnetic resonance imaging (MRI)

Chest and abdominal radiography

A great deal of information can be obtained from a plain chest radiograph. Unless very small, most primary and metastatic lung tumours can be detected. Occasionally, however, the radiograph fails to show the full extent of the lesion and CT scanning is needed.

Plain abdominal radiographs are of little value and most investigations for suspected tumours use barium contrast agents. A **barium meal** is used in studies of the stomach and duodenum. Granules that will generate carbon dioxide are also given, providing a double contrast between air and the barium. A **barium enema** is used to provide radiographic images of the colon. The patient is first given laxatives to empty the colon. At the examination barium and air are introduced into the rectum by a catheter to provide a double-contrast view.

Ultrasonography

> *Ultrasonography is cheap, simple and safe*

Most people will be aware of the use of ultrasound in monitoring pregnancy. The transducer is applied to the abdominal surface with a contact gel and abdominal structures can be visualised, hence the method has some application for the detection of tumour masses. Ultrasound can be used to direct percutaneous needle biopsy. A further application in oncology is for monitoring response to treatment (between chemotherapy treatment cycles for example).

The organs accessible to ultrasonographic examination include the thyroid, heart, liver and spleen. Pelvic structures and the pancreas can be visualised if the bladder is well filled, although some structures may be obscured by gas in the bowel. The technique is particularly valuable in discriminating solid tissues from fluid-filled cysts. Ultrasound is poorly transmitted through air and is therefore unsuitable for examination of the lungs and gastrointestinal tract. The method cannot be used to investigate any structures underlying bone because all the sound is reflected back by the bone.

A variant of the technique using **Doppler ultrasound** can be used to detect changes in the frequency of sound waves caused by movement. Its main application is in assessing the presence and direction of blood flow. This can be helpful in discriminating liver metastases (with a relatively poor blood supply) from angioma.

Ultrasound transducers are small enough to be inserted into a body orifice or surgical incision. The nearer the transducer is to its target, the more precise the image obtained. **Transrectal** ultrasonography is used to evaluate enlargement of the prostate and **transvaginal** ultrasonography to evaluate

Angioma: a benign tumour of blood vessels.

Radioisotope, radionuclide: unstable radioactive material that emits radiation as it decays.

Ultrasonography: different tissue structures reflect or absorb high-frequency sound waves (ultrasound). The detection of the reflected sound, or echo, can give some indication of the nature and shape of the tissue that was in its path. Ultrasound waves are emitted and received by a transducer and the echoes are converted to a moving television image.

cervical and ovarian lesions.

Radioisotope scanning

The main application of radioisotope scanning is detection of early bone metastases. Bone metastases cause increases in blood flow and new bone formation which will appear as 'hot spots' on the bone scan when a technetium-labelled phosphate tracer is used (Fig. 13.10). Not all bone metastases show up well, particularly if blood flow is impaired or if the tumour is mainly osteolytic (bone dissolving). This is often the case with metastatic thyroid, kidney and colonic cancers, and multiple myeloma.

Radioisotope scanning uses a small-dose radioactive tracer to detect metastases

Multiple myeloma: a malignancy of plasma cells characterised by continuous synthesis of immunoglobulins; may be detectable in the urine as Bence–Jones protein. Most cases occur in people over 60.

(a)   (b)

(c)

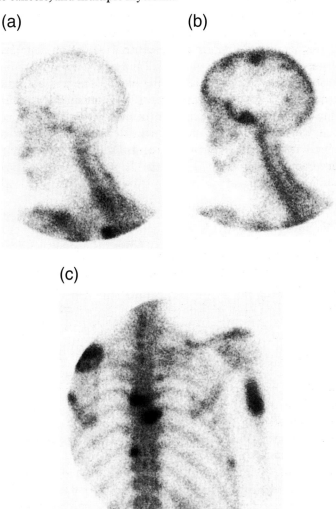

Fig 13.10 ^{99}Tc radionuclide scans. (a) Left lateral view of a normal skull. (b) Left lateral view of the skull of a 67-year old woman with adenocarcinoma of the oesophagus. Dense deposits indicate the presence of metastatic tumour. (c) Posterior view showing metastatic tumour in the spine and arm of a 55-year old woman with breast cancer.

Different isotopes can be employed in combination with other molecules, for example monoclonal antibodies, to target particular tumour types.

Computed tomography

CT scanning can be used to form an image from any part the body. The method is used for the detection of benign and malignant solid or cystic tumours, giving much more detail and sensitivity than conventional radiography. Specificity for distinguishing the type of tumour is relatively poor, and proper identification often depends on examination of a biopsy. Mapping by CT scanning is frequently used to ensure that biopsy tissue is taken from the right area.

CT investigations are time-consuming and expensive and expose the patient to a much higher radiation dose than conventional radiography. Interpretation of the images obtained depends on the skill and experience of the radiologist. Consequently the method is not a first-line investigation and, in oncology, is most frequently used as a staging procedure. It has an important role in the evaluation of tumours within the chest, particularly mediastinal masses which are very difficult to demonstrate by other means. It is also suited to the detection of retroperitoneal structures such as tumours of the kidneys, adrenals and associated lymph nodes.

Magnetic resonance imaging

The major advantage of MRI is that it does not employ ionising radiation, although resolution of small lesions may not be as good as with CT. It is extremely good at visualising soft-tissue tumours – MRI is at least as good as, and preferable to, using CT in these applications. The disadvantages are mainly related to the cost of the equipment and the long scanning times (30–40 minutes). These affect image quality because body movement is inevitable. Imaging of the gut is hampered because of the lack of a suitable contrast agent.

This technique is particularly valuable for imaging the central nervous system because of its ability to distinguish grey and white matter. It also provides good contrast between blood vessels and surrounding structures. Excellent detail of pelvic organs such as the bladder, prostate and uterus can be obtained.

Lymphography

Lymphography is used to identify primary and metastatic tumour deposits in the lymph nodes. Contrast material is injected into the lymphatics in the dorsum of the foot and drains to the pelvic, iliac and para-aortic lymph nodes which take on an opacified appearance under X-rays, especially if involved by tumour. The method is invasive and, with the availability of CT scanning and MRI, is now less frequently used. It remains useful for staging tumours in the pelvis because it yields fine anatomical detail (CT scanning shows only node enlargement). One advantage is that the contrast agent remains in the lymphatics for many months, allowing sequential examinations.

CT is primarily used for tumour staging

Computed tomography (CT) scanning: a radiological method in which a narrow beam of X-rays is scanned across the body in a linear fashion. Different tissues have different absorption characteristics, and unabsorbed X-rays are detected. Multiple absorption measurements are used to construct tomographic planes (slices) of the body by computer. A cross-sectional image can be displayed at any defined depth in different planes.

Radionuclide scan: a radioactive tracer is injected into the body and subsequent decay is detected by means of a gamma camera. The uptake of the tracer in the body depends on blood supply and biological activity.

MRI is used to evaluate soft-tissue tumours and tumours in the brain and spinal cord

Lymphography is used to provide radiographic images of the lymphatic system

▲ **Key points**

Imaging methods in oncology

Plain chest radiography:
▲ Can show primary tumours and metastases in lungs and bones
▲ Small lesions can be missed if obscured by rib cage

Barium contrast:
▲ Barium meal used to study stomach and duodenum
▲ Barium enema provides double contrast view of whole colon

Ultrasonography:
▲ Distinguishes between tumours and cysts
▲ Not suitable for examination of structures underlying bone or air-filled areas
▲ Useful for monitoring treatment response

Radioisotope bone scanning:
▲ Early indication of metastases

CT:
▲ Far superior to conventional radiography
▲ Staging procedure
▲ Useful for evaluation of chest and retroperitoneal tumours

MRI:
▲ Does not use ionising radiation
▲ Used for benign and malignant tumours in brain and spinal cord, soft-tissue tumours
▲ Evaluation of pelvic structures

Lymphography:
▲ Invasive, largely superseded by CT and MRI

Cytology: evaluation of cell structures using a microscope. Cells can be smeared or centrifuged onto a glass slide, fixed and stained with dyes with selective affinities for the cell nucleus and cytoplasm.

Histology: evaluation of complete tissues using a microscope. The overall architecture of cells and surrounding connective tissues can be seen. Tissues must be thinly sliced with a microtome before staining.

Magnetic resonance imaging (MRI): exploits inherent differences in the magnetic properties of tissues to provide a differential image. The source of the signal is the hydrogen atom, which is present in all the molecules of the body. When a patient is placed in a uniform magnetic field all the hydrogen nuclei are aligned in the direction of the magnetic field. A radio pulse is then applied, at a precise frequency which causes the hydrogen nuclei to resonate. The hydrogen nuclei continue to resonate for some time, giving up energy, before returning to their original positions. The time taken for the hydrogen nuclei to return to their original positions is called the relaxation time and the energy lost forms the basis of the MRI signal. Different tissues in the body display different relaxation times and signal intensities, depending on the amount of water they contain.

Laboratory investigations

Biopsy

Biochemical markers and imaging techniques play an invaluable role in identifying and determining the location of tumours but if any treatment is planned it will usually be necessary to sample some tumour cells and examine them under the microscope.

Modern techniques have greatly reduced the need for open surgical biopsy. Cells can now be sampled from virtually any part of the body through a thin flexible needle, guided by palpation, ultrasound and CT scanning or MRI. This permits accurate diagnosis of both primary and metastatic deposits and allows planning of the most appropriate therapeutic intervention.

In most cases the biopsy material will be subjected to microscopic evaluation, although cells and tissues can also be submitted for biochemical analysis of tumour markers (see p. 410). Laboratory methods for the microscopic examination of cells are **cytology** and **histology**; the difference lies in the nature of the cell sample received. By needle aspiration only loose cells are sampled, and structures such as connective tissues, lymphatics and blood vessels will not be present. Microscopic assessment will be confined to the cytological examination of the cells. Larger tissue biopsies offer the opportunity to determine the extent of tumour spread by histology.

Cytology

Cancer and precancerous changes in cells often cause changes in size and shape

Cancer and precancerous changes in cells are usually accompanied by some change in cellular morphology, visible under the microscope. Cytology is a relatively non-invasive and inexpensive way of obtaining a diagnosis. Cells are obtained for cytology by exfoliation or fine-needle aspiration.

Exfoliative cytology

In the normal process of epithelial renewal cells are continually removed from the surface as they degenerate and are replaced from below by cell division. This means that body fluids such as sputum and urine will usually contain some cells. When the epithelium contains a cancerous or pre-cancerous lesion these cells will also be sloughed into the body fluid. Exfoliative cytology is the microscopic examination of cells present in body fluid. With large volumes of fluid such as urine the fluid should be centrifuged or filtered in order to concentrate or isolate the cells. Urine and sputum cytology is useful for diagnosis of bladder and lung cancers. In some locations it is possible to directly brush or scrape cells from the surface epithelium. This is the method used for cervical screening (see Chapter 16).

Fine-needle aspiration cytology

This technique is commonly used in the preoperative assessment of breast lumps, lymph nodes, palpable abdominal masses, prostatic enlargement, thyroid tumours and other lesions in the neck. These sites are near to the body surface and thus easily accessible. However, with CT or MRI guidance almost any site in the body can be sampled. Guided needle aspiration is most often used to assess the nature of suspicious deposits in the lungs, liver, pancreas, bowel, kidney and mediastinum.

The procedure does not always require local anaesthesia, although it can be helpful, particularly when deeper lesions are to be assessed under CT guidance. Aseptic technique is of obvious importance. Normally cells are removed, smeared on to a slide, and fixed and stained for microscopic examination within minutes. If necessary, the procedure can be repeated without having to arrange another appointment.

Histology

Histology is the microscopic examination of cells and tissues

In most cases cytological diagnosis of cancer or precancer must be confirmed by histology. This allows assessment of the types of cells involved, their location and, in the case of cancer, the degree of local invasion.

A core of tissue for histology can be obtained using a wide-bore needle (a

> ▲ **Key points**
>
> ## Applications of fine-needle aspiration cytology
>
> | Tissue | Identifiable conditions |
> | --- | --- |
> | Breast | Fibroadenoma, cysts, malignancy |
> | Lymph nodes | Secondary carcinoma, reactive nodes, abscess and infections, Hodgkin's disease, non-Hodgkin's lymphoma |
> | Salivary glands | Infected or inflammatory, various tumours characterised by mucus production |
> | Thyroid gland | Inflammatory diseases and benign tumours, anaplastic carcinomas |
> | Prostate gland | Hyperplasia, inflammation, carcinoma |
> | Lungs | Inflammatory lesions, primary carcinoma, secondary tumour deposits |
> | Pancreas | Carcinoma, chronic pancreatitis |

Immunocytochemistry: a method of demonstrating cell components by the use of specific antibodies. Binding of antibody to its antigen can be visualised using fluorescent dyes or enzymatic marker systems.

In-situ **hybridisation:** a method of detecting specific DNA sequences in cells by the use of probes consisting of the complementary nucleotide sequence. Hybridisation of the probe to its target can be visualised by radionuclides or enzymatic marker systems.

'Trucut' needle for example). Originally this method was employed 'blind' to obtain liver and kidney biopsies, but with CT or MRI mapping the needle can be placed accurately: this increases the number of body sites that can be sampled.

Tissue may also be obtained using wire diathermy (a heated wire loop). This method is commonly used to excise cervical lesions and to remove polyps in the bowel.

Tissue can also be obtained through an open incision at operation. Although this is less frequently used as a primary diagnostic procedure, any tumour resected for treatment will automatically be submitted for histological assessment, mainly to ensure that all the tumour has been removed.

The histological technique is also used to demonstrate tumour markers (see below) within the cells themselves. This refinement, known as **immunocytochemistry**, is invaluable in determining the precise origin of tumour cells; sometimes the tissue of origin can be difficult to establish on morphological criteria alone, particularly if the cells are anaplastic. The most appropriate treatment, and determination of prognosis, is often dependent on accurate identification of tumour type.

Histological examination can also give some indication of tumour grade, which is helpful as a prognostic indicator. Generally tumour grade is estimated by morphological criteria such as alteration in cell size and shape and the number of mitoses (cells undergoing division) in the tumour mass. Markers of cell proliferative activity can be identified by immunocytochemical techniques.

It is possible to detect genetic alterations in the cells by a technique known as *in-situ* hybridisation. The detection of oncogene activation (for example *c-myc*) or tumour suppressor gene inactivation (for example *p53*) can be useful prognostic indicators in types of cancer. Both immunocytochemistry and *in-*

situ hybridisation can be employed on cytological preparations.

Tumour markers

Tumour markers are usually enzymes or hormones (Table 13.2): some malignant tumours produce proteins in such large quantities that there are measurable changes in their concentration in the blood. Not all tumours produce marker proteins. The more rare testicular cancers and choriocarcinomas produce relatively specific markers, but production of specific proteins by the more common tumours such as breast, lung and colorectal cancers is much more variable. In some circumstances the concentration of the marker in the blood correlates well with the size of the tumour.

The diagnostic application of many markers is limited by lack of specificity: some markers are produced by a range of both benign and malignant conditions as well as by normal tissues. Consequently the diagnostic application of tumour markers is limited. The most important application is in monitoring patients after treatment for evidence of recurrence (in patients whose tumours were known to produce markers). There is still a chance of cure even after recurrence of some testicular or ovarian germ cell tumours.

One important class of tumour markers is known as the onco-fetal antigens. These arise because cancer cells become less differentiated: they lose their tissue-specific functions and come to resemble fetal precursor cells; consequently they produce proteins that are more appropriate for fetal cells.

Occasionally cancer cells produce proteins that are inappropriate for their tissue of origin. Examples are small-cell bronchial cancers which produce ADH (antidiuretic hormone) or ACTH (adrenocorticotrophic hormone). These are referred to as ectopic hormones. Some cancer cells retain the characteristics of their tissue of origin, even when widely disseminated, and continue to elaborate a specific protein. Identification of protein can be a means of determining the origin of the cancer cells.

Table 13.2 Tumour markers and associated cancers

Tumour marker	Cancer type
Onco-fetal antigens:	
Carcino-embryonic antigen	Colorectal, breast, pancreas
α-fetoprotein	Germ cell tumours, primary liver cancer
CA-125	Ovarian cancer
Placental products:	
Human chorionic gonadotrophin	Choriocarcinoma, teratoma
Placental alkaline phosphatase	Ovarian cancer, testicular cancer (seminoma)
Ectopic hormones:	
ACTH, ADH	Small-cell carcinoma of bronchus
Calcitonin	Medullary carcinoma of thyroid

Tissue-specific antigens:	
Prostate-specific antigen	Prostate cancer
Thyroglobulin	Thyroid cancer
Enzymes:	
Alkaline phosphatase	Osteosarcoma
Prostatic acid phosphatase	Prostate cancer
Lactic dehydrogenase	Neuroblastoma

Haematology

A full blood count showing iron-deficient anaemia will arouse suspicion of bleeding. A common cause of rectal bleeding which may go unnoticed by the patient is colonic cancer. Widespread infiltration of the bone marrow by cancer becomes apparent in the presence of immature red and white blood cells in the blood (leukoerythroblastic anaemia). This is typical of advanced adenocarcinoma, such as might arise from the breast.

If bone marrow infiltration is suspected, **bone marrow aspiration** or **trephine** biopsy may be carried out as a staging procedure. Bone marrow aspiration provides a marrow smear for microscopic examination of the blood-forming cells. Cell types can be identified on the basis of their morphology but immunological markers can also be used for definitive cell typing. Bone marrow aspiration is used in the diagnosis of leukaemia: acute leukaemia usually causes increased cellularity and large numbers of abnormal lymphoid or myeloid precursor (blast) cells; chronic myeloid leukaemia causes an increase in myeloid precursors. A trephine provides a solid core of tissue suitable for histological examination of the overall architecture. This procedure may be used to evaluate bone marrow infiltration in a variety of cancers, particularly Hodgkin's disease and other lymphomas.

Liver enzymes

Liver enzymes may be estimated to support a clinical suspicion of liver metastases. Tumour involvement can cause, for example, raised blood levels of alkaline phosphatase. The measurement of liver enzymes in blood for evaluation of liver metastases has now largely been superseded by imaging methods, particularly ultrasonography.

Treatment of cancer

Can cancer be cured?

The ability to cure cancer depends on the type of tumour and how far it has spread (tumour stage). Some cancers are extremely slow-growing and are readily treated but other types behave very aggressively and always produce metastases. There is individual variation in how quickly a cancer progresses.

Acute leukaemia: characterised by very immature stem cells.

Blast cell, stem cell: a precursor cell with the capacity for replication and differentiation.

Chronic leukaemia: the stem cells have progressed further along their pathways of differentiation and maturation.

Lymphocytic leukaemia: arises from the precursors for the lymphocytes.

Myeloid leukaemia: arises from myeloid cell lines responsible for the production of blood cells except lymphocytes.

Review question 5

Which features of tumour pathology are helpful as prognostic indicators?

The most important cause of deaths from cancer is metastatic spread

Generally, the more advanced the cancer, the more aggressive the treatment needs to be. Sometimes very aggressive treatments will be given at an early stage in an attempt to achieve a pre-emptive 'knock-out'. With some exceptions (basal cell carcinoma of the skin for example), many cancer treatments do not achieve 100% cure – it is more usual to assess treatment effectiveness in terms of 5- or 10-year survival. For many people the aim will be to achieve a personal cure. This recognises that it is almost impossible to eradicate every single cancer cell in the body, and eventually the condition will recur. As most symptomatic cancers are seen in older people, the treated patient may die of another cause before the cancer recurs. After all, no one is immortal although, paradoxically, cultured cancer cells display every appearance of being just that.

The principal approaches to treatment of cancer are surgery, radiotherapy and chemotherapy. Other approaches have been tried, or are in development, but their use is currently confined to research protocols and clinical trials.

Surgery

Modern treatments for cancer are based on a two-pronged approach: local control coupled with systemic therapy

For many years the treatment of cancer was based on the premise that cancers spread radially, first by tissue invasion, then to the lymph nodes and then to other parts of the body. Surgical resections included wide margins of normal tissues and lymph nodes because these were deemed to be at risk of tumour invasion. For example, breast cancers were routinely treated by radical mastectomy (removal of the whole breast together with pectoral muscles and axillary lymph nodes).

It is now recognised that extensive surgical procedures are not always necessary. By the time of surgery, tumour cells may already have spread to other parts of the body, producing very small, but undetectable, metastatic deposits (micrometastases). It would be impossible to excise all tissue that could become involved by tumour and the principle of treatment is to use a combination of local and systemic control. Surgery and radiotherapy are used to treat the primary tumour and local lymph nodes, and systemic therapies (such as cytotoxic drugs) are used to counter metastases.

Occasionally a cancer may be so advanced that complete removal by surgery is impossible for functional or cosmetic reasons. In this circumstance as much tumour as possible is removed by surgery, and the remainder is treated with radiotherapy or systemic agents. In advanced tumours with obvious metastases treatment is aimed at palliation rather than cure – this might still involve surgery to reduce the tumour bulk or to relieve obstruction.

Radiotherapy

About half of all patients in Western countries with cancer are treated with radiotherapy

Radiotherapy may be used as the principal means of local control, or as an adjunct to surgery. It is also used for palliative pain relief in people with metastatic cancer.

Types of radiotherapy

Radiotherapy is employed externally (**external beam therapy**) or internally (**brachytherapy**) by placing radioactive implants inside or immediately adjacent to the tumour area. The two approaches can be combined – combination is the treatment of choice for advanced cervical cancer. Brachytherapy alone is sometimes used to treat inoperable tumours of the tongue and floor of the mouth; similarly, radioactive wires or needles can be inserted into lymph nodes or a breast lump.

Principles of radiotherapy

All radiotherapy relies on the use of ionising radiation, which is destructive to tissues – X-rays and γ rays produce breaks in the DNA of both healthy and malignant cells. Single-strand breaks are of little consequence because they can easily be repaired using the undamaged complementary strand as a template; however, if breaks occur in both strands the template is lost, the DNA cannot be repaired, the cell cannot replicate and dies.

The effects of radiotherapy are seen more quickly in sites of rapid cell turnover. Unfortunately this means that normal cells in sites of rapid turnover are also susceptible to radiotherapy, producing unpleasant side-effects such as gastrointestinal disturbance and anaemia.

During radiotherapy normal cells will inevitably be killed along with the tumour cells. Normal cells often recover faster than tumour cells, and this difference can be exploited by separating the treatment into a series of small doses (Figure 13.11) to allow for normal tissue recovery; this is called **fractionation**. Each dose is calculated to kill half the remaining tumour cells.

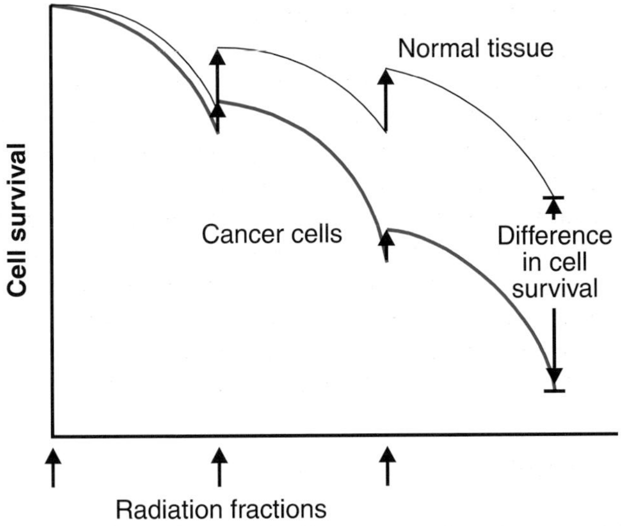

External beam radiotherapy: uses X-rays from a linear accelerator or γ rays produced by radio-cobalt units. Linear accelerators produce a more precise beam, and may produce electrons which are better for treating more superficial tumours of the skin. The X-ray doses are unlike those delivered by conventional diagnostic radiography, being about half a million times greater.

Radioactive implants, brachytherapy: used to deliver high doses of radiation locally, either by inserting needles directly into the tumour or by placing the radioactive source into a body cavity close to the tumour area. Radioactive sources are encapsulated in applicators, or embedded in tissues as wires or needles.

Figure 13.11 Dose fractionation in radiotherapy. Dose fractionation exploits differences in the recovery capacities of normal tissues and cancer cells. A large cumulative dose can be used if it is split into a series of smaller doses, achieving a greater cell kill in the tumour with relative sparing of normal tissues.

Astrocytoma: the most common primary malignancy in the brain, arising from astrocytes, the supporting 'connective tissue' cells.

Seminoma: arises from testicular germ cells and comprises about 40% of testicular cancers. About 10% of patients have a history of undescended testis.

It is important to continue radiotherapy until the tumour is totally eradicated: there is a high chance of tumour recurrence even if only a few cells remain. The progress of tumour shrinkage during a course of radiotherapy can be monitored by various imaging techniques (e.g. ultrasonography) and, if appropriate, by the disappearance of tumour marker.

Cancer cells vary in their radiosensitivity depending on their tissue of origin: a relatively low dose of 25 Gy may be adequate to control a seminoma whereas doses of over 70 Gy are needed to control an astrocytoma of similar size.

Curative radiotherapy

Radiotherapy is the treatment of choice for some types of cancer (examples are basal cell and squamous cell carcinomas of the skin). In these, radiotherapy yields better cosmetic results than surgery and has comparable (nearly 100%) 5-year survival rates.

Radiotherapy is also successful as the sole treatment in some cancers of the larynx and nasopharynx, Hodgkin's disease, bladder cancer, early prostate cancer, cancer of the anus, early lung cancer, some brain tumours and thyroid cancer. Cancers of the nasopharynx and the posterior tongue are treated in this way because they are inappropriate for surgery. In cancer of the larynx, radiotherapy may be preferable to surgery as it may preserve the person's natural voice. Sometimes the age and frailty of the patient may preclude surgical treatment.

Some cancers (some types of kidney cancer, colorectal adenocarcinoma and malignant melanoma) are not radio-sensitive and other approaches result in better survival.

Palliative radiotherapy

In some circumstances radiotherapy is employed as a treatment even when there is no hope of a cure, usually to reduce pain or control bleeding. Bone metastases are a principal cause of pain in advanced cancers, which can be treated by radiotherapy. Some cancers can spread to produce painful and disabling compression of the spinal cord. Radiotherapy can be used to control bleeding and discharge in advanced cervical cancer. Brain metastases and venous or lymphatic obstruction are also indications for palliative radiotherapy.

Maximising radiotherapy

The development of CT and MRI scanning has allowed accurate location of tumours and precise targeting of the radiotherapy beam. Radiation fields can be shaped and shielded to maximise exposure to the tumour while sparing the surrounding tissues, allowing higher doses to be used.

Accurate tumour localisation by CT and MRI scanning has revolutionised the application of radiotherapy

Trials are under way to assess the effect of shortening the time between sequential radiotherapy treatments with a view to reducing regrowth of cancer cells between treatment sessions. This is known as **accelerated fractionation** and involves delivery of several small doses of radiation each day. Encouraging results have been obtained in the treatment of non-small-cell carcinoma of the bronchus and advanced head and neck cancers.

A possible cause of failure of radiotherapy is the oxygen potential of the target cells. Malignant tumours often have a poorly organised vascular supply, causing some cells to be hypoxic and hypoxia is believed to confer resistance to radiation. It is possible to increase the oxygen uptake of cancer cells by placing the patient in a hyperbaric chamber or to increase the oxygen potential within the tumour using drugs. These approaches are still experimental and it is too soon to say whether they offer any survival advantage.

> *Susceptibility of cells to radiation depends on how well oxygenated they are*

Table 13.3 Indications for radiotherapy: radiocurable cancers

Tumour type	Comments	5-year survival
Basal cell	Treatment of choice	Over 95%
Squamous cell	Good cosmetic result	
Larynx, nasopharynx	Treatment of choice	Over 90% when localised
Thyroid	Radioiodine uptake, multimodal treatment	75–90% when well differentiated
Breast	Combined with surgery, adjuvant chemotherapy or tamoxifen	70% overall
Cervix	Treatment of choice in advanced cases	25–30% for stages III/IV
Bladder	Treatment of choice	10–75% depending on stage and grade
Penis	Preferable to surgery	Excellent in node-negative cases
Rectum	Adjuvant postoperative	Related to Dukes' stage
Anus	Replacing surgery as treatment of choice	Related to grade and patient age
Hodgkin's disease	Treatment of choice in early cases, with chemotherapy in advanced disease	85% in early cases
Multiple myeloma	Total body irradiation	Variable, up to 50%
Leukaemia	Cranial prophylaxis systemic with marrow transplantation	Variable according to age, cell type and haematology
Paediatric	Treatment of choice for brain tumours; chemotherapy indicated for most non-cerebral tumours	

Adapted from Tobias, 1992.

Chemotherapy

Chemotherapeutic agents arrest cell division by interfering with the synthesis or function of DNA and killing the cells: the drugs are **cytotoxic**. Both normal and cancer cells can be killed by cytotoxic drugs. Generally, cancers contain a higher proportion of dividing cells than normal tissues and hence chemotherapy preferentially affects the cancer cells. However, some tissues, such as bone marrow and epithelium in the gut and skin, are vulnerable because the normal cells have high turnover rates. As a consequence many chemotherapeutic treatments have associated side-effects of bone marrow suppression (myelosuppression), nausea and vomiting and hair loss (alopecia).

The loss of normal cells, particularly of the bone marrow, dictates the maximum dose that can be used: most regimens are administered cyclically to allow for normal tissue recovery. Fortunately normal bone marrow cells divide more rapidly than malignant cells and thus recover more quickly. During treatment bone marrow suppression and recovery is monitored by regular blood counts, with the aim of repeating the cycle before the cancer cells have a chance to recover. Therapy is designed to achieve the maximum toxic dose to the cancer cells with the minimum of damage to normal cells.

Generally, treatments are separated by intervals of 3–4 weeks: the white blood cell count is at its lowest about 10 days after treatment, and recovery is usually sufficient in 3 weeks. Some cancers are very sensitive to cytotoxic drugs but others are only slightly so. Repeated cycles are used to deplete the tumour steadily, but a point can be reached when resistance occurs.

In common with radiotherapy, chemotherapy is used with curative or palliative intentions but, unlike most forms of radiotherapy, chemotherapy offers a systemic therapy that can reach both known and occult deposits of cancer cells. Chemotherapy can be used alone for the treatment of systemic cancers such as lymphomas or as an adjunct to surgery or radiotherapy.

Choriocarcinoma (female): a highly malignant, invasive cancer arising from implanted fetal cells in the uterus or site of an ectopic pregnancy.

Ewing's sarcoma: an aggressive cancer arising in the long bones or pelvis. Most common in adolescence.

Wilms' tumour, nephroblastoma: a cancer of the kidney, most common in children. Can form very large abdominal masses and metastases in lungs, liver, bone and brain.

Some tumours are so sensitive to chemotherapy that a cure is possible; these include female choriocarcinoma, acute leukaemia in children, Hodgkin's disease and some other lymphomas, testicular and ovarian cancers, Ewing's sarcoma and Wilms' tumour. Very often these cancers are widely disseminated at the time of diagnosis and cannot be treated by other means.

Few of the common cancers (e.g. lung, breast and colorectal cancers) are cured by chemotherapy but adjuvant treatment can offer significant survival advantages. Adjuvant chemotherapy is most often used after surgery as a means of treating secondary deposits or latent micrometastases. It is possible to use **neoadjuvant** therapy to shrink the tumour before surgery or radiotherapy. Chemotherapy can also be used for pain relief.

Biological principles of chemotherapy

Cytotoxic drugs interfere with the cell growth cycle (see Chapter 4) generally or at specific phases (Figure 13.12).

The **phase-specific** drugs are antimetabolites that can block cellular reactions in specific parts of the growth cycle. Because the cells in a tumour

> ## ▲ Key points
>
> ### Cancers curable by chemotherapy
>
> ▲ Acute leukaemia
>
> ▲ Hodgkin's disease
>
> ▲ Lymphoma (high grade)
>
> ▲ Testicular cancer
>
> ▲ Some cancers of childhood and adolescence: Ewing's sarcoma, Wilms' tumour
>
> ▲ Female choriocarcinoma

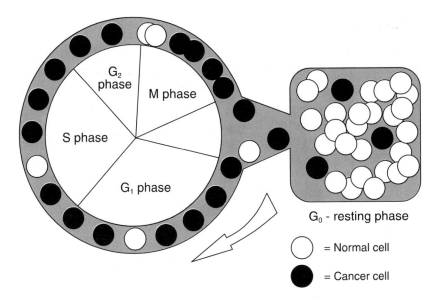

Figure 13.12 Principles of chemotherapy. At any one time more cancer cells enter the growth cycle and go through cell division than normal cells. The aim of chemotherapy is to take advantage of this growth differential by targeting cytotoxic drugs at cells in various phases of the growth cycle.

> ▲ **Key points**
>
> **Principles of combination chemotherapy**
>
> ▲ Combination chemotherapy minimises tumour resistance
>
> ▲ Separation of doses allows recovery of normal tissues
>
> ▲ Each drug in the combination should be effective as a single agent
>
> ▲ Employ agents that operate at different phases of the growth cycle
>
> ▲ Use drugs that do not overlap in toxicity

will be in different phases of the growth cycle at any one time the drugs must be given in multiple repeated fractions. The phase-specific drugs include asparaginase (G_1 phase-dependent), mercaptopurine and methotrexate (S phase), bleomycin (G_2 phase) and the vinca alkaloids (M phase).

The **non-phase-specific** agents operate at any stage of the growth cycle. Their effectiveness is less dependent on a schedule of fractionated doses than on the absolute dose given. Typical drugs of this type are alkylating agents such as melphalan and mechlorethamine (nitrogen mustard), nitrosoureas and most antibiotics with antitumour activity.

Although initial applications of chemotherapy used single agents the modern practice is to use a combination of agents. Many of the drugs appear to have synergistic effects, enabling lower doses to be used with less toxicity and at the same time reducing tumour resistance. The ideal is to use drugs that have different mechanisms of action, with different toxicity profiles. Each agent used should have proven independent cytotoxic activity. In practice, many effective combination therapies are formulated on an empirical basis.

Cytotoxic drugs are classified according to their mode of action or chemical similarities.

The **alkylating agents** (for example, nitrogen mustard) exert their cytotoxic effect by forming covalent bonds with DNA, causing cross-links and breaks in the DNA. The use of nitrogen mustard as a chemotherapeutic agent dates from 1946 when it was shown to induce regression of lymphomas. The agent is highly toxic and is associated with production of lung fibrosis, male infertility and second cancers (acute myeloid leukaemia in patients treated for Hodgkin's disease). Various derivatives of nitrogen mustard have been developed that have less short-term toxicity. These include melphalan, chlorambucil and cyclophosphamide.

The **nitrosoureas** (e.g. *cis*-chloroethylnitrosourea (CCNU) and lomustine) have a mechanism of action similar to that of the alkylating agents. They are lipid soluble and will cross the blood–brain barrier and so are used in the treatment of intracranial tumours. They are also used in the treatment of small-cell lung cancer and lymphoma.

The **platinum-containing** drug cisplatin behaves much like an alkylating agent. It is taken up by the ovaries and testes and is very useful for treating cancers of these organs.

The **antimetabolites** are structural analogues of molecules normally required for cell function and replication. Because the differences in their molecular structures are very subtle the cell is 'fooled' into using the non-functional analogue. Drugs of this class include the folic acid antagonist methotrexate (folic acid is required for the synthesis of purines), the pyrimidine antagonist 5-fluorouracil (5-FU) and the purine antagonist 6-mercaptopurine. These agents inhibit the assembly of purine and pyrimidine bases into DNA and RNA. Methotrexate is often used for treating acute lymphoblastic leukaemia, non-Hodgkin's lymphomas, breast cancer and some sarcomas, 5-FU is active against adenocarcinomas of the breast, ovary and large intestine and 6-mercaptopurine is used in the treatment of leukaemias.

The **vinca alkaloids** are derivatives of the periwinkle plant and include vinblastine, vincristine and vindesine. These drugs disrupt assembly of the mitotic spindle by binding to tubulin, a protein component of microtubules. Normally the mitotic spindle is assembled from microtubules immediately before cell division. Vincristine is useful in combination chemotherapy. Vinblastine is used in similar circumstances to vincristine and is useful in treating some testicular teratomas.

The **taxoids** are a new class of drugs with a taxane ring in their chemical structure. These agents were discovered by screening natural products for potential use as anticancer agents. The first drug in the series, paclitaxel (Taxol), was isolated from the bark of the Pacific yew tree (*Taxus brevifolia*) and is licensed in some countries for the treatment of ovarian cancer. A second drug, docetaxol, is a semi-synthetic derivative of an extract of needles from the European yew (*Taxus baccata*). This agent is more potent than paclitaxel.

In clinical trials, docetaxol has shown promising results in the treatment of non-small-cell lung cancers, particularly those that are intractable to treatment by other regimens. Very good response rates have been reported for gastric, breast, ovarian, head and neck, pancreatic and small-cell lung cancers, malignant melanoma and soft-tissue sarcomas. Responses can be achieved even after first-line chemotherapy has failed to control the cancer.

The **antibiotics** include the anthracyclins (for example doxorubicin, daunorubicin and epirubicin), dactinomycin, bleomycin and mitomycin.

Antibiotics have different activities. For example, bleomycin intercalates with DNA, generates free radicals, and complexes with iron, causing breakage of DNA and cell death. It is active in the G_2 phase of the cell cycle. This agent is commonly used with others to treat testicular tumours, head and neck cancers and lymphomas. The anthracyclins are usually given intravenously and are useful for the treatment of acute leukaemias, lymphomas, Hodgkin's disease, small-cell lung cancer, sarcomas and cancers of the stomach, bladder, ovary and liver.

The **miscellaneous agents** possess a variety of activities and include procarbazine, hydroxyurea, hexamethylmelamine and L-asparaginase. Procarbazine is especially useful for treatment of Hodgkin's disease and brain tumours.

Administration of chemotherapy

The usual mode of administration is intravenous. Some agents are available as oral preparations, but it is less easy to calculate the proper dose and to monitor compliance. Drugs can be instilled into the pleural or pericardial space in order to control effusions, or infused directly into an artery, for example the hepatic artery (liver metastases) or carotid artery (head and neck cancers).

In acute lymphoblastic leukaemia there is a risk of relapse involving the brain and spinal cord. Injections of methotrexate are now given into the spine (intrathecal injection) to combat this, usually in combination with cranial radiotherapy. This strategy has contributed to the significant improvements in survival over the last 20 years or so (Figure 13.13), the other main factors being the use of chemotherapy in optimal combination regimens and more effective means of combating infection.

Complications of chemotherapy

The principal problem of chemotherapy is to achieve an acceptable therapeutic ratio (tumour cell death:normal cell death). Most of the drugs used cause bone marrow toxicity, evident as thrombocytopenia and neutropenia. This is the main dose-limiting factor because of the risk of bleeding or life-threatening infection.

The aim of chemotherapy is to maximise tumour cell death without causing unacceptable toxicity in normal tissues

A side-effect of most cytotoxic drugs is **emesis** (nausea and vomiting). This can be reduced by administration of antiemetics. With moderately emetic regimens (such as combination therapy of cyclophosphamide, methotrexate and fluorouracil) intravenous dexamethasone and metoclopramide are given before or after chemotherapy, with oral dexamethasone if necessary. With highly emetic regimens (containing high doses of doxorubicin and cisplatin for example) intravenous ondansetron can be administered in addition to intravenous and oral dexamethasone.

Neutropenia: low neutrophil count in blood.

Thrombocytopenia: deficiency of platelets in the blood circulation.

Some cytotoxic drugs cause diarrhoea and patients may need codeine phosphate to help with this in subsequent treatments.

Another problem is mucositis (loss of the buccal mucosa), and oral hygiene is very important at this stage to avoid infection.

Kidney damage is associated with some cytotoxic drugs (e.g. cisplatin) and it is essential that a high urine output is maintained using intravenous fluids before and after treatment to minimise this effect.

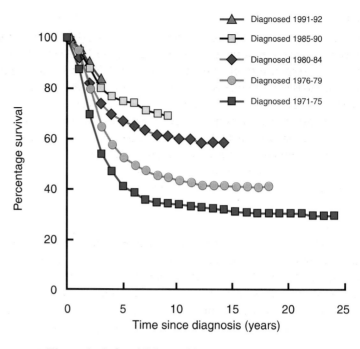

Figure 13.13 The outlook for children with acute lymphoblastic leukaemia has improved appreciably with the advent of new chemotherapy regimens. The 10-year survival rate of children diagnosed in 1971–75 was about 34%, but this had increased to about 60% for children diagnosed a decade later, and is still increasing. (Adapted from Eden, T. (1994) *MRC News*, **63**, 16–19.)

Pulmonary and cardiac toxicity are possible, particularly if the patient has previously received radiotherapy to the mediastinum or left breast (causing cardiomyopathy).

The vinca alkaloids cause a peripheral neuropathy that can persist for many years. This is first noticed as a loss of tendon reflexes and numbness of the fingers and toes. The dose should be lowered or alternative drug combinations sought. Vinblastine is less neurotoxic than vincristine but causes more bone marrow suppression.

A psychologically important side-effect is alopecia. Usually only the head hair is lost and this is reversible. Cooling of the scalp during and after treatment induces vasospasm so that less drug reaches the hair follicles. Hair loss is likely with the anthracyclins, cyclophosphamide, mustine and vincristine.

Combination chemotherapy usually causes some degree of infertility. Male infertility is often reversed in a year or two of finishing treatment, although sperm counts remain low for much longer. However, most men treated by combination chemotherapy for Hodgkin's disease remain permanently infertile. Loss of ovarian function after combination chemotherapy is more likely the nearer the patient is to her natural menopause. In any event subfertility is common and the menopause is often premature.

▲ **Key points**

Chemotherapy toxicity

▲ Dose limiting bone marrow suppression evident as thrombocytopenia and neutropenia

▲ Nausea, vomiting, constipation or diarrhoea

▲ Oral ulceration

▲ Alopecia

▲ Nephrotoxicity, cardiotoxicity and pulmonary toxicity associated with some agents

Tumour resistance

Some tumours appear to develop resistance to cytotoxic drugs as the therapy progresses. In small-cell lung tumours for example 80% of new patients may show a clear response to chemotherapy and 50% will undergo complete remission. However, the disease recurs in most cases, and despite further chemotherapy the 2-year survival is only about 10%. There are probably several reasons for this: new mutations will occur with time which may not be so responsive to chemotherapy; all tumours consist of heterogeneous clones of cells in various mutated states and it is probable that these clones exhibit differential susceptibilities to chemotherapy, so that when the most sensitive clones are eradicated the least sensitive cells are left behind.

Long-term survival after chemotherapy can be limited by resistance of some cells within the tumour population

Secondary cancers

Many cytotoxic drugs are themselves carcinogenic. Long-term treatment can result in the production of other cancers, most notably acute leukaemia which has a peak incidence 3–5 years after the initial therapy. Other solid tumours can develop, but usually after a longer interval. Although the relative risk of developing leukaemia can be more than 100 times that of the untreated population, the benefit of the treatment far exceeds the risk of second cancers.

Gynaecomastia: excessive breast development in males.

Orchidectomy, orchiectomy: surgical removal of testis.

Hormonal therapy

Sex hormones and antagonists are mainly used for the treatment of prostate and breast cancer. Cells in both these organs are highly responsive to androgens and other sex hormones which behave as growth promoters. The rationale behind therapy is to achieve regression of a tumour by depriving it of hormonal stimulation.

The prostate gland and tumours arising from it are sensitive to androgens produced by the adrenal glands and testes. One of the first strategies employed was to remove this stimulus by orchidectomy. Alternatively, androgenic stimulation of prostate cancer cells can be modified by oestrogen. This is effective, but carries possible cerebrovascular and cardiovascular complications because it alters platelet aggregation. A further complication is gynaecomastia.

Newer therapies centre on the use of the antiandrogen drugs cyproterone acetate and flutamide. These drugs inhibit testosterone production and the formation of hormone–receptor complexes in the prostate cells and can be just as effective as orchidectomy or oestrogen therapy. In advanced prostatic cancer the cells may no longer all be hormone sensitive and second-line cytotoxic chemotherapy or radiotherapy treatments may be necessary.

In breast cancer the most common hormonal treatment is with the antioestrogen drug tamoxifen. This has been shown to increase survival in surgically treated patients, particularly in post-menopausal women and patients shown by biochemical assay to have tumour cells with oestrogen receptors. Another drug, aminoglutethimide, inhibits oestrogens produced (from androgens) in the peripheral tissues. This is a second-line choice for post-menopausal women.

Review question 6

Why are different approaches (e.g. surgery, radiotherapy, chemotherapy) necessary for the treatment of cancer?

Other approaches

A number of other approaches are possible in the treatment of cancer but presently none is widely used for routine treatment. One approach, which has received widespread publicity as the 'magic bullet', employs monoclonal antibodies to target tumour cell antigens. The antibody can be linked to a cytotoxic agent to achieve a highly localised cell kill. In practice monoclonal antibody therapy has been disappointing: the antibody is recognised as 'foreign' and eliminated by the immune system before any significant tumour cell kill is achieved.

Another approach is to employ biological response modifiers to stimulate immune system cells to attack the cancer cells. One of these agents, interferon, has been used to induce long-term remission in hairy cell leukaemia (an uncommon form of leukaemia mainly affecting middle aged men) and to maintain remission in multiple myeloma. Only a small minority of patients appear to benefit from the treatment.

Interleukin-2 can activate the patient's killer T lymphocytes. Trials of this agent have demonstrated cancer remissions, particularly in renal cancer and melanoma, but the treatment is highly toxic.

Screening for cancer and precancer

Screening aims to detect precancerous or preinvasive lesions in asymptomatic people

One of the first cancer screening programmes in the UK was aimed at the early detection of lung cancers. This failed because the treatment and mortality in the screen-detected cases was little different from people with symptomatic cancers. Current mass screening programmes are intended to detect and treat precancerous cervical lesions and early breast cancers. A number of trials are in operation to extend screening for other types of cancer. In certain situations mass screening of the general population is unwarranted but at-risk populations are screened. An example is screening for bladder cancers in workers in some occupations.

The ideal situation in cancer screening is to expose the disease at a precancerous stage and then offer an effective treatment. This can be achieved in cervical screening, and many lives have been saved by the screening programme.

Screening for breast cancer occupies an intermediate position in which precancerous stages cannot be recognised, but preinvasive cancers *can* sometimes be detected and treated. Most screen-detected breast cancers are already invasive but breast screening has been shown to reduce mortality from breast cancer and, because screen-detected cancers are usually smaller, it is possible to use more conservative treatments for local control of the disease.

In other cancer types (such as lung, prostate and ovarian cancers) the screening methods available are limited to the detection of invasive cancer. In these cases, treatment of the screen-detected cancers is at a late stage in the natural history of the disease.

It cannot be expected that the detection of invasive cancers will substantially reduce mortality rates. A tumour of 1 cm may contain 10^9 or more cells, which could mean that some of the slower-growing breast cancers have taken about 15 years to reach a palpable size (assuming a doubling time of 2–5 months). Earlier detection by mammography when a few millimetres in size is only equivalent to a few cell doublings: by this stage tens or even hundreds of millions of cancer cells will be present (Figure 13.14). While this means that the diagnosis can be advanced by a year or two, the possibility remains that the cancer has already disseminated elsewhere so there is little or no difference in the eventual outcome.

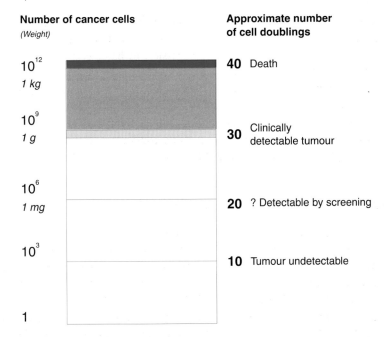

Number of cancer cells
(Weight)

Approximate number of cell doublings

10^{12}	**40** Death
1 kg	
10^9	**30** Clinically detectable tumour
1 g	
10^6	**20** ? Detectable by screening
1 mg	
10^3	**10** Tumour undetectable
1	

Figure 13.14 Logarithmic growth of cancer cells. Screening may come too late in the life history of some cancers to make any significant difference to the outcome. A tumour weighing 1 g may be 1 cm in diameter and could just be detectable clinically. At this stage it will contain in excess of 10^9 cells and will already have completed three-quarters of its growth, assuming exponential growth to about 1 kg (about 40 doublings) which is the maximum size compatible with life. In terms of the number of cell doublings, screening for cancer (not precancer) is only a small advance before the tumour becomes clinically apparent. Even so, if the gain in detection occurs before the tumour has metastasised the chances of successful treatment are markedly improved.

It therefore seems desirable to try to detect conditions leading to cancer as early as practicable: the treatment of precancerous lesions is usually much more successful than treatment for cancer. However, this presents problems: the detection of a tumour at an early stage could mean that many people would receive unnecessary treatment because it is possible that a precancerous lesion will revert to normal. Paradoxically, as the chances of successful treatment become more certain, the need for the treatment becomes more questionable.

Undoubtedly the lives of many people will be saved by intervention at an

Not everyone who has a precancerous lesion develops invasive cancer

early stage. In the case of early cervical abnormalities most treatments are relatively quick, inexpensive and without significant long-term physical effects. The inevitable over-treatment of a small minority of women is not catastrophic in view of the benefits gained for the majority of women who would otherwise go on to develop invasive cancer. With other cancer types, even if the technology to distinguish a precancerous phase were available, the current treatment options are much more extensive, involving surgery, radiotherapy or chemotherapy, all of which are associated with more severe adverse physical and psychological effects. Any new advances in screening technology that result in the downstaging of screen-detected disease to a precancerous phase will have to be accompanied by similarly impressive advances in therapy.

Even with more effective methods of detection and treatment, it does not necessarily follow that screening for cancer will benefit everyone. The incidence of most cancers increases with age. A typical example is prostate cancer, 95% of cases occurring in men older than 65 years of age. A man of this age with non-metastatic prostate cancer would be expected to survive 8 years, which is his life expectancy anyway. In this circumstance screening does not prevent death; it only influences what the person dies from. The greatest potential for cancer screening is in the prevention of premature death (defined as death below the age of 65) and in this respect some screening programmes succeed (for example prevention of death from cervical cancer) but others (prostate cancer included) are limited by technical problems.

To some extent, screening for cancerous conditions is born out of frustration: there is no known means of preventing breast, ovarian and prostate cancers. Prostate screening presently has no proven reduction in mortality, and some patients could be harmed by treatments that in fact they did not need. Refinement of the screening tools and methods of predicting who has an aggressive tumour and would benefit from early and aggressive treatment, and who has not, are needed.

Progress is being made, and in some cancer types specific changes in oncogene and tumour suppresser gene expression have been characterised for precancerous, preinvasive and invasive stages. As yet these markers are of limited predictive value, but this position could be improved with further advances in our understanding of tumour molecular biology. An understanding of what it takes to make a precancerous lesion regress to normal would be of enormous advantage.

All of the approaches to screening are, by their nature, technological 'fixes', bringing their own problems and costs. Primary prevention of cancers (for example, by the cessation of tobacco smoking or by modifying diet or lifestyle and behavioural risk factors) will do more to prevent early deaths than all the currently devised screening programmes will ever do.

ANSWERS TO REVIEW QUESTIONS

Question 1

Why have deaths from cervical cancer fallen?

The main factor (from the 1960s) is the availability of cervical screening. This has arrested the disease process in its early stages, usually before cancer has developed.

Assess the potential for reducing deaths from cancer or improving survival

Question 2

1.   The historical picture, over the past 20 years:

Cancer site	Primary prevention	Screening	Treatment
Lung	1	0	1
Breast	0	1	3
Colorectal	0	0	1
Cervix	0	3	1
Prostate	0	0	2
Stomach	4	1	1
Skin	0	0	1

2.   The potential for improvement over the next decade:

Cancer site	Primary prevention	Screening	Treatment
Lung	5	1	1
Breast	1	3	3
Colorectal	3	3	2
Cervix	2	5	1
Prostate	1	3	2
Stomach	3	1	1
Skin	5	0	1

Lung cancer
Only in recent years have some sectors of the population taken heed of the message to stop smoking, and this has yet to be translated into marked reductions in deaths from lung cancer. Although screening for lung cancer has been tried, this had no impact on survival or mortality rates. Treatment of lung cancer has made few substantial differences because a large proportion of the cancers are inoperable. There has been a small improvement in survival

after chemotherapy for small-cell lung cancers. The potential for reducing deaths from lung cancer by primary prevention is enormous: before the introduction of smoking this was a very rare disease (see Chapter 1).

Breast cancer

The risk factors for breast cancer are mainly unalterable and therefore have not significantly influenced survival rates. Geographic differences in breast cancer suggest that diet may play a minor role; a reduction in the frequency of the disease could accompany the current recommendations for lower fat diets. Screening has only recently been introduced on a national basis in the UK and its influence has not yet been reflected in the statistics. Some advances in the systemic treatment of breast cancer have been shown to increase survival (see Chapter 15).

Colorectal cancer

Dietary factors are believed to play a part in the development of colorectal cancer and a move towards low-fat high-fibre diets could reduce its incidence in developed countries. Screening has not been successful in the past, although there is now some potential for improved early diagnosis. Non-surgical means of treating colorectal cancer have so far made little impact on survival (see Chapter 17), but there is scope for improvement.

Cervical cancer

There is evidence that this is a sexually transmitted disease and so there is great potential for reducing its incidence. The health education messages aimed at reducing the spread of AIDS may also have some impact on the incidence of cervical cancer. Screening is extremely effective in identifying this disease in its asymptomatic precursor stages. The main limitation to its success in the UK is poor response. With improved attendance there is great potential to reduce further the incidence of invasive cervical cancer (see Chapter 16).

Prostate cancer

The cause of prostate cancer is unknown. Epidemiological studies have shown an association between consumption of saturated animal fats and prostate cancer: there is therefore a small possibility that primary prevention may be useful. In the USA screening forms part of routine health checks for middle-aged and older men, but has produced no consistent reduction in deaths from the disease. More sensitive and specific screening tests, as well as better treatments, are needed for this disease (see Chapters 10 and 18).

Stomach cancer

Deaths from this type of cancer have fallen dramatically in most Western countries, but the change in less developed countries is not as impressive. This suggests that environmental factors are of importance in causing the disease. One factor is infection with *Helicobacter pylori* (see Chapter 19).

Improvements in general hygiene have meant that the organism is less likely to be transmitted by the faecal–oral route. There is thus some potential for primary prevention. In some areas of high incidence (e.g. Japan) radiographic screening is used, but the low detection rate means that the method is inefficient for screening of low-incidence populations.

Skin cancer

Over the past 30 years the incidence of both melanotic and non-melanotic skin cancers has increased in most Western countries. A probable factor underlying this trend is the fashion for a tanned body, achieved by the use of sunbeds and intensive bursts of sunlight. Numerous government campaigns aim to promote sensible exposure to UV light through public information and awareness activities: in other words, primary prevention.

Why were the *Health of the Nation* objectives chosen and how might they be achieved?

Question 3

The cancers targeted are those that are considered most amenable to prevention by modification of risk factors or screening (see Review question 2). Rates of lung and skin cancers could be reduced by primary prevention: reducing smoking and excessive exposure to the sun, respectively. Screening is particularly effective in preventing cervical cancer and is also useful in the early detection of breast cancers, improving both morbidity and mortality. The greatest challenge lies in persuading the public to carry out primary prevention measures and to attend screening.

Why are changes in proto-oncogenes and tumour suppressor genes of fundamental importance to the development of cancer?

Question 4

Cancers necessarily involve changes at the genetic level – some of which can even be inherited. Two distinct categories of genes which regulate normal cell growth and proliferation have been identified – the proto-oncogenes and the tumour suppressor genes. These two classes of genes differ in the way in which they contribute to the neoplastic transformation of a cell.

Cancers can arise through the aberrant expression of proto-oncogenes – when this occurs the gene is said to have become an oncogene. Oncogenes act dominantly to promote uncontrolled cell division. In contrast, the usual role of the tumour suppressor gene is to regulate the extent of cell growth by inhibiting cell division. Therefore, the loss of tumour suppressor gene activity through genetic damage will result in a loss of this controlling mechanism and lead to uncontrolled cell growth.

Which features of tumour pathology are helpful as prognostic indicators?

Question 5

The most valuable prognostic indicators are tumour stage and grade. Tumour stage refers to the degree of spread of the tumour. Involvement of local lymph nodes and the presence of distant metastases indicate a poor prognosis. Tumour grade refers to the degree of differentiation of the tumour cells. A well differentiated tumour (one that retains cell morphology and function) is associated with a better prognosis than an undifferentiated (anaplastic) cancer. Aneuploidy (change in chromosomal number) and the mitotic index (an indication of cell proliferation) are helpful factors in determining the tumour grade.

The identification of oncogene activation or deletion of tumour suppressor genes can serve as a prognostic marker, but is less frequently used. The activation of the *c-myc* oncogene is believed to be a poor prognostic indicator for some cancers, as is the loss of *p53* tumour suppressor activity.

Question 6

Why are different approaches (e.g. surgery, radiotherapy, chemotherapy) necessary for the treatment of cancer?

Although many cancers arise locally they need to be treated both locally and systemically. Even if metastatic deposits are not evident cancer cells may already have seeded in other parts of the body.

Surgery remains the mainstay of treatment, particularly for the local control of cancer. Other than for the removal of lymph nodes it is only of limited application for the treatment of widespread or metastatic disease.

Chemotherapy offers the advantage that delivery of the cytotoxic drugs is body-wide and so tumour cells can be reached wherever they are. At the same time this is a disadvantage, because normal cells are also susceptible to therapeutic doses. Cancers differ in their susceptibility to chemotherapeutic agents, although it is often possible to devise a cocktail of drugs which will deliver the optimal therapeutic advantage.

Radiotherapy offers an intermediate approach for local and systemic treatment. It is possible to employ total body irradiation, although this is usually reserved for the treatment of some lymphomas. More frequently, radiotherapy is used for local control as an adjunct to conservative surgery. Both radiotherapy and chemotherapy can be used to debulk tumours before surgery. Radiotherapy and chemotherapy are also of value as palliative treatments.

The growth of some cancers is stimulated by specific hormones (for example oestrogen in breast cancer and androgens in prostate cancers). In these instances it is often possible to limit tumour growth, both locally and systemically, by the use of **hormone antagonists**.

References

Cheng, H.H., Day, N.E., Duffy, S.W. *et al.* (1992) Pickled vegetables in the aetiology of oesophageal cancer in Hong Kong Chinese. *Lancet*, **339**, 1314–18.

Muir, C.S. (1990) Epidemiology, basic science, and the prevention of cancer: implications for the future. *Cancer Res.*, **50**, 6441–8.

Tobias, J.S. (1992) Clinical practice of radiotherapy. *Lancet*, **339**, 159–63.

Further reading

Harris, C.C. and Hollstein, M. (1993) Clinical implications of the *p53* tumour-suppressor gene. *N. Engl. J. Med.*, **329**, 1318–27.

Hoffbrand, A.V. and Pettit, J.E. (1993) *Essential Haematology*, 3rd edn, Blackwell Scientific Publications, Oxford.

Horwich, A. (1992) Radiotherapy update. *BMJ*, **304**, 1554–7.

Lever, J.V., Trott, P.A. and Webb, A.J. (1985) Fine needle aspiration cytology. *J. Clin. Pathol.*, **38**, 1–11.

Mead, G.M. (1992) *Current Issues in Cancer*. BMJ Publishing group, London.

Rubens, R.D., Towlson, K.E., Ramirez, A.J. *et al.* (1992) Appropriate chemotherapy for palliating advanced cancer. *BMJ*, **304**, 35–40.

Sikora, K. and Halnan, K.E. (1992) *Treatment of Cancer*, 2nd edn, Chapman & Hall, London.

Souhami, R. and Tobias, J. (1995) *Cancer and its Management*, 2nd edn, Blackwell Scientific, Oxford.

Withers, H.R. (1992) Biological basis of radiation therapy for cancer. *Lancet*, **339**, 156–9.

Zur Hausen, H. (1991) Viruses in human cancer. *Science*, **254**, 1167–73.

14   Lung cancer

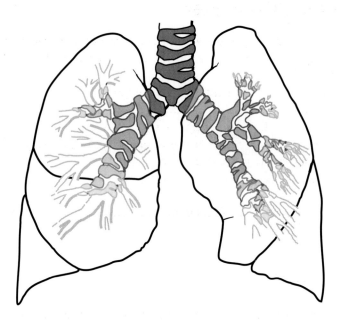

In most developed countries lung cancer is the most common cause of death from cancer. The vast majority of cases are caused by smoking and could therefore have been prevented. Other causes include exposure to asbestos, ionising radiation and industrial pollution, but together these account for only about 10% of cases. Unfortunately lung cancer, once established, is very difficult to treat successfully, and survival is relatively poor.

Most lung cancers are detected by the symptoms of weight loss, cough, blood in the sputum, shortness of breath, or pain in the chest. At this stage the cancer is well advanced. It is not unusual for some cancers to become evident by symptoms arising from metastatic spread. Attempts to detect the disease at an earlier stage by screening, using chest radiography or sputum cytology, have failed to show any survival benefit.

The diagnosis of lung cancer can be confirmed by sputum cytology but bronchoscopy is more reliable. Curative surgical treatment is appropriate in only a minority of patients, but there is a role for surgery as a palliative measure. Similarly, radiotherapy is not usually curative but can prolong survival in patients who are unfit for surgery, and is used as a palliative measure to control bone pain.

Chemotherapy is of little benefit for the more common non-small-cell cancers, but increases survival by several months in patients with small-cell cancers, for whom no other treatment is effective.

Pre-test

- **How common is lung cancer?**
- **What is your own risk of developing lung cancer?**
- **What is the average survival of newly diagnosed and treated patients?**
- **What treatments are available for lung cancer?**
- **What can be done to prevent the disease?**

Aims of this chapter

By the end of this chapter you will have increased your knowledge of:
◆ The epidemiology of lung cancer: who is affected and the risk factors involved
◆ Pathology of the different types of lung cancer
◆ Methods available for diagnosis and treatment

In addition, this chapter will help you to:
◆ Explain why lung cancer has been transformed from a very rare disease into a major public health problem
◆ Evaluate the possibilities for primary or secondary prevention of lung cancer
◆ Understand the difficulties in treating lung cancer and reasons for poor survival

Introduction

In most industrialised countries lung cancer is the most common cause of death from cancer among men. In the USA and in some regions of the UK lung cancer has recently overtaken breast cancer as the most common cause of cancer death among women. Because survival rates for lung cancers are so low, mortality rates are a reasonable reflection of the incidence of the disease.

There is no doubt that smoking is a major risk for the development of lung cancer. A minority of cases are caused by other factors, usually airborne agents, but even then the risk of developing the disease is made much worse by smoking. The mortality rates for men and women differ because of historic gender differences in the social acceptability of smoking. It is worrying that the incidence of lung cancer is still rising, particularly among women and, because of the increase in smoking by teenage girls, the upward trend in female mortality from the disease is likely to continue.

Most patients present with symptoms late in the course of the disease, by which time the cancer is usually incurable. As the major risk factor for developing lung cancer is smoking, the most obvious approach to the problem is one of prevention. This has been recognised by the British government's *Health of the Nation* strategy, which focuses on targets to reduce the prevalence of cigarette smoking.

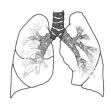

More than 85% of lung cancers are directly attributable to smoking, and most cases are incurable

Bt the time symptoms develop, about 70% of patients with lung cancer already have metastases

Epidemiology

At the beginning of the twentieth century lung cancer was a very rare cause of death. Unfortunately, this picture has changed and lung cancer is now the leading cause of death from cancer. In England and Wales lung cancer accounts for 17% of all new cases of cancer and 25% of all cancer deaths. About half of the deaths occur in people in middle age (35–69 years).

In the UK the mortality rate from lung cancer among men has gradually declined since the early 1970s. In contrast, death rates for women are increasing, albeit from a lower base (Figure 14.1).

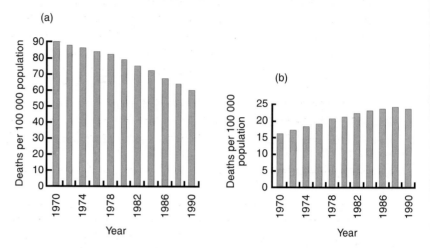

Figure 14.1 Deaths from lung cancer in (a) men and (b) women under 75 years in England, 1970–1990. Mortality from lung cancer in men has steadily declined since 1970. Rates in women are 30–50% of those for men, but the gap is narrowing, reflecting the fact that more women are smoking. Although overall prevalence of smoking is in decline (see Chapter 2), this is not true for all sectors of the population and lung cancer will remain with us for a long time. (Source: OPCS.)

Aetiology

Smoking

> *Risk of lung cancer increases with the duration of smoking and the number of cigarettes smoked*

Epidemiological evidence overwhelmingly suggests that smoking is a major cause of lung cancer. The risk of lung cancer increases rapidly in people who smoke up to 25 cigarettes a day, but above this level the increase in risk is less dramatic. The risk of lung cancer is not as great with low-tar/nicotine and filter cigarettes as with the high-tar/nicotine unfiltered equivalents, suggesting that the tar contains most of the carcinogens responsible for lung cancer. Generally, 'average' smokers increase their risk of lung cancer around tenfold, and heavy smokers (more than 40 cigarettes a day for several years) 20-fold. Pipe and cigar smoking carry smaller risks for developing lung cancer.

> *After a person has stopped smoking for 10 years or more, their lung cancer risk is comparable to that of people who have never smoked*

A critical factor is the duration of smoking, and it is no coincidence that the recently experienced high incidence of lung cancer is associated with people who have had the opportunity to smoke throughout their adult lives. Cessation of smoking leads to a fall in the risk from lung cancer in 5–10 years. After 15 years of abstinence the risk approaches that for people who have never smoked. The effects of passive smoking have been studied only relatively recently but the indications are that there is some elevation of risk, particularly for family members who live in the same household as a smoker.

The association with cigarette smoking is also dramatically illustrated by comparing the lung cancer statistics in men and women. When smoking first became popular in the early 1900s it was predominantly a male practice. After a 30–40 year latency, increases in lung cancer became apparent in men. 'Scare' stories about cigarette smoking began to appear in the 1960s, and may have been responsible for small reductions in men taking up smoking and in changing habits towards filtered and low-tar/nicotine brands. Slowly, in the 1970s, male deaths from lung cancer began to decline (see Figure 1. 2).

Around the time of the Second World War it became much more socially acceptable for women to smoke – and we are still seeing the consequence of this in terms of rising mortality rates from lung cancer in women. A further worrying aspect is that the geographical distribution of lung cancer is changing; the incidence is increasing in many parts of the world, including the less developed countries.

There is evidence that the health education message is getting through to smokers in developed countries, as shown by decreases in the annual per capita consumption of tobacco, but this is not the case in less developed countries, which are increasingly the marketing target of the tobacco companies. On a world-wide basis, the attrition from cigarette-related disease is set to increase further. Even in developed countries much education is still needed: the decline in tobacco consumption is mostly because of people giving up, and the number of people who take up the habit remains relatively unchanged (see Figure 2.8).

The epidemiological evidence supporting a causal link between smoking and lung cancer is now (late 1996) supported by solid scientific evidence. It has been shown in cell culture studies that a metabolite of cigarette smoke, BPDE (β-dihydroxy-epoxy-tetrahydrobenzo(a)pyrene) binds to DNA at the site of the *p53* tumour suppressor gene (this gene is mutated in about 60% of lung cancer cases). The most common mutations to the *p53* gene in lung cancers are at the nucleotide sequence positions 157, 248 and 273. These happen to be the same positions at which BPDE preferentially binds; in other words it is very probable that BPDE is the original cause of *p53* mutation in lung cancer. There may well be other agents in cigarette smoke that can cause genetic damage to cells in the lungs and other organs of the body.

HEALTH OF THE NATION

Targets on smoking

▲ Reduce the death rate for lung cancer in people under the age of 75, by at least 30% in men and at least 15% in women, by the year 2010 (from 60 per 100 000 men and 24.1 per 100 000 women in 1990)

Prevention measures to decrease the mortality from lung cancer might include:

▲ Health education about the effects of smoking

▲ Actions to stop people from taking up smoking

▲ Helping people to give up smoking

▲ Protecting non-smokers from passive smoking

▲ Preventing occupational exposure to other agents involved in lung cancer (e.g. asbestos)

Environmental and industrial agents

Lung cancer in non-smokers must be caused by other factors – industrial and other airborne pollutants are believed to be possible risk factors, mainly on the basis of epidemiological evidence that shows differences in lung cancer mortality rates in urban and rural areas, independent of any differences in smoking habits in these areas. In particular, people living or working in the vicinity of gas retorts and coke ovens appear to be at greater risk. However, because of the stringent restrictions on air pollution levels that are now in place in most developed countries, it is likely that general air pollution will continue to have only a minor impact on the prevalence of lung cancer in these countries.

The strength of the association between smoking and lung cancer far outweighs all other factors

Smokers with a history of heavy and prolonged exposure to asbestos have a 50-fold excess risk of lung cancer

Exposure to asbestos is another important factor associated with lung cancer, especially when this is coupled with cigarette smoking. A rare kind of lung cancer, mesothelioma, is associated with people who work with asbestos, or who live in surroundings where it is used. Asbestos can also cause the more common types of lung cancers, particularly when associated with cigarette smoking. The so-called 'blue asbestos' derived from crocidolite ore is much more dangerous than the 'white' asbestos derived from chrysotile. The size of the fibres is crucial in determining carcinogenic potential; blue asbestos fibres are so much more dangerous because they are small and straight and can penetrate far into the deepest recesses of the lung. The white fibres are curly and larger and are far more likely to be cleared by the respiratory mucus.

Ionising radiation

Radon can seep into buildings from the ground below

Radon: a gas produced from the natural decay of uranium. Uranium is present in small amounts in many common rocks and minerals, including granite.

The most common naturally occurring ionising radiation is radon. The highest levels are seen where there are large deposits of granite, such as in Cornwall, but these areas are not particularly associated with a high incidence of non-smoking-related lung cancer. People who are exposed to very high levels of radon, such as miners, are at increased risk, particularly if they are also smokers. High concentrations of radon occasionally accumulate inside buildings, particularly if the walls and windows are well insulated.

Family history and genetics

There is a genetic component to lung cancer: not all people who smoke 40 cigarettes a day develop the disease

Some people appear to be more susceptible to the effects of cigarette smoking than others: one person may smoke heavily and not develop lung cancer while another may smoke only 15 cigarettes a day and contract the disease. Of probable importance is a person's ability to metabolise some of the products of cigarette smoke. Levels of the enzyme aryl-hydrocarbon-hydroxylase are raised in patients with lung cancer, and it is suggested that this enzyme converts the polycyclic hydrocarbons of cigarette smoke into carcinogenic substances. Some people may be genetically predisposed to have higher levels of this enzyme than others.

Exposure to birds

A possible link between lung cancer and the keeping of pet birds, especially pigeons, has been postulated. However, the epidemiological studies purporting to show such a link have been poorly designed and have not taken account of the influence of cigarette smoking by pigeon-fanciers.

Pathology

Most lung cancers arise from the bronchial epithelium

About 95% of primary lung cancers arise from the epithelial cells lining the bronchi, bronchioles and alveoli. Consequently these cancers are referred to as **bronchogenic** or **bronchial** carcinomas. The remaining cancers arise from the glands (**bronchial gland** carcinoma) or the pleural membrane (**mesothelioma**).

There are four major histological types of bronchogenic carcinoma: **squamous cell carcinoma, adenocarcinoma, large-cell carcinoma** and **small-cell carcinoma**. Further sub-categories are based on the morphological appearances of the cells, together with some rare types including carcinoid and bronchial gland tumours (see Table 14.1). Sometimes mixed patterns are seen, with elements of both small-cell carcinoma and areas of differentiated squamous cell or adenocarcinoma. All of these cancers are believed to arise from a common bronchial precursor cell, differentiation proceeding along different pathways and giving rise to the mixed patterns. For treatment and prognostic purposes the only real distinction to be made is between small-cell carcinomas and the other types, collectively referred to as non-small-cell carcinomas.

Table 14.1 Classification of lung tumours (WHO, 1981)

1 Squamous carcinoma (epidermoid carcinoma)
2 Small-cell carcinoma: • Oat-cell carcinoma   • Intermediate cell type   • Combined oat-cell carcinoma
3 Adenocarcinoma: • Acinar adenocarcinoma   • Papillary adenocarcinoma   • Bronchoalveolar carcinoma   • Solid mucin-producing carcinoma
4 Large-cell carcinoma: • Giant-cell carcinoma   • Clear-cell carcinoma
5 Adenosquamous carcinoma
6 Carcinoid tumour
7 Bronchial gland carcinoma: • Adenoid cystic carcinoma   • Mucoepidermoid carcinoma   • Others
8 Others

Non-small-cell carcinomas

Squamous cell carcinoma

The most common form of lung cancer, squamous cell carcinoma (also known

Keratin: a hard protein produced by squamous cells. Found on the surface of the skin, but can also be produced in the respiratory tract and cervix in sites of squamous metaplasia. Tumours derived from squamous cells (keratinocytes) produce the protein.

as epidermoid carcinoma), accounts for 40% or more of lung cancers. This type is most closely correlated with smoking. The tumour is often well differentiated and in the early stage can be relatively slow growing. It usually arises in the large bronchi, eventually causing bronchial obstruction. By the time symptoms develop this type of tumour may have taken 8 years to grow from the initial malignant change.

Histologically, the tumours can be well or poorly differentiated according to the presence of keratin: when keratin is prominent the tumour is a well differentiated tumour. Cell nuclei are often enlarged and pleomorphic. There is often evidence of intra- and extracellular production of mucin.

Adenocarcinoma

Adenocarcinoma accounts for 10–20% of all lung cancers and is found in both smokers and non-smokers. It is the most common type of tumour in non-smokers, and is more common in women (both smokers and non-smokers). This type of lung cancer appears to be increasing in frequency, and in some countries (for example the USA and Japan) is more common than squamous cell carcinoma.

Many of these tumours are situated at the periphery of the lung. Because of this they do not cause significant obstruction of the airways and often remain clinically silent until symptoms are caused by metastases. The growth rate can be slow, taking up to 25 years to reach 2 cm in diameter. Histologically, adenocarcinomas are characterised by mucin production, seen both intracellularly and extracellularly, and by a papillary pattern of tumour cells. They are often rich in cytoplasmic organelles and bear some morphological similarities to Type II pneumocytes which line the alveoli and secrete surfactant.

Large-cell carcinomas

The large-cell carcinomas account for up to 25% of lung cancers. These tumours are often highly malignant, poorly differentiated and disseminate widely. They often appear in heavy smokers and patients rapidly die after only a short history of symptoms. Histologically, the tumour comprises large polygonal cells with large pleomorphic multilobed nuclei and numerous mitoses; there is also a clear-cell type with watery cytoplasm. All large-cell tumour cells contain mucin in their cytoplasm. These cancers are probably squamous cell or glandular cancers, but have become too anaplastic to make the distinction.

Small-cell carcinoma

Some 20–30% of lung cancers are small-cell carcinomas, also known as **oat-cell carcinoma**. This type of tumour is particularly invasive as the cells are poorly differentiated (anaplastic), growing within only 3 years of the initial malignant change. It is the only type of lung cancer that responds to chemotherapy. Distant metastases are present in 90% of patients with this tumour at the time of presentation, and therefore surgical intervention alone would not be curative.

A small proportion of these tumours produce ectopic hormones similar to ACTH, ADH and occasionally parathyroid hormone. These exert their appropriate metabolic effects and may be the cause of presenting symptoms. Histologically, the cells are distinctive with oval or elongated nuclei and very little cytoplasm. Frequent mitoses can be seen and the chromatin is often granular. Cell marker studies support a neuroendocrine origin.

Malignant mesothelioma

Malignant mesothelioma is a rare cancer arising from mesothelial cells that form the serous membrane covering the outside surfaces of the lungs. These cancers spread rapidly by seeding surfaces within the pleural cavity, eventually encasing the lung in a shell of tumour cells. Penetration of the tumour into the lung is relatively infrequent and metastatic spread is also uncommon. However, the prognosis is very poor and few patients survive beyond a year after diagnosis.

Mesotheliomas are related to exposure to asbestos, usually many years in the past. The greatest risk is attached to heavy occupational exposure, although cases have been reported in people who live close to an asbestos factory or in the same household as an asbestos worker. Mesothelioma occurs independently of cigarette smoking: in contrast to bronchial carcinoma there is no extra risk attached to smoking. A small minority of mesotheliomas appear to be unrelated to asbestos exposure, but the cause is unknown.

> *Malignant mesothelioma is usually caused by exposure to asbestos, and is unrelated to smoking*

Spread of lung cancer

Local spread
Bronchial tumours spread locally by invading the bronchial walls and into the surrounding lung tissues. A common feature is peribronchial spread: the tumour tracks along the outside edge of the bronchial wall to distant parts of the lung. In advanced disease the tumour often extends directly into the pleura and mediastinal structures. The superior vena cava can become obstructed by tumour, causing early morning headache, facial congestion and oedema of the upper limbs. Oesophageal involvement produces progressive dysphagia and spread to the pericardium will produce effusion and malignant dysrhythmias. Invasion of nerves, including the cervical sympathetic chain, the brachial plexus and laryngeal nerve, are also features with characteristic symptoms.

Lymphatic spread
Lung cancers spread to the ipsilateral and contralateral peribronchial and hilar lymph nodes.

Haematogenous spread
Given the rich blood supply of the lung it is hardly surprising that blood-borne metastases are common. The usual sites of secondary tumours are the

Leukoerythroblastic anaemia: anaemia characterised by depletion of both red and white blood cells.

bones, causing severe pain, pathological fractures and, as the bone marrow is extensively replaced by tumour, leukoerythroblastic anaemia. Bone metastases are most common in the ribs, vertebrae, humerus and femur. The liver frequently becomes involved, giving rise to hepatomegaly and symptoms of jaundice. Secondary deposits in the brain may be responsible for changes in personality or epilepsy.

Secondary tumours

The lungs are a favoured site for metastatic tumour deposits from other tissue sites: usually the kidney, bone, breast, prostate, gastrointestinal tract, cervix or ovary. Secondary deposits are usually detected radiologically as round nodules 1.5–3 cm in diameter. They develop in the parenchyma, and are often asymptomatic.

Metaplastic and dysplastic changes in the airways could be precursor lesions of lung cancer

Histological examination of squamous cell carcinoma often reveals hyperplastic, metaplastic, or dysplastic changes in areas adjacent to the tumour. This has stimulated some speculation that a sequence of precursor changes might precede the development of invasive lung cancer, in much the same way that dysplastic changes are recognised as precursor lesions for cervical cancer (see Chapter 16). Recognition of these lesions could allow earlier diagnosis and treatment, thereby preventing the progression to invasive cancer.

The sequence is believed to involve progression from hyperplasia, through metaplasia, dysplasia and carcinoma *in situ*, to invasive cancer. However, some of these 'precursor' changes are seen in other conditions, but they are not associated with increased risk of lung cancer. These include asthma and severe influenza, in which squamous metaplasia is often extensive. It may be that the metaplastic change is simply a marker for tissue repair after damage. Another problem is that these changes, if indeed they do represent precursor stages, are not easily detected by the currently available methods for diagnosis.

Lung cancer staging

In common with other types of cancer the size and spread of lung cancers are assessed by the TNM system. Tumours of less than 3 cm and confined to the lung are classified as Stage I, larger tumours and those with lymph node involvement are grouped into Stages II or III. All tumours with metastases are Stage IV. Surgical resection is considered for the treatment of all Stage I and II and some Stage III cancers. The more advanced cases, or patients who are not fit for surgery for other reasons, would be considered for radical radiotherapy. Chemotherapy is the treatment of choice for inoperable small-cell lung cancers.

Genetic alterations

One of the most frequent cytogenetic alterations seen in lung cancer is deletion of part of the short arm of chromosome 3. This region probably contains tumour suppressor genes although these have yet to be identified. Mutations of the *p53* tumour suppressor gene have been identified in tumour cells from patients with non-small-cell and small-cell lung cancers: this alteration does not appear to be associated with survival differences.

In contrast, mutations to the *K-ras* oncogene (see Chapter 13) have been found in about 20% of non-small-cell adenocarcinomas, but not in small-cell lung cancers. The presence of the mutation is an indicator of poor prognosis. The *K-ras* mutations are much more common in tumours from smokers. Oncogenes of the *erb-B* and *myc* families are also abnormally expressed in lung cancer patients. *Myc* amplification correlates with more aggressive tumours and poorer survival.

Other lung pathologies related to cancer

Drugs or radiation used in the treatment of primary or secondary lung cancers can lead to changes in the lungs, restricting their function. Most notable is the production of fibrosis in the alveolar wall, which is associated with the use of chemotherapeutic agents such as bleomycin, chlorambucil, melphalan and methotrexate. In some cases lung fibrosis occurs many years after successful therapy. Radiation damage can produce acute symptoms of dyspnoea and cough with fever, usually within 6 months of irradiation to the chest wall.

The bronchial obstruction caused by a tumour will initially impair the clearance of mucus secretions. This area of stagnation will often become the site of recurrent infection and persistent inflammation. The effect of this is to damage the walls of the airway so that there is a loss of support. This causes the permanent dilation of the airway called **bronchiectasis** (see Chapter 5). In this condition normal epithelium is replaced by chronic inflammatory granulation tissue, causing bleeding. Patients with bronchiectasis have symptoms of recurrent cough and haemoptysis, and often expectorate copious quantities of infected sputum. Repeated episodes of infection can lead to fibrosis and abscesses. Eventually obliteration of lung tissue by the tumour itself or by the bronchiectatic sequelae can lead to respiratory failure.

Clinical features

A variety of clinical symptoms become apparent according to the type of tumour and its degree of spread. In many cases patients remain asymptomatic until the tumour spread is well advanced.

Most lesions arise in the bronchi rather than the alveoli or the periphery of the lung. As a consequence symptoms may include or be related to partial lung collapse (emphysema or atelectasis), mucosal ulceration and bronchitis, pneumonia or repeated bronchiectatic infection, cough, wheeze, obstructive dyspnoea, chest pain, fever, haemoptysis or fatal haemorrhage.

Peripheral tumours can cause pain in the chest wall, cough, pleuritic pain, pleural effusion and restrictive dyspnoea. Cancers in this site are more likely to be asymptomatic until there is significant local spread or metastases. Venous

▲ Key points

Principal types of lung cancer

Squamous cell carcinoma:
- ▲ Most common type of lung cancer
- ▲ Strong association with smoking
- ▲ Often arise centrally in major bronchi
- ▲ Believed to be preceded by precancerous metaplastic or dysplastic changes

Adenocarcinoma:
- ▲ Weaker association with smoking than the squamous cell type
- ▲ Usually peripherally located
- ▲ Slow-growing, but metastases occur at an early stage

Large-cell carcinoma:
- ▲ Undifferentiated tumours
- ▲ Poor prognosis, early metastases, often involving central nervous system

Small-cell carcinoma:
- ▲ Strong association with cigarette smoking
- ▲ Usually centrally located
- ▲ Often secrete polypeptide hormones (e.g. ACTH, calcitonin)
- ▲ Poor prognosis, usually inoperable but sensitive to chemotherapy

Some symptoms become evident because of local invasion or metastases

congestion is common, particularly when the superior vena cava is involved by tumour.

Invasion of the pericardium, mediastinum, oesophagus, thoracic inlet and ribs may be associated with lung cancer. In turn damage can be caused to the brachial plexus and sympathetic plexus, resulting in severe pain in the arm and ulnar nerve palsy. Common sites of metastasis are the liver (30% of cases), brain (20%) and bone (20%).

Many tumour types, but particularly small-cell tumours, produce endocrine hormones not normally associated with the lung tissues. This excessive production of hormones can lead to a number of systemic effects, for example, ADH leads to hyponatraemia, ACTH to Cushing's syndrome, parathyroid hormone to hypercalcaemia, calcitonin to hypocalcaemia, gonadotrophins to gynaecomastia and serotonin to the carcinoid syndrome. The inappropriate elaboration of these hormones and their symptoms are described as a **paraneoplasia syndrome**.

In the late stages of the disease patients experience symptoms of nausea and vomiting, cachexia, hypercalcaemia and pain. The causes of nausea and vomiting include gastrointestinal disturbances because of compression or obstruction from the tumour mass, or liver metastases. Secondary deposits in the brain increase intracranial pressure and disturb the CNS. Nausea and vomiting can also be experienced as a consequence of hypercalcaemia, secondary to bone involvement or increased bone resorption. Finally, these symptoms can also be produced by treatment, notably chemotherapy, radiotherapy and administration of narcotics.

Loss of appetite, with ensuing loss of weight, is a significant cause for concern in patients with lung cancer. The causes of anorexia may be the cancer itself, reactions to treatment or complications arising from treatments including obstruction, infection, nausea and vomiting and diarrhoea. Weight loss often predicts a poor prognosis or response to treatment. Patients easily become fatigued and depressed.

Hypercalcaemia (serum calcium >11 mg/dl) affects up to 15% of patients, but is rare in those with small-cell lung cancer. It is produced when bone resorption exceeds bone formation. This typically accompanies bone metastases, but can also be associated with solid tumours that have not metastasised. In this instance the tumour cells release substances (for example parathyroid hormone-related protein) that act systemically to increase bone breakdown. The symptoms of hypercalcaemia include nausea and vomiting, anorexia, constipation, lethargy and drowsiness. Late changes include confusion, coma, hypertension and bradycardia. The most effective treatment is to treat the malignancy, but in refractory tumours the goal is to decrease bone resorption and at the same time increase renal calcium excretion. Treatment can include rehydration and a review of medication, or more aggressive intervention with calcitonin or etidronate.

Cancer pain can be either localised, as is often the case with bone metastases, or generalised and referred to distant sites. Bone pain can be managed by NSAIDs. Visceral pain is often described as cramp-like, deep aching or

---

Symptoms may be produced by excessive production of hormones

▲   **Key points**

Clinical features of lung cancer

▲ Cough, caused by blockage of airways and infection
▲ Chest pain, caused by involvement of pleura and chest wall
▲ Haemoptysis (with cough), caused by ulceration of tumour in the bronchus, can result in fatal haemorrhage
▲ Chest infection – bronchitis, pneumonia or repeated bronchiectatic infection
▲ Malaise, weight loss, shortness of breath, hoarseness
▲ Further symptoms due to local invasion or metastasis
▲ Paraneoplasia – endocrine-associated symptoms in some small-cell cancers

squeezing. In patients with lung cancer this usually arises from the thoracic or abdominal viscera if liver metastases are present. Narcotic analgesics such as morphine, hydromorphine or fentanyl are most appropriate for managing this type of pain. There is no ceiling effect with these drugs and doses should be appropriate to the response.

Diagnosis

Diagnostic methods are currently limited to the detection of invasive cancer. In a few situations precursor or *in-situ* lesions can be detected, but not reliably. Although strategies for prevention of smoking are the best way of reducing the large numbers of deaths from lung cancer, this will not help the millions of people who are currently smokers or who have only recently given up. On a world view, substantive decreases in the deaths from this disease will not be seen for many years – there is still a need for methods of early diagnosis and more effective treatments.

The diagnosis of lung cancer is currently based on the clinical findings, together with bronchoscopy, radiological imaging methods or laboratory tests. Physiological performance can be assessed by lung function tests.

Radiology and MRI

The initial diagnostic procedure would usually involve chest radiography to allow visualisation of the tumour and assessment of its size, location and secondary features such as infection and partial lung collapse. The method is relatively insensitive, and tumours typically need to be larger than 1 cm in size before they can be detected.

Both CT scanning and MRI can also be employed to visualise and assess the involvement of tumour locally and as metastases in organs such as the brain. CT scanning detects tumours of smaller size, but is inappropriate as an initial diagnostic procedure because it is time-consuming and relatively expensive. MRI has advantages over CT scanning in visualising mediastinal lesions that are close to blood vessels. Discrete tumour deposits in the chest or distant metastatic deposits can also be detected by the use of radioisotopes, usually gallium-35.

Bronchoscopy

This is the principal means of confirming diagnosis and involves introducing a flexible fibreoptic bronchoscope into the nasal passage and passing it down into the bronchial tree. Bronchoscopy allows visualisation of the bronchial surfaces and the taking of small tissue biopsies from abnormal-appearing areas. The method is sensitive enough to detect tumours not seen by radiographic methods, although early stage cancers (carcinoma *in situ*) may be missed. The reason is that these tumours are often small and only a few cell layers thick, so that no abnormality is visible when examined by conventional white-light bronchoscopy.

These problems have led to the development of fluorescence bronchoscopy, which uses fluorescent porphyrin drugs that are taken up and retained by tumours. When these substances are excited by violet light, red fluorescence is emitted. To date the diagnostic applications of these methods are limited by side-effects of the drug. However, there is evidence that the use of fluorescent drugs is not essential because dysplastic and carcinoma *in situ* cells exhibit spectroscopic changes of their own when examined by laser fluorescence.

Lung function tests

Tests of lung function are used as preoperative respiratory performance measures and offer a crude assessment of the degree of lung involvement. The decision to perform a partial or complete lung resection is influenced by the respiratory capacity.

Laboratory investigations

Sputum cytology

Malignant epithelial cells can be detected in the sputum; some cellular changes can be detected before a clinically evident tumour occurs. Detection rates (sensitivity) can be in the order of 85% for squamous lung cancers but more peripherally located adenocarcinomas are less easily detected.

Unfortunately, cytological methods are very insensitive for the detection of premalignant or *in-situ* lesions because they do not rapidly exfoliate and the yield of cells in sputum is very low. Even when atypical cells are identified by cytology, only about 10% of patients develop cancer on follow-up. Trials have shown that sputum cytology is ineffective at reducing mortality from lung cancer when used as a screening method.

The diagnosis is confirmed by histology of tissues taken specifically for biopsy purposes or from the surgically resected lung.

Treatment

The prognosis for patients with lung cancer is generally very poor

The 5-year survival rate for lung cancer is less than 10%

Attempts to cure patients of lung cancer rely on surgical intervention. In most patients the cancer is so advanced that it is considered inoperable, and therefore the main aim of treatment is palliation. Most tumours are inoperable because they have spread beyond the lung or because they involve major airways, invade major blood vessels, involve nerves supplying the vocal cords, have caused pleural effusion or have spread to local lymph nodes.

The important prognostic factors are the stage and histological grade of the tumour. In lung cancers, the type of tumour is also an important influence on treatment and outcome. Generally patients with small-cell carcinomas do worse than those with other types of lung cancer. Almost invariably these tumours are inoperable and are treated with chemotherapy and radiotherapy.

Complete or partial surgical resection of the lung in selected patients with early disease (8–15% of patients) can result in a 50% 5-year survival rate, compared with the overall 5-year survival rate of less than 10% for all types of lung cancer. Early disease is defined as a localised solitary tumour of less than 4 cm in diameter which does not involve lymph nodes and is without metastases (Stage T1–T2, N0, M0). These cases of early disease are more likely to be detected as an incidental finding on chest radiograph or sputum analysis, rather than as symptomatic disease

Surgical resection is usually confined to one lobe of the lung (lobectomy): total resection of the whole lung is not common. Although the lesser resection has the advantage of preserving lung tissue, its disadvantage is that there is a risk of recurrence (in up to 25% of patients) in the remaining lobe, generally within 2 years of surgery. The prognosis is much better for patients who do not suffer relapse in the first 4–5 years. However, the mortality rate from surgery can be high, with 10% of patients dying within 30 days.

Radiotherapy

Radiotherapy is used as a standalone treatment, as an adjunct to surgery or as a palliative measure. Most commonly the treatment is employed in fractionated doses over a period of 3–4 weeks, with 4–5 sessions per week and a total dose of 55–65 Gy. Survival can be as good as that obtained by surgery in patients with slow-growing squamous cell tumours. It is the treatment of choice in patients who cannot be operated on because of poor lung function.

Patients suffer the usual side-effects associated with radiotherapy: pain, tiredness, nausea, anorexia, skin lesions and hypersensitivity, decreased concentration and cough. Properly applied, the treatment carries no immediate mortality risk. Radiotherapy is usually specifically aimed at the site of the primary tumour but the widespread lung deposits often associated with small-cell carcinomas are less suitable for treatment. In these cases radiotherapy is used in conjunction with chemotherapy. Prophylactic cranial irradiation significantly reduces the incidence of brain metastases of small-cell lung cancers but does not significantly improve overall survival.

Radiotherapy is the most effective treatment for palliation of haemoptysis, bronchial obstruction or obstruction of the superior vena cava. Bone pain can also be relieved by radiotherapy.

Chemotherapy

Chemotherapy can be offered as a palliative therapy but the significant side-effects associated with the treatment must be weighed very carefully against the possible benefits. Side-effects include hair loss, lethargy, anaemia, lowered immunity and increased bleeding. Most chemotherapeutic approaches use drugs in combination, aimed at cells in different stages of the growth cycle.

The main use of chemotherapy is for the treatment of small-cell lung cancers. One treatment protocol uses cisplatin, doxorubicin, etoposide and ifosfamide.

▲ **Key points**

Treatment of lung cancer

▲ By the time symptoms develop most lung cancers cannot be cured

▲ Early detection of lung cancer by screening is not currently feasible

▲ A cure may be attempted in some early non-small-cell cancers by surgical resection

▲ Survival in cases of small-cell cancer can be prolonged by a combination of radiotherapy and chemotherapy

---

Review question 1

Explain why lung cancer continues to be a major public health problem.

Chemotherapy cannot cure lung cancer, unless combined with surgery or radiotherapy

> *Small-cell lung cancers are the most sensitive to chemotherapy, but even these soon become resistant*

Initial success in shrinking tumours and relieving symptoms can be very high (80–90%) in small-cell carcinomas but is less successful in the long term; most treated patients with small-cell carcinoma die within a year. Chemotherapy can also help to relieve pain, reduce breathlessness, improve mobility and slow weight loss. A small proportion of patients achieve several years of remission. Without treatment, the median survival for newly diagnosed patients with small-cell lung cancer is 1–3 months.

ANSWERS TO REVIEW QUESTIONS

Question 1

Explain why lung cancer continues to be a major public health problem

The main influences on the incidence and mortality rates for all types of cancer are the ability to prevent the disease, or diagnose it at an early stage, and treat it effectively. With respect to lung cancer there has been a spectacular failure on all counts. The greatest potential for reducing lung cancer deaths is primary prevention. Here, the message appears to be quite simple – do not smoke.

There are many problems in getting that message across, not least of which are the attitudes and vested interests of the tobacco companies, taxation revenue implications for the government, and issues around the individual freedoms of people to live their lives as they wish. A major problem remains in the less developed counties, where tobacco companies concentrate their marketing efforts.

The factors governing smoking are extremely complex: many smokers are aware of the risks but continue the habit. Modification of these factors strikes at the heart of how society is organised and will not come about overnight, or even in the lifetimes of many readers of this book. A realistic way forward is to ensure that the message about the dangers of smoking is given at every opportunity, and to help those that want to give up the habit in every way possible.

The second strategy is that of secondary prevention. This usually means screening, but currently lung cancer can not be reliably detected at an early asymptomatic stage.

Despite the advances in surgery, chemotherapy and radiotherapy over the past 40 years the impact on lung cancer mortality has been negligible. Perhaps the most notable achievement is the use of chemotherapy and radiotherapy in small-cell lung cancers, but at best these treatments achieve only a modest increase in survival. Today, most people with lung cancer can expect to die of their disease, just as people did 40 years ago. The only real difference is that 40 years ago there were far fewer cases, because cigarette consumption had not yet reached its peak.

Further reading

Austoker, J. (1994) Smoking and cancer: smoking cessation. *BMJ*, **308**, 1478–82.

Editorial. (1991) Screening for lung cancer. *J. Surg. Oncol.*, **46**, 1–2.

Hinson, J.A. and Perry, M.C. (1993) Small cell lung cancer. *CA Cancer J. Clin.*, **43**, 216–25.

Ihde, D.C. (1992) Chemotherapy of lung cancer. *N. Engl. J. Med.*, **327**, 1434–41.

Martini, M. (1993) Operable lung cancer. *CA Cancer J. Clin.*, **43**, 201–14.

Peto, R. (1994) Smoking and death: the past 40 years and the next 40. *BMJ*, **309**, 937–9.

Various (1993) Conference extracts on 'Innovations in the multimodality therapy of lung cancer'. *Chest*, **103**, Suppl 1.

15 Breast cancer

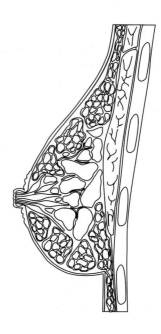

In some developed countries breast cancer can affect up to one in ten women. The strongest risk factor for the disease is family history and there is currently no means of primary prevention. Despite advances in medical treatment there has been little real progress in reducing mortality from this disease although it is to be hoped that routine mammographic screening will have some impact.

Over the past decade it has been recognised that breast cancer should be regarded as a systemic disease, and that many women have latent micrometastases at the time of presentation. Treatment of the primary breast tumour is nowadays aimed at local control; the radical and disfiguring surgical procedures of the past will not be necessary for all women with breast cancer. Where these are required a range of reconstructive procedures are available that improve the cosmetic result.

For many women adequate local control can be achieved by the combination of 'lumpectomy' or partial mastectomy with radiotherapy. A systemic approach to treatment in the younger woman will probably include adjuvant chemotherapy. In a woman who has reached the menopause and has an oestrogen receptor-positive tumour, adjuvant treatment with the antioestrogen drug tamoxifen is likely to improve survival prospects.

Pre-test

- **What are the chances of a woman living in the UK developing breast cancer?**
- **What are the chances of dying from breast cancer?**
- **Does the risk of breast cancer differ in various parts of the world?**
- **What factors are believed to cause or influence the development of breast cancer?**
- **What symptoms accompany breast cancer?**
- **What treatments are available for breast cancer?**
- **Can people be screened for breast cancer before they become aware of any symptoms?**

Aims of this chapter

By the end of this chapter you will have increased your knowledge of:
- The epidemiology of breast cancer, the age at which the disease is most likely to occur and geographical differences in incidence and mortality
- The genetic and environmental factors involved in the development of breast cancer
- The various types of breast cancer, where they arise and the parts of the body to which they spread
- How breast cancer is diagnosed and the measures that can be taken to detect the condition at an early stage
- The factors that influence survival
- How breast cancer is treated

In addition, this chapter will help you to:
- Suggest reasons for the historical and geographical differences in rates of breast cancer
- Assess the role of reproductive hormones in breast cancer and the potential of endocrine therapy as a means of systemic control
- Describe the different approaches to treatment, their indications and implications
- Describe the ways in which prognosis can be assessed
- Analyse the *Health of the Nation* strategy for reducing deaths from breast cancer and how the targets can be met

Introduction

About 25 000 new cases of breast cancer are diagnosed each year in the UK and 15 000 women die from the disease – the disease affects one in 12 women in the UK. Despite advances in medical treatments the mortality rate from the disease has not markedly declined in recent years. The changes in medical treatments involve more conservative surgery and adjuvant chemotherapy or hormonal treatment. The prospects for preventing the disease are limited because there is no known single cause and many of the risk factors that have been identified are not easily altered.

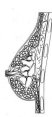

Breast cancer is the most common cause of death from cancer among women in the UK

Recent advances have been made in our understanding of the genetics of breast cancer. Many women with breast cancer have a family history of the disease. Most inherited genetic alterations that are responsible for the development of breast cancer involve one of two genes, *BRCA1* and *BRCA2*. It is likely that a wide variety of mutations can occur in these genes, which would make it very difficult to identify women with a predisposition for breast cancer on the basis of finding a single specific genetic defect. Moreover, most breast cancers occur as sporadic events and, although there may be some mutations to the *BRCA* genes, it is more likely that there will be alterations in other genes.

Women do not respond in the same way to breast cancer: one will present with a 1.5 cm lump in her breast, have a mastectomy, and go on to live another 30 years. Another, with a similar presentation, will rapidly die from metastatic disease. In some women metastases will spread to the lungs or liver, in others the bones or brain will be affected. At present the factors governing these differences are not known.

The *Health of the Nation* strategy for reducing mortality from breast cancer focuses on mammographic breast screening. In most cases screening detects only breast changes after they have become invasive: it is not very effective at detecting preinvasive malignant changes (compared with cervical screening, for example). This restricts the potential of the method to reduce the number of deaths from breast cancer. Even so, screen-detected breast cancers are usually smaller and at an earlier stage and hence some improvement in morbidity and mortality statistics is possible by regular screening.

Epidemiology

Other countries have similar breast cancer incidence rates but lower mortality rates than in the UK

There is a significant geographical variation in both the incidence and mortality from breast cancer (Figure 15.1). Generally, incidence of the disease is lower in the less developed countries. In developed countries there is variation in mortality from breast cancer. For example, there are greater numbers of cases of breast cancer in Sweden and the USA than the UK, but deaths from the disease are fewer. Why this should be so is not clear, since the available treatments do not differ substantially in these countries. The disparity is most probably caused by women delaying presenting with the disease: as with many cancers, survival is related to the tumour stage at the time of diagnosis. The overall 5-year survival rate is about 64%, but the disease often recurs within 20–25 years. Two-thirds of all women who contract breast cancer will eventually die from it.

Countries in which breast cancer incidence rates were historically low now have the largest increases. This may be because of a combination of better diagnosis and reporting, longer life expectancy, conversion to a more affluent way of life and better diet.

Migration studies (in Japanese women who migrated to Hawaii for example) show that immigrants tend to take on the rate in the host country. This suggests that environmental factors may be of some importance in the development of breast cancer (Figure 15.2).

Risk factors

Breast cancer is more common in post-menopausal women

The cause of breast cancer is not understood and currently there is little prospect for preventing the disease by altering lifestyle or behavioural factors. Generally, the incidence rises with age. The greatest risk for developing the disease appears to be a positive family history (Table 15.1).

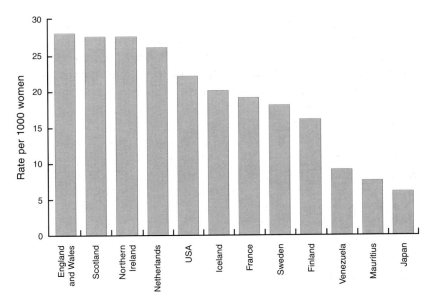

Figure 15.1 Geographical variation in deaths from breast cancer. The highest mortality rates for breast cancer are seen in the UK. Low incidence and mortality rates are found in Japan and in less developed countries. (Source: Forrest, 1986.)

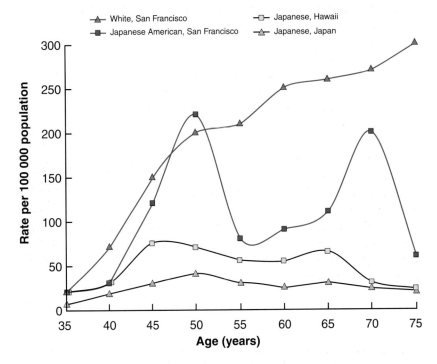

Figure 15.2 Annual incidence of breast cancer in Japanese and American women. In American white women incidence of breast cancer increases with age. In Japan there is a comparatively low incidence of breast cancer. Incidence rises dramatically in Japanese migrants to the USA, particularly in menopausal and older age groups. (Source: Buel J. (1973) *J. Natl. Cancer Inst.*, **51**, 1479–53.)

Table 15.1　Relative risk estimates for breast cancer

Risk factor	Relative risk
Age at first live birth (years)	
< 20	1.00
20–24	1.55
25–29	2.12
30	2.71
No birth	2.31
Family history of breast cancer	3.11
Age at menopause (years)	
< 44	0.58
25–49	0.63
> 50	0.91
Age at menarche (years)	
< 11	1.00
12–13	1.28
14–15	1.10
16	0.98
Socioeconomic group	
I	2.07
II	1.33
III	1.11
IV	1.00

A relative risk of 3.11 (e.g. a positive family history of breast cancer) indicates that for every 100 patients who do not have a family history of the disease, there will be 311 with a family history. Data from WHO Collaborative Study, 1990

Age

The incidence of breast cancer rises from about 10 per 100 000 women under 30 years of age to 150 per 100 000 aged 50 and 200 per 100 000 women aged 65 years (Figure 15.3). The incidence and mortality rates have shown increases since 1951 in most age groups except 15–44 years. Most population studies point towards a poorer survival in women diagnosed with breast cancer under 35 years of age. In this age group it is estimated that 8–20% fewer patients are cured of breast cancer than in other pre-menopausal patients aged 40–49. The poorer prognosis appears to be independent of other prognostic factors such as tumour size, lymph node status, histological grade or hormone receptor status. The biological explanation for the difference is uncertain and may be explained by delays in diagnosis and treatment.

Encouragingly, there is now evidence that mortality from breast cancer in England and Wales is beginning to decline (Figure 15.4). This has occurred across the age range but is particularly apparent in younger women (aged 20–49). The reasons are unclear, but contributory factors could be earlier medical

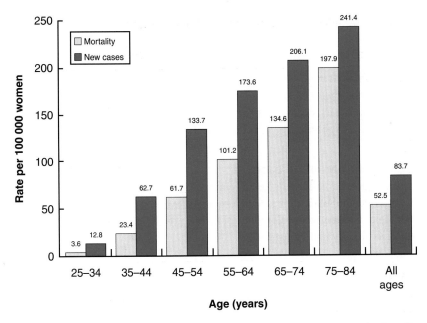

Figure 15.3 Incidence of and mortality from breast cancer. Breast cancer is virtually unknown in women under the age of 25 years. Thereafter the incidence and mortality increase. (Source: OPCS.)

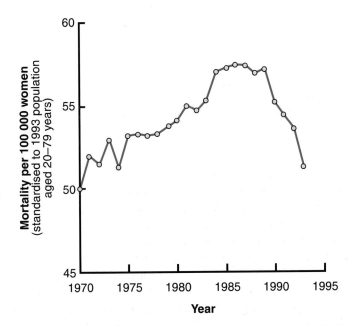

Figure 15.4 Since 1989 mortality rates from breast cancer have declined in England and Wales. (Adapted from Beral, V. *et al.* (1995) *Lancet*, **345**, 1642–43.)

attention and improvements in treatment. The fall has been too sudden to reflect a decrease in the number of women developing the disease. Although a national breast screening programme is now in place much of the reduction in mortality has occurred in women who have not been screened because they are too young.

Family history

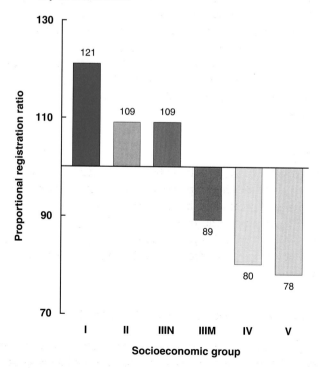

Breast cancer very often runs in families

A further risk factor is family history. Women who have first-degree relatives (mother, aunt, sister) are at higher risk, especially if more than one relative is affected, or if the breast cancer occurred before the menopause or was bilateral.

History of breast disease

Most women who have a history of fibrocystic disease are not at increased risk of breast cancer

Unless accompanied by epithelial hyperplasia, fibrocystic disease of the breast is not associated with increased risk of breast cancer. A much more significant risk is recurrence, or development of tumour in the other breast, in a woman who has already had breast cancer.

Social class

Epithelial hyperplasia: overgrowth of cells within the proliferated ducts and lobules of fibrocystic disease. In most cases the cells are cytologically normal (hyperplasia of usual type), but in the less frequent atypical hyperplasia cells have abnormal appearance. Associated with increased risk of breast cancer.

Fibrocystic disease: a benign overgrowth of breast lobules, ducts and fibrous connective tissues.

The incidence and mortality statistics for England and Wales demonstrate a variation in risk with social class: women in higher socioeconomic groups have a slightly increased risk of developing the disease, although women of lower socioeconomic status are more likely to die from the disease (Figure 15.5). Non-white women are less likely to develop the disease, but those who do are more likely to die from it.

Figure 15.5 Women from higher socioeconomic groups in England and Wales are at greater risk of developing breast cancer: for every 78 women in socioeconomic group V who develop breast cancer, there are 121 women in group I.

These patterns probably reflect cultural and social differences. Well educated women are more likely to recognise the significance of any signs or symptoms and seek early medical attention, thereby improving their survival. Cultural factors involving contraception, family size and dietary habits could influence the risk of developing breast cancer. Religious beliefs and social taboos about intimate areas of the body can delay presentation for medical attention.

Oestrogen-related risk factors

Other main risk factors are related to oestrogen exposure. This hormone is known to play a role in both human and animal carcinogenesis. For this reason concerns have been raised about a possible role for oral contraceptives and HRT in breast cancer.

The risk of breast cancer is associated with duration of exposure to oestrogen

Those women who undergo menopause early (before the age of 50 years) have a lower risk than women whose menopause is late. The age of menarche is relatively unimportant. Paradoxically, in view of the oestrogen influx during pregnancy, women with children have a lower risk than those who do not. The age of first pregnancy is an important factor: the risk being lower the younger the woman was at first birth.

Exposure to oestrogen is influenced by menstrual and reproductive histories

Obesity is a risk factor for breast cancer in post-menopausal women. This may be related to the storage of oestrogens in adipose tissue. Oestrogens can act as tumour promoters and may be released over a longer period than in non-obese women. There may also be some association with fat consumption (diets in developed countries are different from those in other countries, where the incidence of breast cancer is lower). These studies are inconclusive, and are complicated by differences in pregnancy rates in developed and less developed countries. High alcohol consumption (more than two units a day) has also been associated with increased risk of breast cancer. The mechanism is uncertain: alcohol can be a contributory factor in obesity and may elevate oestrogen levels.

Obesity is a risk factor because oestrogen is stored in adipose tissue

Pregnancy

Young women who are diagnosed with breast cancer during pregnancy or within a few years of pregnancy have a poorer prognosis than women of a similar age who have not been pregnant. The shorter the time between a pregnancy and diagnosis of breast cancer, the greater the risk of dying from the disease. This increased risk persists for 3–4 years after pregnancy. The reasons for this are unknown, but could be related to hormonal or immunological changes during pregnancy.

Women who are pregnant at the time of diagnosis are more than twice as likely to die of breast cancer

Oral contraceptives and breast cancer

If the hormones in oral contraceptives acted as tumour promoters any adverse effects should be revealed by a dose response associated with duration of use. When oral contraceptives were first introduced in the UK in the late 1960s they were taken mainly by older women who had completed their families. So far, there is no epidemiological evidence to suggest that these women are at

Oral contraceptive use is not associated with a markedly increased risk of developing breast cancer

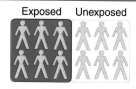

Exposed   Unexposed

Nurses' Health Study

▲ Involved 121 700 nurses aged 30–55 years in 1976

▲ Questionnaire every 2 years on current use of hormones, duration and type of preparation

▲ Follow-up 725 550 woman-years

▲ Cases of invasive breast cancer: 1935

▲ Relative risk of breast cancer 1.46 for women taking HRT for more than 5 years, compared with postmenopausal women who had never used hormones

From Colditz *et al.*, 1995.

The risk of breast cancer for women on long-term HRT may be increased

---

Review question 1

A 30-year-old primary school teacher discovers a lump in her breast. She has no children, and her mother recently died from breast cancer at the age of 65. An aunt also died from the disease at the age of 45 some years ago. What is the likelihood that the lump is caused by breast cancer?

The knowledge that breast cancer aggregates in certain families has led to an intensive search for the genes responsible

---

increased risk of developing breast cancer.

As oral contraceptives were not available for use when these women were young these findings may not be representative of current patterns of use. Information is now becoming available on breast cancer risk in women who initiated oral contraceptives before the age of 25. These studies suggest that long-term use (more than 8 years) could increase the risk of breast cancer occurring at an early age. However, the studies lack consistency and statistical power, mainly because the number of young women available for study is small (the risk of breast cancer in women under 35 in the UK is about one in 500).

Studies of oral contraception in women with a family history of breast cancer have not produced conclusive results, some studies showing excess risk, and others not. Women who have existing benign disease and take oral contraceptives do not appear to be at markedly greater risk than similar women without benign disease.

Overall, epidemiological studies suggest that any effects of oral contraceptives are subtle. If anything, long-term oral contraception may promote the earlier appearance of breast cancer in women who would anyway go on to develop the condition, and does not cause an increase in the absolute number of women affected.

Breast cancer risk and HRT

There has been some debate about the possibility that HRT increases the risk of breast cancer. The problem is that HRT has changed over the years, and reliable information about the more common combined therapy (oestrogen and progestagens) is only now becoming available. Evidence from the Nurses' Health Study shows an increase in risk of about 50% for long-term (more than 5 years) use of HRT. The addition of progestins to the therapy does not appear to change the risk, compared with oestrogen alone. Most epidemiological studies indicate that shorter durations of use are not associated with increased risk.

The risks of HRT have to be weighed against its advantages in reducing CHD and osteoporotic fractures. These effects probably give rise to a net gain in years of life. Even so, because of the possibility that oestrogens stimulate tumour growth it is probably prudent for women who have had breast cancer, or who have a family history of the disease, to avoid HRT.

Genetics

Some families are devastated by an inherited form of breast cancer that strikes women when in their thirties or forties. This pattern of breast cancer accounts for only about 5% of all breast cancer cases, and is believed to involve highly penetrant dominant genes. In some of these families the high incidence of breast cancer is accompanied by a clustering of ovarian cancers. The two cancer types can even occur in the same woman.

Genetic linkage analysis of affected family members has revealed the presence of an inherited susceptibility gene for these cancers on the long arm of chromosome 17 (17q12–q21). This gene, called *BRCA1*, comprises 23 exons spread over 100 kb of genomic DNA. The gene product has not yet been identified, but is predicted to be a DNA-binding protein of about 1860 amino acids.

More than 100 different types of mutation have now been found in *BRCA1*, many of which are confined to one or two families. A common mutation is a frame-shift at position 185, involving the deletion of adenine and guanine (185delAG). Most notably, the mutation is found in Ashkenazi Jews (of Eastern European origin) at an estimated frequency of about one in 100 women. This compares with an estimated frequency of one in 833 for all *BRCA1* mutations in non-Jewish women. Nearly half of the families with early-onset cancer carry a mutation in the *BRCA1* gene, and virtually all families with both breast and ovarian cancer clustering show linkage to the defective *BRCA1* gene.

> *BRCA1 mutations account for 30–50% of inherited breast cancers*

Another cancer susceptibility gene, *BRCA2*, has recently been found in a region on the long arm of chromosome 13 (13q 12–13). Mutations in this area probably account for as many cases of inherited breast cancer as the *BRCA1* gene but there does not appear to be such a strong association with ovarian cancer. Together, *BRCA1* and *BRCA2* mutations account for most, but not all, familial cases of breast cancer and it is therefore likely that there are other susceptibility genes that remain to be identified.

Breast cancers caused by either *BRCA1* or *BRCA2* mutations are characterised by early age of onset (usually before 40 years), disease in both breasts, and another affected woman in the family. Although the mutations can be detected by linkage analysis in the affected families, there are problems about what to do when such a genetic abnormality is found. In high-risk families a woman who has the gene mutation has an 85% risk of developing breast or ovarian cancer during her lifetime, and her risk of developing ovarian cancer during her life may be 50%. This places the woman in the unenviable position of having to decide whether to have both breasts and her ovaries removed as a precautionary measure. Alternatively, she may elect for careful surveillance in the hope of early detection of cancer, although both options have their problems. It has been reported that cancer can arise in residual epithelial cells even after breast or ovarian surgery. Mammography and clinical examination in women under the age of 40 are not wholly reliable for the detection of breast cancer and there are no screening methods of proven reliability for ovarian cancer.

> *Genetic linkage analysis can be used to trace the inheritance of BRCA mutations in high-risk families*

Conversely, a result showing that a woman has not inherited a mutant gene does not clear her of risk of breast cancer. She faces the same risk of breast cancer as any other woman and it is still possible for her to acquire *BRCA* mutations – or indeed mutations in other genes that confer susceptibility to breast cancer.

It is possible that mutations to the *BRCA1* gene can occur as sporadic events, but this is probably rare in non-inherited breast cancers: most are caused by multiple mutations in a number of common genes. Other genetic alterations in breast cancer involve amplification or expression of oncogenes. Amplification of *erbB*, *HER2* (*erbB-2*) and *erbB-3* oncogenes is seen in about

> *The BRCA genes are not the only genes involved in breast cancer susceptibility*

two-thirds of breast cancer cases. Over-expression of *HER2* (*erbB-2*) appears to be associated with poor prognosis. The protein product probably corresponds to a growth factor receptor, expressed on the cell surface, which renders the cell more susceptible to growth stimulation.

High tumour concentrations of the *HER2* gene product have also been found in post-menopausal patients with a family history of breast cancer. This is in contrast to the inherited *BRCA1* gene mutations that are predominantly associated with breast cancer in younger women. Although few mutations have been found in the *HER2* gene itself, it is likely that mutations occur in a nearby region of the chromosome which regulate the expression of the *HER2* gene product. Other alterations involve the oncogenes *c-myc* and *H-ras*. The *p53* tumour suppressor gene may also become deleted or mutated.

> *Tumours from women with a family history of breast cancer have high levels of HER2 protein*

Review question 2

What are the known risk factors for breast cancer?

> *Breast cancers usually arise in the milk-producing glands and ducts*

Pathology

The most common adenocarcinomas of the breast arise from the **terminal ductal lobular units** (Figure 15.6): the milk-secreting glands (lobules) and the terminal portion of a branching duct system that transports the milk to the nipple. The tumours are classified as either **invasive lobular** or **invasive ductal** carcinoma. The preinvasive forms, confined entirely within the lobules or ducts, are **lobular carcinoma *in situ*** (LCIS) and **ductal carcinoma *in situ*** (DCIS). At one time DCIS was unusual but it is now commonly detected by routine mammographic screening. The incidence of lobular carcinoma *in situ*, which is not usually diagnosed by mammography, remains much the same.

> **▲ Key points**
>
> **Genetic alterations in familial breast cancer**
>
> ▲ Mutations in *BRCA1* account for 30–50% of inherited breast cancers and are associated with ovarian cancer
>
> ▲ More than 100 mutations of *BRCA1* are known, but the 185delAG mutation is more common in Ashkenazi Jews
>
> ▲ Mutations in *BRCA2* account for as many cases of breast cancer as *BRCA1*, but are not associated with ovarian cancer

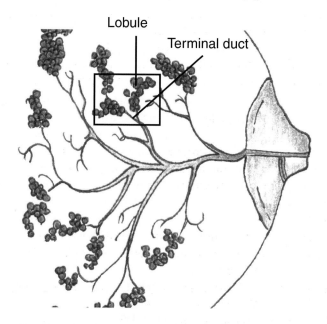

Figure 15. 6 Invasive adenocarcinoma of the breast arises from the terminal ducts and lobular units.

Some rarer categories of breast cancer are medullary, mucinous, papillary and tubular carcinomas. Together they account for less than 10% of breast cancers.

Relationship between *in-situ* and invasive breast cancers

As the name suggests, *in-situ* breast cancers (LCIS and DCIS) are made up of cancerous cells that have not yet progressed to invasive cancer. All *in-situ* cancers have the potential to progress to invasive cancer, but not all do so. Lesions of DCIS can be classified on the basis of general morphological (into **comedo** or **non-comedo** lesions) and cellular appearances (according to tumour stage), which helps to predict which lesions are more likely to recur in women treated by breast-conserving surgery.

In one study of DCIS (Silverstein *et al.*, 1995) the greatest risk of recurrence was attached to high-grade lesions with comedo-type necrosis, for which recurrence rates were of the order of 40% at 8 years. This compares with about 7% in women with low-grade non-comedo lesions. Nearly 50% of recurrences were invasive cancers.

Poor survival from breast cancer is related to tumour recurrence and metastatic disease. These characteristics are extremely variable and may occur quickly in some patients, while in others they may not occur until many years after local treatment, if at all. **Local** spread is into the adjacent breast tissue, and can include the skin or the underlying pectoral muscles. More distant spread is by the lymphatics or blood circulation. **Lymphatic** spread refers to the dissemination of tumour cells by the lymphatic drainage system (Figure 15.7). Involvement of lymphatics draining the skin by tumour gives rise to a characteristic puckering or **peau d'orange** effect. The most commonly involved lymph nodes are the axillary and internal mammary nodes. **Vascular** spread is commonly, but not predictably, to the bone, lungs, liver pleura and ovary.

Staging and prognosis

Breast cancers are classified according to the size of the tumour (T) and its involvement in the chest wall or the skin, the involvement of lymph nodes (N) and the occurrence of metastases (M): this is known as the TNM staging classification system.

- **Stage 0:** carcinoma *in situ*
- **Stage I:** mobile tumour of 1 cm and confined to the breast
- **Stage II:** as Stage I, but with some nodal involvement or larger tumours (2–5 cm). No known metastases
- **Stage III:** locally advanced tumour (e.g. attached to chest wall). Lymph nodes involved. No known metastases
- **Stage IV:** distant metastases present

Survival is best if the lymph nodes are not involved and there are no detectable metastases (Figure 15.8).

▲ Key points

Oncogene alterations in breast cancer

- ▲ The *erbB* group is amplified or over-expressed in 60% of cases
- ▲ Amplification of *erbB-2* (*HER2*) is a marker of poor prognosis; gene product corresponds to a growth factor receptor protein
- ▲ *c-myc* may be amplified or over-expressed
- ▲ *H-ras* may be amplified or over-expressed

▲ Key points

Types of breast cancer

Pre-invasive:
- ▲ Ductal carcinoma *in situ*
- ▲ Lobular carcinoma *in situ*

Invasive:
- ▲ Ductal carcinoma
- ▲ Lobular carcinoma
- ▲ Medullary carcinoma
- ▲ Mucinous carcinoma
- ▲ Tubular carcinoma
- ▲ Papillary carcinoma

The further a tumour has spread, the worse the prognosis

Comedo ductal carcinoma *in situ*: morphological type of *in-situ* carcinoma of the breast, in which the central area of the lesion contains necrotic debris. This is surrounded by large, irregularly shaped cells in solid clumps.

Non-comedo ductal carcinoma *in situ*: includes other tumour growth patterns such as cribriform (contains spaces or holes, like a sieve) or micropapillary (small projections).

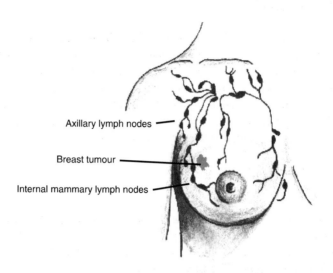

Figure 15.7 Local spread of breast cancer. Breast cancer cells invade lymphatic channels and typically spread to the axillary lymph nodes. Internal mammary lymph nodes may also become involved by tumour.

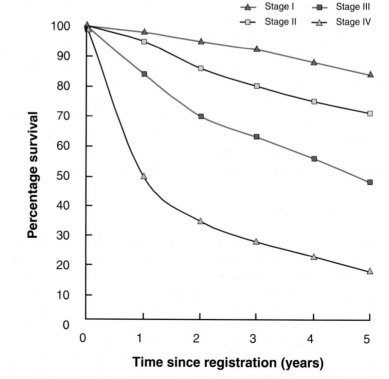

Figure 15.8 Breast cancer survival by stage. Women with Stage I disease have a better prognosis than those with later stage disease.

▲   Key points

Breast cancer survival

- ▲ Overall 5-year survival about 64%
- ▲ Overall 20-year survival about 25%
- ▲ Stage I disease-free 5-year survival 84%
- ▲ Stage II disease-free 5-year survival 71%
- ▲ Stage III disease-free 5-year survival 48%
- ▲ Stage IV disease-free 5-year survival 18%

Histological grade

Histological grade refers to the degree of differentiation of the tumour cells and is based on criteria such as gland formation, the size and shape of the cell nuclei and the number of dividing cells. The grade can be used to predict the aggressiveness of the tumour and its potential for metastasis. Few non-screen-detected breast cancers are well differentiated (grade 1, 10-year survival 85%); moderately and poorly differentiated tumours correspond to grade 2 (10-year survival 60%) and 3 (10-year survival 45%), respectively.

A further prognostic factor is based on histological grade

Differentiation: cells are said to be differentiated when they carry out specific functions in a particular type of tissue.

Fat necrosis: localised area of inflammation following trauma and collapse of adipose tissue.

Fibroadenoma: a benign localised proliferation of breast ducts and connective tissues.

Mastitis: a painful, tender enlargement of the breast caused by infection, commonly *Staphylococcus aureus* or *Streptococcus*. Usually associated with lactation.

Diagnosis

Breast cancer is diagnosed after screening or presentation of signs or symptoms, which include the appearance of a lump in the breast, breast pain, swelling of the breast (which may extend under the arm), puckering of the skin and bleeding from the nipple. The presence of a tumour may be revealed by palpation, performed by the woman herself or by her physician. Generally, lumps over 1.5 cm in diameter are revealed by self examination, although with experience lumps of about 1 cm diameter can be palpated. This contrasts with the 2–5 mm tumours that can be detected by mammography.

Not all breast lumps are malignant: about 30% have no detectable disease. The most common reason for a lump is fibrocystic disease, accounting for about 40% of breast lumps. It is estimated that about 10% of women develop fibrocystic lumps at some stage, and the number in whom lumps never become clinically apparent but are found at post mortem is higher. Fibrocystic disease accounts for nearly half of all surgical operations on the female breast: very often these lumps are excised to confirm the diagnosis by histology. Some 'lumps' may turn out to be fluid-filled cysts, perhaps arising from an infection.

The most common benign tumour of the female breast is fibroadenoma, accounting for about 7% of breast lumps. This can occur at any age but is more common in women under 30. Other benign disorders include mastitis and fat necrosis, which together account for about 13% of breast lumps.

Only one in ten breast lumps are caused by cancer

Imaging methods

A woman who has a palpable breast lump will usually be referred for mammography (Plate 1). Both breasts will be examined even though a lump may have only been felt in one: sometimes cancers are also detected in the non-symptomatic side. In older women it is relatively easy to discriminate cell proliferation or calcification against a background of fibrofatty tissue but this becomes much more difficult in younger women (below 40 years), in whom the breast contains a much higher proportion of glandular tissue.

Discrimination between benign and malignant tumours is usually possible because of differences in shape and radiodensity: benign tumours usually have regular margins whereas malignant tumours are more likely to be irregular in shape. Malignant tumours often contain small foci of calcification

The initial diagnostic tests usually involve an imaging technique such as mammography or ultrasound

Benign and malignant tumours usually have different mammographic appearances

Mammography: radiological examination of the breast using low-energy photons in the 25–35 kV range. The breast must be compressed between perspex plates in order to optimise image quality and minimise the radiation dose.

(**microcalcification**), which sometimes are the only sign of malignancy (Figure 15.9). Most breast cancers are detectable by mammography, but there is a risk of both false-positive and false-negative results.

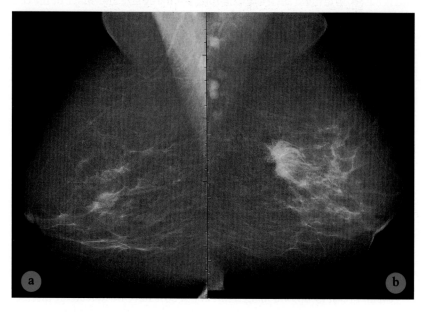

Figure 15.9 Mammograms of (a) normal breast and (b) of breast tumour with irregular outline and some microcalcification.

Ultrasonography is used to discriminate breast cysts and to investigate younger women in whom mammography is uninformative

Ultrasonography is useful for the examination of dense breast tissues, but does not detect microcalcifications very well. It can provide excellent discrimination of (completely benign) breast cysts (Figure 15.10). The breasts are usually scanned in a radial motion so as to follow the line of the ducts. The examination is a real-time dynamic process although results can be reviewed on a video recording.

Laboratory diagnosis

Ultimately, the diagnosis is confirmed by microscopic examination of the cells

Cells can be obtained by needle aspiration, wide-bore needle biopsy (Trucut needle) or by surgery. The simplest technique is fine-needle aspiration, often performed with mammographic guidance to ensure the correct area is sampled. The technique is performed under local anaesthesia by inserting a 21-gauge needle into the lump and evacuating fluid and cells. The contents are expelled on to a microscope slide, fixed, stained and examined. Intact tissue is not removed by this technique, and the individual cells are evaluated according to their cytological characteristics. This method can be less reliable than histological examination of intact tissue.

Histological examination is used for diagnosis and tumour staging

Histological diagnosis can be made on tissue removed at surgery or by Trucut needle biopsy. This is the most accurate form of diagnosis because it is possible to see the cytological characteristics of the cells and the degree of invasion

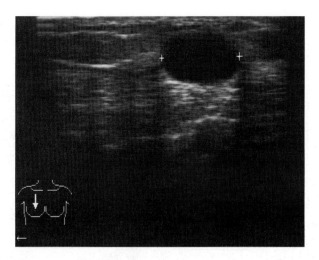

Figure 15.10 Ultrasonographic image of breast tissue, showing a cyst with typical rounded appearance.

outside the glands or ducts. Histology is also the most appropriate technique for assessing the presence of malignancy in surgically removed axillary lymph nodes.

Prognostic factors

The main prognostic factors are tumour stage, grade and size (Figure 15.11). These factors, together with the pre- or post-menopausal status of the patient, influence selection for adjuvant chemotherapy, endocrine therapy or radiotherapy. Younger women (under 35 years of age) usually have a poorer prognosis than older women with cancers of similar stage (Table 15.2), possibly because their tumours are unlikely to be oestrogen receptor-positive, and will therefore be unresponsive to hormonal therapy.

Prognosis depends on how far the cancer has spread before it is diagnosed and treated

Currently the most effective means of staging involves surgical removal and histological examination of the axillary lymph nodes. Lymph node involvement can also, but not invariably, be detected by radiographic means. Node-positive women are more likely to die from breast cancer and therefore will usually be given adjuvant therapy. There is also some advantage in giving adjuvant therapy to node-negative patients. However, most node-negative patients will not die of their disease, and adjuvant therapy would represent over-treatment of many women. Unnecessary chemotherapy should be avoided because the side-effects are distressing and hazardous.

It would be useful to identify the node-negative women who will eventually die from breast cancer (some 20–30%) so that they could benefit from adjuvant therapy. Unfortunately this is not possible by morphological methods and, to date, most attention has been on the determination of steroid hormone receptor status. Research is in progress to evaluate other possible prognostic markers such as cellular oncogenes, oncogene products, and various growth factors.

A minority of node-negative women with breast cancer do badly, but it is difficult to identify who these women are

Review question 3

What are the possible disorders, other than breast cancer, in a woman who presents with a lump in her breast?

Review question 4

What symptoms might be present in breast cancer?

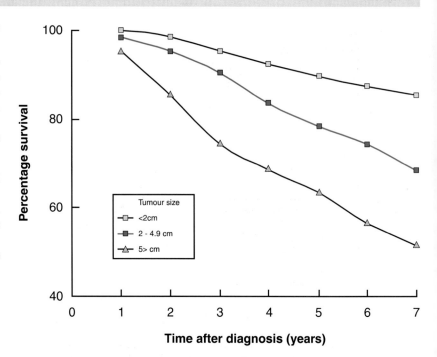

Figure 15.11 Tumour size and survival rates. Breast cancer survival is related to the size of the tumour at diagnosis. Tumour size (cm): < 2; 2–4.9; >5. (Adapted from Miller *et al.*, 1994.)

Table 15.2   Patient age and survival

Age (years)	Local recurrence		Distant metastases	
	5 year	10 year	5 year	10 year
< 35	64	49	76	63
35–65	76	63	83	72

All figures are percentages without disease.
Data from Miller *et al.*, 1994.

Steroid hormone receptors

Estimation of steroid hormone receptors is undertaken to determine whether hormone therapy would be beneficial

The presence of oestrogen and progesterone receptors shows a good correlation with patient response to endocrine therapy, and their determination may be used as a basis for the selection of patients for such therapy. These receptors are most frequently found in invasive lobular carcinoma, and the rarer mucinous and tubular carcinomas. The incidence of receptor positivity increases with age, which may explain why older women usually have a better response to endocrine therapy. Patients with oestrogen receptor-positive tumours survive longer than those without, because their response to endocrine therapy is better (Figure 15.12). Relapse-free survival also appears to be strongly associated with the presence of progesterone receptors.

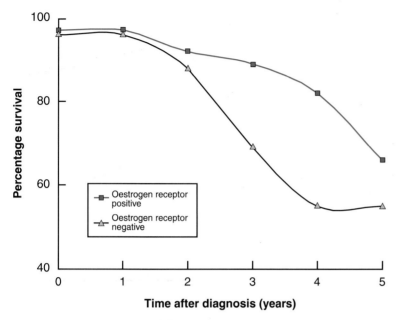

Figure 15.12 Oestrogen receptor status and survival. The overall 5-year survival rate for women who are oestrogen receptor-positive and who have been treated with hormonal therapy (tamoxifen) approaches 70%. The comparable rate in oestrogen receptor-negative women is just over 50%. (Adapted from Miller *et al.*, 1994.)

Growth factor receptors

Receptors for various polypeptide growth factors may also be expressed in some breast cancers. One of these, the receptor for epidermal growth factor, shows an inverse relationship with oestrogen receptor status. The receptor is over-expressed in 20–40% of breast cancers. It is more likely to be expressed in poor-grade tumours and is thus associated with a worse prognosis. Patients whose tumours contain this receptor are less likely to respond to endocrine therapy.

> *Breast cancer cells that are receptive to growth factors are likely to be fast-growing*

Oncogene amplification

Another growth factor receptor is the product of the *c-erbB-2* (*HER2* or *neu*) oncogene. The gene is amplified in some patients with invasive breast cancer, probably causing over-expression of the growth factor receptor and proliferation of tumour cells. Cell culture studies indicate that over-expression of the oncogene inhibits other genes that transcribe adhesion molecules (E-cadherin and α-2 integrin). This causes disruption of cell adhesion, which is a feature of tumour invasiveness and metastatic potential. In patients with breast cancer amplification of this oncogene correlates with the number of axillary lymph nodes involved by metastatic disease, and is an indicator of poor prognosis.

> *Oncogene activation causes some breast cancer cells to become very responsive to growth factors*

Oestrogen receptor: cell surface receptor for oestrogen. Interaction between the receptor and its hormone modifies DNA activity of the cell and hence its growth and replication.

Cathepsin D

Cathepsin D: a proteolytic enzyme which acts on extracellular proteoglycans and basement membranes.

Cathepsin D is secreted by some human breast cancer cells, particularly in node-positive disease. This enzyme activity is believed to facilitate the spread of tumour cells into surrounding tissues. In addition, cell culture studies show that cathepsin D can stimulate the proliferation of some breast cancer cell lines.

High concentrations of cathepsin D correlate with tumour aneuploidy, but not with other prognostic markers such as oestrogen and progesterone receptor status, tumour size or the age of the patient. In patients with node-negative disease, high tumour levels of cathepsin D appear to be associated with shorter relapse and overall survival times.

Genetic factors

Tumour cells often possess abnormal numbers of chromosomes

Cells with abnormal chromosome numbers are more likely to behave aggressively

High rates of cell proliferation are associated with worse prognosis

The number of chromosomes (ploidy) can be assessed by flow cytometry on the basis of the cellular DNA content. The proliferative capacity of tumour cells can be measured by evaluating the proportion of cells in the synthesis phase (precursor stage to cell division) of the cell cycle by means of thymidine labelling.

About 65% of breast cancers are aneuploid. Ploidy appears to correlate with disease-free survival: diploid lesions are generally better differentiated, steroid receptor-positive and usually follow a less aggressive course. Diploid tumours with a high S-phase fraction (large numbers of proliferating cells) are believed to have a poorer prognosis; in practice, however, studies have shown divergent results.

Thymidine labelling indices are related to prognosis. A high labelling index is associated with decreased disease-free survival, independently of steroid receptor or lymph node status. Patients with high labelling indices benefit from adjuvant chemotherapy.

Although it is hoped that the new biochemical and genetic markers expressed by primary breast tumours can be used as prognostic indicators, to date they have not replaced the traditional morphological features of histological grade, lymph node stage and tumour size.

Treatment

Aneuploid: an abnormal number of chromosomes.

Diploid: the normal number of chromosomes in a somatic cell.

Flow cytometry: cell sorting, using a laser instrument, by size and granularity of the nucleus or cytoplasm. The individual cell types can be measured after labelling with an antibody conjugated to a fluorescent dye.

The traditional view that breast cancer follows a sequence, starting as a localised microscopic lesion that grows and spreads into the regional lymph nodes and spreads to the rest of the body, is not borne out by experience. Despite early and aggressive intervention some women will die from liver or lung secondaries within a year of the original diagnosis. Others can receive conservative surgery, are subsequently found to have invasive cancer in the same breast, and yet still do not produce detectable secondary deposits. These differences suggest that breast cancer is a local manifestation of a systemic failure of growth control.

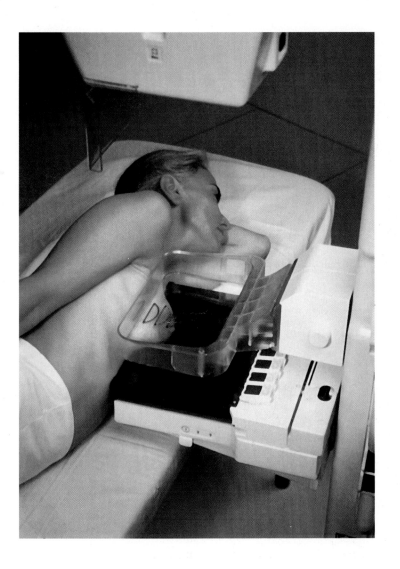

Plate 1 Mammographic equipment (General Electric CGR). Column with compression plates which can be rotated to allow mammography with the patient in standing, sitting or recumbent positions (operator console not shown). The breast is compressed between two motorised plates.

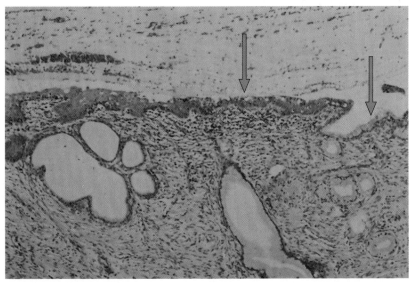

Plate 2 Transformation zone. Stratified squamous epithelium (left arrow) changing to columnar epithelium (right arrow).

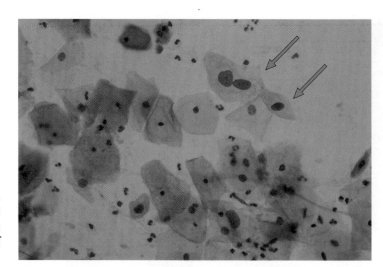

Plate 3 Moderate dyskaryosis. Cells in the top right of the picture (arrowed) have enlarged nuclei compared with relatively normal cells in the middle of the picture.

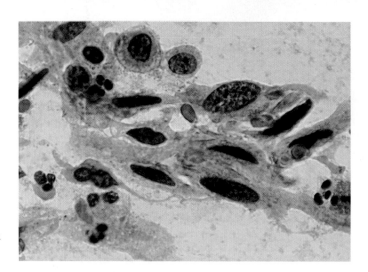

Plate 4 Invasive squamous carcinoma in a cytological smear.

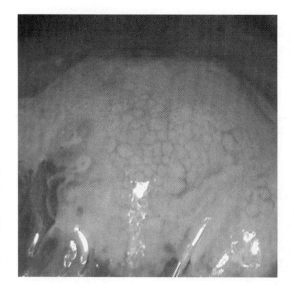

Plate 5 Colposcopy showing aceto-white lesions in CIN with mosaic pattern of underlying blood vessels. (From: Anderson, M., Jordan, J., Morse, A. and Sharp, F. *A text and Colour Atlas of Integrated Colposcopy*, published by Chapman & Hall, London, 1996.)

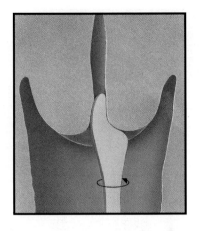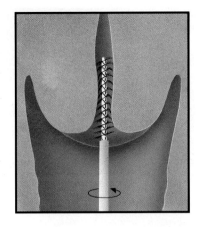

Plate 6 Spatula (left) and endocervical brush (right) for sampling cells from the transformation zone. The spatula or brush must be inserted into the os and rotated.

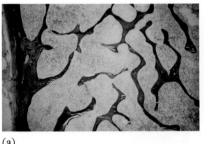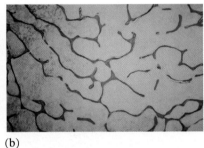

(a) (b)

Plate 7 (a) Iliac crest biopsy showing normal bone. (b) Osteoporotic bone, typical of an older man (over 60 years). Note that, although there is some bone thinning, the overall architecture is disrupted very little. (Supplied by Dr Jean Aaron)

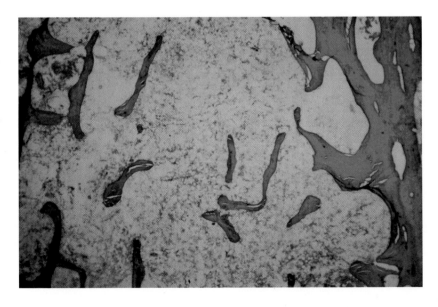

Plate 8 Osteoporotic bone in an older woman (over 60 years). Loss of bone has caused disruption to the overall architecture by shortening of individual trabeculae. (Supplied by Dr Jean Aaron)

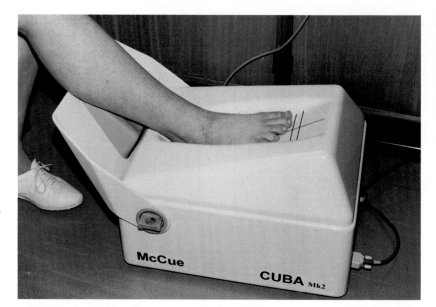

Plate 9 Ultrasound measurement of heel bone. Bone density is calculated by linking the portable instrument to a computer. The procedure is quick but does not offer the accuracy of other methods.

Plate 10 (a) Retinal blood vessels in the normal eye. (b) Proliferative diabetic retinopathy with moderate proliferation of new retinal blood vessels.

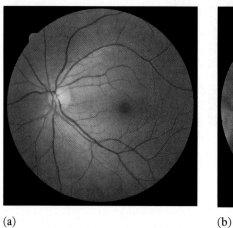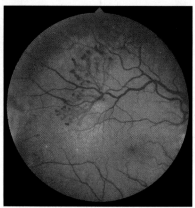

(a)   (b)

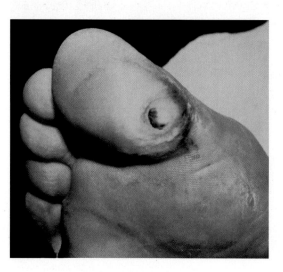

Plate 11 Neuropathic ulcer in the first toe.

Key points

Prognostic factors in breast cancer

▲ Age: breast cancer in premenopuasal women carries a worse prognosis
▲ Lymph node involvement is an indication of poor prognosis
▲ Tumour size
▲ Tumour grade: well differentiated breast cancers are associated with a better prognosis
▲ Oestrogen and progesterone receptor status predicts a good response to hormone therapy and better survival
▲ Ploidy: altered chromosome number is associated with worse prognosis
▲ Epidermal growth factor receptor is expressed in poor-grade tumours with a worse prognosis
▲ Oncogene activation (*HER2*) is an expression of poor prognosis
▲ High levels of cathepsin D carry poorer prognosis
▲ High cell proliferation rates associated with poor prognosis

A two-stage treatment strategy is used to control breast cancer. First, surgery is employed to achieve local control of the tumour. This may be supplemented by radiotherapy, aimed at reducing the risk of local or regional tumour recurrence. The second stage is a systemic therapy, intended to kill tumour cells that have migrated to other parts of the body. Chemotherapy is usual for this purpose in younger women, postmenopausal women being more likely to benefit from hormonal therapy with tamoxifen.

▲ **Key points**

Axillary sampling and clearance

Axillary sampling:
▲ Prognostic indicator (histological assessment of dissected lymph nodes for tumour involvement)
▲ Determines need for systemic therapy
▲ At least four nodes must be removed
▲ Accuracy improves with greater number of nodes sampled

Axillary clearance:
▲ Means of local tumour control
▲ Essential for women undergoing mastectomy and immediate breast reconstruction by tissue expansion
▲ Fewer complications than partial clearance and axillary radiotherapy
▲ Does not affect survival outcome but axillary recurrence difficult to treat and very distressing for patient
▲ Main complication is lymphoedema

> *The decision to give systemic therapy to younger women depends on whether the axillary lymph nodes are involved by tumour*

Systemic therapy will be given when lymph nodes are involved by tumour (Figure 15.13). If the lymph nodes are clear then chemotherapy may be avoided in younger women but older women are likely to receive systemic therapy regardless of whether the lymph nodes are involved, since the hormonal treatment used does not carry the same side-effects and risks as chemotherapy.

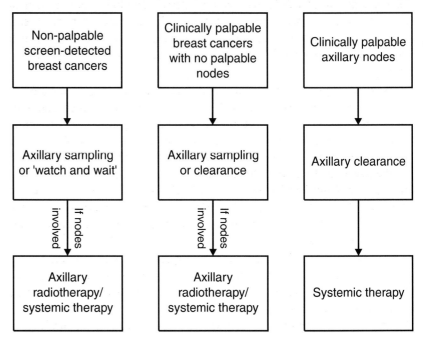

Figure 15.13 Indications for axillary sampling. The best way of determining the need for systemic therapy is to sample the axillary lymph nodes. Axillary clearance provides local tumour control, and can be used to select patients for aggressive systemic treatment based on assessment of the number of nodes involved. Axillary sampling or clearance can be avoided by women with non-palpable breast cancers identified by mammographic screening. In these women the risk of axillary metastasis is less than 10% and therefore axillary sampling, or a 'watch and wait' policy, can be followed.

Axillary clearance: complete surgical removal of all lymph nodes under the arm. This form of treatment is used to prevent axillary recurrence in patients with clinically palpable nodes and those undergoing mastectomy with breast reconstruction.

Axillary dissection: sample extraction of at least four lymph nodes from under the arm, used as a staging procedure. This procedure is most likely to be carried out when there is a clinically palpable breast tumour but no palpable nodes. Patients found to have lymph node involvement will then receive axillary radiotherapy.

Lymphoedema (axillary): lymphatic oedema in the armpit, caused by accumulation of fluid.

Lymph node status is best assessed by surgical dissection or clearance. Lymph nodes are most likely to be involved if the breast tumour is large, symptomatic rather than screen-detected, poorly differentiated or oestrogen receptor negative. Some surgeons argue that axillary clearance is not necessary because control is achievable by systemic therapy; others will clear the lymph nodes and treat with radiotherapy. However, the combination of axillary dissection and radiotherapy is associated with a high risk of lymphoedema. The number of lymph nodes involved by tumour has prognostic significance: 5-year survival is about 90% when no lymph nodes are involved but is reduced to 50% when four nodes are involved and to less than 25% with ten or more nodes.

Surgery

A variety of surgical procedures can be employed for treating breast cancer, ranging from radical to simple mastectomy to breast-conserving surgery involving simply removing the lump (lumpectomy) plus a small cuff of surrounding tissue (wide local excision). Until the late 1960s the only form of surgical treatment was radical mastectomy. The rationale was that breast tumours rapidly spread to the surrounding lymph nodes and thus as much tissue as possible should be removed in order minimise the risk of tumour spread.

It is now recognised that spread to other parts of the body (micrometastases) may have taken place by the time of diagnosis and treatment; thus the emphasis is now on local control by conservative treatments, supplemented by systemic therapies. The extent of surgery required is based on the probable cosmetic result and the likelihood of local recurrence. Factors influencing these aspects are the size of the tumour, its location in the breast, the size of the breast and the presence of multifocal or extensive *in-situ* disease. Some tumours are viewed as inoperable, usually those that are no longer mobile (tumour is fixed to the chest wall or presence of fixed axillary nodes) or where there are obvious systemic metastases.

It has been suggested that the timing of surgery with respect to the woman's menstrual cycle may influence survival prospects. A small survey has shown that surgery during the second part of the menstrual cycle (13–32 days after the last menstrual period) appears to increase survival: 10-year survival was 84% for these, whereas the figure was only 54% for women who underwent surgery earlier in their cycle.

It is believed that tumour cells are less likely to be disseminated when oestrogen is opposed by progesterone, as occurs during the second half of the cycle. This may be due to differences in the adhesiveness of the cells, and in the oestrogenic stimulation of tumour-promoting growth hormones and proteases. Prospective studies are currently under way to evaluate this phenomenon properly.

There is little evidence for any significant differences in survival between simple or radical mastectomy and the local removal of tumour. Some 5–10% of women suffer local recurrence whatever form of surgery is employed. Survival prospects can be improved by adjuvant therapy. Although normally given when there is reason to suspect metastatic disease, adjuvant therapy also appears to be beneficial for women with early breast cancer in whom metastases cannot be identified.

About 50% of patients who present with symptomatic breast lumps already have metastases in the lymph nodes, usually the axillary lymph nodes, but spread to the internal mammary lymph nodes can take place. Clearance of axillary lymph nodes is an effective method of local tumour control, but is associated with the side-effects of lymphoedema, pain, swelling of the arm, arm numbness and limitations to shoulder movement. Surgical removal or radiotherapy of involved axillary lymph nodes does not seem to confer any

---

The primary treatment for breast cancer is usually some form of surgery

Breast-conserving surgery: surgical removal of tumour with a variable amount of surrounding breast tissue. A lumpectomy aims to remove the smallest amount of tissue possible, consistent with complete removal of the tumour mass. In a wide local excision or segmental mastectomy the aim is to remove the palpable tumour with a margin of tissue that is microscopically free of tumour of at least 1 cm. Generally, the wider the excision margin the poorer the cosmetic result.

Modified radical mastectomy: removal of the breast together with the underlying pectoralis major fascia (connective tissue covering) but not the muscle itself. Axillary lymph nodes are also removed. Provides a better cosmetic and functional result than unmodified radical mastectomy.

Radical mastectomy: removal of the entire breast including division of the pectoralis major and minor muscles. This operation also includes dissection of the axillary lymph nodes.

Simple mastectomy: removal of the breast without dissection of axillary lymph nodes.

Survival can be improved by systemic control: adjuvant chemotherapy or endocrine therapy

Treatment of the axilla does not markedly affect long-term survival

*The demand for more
conservative surgery has led to
increased use of
supplementary radiotherapy*

significant survival benefit because lymph node involvement is an expression, rather than the cause of, poor prognosis.

Lymphoedema

Some women experience lymphoedema after breast surgery. This is more likely to occur in those who have undergone axillary dissection or clearance or a course of radiotherapy. The main ways of controlling lymphoedema are exercise, massage and the use of pressure sleeves.

The exercises comprise a number of movements such as those involved in brushing the hair, fastening a brassière and towelling the back. Squeezing and relaxing the hands, arm swinging and exercises with ropes and pulleys are also useful.

Pressure sleeves work by compressing the swollen tissue and preventing fluid from building up. It is important that the sleeves fit so that blood flow is not severely restricted. Massage is an excellent way to stimulate lymph flow. Best results are achieved by gentle hand massage. Deep massage is counter-productive because this stimulates blood flow and hence the amount of fluid produced.

Radiotherapy

Conservative surgery and radiotherapy

Radiotherapy is usually combined with the more conservative surgical treatments. An example is the combination of lumpectomy and irradiation, which is usually applicable for tumours of less than 3 cm in size, except where the tumour underlies the nipple or there is suspicion of axillary lymph node involvement.

Conservative surgical procedures remove the tumour with only a small margin of normal-appearing tissue. Some isolated tumour cells could remain in the breast tissue so radiotherapy is aimed at eliminating any tumour cells left behind. Another indication for radiotherapy is elimination of any associated *in-situ* cancers.

Radiotherapy is usually applied 7–10 days postoperatively, in dose fractions over a period of up to 6 weeks to give a total dose of 40–50 Gy. Localised radiotherapy (brachytherapy) can be given instead or with external beam therapy, but is not commonly used in the UK.

Irradiation of the axilla is as effective as surgical clearance in preventing recurrence in the axillary nodes. The disadvantage is that the prognostic information given by the surgical method will not be available.

Treatment of DCIS

Mastectomy is virtually 100% effective in curing DCIS but it seems over-cautious to treat these non-invasive cancers by mastectomy when some already invasive cancers are managed more conservatively. A number of trials are under way in Europe and the USA to evaluate more conservative approaches for treatment of DCIS.

In the National Surgical Adjuvant Breast and Bowel Study (Fisher *et al.*, 1993, 1995) subsequent non-invasive cancers were found in 10.4% of patients treated by lumpectomy alone, and invasive cancers in a further 10.5%. In contrast, non-invasive cancers were found in 7.5%, and invasive cancers in 2.9% of patients treated by lumpectomy and radiotherapy (see p. 471). It is too soon to say whether the combined therapy will translate into a survival advantage: it could be that the additional radiotherapy merely delays tumour development or recurrence. It will be some years before the most appropriate treatment for DCIS emerges, but lumpectomy alone with narrow excision margins, is probably inadequate. Different subsets of DCIS (defined by grade or comedo-type necrosis) may also require different treatment.

Mastectomy and radiotherapy

Radiotherapy is used after modified radical mastectomy to reduce the risk of tumour recurrence involving the chest wall or the axillary, supraclavicular and internal mammary lymph nodes. This approach was believed to result in improved survival compared with modified mastectomy alone, but recent randomised trials have failed to demonstrate this.

> *Radiotherapy after mastectomy is not commonly used*

Adjuvant therapy

Adjuvant therapies have been shown to reduce short-term mortality rate in women with lymph node metastasis. The choice of adjuvant treatment, if any, in women without lymph node involvement remains more problematic because of their relatively good prognosis: only about 20% will relapse within 5 years. Given the toxicity of chemotherapy and its limited potential for reducing the odds of death, if all were treated many women would be treated unnecessarily for little or no benefit. However, tamoxifen therapy has fewer side-effects and is considered an acceptable form of treatment.

> *Adjuvant therapies are aimed at killing or blocking the growth of breast cancer cells wherever they are in the body*

Endocrine therapy

The principle of endocrine therapy is to block the oestrogenic stimulation of breast cancer cells., which is most likely to occur when the tumour cells have many oestrogen receptors. Oestrogen receptor status can be determined by biochemical or histochemical methods: about 40% of all breast cancers are positive. Growth stimulation in these cancers may be inhibited either by eliminating most oestrogen at source (by ovarian ablation) or by blocking the binding of oestrogen to its receptor.

Among premenopausal and perimenopausal women ovarian ablation is an effective adjuvant treatment, producing improvements in recurrence and survival rates of about 25%. Ovarian ablation may be achieved by means of surgery, radiotherapy or chemotherapy. Treatment will induce the menopause with its attendant symptoms of hot flushes, vaginal dryness, psychological changes and, in the longer term, osteoporosis.

The antioestrogen drug tamoxifen is an effective adjuvant therapy in the treatment of breast cancer, particularly for post-menopausal women. The annual

> *Tamoxifen blocks the stimulatory effect of oestrogen on breast cancer cells*

recurrence rate in early breast cancer (stage I or II) is reduced by about 25%, and mortality by about 17%, when tamoxifen is given, compared with surgery alone.

An alternative is to remove the prime source of oestrogen

Oestrogen receptor-positive tumours are more likely to be found in older patients, but tamoxifen can be effective in all age groups. Between 45 and 60% of older women respond to tamoxifen therapy. Only about 5–10% of women with oestrogen receptor-negative status show any response.

A possible disadvantage of tamofixen is that it has some oestrogenic activity of its own (in other words, it behaves as a partial agonist) and hence may not completely inhibit cell proliferation. More effective antioestrogens are currently entering clinical trials, based on the oestradiol molecule itself but with substitutions at different positions within the steroid structure. These pure antioestrogens have been shown to inhibit the proliferation of breast cancer cells in culture, even including those that have become insensitive to tamoxifen. Large phase III clinical trials will be needed to evaluate the toxicity profiles of the new drugs and whether they have any clinical advantages over tamoxifen. Also under evaluation are a new class of specific aromatase inhibitors (anastrozole or 'arimidex'). These work by inhibiting the synthesis of oestrogen from adrenal androstendione, which is the major source of oestrogen in postmenopausal women. A number of clinical trials are underway aimed at comparing the benefits of aromatase inhibitor alone and in combination with tamoxifen for the treatment of postmenopausal breast cancer.

Chemoprevention of breast cancer

It is hoped that tamoxifen can prevent breast cancer in women at high risk

Tamoxifen therapy has potential for preventing breast cancer in women who have a high familial risk. Randomised clinical trials are currently under way, but it will be many years before its effectiveness is known because of the long time intervals involved in the development of breast cancer. Additional benefits might arise because tamoxifen reduces the risk of CHD by reducing overall blood cholesterol concentrations. The drug is also believed to provide protection against osteoporosis.

Acute side-effects of tamoxifen include hot flushes, altered libido, vaginal dryness, menstrual disturbance, weight gain and gastrointestinal upset. More seriously, there appears to be an increased risk of endometrial cancer with long-term tamoxifen therapy (3–5 years). A rare complication is retinopathy; treatment should be stopped if any visual disturbance is reported. In some animals liver cancers have been induced with tamoxifen doses comparable to those used in humans, although there is insufficient information on whether the drug exerts similar effects in human subjects. In patients with breast cancer the risks are justified by the gains in survival.

The benefits are less certain for those healthy postmenopausal women taking tamoxifen as a possible protection against the development of breast cancer. Many women, even those classified as high risk, will never go on to develop breast cancer and so will have been given treatment needlessly. This can be justified if there are no adverse side-effects, but the decision is more difficult if the agent intended to prevent disease also has potential to produce disease.

Most of the tamoxifen-associated endometrial abnormalities so far reported have been benign processes such as epithelial metaplasia, hyperplasia and the production of polyps. The risk of developing symptomatic endometrial cancer is estimated at 20 women per 10 000 per year.

Randomised clinical trials of tamoxifen chemoprevention are currently under way in the USA, the UK, Italy and Australia. In the USA trial the intention is to recruit 16 000 healthy women at high risk of developing breast cancer and randomise them to receive 20 mg tamoxifen daily for five years or placebo. High risk is defined as any woman over the age of 35 who is estimated to have at least a 1.7% chance of developing breast cancer – a woman with a first-degree relative who has developed the disease, or any woman over the age of 60.

Because of concerns over the safety of tamoxifen with respect to endometrial abnormalities, 111 women (61 receiving tamoxifen and 51 placebo) in the British trial have been investigated by transvaginal ultrasonography and endometrial biopsy. This showed an excess of endometrial abnormalities in the group receiving tamoxifen. The recommendation is to conduct regular screening for endometrial abnormalities by transvaginal ultrasonography and, where indicated, histological assessment of endometrial biopsy. This should apply to both women with primary breast cancer and those receiving tamoxifen in prevention programmes.

> *Inevitably, tamoxifen will be given to women who would not develop breast cancer anyway*

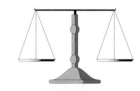

National Surgical Adjuvant Breast and Bowel Project

Lumpectomy vs. Lumpectomy with radiotherapy for treatment of DCIS

▲ Studied 391 women with DCIS randomised to lumpectomy alone, and 399 to lumpectomy with radiotherapy (50 Gy)
▲ Median follow-up 43 months (range 11–86 months)
▲ In lumpectomy group, incidence of non-invasive cancers 10.4%, invasive cancers 10.5%, vs. 7.5% and 2.9% in lumpectomy with radiotherapy group
▲ Lumpectomy alone inadequate in preventing subsequent need for mastectomy

Source: Fisher *et al.*, 1993.

Tamoxifen for the prevention of breast cancer

Point	Counterpoint
Tamoxifen has been used since 1971 to treat 3 million women with breast cancer, delaying relapse and prolonging survival in 20–30%	Treatment of disease justifies some risk but this might not be acceptable for healthy women in whom there is currently no proven benefit
Could prevent breast cancer in pre- and postmenopausal women at high risk	Most benefits proven in post-menopausal women only
Tamoxifen reduces incidence of breast cancers induced by chemical carcinogens in rats	The animal model and the chemical carcinogens may not be applicable to humans
Tamoxifen reduces incidence of breast cancer in contralateral breast by 39%	Tamoxifen increases mortality in postmenopausal women who develop contralateral cancer during treatment
Prevents coronary heart disease by lowering plasma cholesterol and fibrinogen	Not all studies in agreement, reduction in total cholesterol without increase in HDL may not be protective

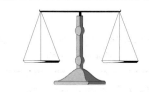

Breast cancer prevention trials

Tamoxifen vs. placebo

▲ Double-blind randomised trials initiated in the UK, USA, Italy and Australia

▲ Eligibility: any woman over the age of 35 estimated to have a risk of 1.7% or greater of developing breast cancer (e.g. at least one first-degree relative who has breast cancer), or any woman over 60 years

▲ Treatment group given 20 mg tamoxifen daily for 5 years

▲ Tamoxifen may prevent or delay development of breast cancer in healthy pre-and post-menopausal women at high risk

▲ In a subgroup of 111 women (61 given tamoxifen), 39% in tamoxifen group had histological evidence of endometrial abnormalities (cf. 10% in control group) after mean of 22 (range 3–75) months

▲ Data not yet available for breast cancer delay or prevention

Source: Kedar et al., 1994.

Oestrogenic effects can reduce bone loss	No study has yet documented decrease in bone fractures
Tamoxifen 20 mg daily has low toxicity	Tamoxifen 40 mg daily increases risk of endometrial cancer fivefold. Potential for over-treatment – most treated women will not develop breast cancer anyway

(Powles, 1992)   (Fugh-Berman and Epstein, 1992)

Author's view

The risks and benefits for women before the menopause are likely to be different from those after it. Breast cancers in premenopausal women are often more aggressive, and this is probably at least in part because of a relative lack of oestrogen receptors: tamoxifen could not be expected to prevent these cancers. Tamoxifen induces menopausal symptoms, which represents a burden for the younger woman in addition to the risks of endometrial abnormalities and other pathologies. There is also some uncertainty over how long prevention would have to be maintained: most women with breast cancer are treated for up to 5 years. Will the premenopausal woman have to take the drug for the rest of her life (current trials are limited to 5 years) and what then are the risks of other pathologies? Once tamoxifen is discontinued, the breast cancer risk might be reasserted, merely delaying rather than preventing the disease. Any cancers that the drug failed to prevent would by definition be tamoxifen-resistant and probably more aggressive.

In high-risk postmenopausal women, tamoxifen could represent a worthwhile precaution, particularly if they have had a hysterectomy. In women inheriting the *BRCA1* or *BRCA2* genes, tamoxifen may be preferable to prophylactic bilateral mastectomy.

Chemotherapy

A large number of trials have been designed to assess the effectiveness of chemotherapy as an adjuvant therapy in breast cancer. A variety of regimes are available, ranging from 1 week of single agent chemotherapy, to a year or more of multiple agent polychemotherapy. The treatments can be given before or after surgery.

Preoperative treatment is given to shrink the size of the tumour to enable more conservative surgery. It is also believed that chemotherapy can 'sterilise' the tumour and reduce the risk of tumour spread during excision. At present, postoperative treatment is more common.

The long-term use of combined cytotoxic agents (polychemotherapy) is more effective than single-agent chemotherapy. The most common regimen

Chemotherapy is used to kill cancer cells that have dispersed

is CMF (cyclophosphamide, methotrexate, 5-fluorouracil), repeated every 21–28 days and continued for 6–12 months. Other regimens include the anthracyclins doxorubicin and epirubicin. The recurrence-free survival advantage in women of all ages given CMF chemotherapy is estimated at 8–10% after 10 years. The improvement is more definite for node-positive patients. Survival in node-negative patients would in any case be expected to be better and adjuvant chemotherapy would not have such a great impact.

The benefits of chemotherapy are greatest in premenopuasal women although there is a small additional benefit when combined with tamoxifen treatment in node-positive postmenopausal women. In the USA patients at very high risk of recurrence (with ten or more tumour-involved axillary lymph nodes) may be offered high-dose chemotherapy. Dose-limiting bone marrow toxicity is overcome by autologous transplantation. This treatment is associated with a mortality rate of about 5% but overall appears to increase time to relapse and to have a small survival benefit.

Prostheses

Breast surgery can be disguised, but the patient will always be aware of her body's change. Prostheses can be worn inside the brassiere: these are made from silicone with a skin-coloured covering of a size and shape to match the other breast. Prostheses are indistinguishable under clothing. In the first 6 weeks after surgery a lightweight prosthesis can be provided to restore shape while exerting minimal pressure on the scar. After 6–8 weeks (sometimes longer if radiotherapy was given) a final prosthesis can be fitted.

Breast reconstruction

Breast reconstruction has become an important element of treatment, although the procedures themselves are substantial surgical operations. The aim of reconstructive surgery is to construct a breast mound and achieve symmetry with the remaining breast. In a woman with large breasts it may be preferable to reduce the size of the remaining breast so as to achieve symmetry with the reconstructed breast. The nipple and areolar complex may also be rebuilt.

Reconstruction can be carried out at the time of surgical treatment or delayed: often a better cosmetic result is obtained with immediate reconstruction, using the breast skin that is not involved by cancer. Reconstruction will probably be delayed if the woman is to receive radiotherapy or adjuvant chemotherapy but this is not always absolutely necessary. Very often women who initially express a desire for reconstructive surgery but in whom reconstructive surgery is delayed do not pursue the option with the passage of time. This may be because they have adjusted to their physical change and fear additional surgery.

Silicone implants

A silicone implant comprises silicone gel encased within a thin silicone

---

▲ Key points

Chemotherapy in treatment of breast cancer

▲ Combined therapy is more effective than single agent therapy

▲ CMF (cyclophosphamide, methotrexate, fluorouracil) is the most widely used regimen in the UK

▲ Most useful as adjuvant therapy in younger women (under 50 years)

▲ Effect may be due to induction of menopause

▲ Older women may still benefit from chemotherapy and tamoxifen

---

Autologous bone marrow transplantation: removal and storage of bone marrow before chemotherapy. The bone marrow is returned to the patient when drug treatment is completed.

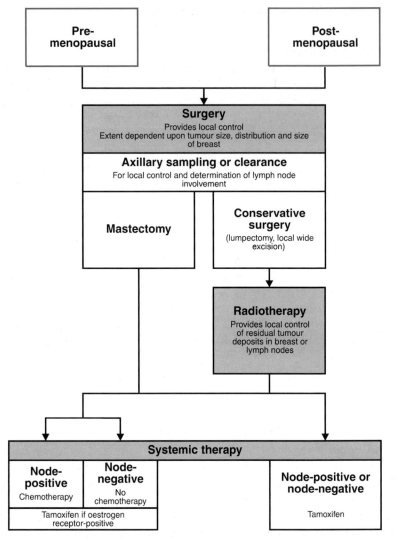

Figure 15.14 Unless inoperable, surgery is the preferred treatment for the local control of tumour in women with breast cancer. Conservative surgery, particularly for screen-detected *in-situ* disease, is usually accompanied by radiotherapy. Systemic therapy will control local recurrence as well as more distant metastases. Evaluation of lymph node status is to determine prognosis and assess the necessity for systemic therapy. Hormonal therapy benefits postmenopausal women, regardless of lymph node status. Chemotherapy and hormonal therapy may be given singly or in combination to both premenopausal and postmenopausal women. The benefits of chemotherapy are greatest in premenopausal women, tamoxifen being of greatest benefit in women (usually, but not necessarily, older women) with oestrogen receptor-positive tumours.

Breast reconstruction can achieve good cosmetic results but patient expectations should not be raised

envelope. This feels soft and its movement mimics that of the real breast tissue. Silicone implants usually give a good cosmetic result although fibrous scar tissue can form around the implant, making it feel hard and rigid. Concerns have been expressed about the safety of silicone implants in circumstances where the gel has leaked into the surrounding tissues.

Tissue expansion

An alternative method of reconstruction in women with large breasts is tissue expansion. An inflatable silicone bag is inserted under the chest muscle and is gradually expanded by introducing a sterile saline solution through a valve. This is done under local anaesthesia on a weekly basis over 2 months or so. When the breast has become slightly larger than the natural breast the valve is removed. After a further 3 months the bag is removed and a permanent silicone prosthesis inserted in a second operation. Although tissue expansion takes some months to complete the procedure results in a good cosmetic result.

Use of flaps

Other methods involve the use of muscle and skin flaps (myocutaneous flaps). A flap of muscle (latissimus dorsi) and skin from the back, directly behind the operated breast, is rotated and moved just below the armpit into the chest wall. A silicone implant will usually also be needed to match the size of the other breast. Scarring consists of a horizontal or diagonal scar on the back together with an oval scar around the breast. Alternatively, a flap of skin and abdominal muscle (rectus abdominis) may be rotated and moved upwards to the breast area. There is usually sufficient tissue in this area to avoid the need for a silicone implant but there could be complications of delayed healing, damage to the blood supply, and necrosis.

Reconstruction of nipple and aureole

Nipple and areolar reconstruction is usually carried out a few months after breast reconstruction to allow the breast to settle into its permanent position. The operation involves skin grafts taken from behind the ear or part of the nipple from the normal breast. Skin for the darker areolar region can be taken from the groin. This is not an easy reconstructive procedure and the results are not perfect. Tattooing of the nipple and areolar complex can improve pigmentation. Alternatively, colour-matched prosthetic nipples can be made from silicone, applied with a medical adhesive and worn for a month at a time.

Complications

The most common immediate complication of breast reconstruction is infection, particularly if an implant has been used. This will require the removal of the implant and therefore most centres now administer prophylactic antibiotic treatment. A longer term complication is fibrosis which causes pain and discomfort. There is also the possibility of implant rupture and all silicone implants bleed a small amount of the gel. Concern has been expressed that the silicone is carcinogenic or may cause autoimmune connective tissue disease. To date, studies have failed to confirm such associations. Patients who have undergone flap reconstruction will have permanent scarring at the donor site.

▲ Key points

Types of breast reconstruction

Silicone implant:
- ▲ Suitable for women with small breasts
- ▲ Can be inserted at time of initial mastectomy

Tissue expansion and implant:
- ▲ For women with larger breasts: an expander is placed under chest wall muscles and inflated over a period of months
- ▲ Expander eventually replaced with implant

Muscle and skin flaps:
- ▲ Latissimus flaps usually require an implant to create a breast mound
- ▲ Abdominal flaps are bulkier and do not require an implant
- ▲ Only suitable method for women who have received radiotherapy

Psychosocial aspects of breast cancer

Psychological problems can be expected in women with breast cancer at every stage of their diagnosis, treatment and rehabilitation

The experience of breast cancer and any disfigurement caused by mastectomy can be devastating for the woman and her partner. The breasts are associated with femininity, sexual attractiveness and nurturing behaviour.

The initial discovery of a lump in the breast undoubtedly subjects a woman to emotional stress. Anxiety will be heightened while waiting for appointments and test results. If malignancy is confirmed even greater stress will be created around uncertainties about the future. Fear of death is often rivalled by fear of the treatment and the disfigurement it may cause.

People react to a diagnosis of cancer in different ways. A variety of coping styles have been identified:
*   Positive or confronting attitude
*   A fatalistic approach
*   Feelings of hopelessness or helplessness
*   Personal denial or avoidance

Patients with a positive or confronting attitude tend to exhibit lower levels of anxiety and depression than those who have feelings of hopelessness and helplessness. The type of treatment undertaken has some influence on a person's psychological state, particularly with regard to the preservation of female identity which can be undermined by the loss of a breast.

Breast conserving surgery helps to preserve female identity and body image

Many patients report feelings of social isolation. Support by partner and family can do much to allay fears and minimise depression. Some women find attendance at a self-help group provides an opportunity to confront and ease their fears through mutual support and shared experiences, and acts as a conduit for anger and dissatisfaction.

Perhaps surprisingly, psychological problems are similar in women treated by mastectomy and those treated more conservatively, such as by lumpectomy and radiotherapy. The possible benefit of less mutilating surgery may be offset by fears that the less radical form of surgery has not removed all the cancerous cells. Involvement in the choice of procedure seems to improve the patient's coping potential and psychosocial functioning.

The attitudes adopted by patients to their cancer do not seem to affect survival rates significantly

Some positive correlation exists between 5- and 10-year recurrence-free intervals and an initial 'fighting spirit' response and seeking of information. However, the biological factors (node involvement, tumour size, age) probably far outweigh any influence of psychosocial factors in determining survival.

Screening for breast cancer

The goal of screening is to reduce mortality by detection of earlier lesions

As there are no obvious causes or modifiable risk factors involved in the development of breast cancer, reductions in mortality can only be achieved by earlier detection and treatment. This is recognised in the *Health of the Nation* targets, which refer only to reducing the mortality from breast cancer by *screening*. The national breast screening programme in the UK is aimed at women most at risk: those of 50–64 years. Screening is repeated every 3 years.

By the time signs or symptoms are detected breast cancer is already invasive, and many women have lymph node metastasis. The aim of screening is to advance the diagnosis, if possible to the pre-invasive phase. It is not possible to detect a precancerous phase by screening or any currently available diagnostic method. One consequence of detection relatively late in the life of breast tumours is that the rate of interval breast cancers is fairly high. In the Swedish two-county trial of breast screening (Tabar *et al.*, 1987) the interval cancer rate was already 45% after 3 years (Figure 15.15).

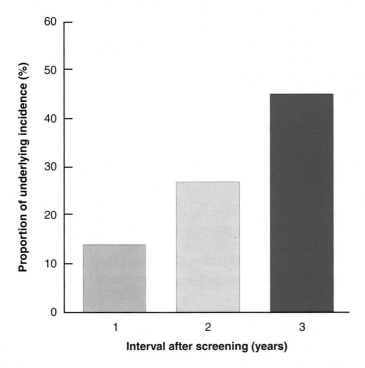

Figure 15.15 Interval cancers expressed as a proportion of the rate in unscreened population (unscreened = 100%). The incidence of breast cancer in screened women increases with time after screening. (Data from Tabar *et al.*, 1987.)

The screening method

Mammographic screening allows the detection of quite small tumours (from about 2 mm): compare this with the 1–2 cm tumours detectable by palpation and by women experienced at breast self-examination. The practice of self-examination does not appear to lead to any significant survival advantage: any tumours detected are already relatively large and in most women their presence would soon become apparent anyway.

Much smaller tumours can be detected by mammography than by any other means

The first evidence that mammography is an effective method for breast cancer screening came with the Health Insurance Plan trials which started in New York in 1964 (Shapiro, Strax and Venet, 1971). This was a randomised study of 62 000 women aged 40–64. The screened women received annual

> *Trials around the world have shown that mammographic screening can reduce breast cancer mortality*

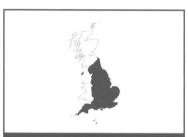

HEALTH OF THE NATION

Target for breast cancer

▲ To reduce the rate of breast cancer deaths among women invited for screening by at least 25% by the year 2000 (from 95.1 per 100 000 population in 1990 to no more than 71.3 per 100 000)

Review question 5

- **What is the most likely treatment for the 30-year-old school teacher (described in review question 1) if she is diagnosed as having Stage I breast cancer?**
- **What is the most likely prognosis after treatment?**
- **Comment on the fact that the lump was originally discovered by breast self-examination. Will the prognosis be improved?**

clinical examination and mammography, and after only a few years it became clear that mortality from breast cancer was reduced in the screened group. This was followed by a second generation of trials initiated in the late 1970s and early 1980s in a number of countries (for example, the Swedish two-county trial (Tabar *et al.*, 1987), Florence District Programme (Paci and Duffy, 1991) and the Canadian National Breast Screening Study (Miller, Howe and Wall, 1981)).

In the UK, initial trials (UK Trial of Early Detection of Breast Cancer, 1988) were conducted in different geographical areas. Women in Guildford and Edinburgh were offered mammography and clinical examination; in other areas of the country they were taught breast self-examination and provided with a self-referral clinic, or no intervention was made.

Although some of the trials were more effective than others, the general consensus was that mammographic screening can reduce deaths from breast cancer in women aged 50–69 years at very little risk. The main concern surrounding mammography is the possibility of developing cancer from exposure to X-rays, calculated at no more than one extra breast cancer per million women screened per year, after a latent interval of 10 years. This should be balanced against the gains of earlier treatment in hundreds of women each year.

There is currently no convincing evidence that mammography has any impact on deaths from breast cancer in younger women. The main reasons for this are that mammography is less sensitive in younger women (because of the more glandular nature of the breast tissue) and that the disease follows a more aggressive course. This may mean that treatment, whether the disease is screen-detected or not, has less impact on mortality in these women. Randomised prospective trials are proposed to assess the benefits of a more frequent (annual) mammographic screen in younger women (aged 40–50).

The overall effectiveness of screening programmes very much depends on compliance: uptake of 70% or more would reduce deaths due to breast cancer by 30–40%. In the UK this would mean that nearly 1300 deaths from breast cancer would be prevented by the year 2000, with an increase in life expectancy of up to 20 years in treated women.

Target population

Most deaths from breast cancer (89% in the UK) are in women over the age of 50. This profile, taken together with the lack of proven benefit of screening for younger women, means that the screening programme should be targeted at women over the age of 50. It may be prudent to initiate screening earlier in women who have first-degree relatives with premenopausal breast cancer. It might become possible to identify high-risk women by genetic testing, perhaps using probes for the *BRCA1* gene and chromosome 13 genes. Even so, genetic screening will not affect the need for mammographic breast screening in the broader population because only about 5% of breast cancers involve inheritance of defective *BRCA* genes.

Very often an upper limit of 65 years is set for screening, not through any technical limitations but because older women are notorious non-attenders. In the UK, older women can still be screened at their own request. It is to be hoped that when several screening rounds have been completed more women over 65 will want to continue: the problem with uptake in women of that age today is that most have no previous experience of screening.

Screening interval

Most breast screening programmes operate on a frequency of 3 years: this is a balance between effectiveness and cost. More frequent screening would probably reduce compliance because the procedure can be uncomfortable. For the attenders, however, the benefits of shorter intervals would be greater because the interval cancer rate is much lower with annual or biennial screening. Trials are under way to assess the practicalities of more frequent screening.

The incidence of interval cancers is a function of the sensitivity of the screening test. Sensitivity is lower in younger women because small cancers are more difficult to detect in young fibroglandular tissue than in the more fatty tissue in the breasts of older women. Sensitivity will also be determined by the number of views taken. Some radiologists have expressed concern that the British programme is based on single-view mammography; evidence from retrospective studies shows that cancer-detection and recall rates are improved by taking two views. Prospective studies are being carried out in the UK to compare the cancer detection and recall rates of single and two-view mammography.

Severity of screen-detected disease

It is not possible to detect precancerous changes by mammography; the best that can be achieved is the detection of cancers in their pre-invasive (DCIS) form (Figure 15.16). Before the advent of screening DCIS accounted for about 5% of breast cancer cases, but now comprises 15–20% of screen-detected cancers. This confirms the success of screening in detecting tumours at an earlier stage.

Screening increases the detection rate of non-invasive breast cancers

Screen-detected cancers are often less advanced than those detected by symptomatic presentation. This is evident using two measures of disease severity: tumour size and the stage of the disease.

The mean diameter of tumours detected by mammography is 1 cm, and some tumours can be detected as microcalcifications of only 2–3 mm. In the Swedish two-county trial of mammographic screening (Day et al., 1989) most of the screen-detected tumours were less than 15 mm in diameter. In contrast, most of the tumours in the unscreened control group were larger than 20 mm (Table 15.3). With repeated screening rounds, the average size of tumours at detection can be expected to be even smaller.

Screen-detected invasive cancers are usually smaller and at an earlier stage

It can also be expected that cancers detected at an earlier stage in their growth will display less spread into surrounding tissues (tumour stage). This was confirmed in the Swedish trial, where the proportion of Stage II or worse

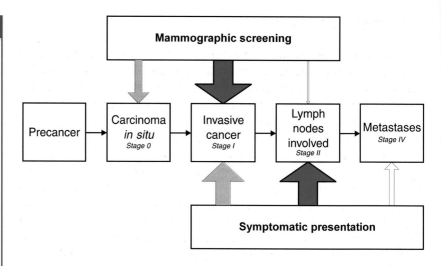

Figure 15.16 Development and detection of breast cancer: 50% of women who present with clinical signs of breast cancer already have lymph node involvement. Mammographic screening advances the diagnosis to an earlier stage in which, as far as can be ascertained, the invasive cancer is confined to the breast. Some 15% or more breast cancers are detected by screening at an even earlier *in situ* stage. The detection of precancer is not yet possible.

cancers was markedly reduced between the initial and subsequent screening rounds (Table 15.4).

Table 15.3   Percentage distribution of invasive breast cancers

	Tumour size (mm)			
	1–9	**10–14**	**15–19**	**>20**
Screen detected (n = 414)	23	29	22	26
Control group (n = 461)	7	15	18	59

Data from Day *et al.* (1989)

Table 15.4   Percentage of Stage II or worse breast cancers

Age (years)	Initial screen	Subsequent screens	Unscreened control group
50–59	33.3	25.0	58.7
60–69	34.3	16.9	58.4

Data from Day *et al.* (1989)

The diagnostic stage

Mammography is not the most specific test available, and women with detected abnormalities will be referred for further diagnosis. Women may be recalled for several reasons, usually because of suspicious findings or, more rarely, because of technical inadequacy of the mammogram. The woman will be assessed clinically and further views may be taken.

Accurate diagnosis requires sampling of tumour cells

If a lesion is palpable further investigation will involve fine-needle aspiration cytology. Impalpable lesions will require further imaging and a fine-needle sample obtained by stereotactic radiological guidance: two radiographs are taken to provide a stereoscopic image which allows calculation of the depth to which the needle should be inserted. Usually a definitive diagnosis can be reached through this combination but occasionally surgical biopsy is needed for histological evaluation. Positive findings of cancer by cytology will obviate the need for biopsy, and from that point any surgical procedure will have a treatment objective.

Before surgery the appropriate area for excision is marked under radiological guidance, usually by inserting a hooked wire, positioned using the nipple as a reference point, or by using a stereotactic device attached to the mammography machine. The surgical specimen will be radiographed and examined by histology to ensure that the tumour had been completely excised.

Treatment stage

The combination of smaller size and more favourable stage distribution in screen-detected tumours often means that more conservative treatment can be offered, with a better chance of success. However, one of the problems associated with the earlier detection of breast tumours concerns the treatment of non-invasive cancers (see p. 469). The detection and treatment of a higher proportion of DCIS are highly desirable and can be expected to have a much greater impact on mortality. Unfortunately, this could be at the expense of over-treatment since there will be some treated women in whom DCIS would not have progressed to invasive cancer. The risk of progression is considered too high to leave DCIS untreated.

Screening experience in the UK

The national breast screening programme was initiated in 1987 in response to the Forrest report, which reviewed the results of mammographic trials around the world. About 4.5 million women aged 50–64 in the UK are eligible for screening every 3 years. This implies an annual workload of 1.5 million women. Initially the woman is identified from computerised family practitioner registers and invited for screening at a fixed site or a mobile unit.

The British breast screening programme covers nearly 5 million women

The success of any breast screening programme is measured by reduced mortality but in the case of the UK programme this will not be known for some time. Supplementary indicators are the compliance rate, the breast cancer

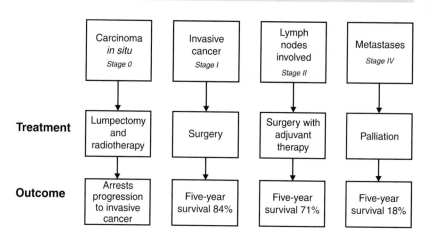

Figure 15.17 The treatment of screen-detected carcinoma *in situ* is most likely to arrest progression to invasive cancer. The treatment of screen-detected Stage I breast cancers carries a better prognosis than treatment of later-stage symptomatic cancers.

> *Repeat screening should result in a decrease in numbers of cancers detected, and those detected will be at an earlier stage*

detection rate, and the malignant to benign biopsy ratio.

In the first round of screening (known as the prevalent round) the cancer detection rate was 63 per 10 000 women screened. In the second round of screening the cancer detection rate fell to 34 per 10 000 women screened. This is to be expected, because in the second round most women are re-attenders and the cancers detected will be interval cancers, rather than cancers that had perhaps existed for several years. In the prevalent round of screening 17.6% screen-detected cancers were at the preinvasive stage (DCIS) and a further 21% were less than 1 cm in diameter. These figures can be expected to improve in future re-attenders. Unfortunately vast numbers of women will at any one time have no detectable abnormalities and will therefore have been subjected to needless investigation and anxiety.

About 7% of those who attend can expect to be recalled for further investigation, and about 1% of the total may require a breast biopsy. At this stage, because of the careful evaluation already undertaken, most biopsies will reveal cancer.

Preliminary analysis of the interval cancer rate in screened women in the UK indicates that the programme is not as effective as had been anticipated from the results of the Swedish two-county trial (Figure 15.18). The reasons for this difference are unclear. The interval cancers would comprise:

- Cancers previously reported as negative because of interpreter error (failure to recognise discrete changes)
- Cancers that were too small to be detected
- Genuinely new cancers arising between screens

The issue of screening sensitivity (false negatives) can be addressed by using two mammographic views rather than one: evidence suggests that up to 20% more women with breast cancer can be detected with this enhanced imaging.

Review question 6

Have all of Wilson's criteria been met with respect to breast cancer screening?

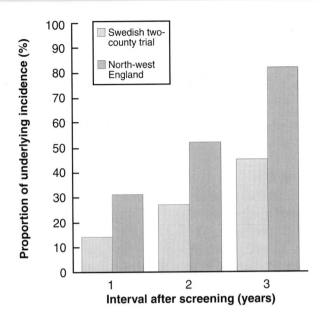

Figure 15.18 Comparison of interval breast cancer rates in the Swedish two-county trial and in north-west England. The interval breast cancer rate in the north-west of England is higher than that anticipated, and after 3 years approaches the underlying incidence rate. (Data from Tabar *et al.*, 1987 and Woodman *et al.*, 1995.)

The currently undetectable or *de novo* cancers could be detected by increasing screening frequency to every 1 or 2 years. Both these strategies have considerable resource implications, but unless implemented it is doubtful whether the *Health of the Nation* target for reducing breast cancer deaths by 25% can be achieved.

Is breast cancer screening worthwhile?

Point	Counterpoint
Mammographic screening can reduce mortality from breast cancer	Mammographic screening is of limited value since most screen-detected cancers are already invasive
Treatment of screen-detected lesions can be less extensive than that required for symptomatic disease, with greater certainty of success	Screen-detected lesions must still be treated aggressively – micrometastases might already have occurred
The treatment of screen-detected preinvasive lesions results in cure rates approaching 100%	Some women will be treated needlessly because the preinvasive cancer might not progress further during their life

▲ **Key points**

Screening and treatment of breast cancer

Screening method:
▲ In the UK most mammography screens consist of a single mediolateral view of the breasts

Diagnostic stage:
▲ Further assessment by clinical examination, additional mammography, ultrasound examination, fine-needle aspiration cytology or surgical biopsy

Treatment stage:
▲ Screen-detected cancers are more likely to be small and treatable by breast-conserving surgery

▲ **Key points**

Breast screening in UK

▲ Nearly 5 million women eligible
▲ Call-recall screening of women aged 50–64 years every 3 years
▲ About 1.6 million women are invited every year
▲ About 70% (1.13 million) actually attend
▲ 79 000 positive mammograms a year (7% of screened women)
▲ 11 300 breast biopsies required (1% of screened women)
▲ 7000 cases of breast cancer in prevalent round (6.2 per 1000 women screened)

Wilson's criteria for mass screening

▲ The disease should be common and serious
▲ The natural history of the disease should be understood
▲ The screening test should be accurate and reliable
▲ Acceptable treatment and the resources for treatment must be available
▲ The treatment should favourably influence the outcome

(After Wilson, 1966)

The mammographic screen is well suited to a mass screening programme	Mammography lacks sufficient sensitivity to detect all pre-invasive conditions reliably. Even if it were possible to increase the sensitivity of the test this would increase the potential for over-treatment

Author's view

There is a need for breast cancer screening and women should attend when offered the opportunity. However, the advantages are not as clear as those of cervical screening (see Chapter 16). Mammographic screening is capable of detecting only breast *cancer*, in contrast to cervical screening which is a screen for *precancerous* conditions. The greatest impact of screening on mortality from breast cancer is by the detection and treatment of preinvasive cancers. Currently, these are only 15–20% of screen-detected lesions. There are still benefits when invasive lesions are detected. The most important prognostic indicator in breast cancer is tumour stage: most women who present with signs or symptoms of breast cancer already have lymph node involvement but this rate is halved by regular screening. The detection of early lesions could be improved by reducing the screening interval to 2 years, and by taking two views.

ANSWERS TO REVIEW QUESTIONS

Question 1

What is the likelihood that the lump is caused by breast cancer?

About 10% of breast lumps are caused by cancer. In a 30-year-old woman without family history the chances of breast cancer are small; the incidence rate at this age is 10 per 100 000 (compared with 200 per 100 000 in women over 65 years). Her family history of breast cancer, however, increases the risk estimate by a multiple of three or four times.

Question 2

What are the known risk factors for breast cancer?

- Age
- Family history (first-degree relatives), especially of bilateral cancers or early onset (premenopausal)
- Genetics: there is a particularly high risk in some families with a clustering of ovarian and breast cancer cases. This is because of inheritance of a mutated gene on chromosome 17, known as *BRCA1*. Mutations

of *BRCA2* are less likely to be associated with ovarian cancer
- Previous history of breast cancer
- Obesity
- Late menopause
- No children or late childbearing
- Exposure to ionising radiation
- High socioeconomic group
- Long-term HRT
- High-fat diets and high alcohol consumption are also believed to be factors in elevating the risk, possibly by causing obesity and adipose tissue production of oestrogenic hormones

What are the possibilities other than breast cancer in a woman who presents with a lump in her breast? **Question 3**

- Fibrocystic disease, which accounts for about 40% of breast lumps
- No disease is found in 30% of apparent breast lumps
- Fibroadenoma, seen in 7% of breast lumps
- Miscellaneous benign disorders, for example inflammatory conditions such as mastitis and fat necrosis. These account for about 13% of breast lumps

What symptoms might be present in breast cancer? **Question 4**

In the early stages the disease is completely asymptomatic and may be detected only by mammographic screening. Even breast lumps of 1 cm and more can go undetected except by the experienced self-examiner or clinician.

Symptoms may include changes in breast size, swelling, pain in the breast (which may extend under the arm), puckering of the skin, discharge or bleeding from the nipple and the presence of a lump.

What is the most likely treatment for the 30-year-old school teacher diagnosed as having Stage I breast cancer? **Question 5**

The surgical treatment is largely dictated by the size of the tumour and the size of the breast. Considering that a Stage I tumour is to be treated breast-conserving surgery or 'lumpectomy' will probably be performed. This may well be followed by radiotherapy.

Given the age of the patient the form of adjuvant therapy that would be considered is chemotherapy. This, however, is usually reserved for more advanced cancers with nodal involvement. Further investigations might include measurement of biochemical prognostic markers. Ovarian ablation might be considered if she is oestrogen-receptor positive, although this (and chemotherapy) depends on whether she wishes to have children.

Tumours of less than 1 cm would not ordinarily be detected by self-examination: those that are detectable by this method would probably soon be felt anyway. There is no conclusive evidence to show that breast self-examination produces a survival advantage but it can be assumed that the sooner the condition is diagnosed and treated, the better. Of far more importance is attendance at mammographic screening. However, a 30-year-old woman would not be eligible for mammographic screening, because of technical limitations in discriminating a small tumour against dense breast tissue.

Question 6

Have all of Wilson's criteria been met with respect to breast cancer screening?

Is breast cancer common and serious? Clearly this is the case; breast cancer is the most common cause of deaths from cancer in women.

Is the natural history of the disease understood? Historically, there has been little opportunity to examine the natural history of this type of cancer. While in theory it should exist, a precancerous phase of this disease cannot be identified at present.

Even the preinvasive phase of breast cancer (DCIS) was seen only rarely before the advent of screening, and therefore there is not a substantial body of knowledge about how frequently and rapidly the lesions progress to invasive cancer. Over-treatment of preinvasive lesions is therefore a possibility.

Is the screening test accurate and reliable? There can be some problems with the specificity and sensitivity of the mammographic screen. In particular, lesions may be missed in younger women because of the increased cellularity of the breast tissues. Lesions may also be missed on single-view mammography, but sensitivity is increased by employing two views. 'Positive' or suspicious findings will need to be confirmed by the more specific cytological or histological investigations.

Are acceptable treatments and resources available? A variety of treatments are available for early breast cancer, but all involve some form of surgery. Acceptability must be viewed in the context that without treatment the woman will die of breast cancer. Within the UK, the aim is to treat 90% of breast cancers within 3 weeks of diagnosis.

Does the treatment favourably influence the outcome? There is no doubt that the treatment of preinvasive breast cancer is highly effective and for most women will eradicate the disease. Higher rates of recurrence are associated with lumpectomy alone if excision margins are narrow. Screening can also advance the diagnosis of invasive breast cancers, which are likely to be smaller and at an earlier stage.

References

Colditz, G.A., Hankinson, S.E., Hunter, D.J. *et al.* (1995) *N. Engl. J. Med.*, **332**, 1589–93.

Day, N.E., Williams, D.R.R. and Khaw, K.T. (1989) Breast cancer screening programmes: the development of a monitoring and evaluation system. *Br. J. Cancer*, **59**, 954–8.

Fisher, B., Constantino, J. Redmond, C. *et al.* (1993) Lumpectomy compared with lumpectomy and radiation therapy for treatment of intraductal breast cancer. *N. Engl. J. Med.*, **328**, 1581–6.

Fisher, B., Anderson, S., Redmond, C.K. *et al.* (1995) Reanalysis and results after 12 years of follow-up in a randomised trial comparing total mastectomy with lumpectomy with or without radiation in the treatment of breast cancer. *N. Engl. J. Med.*, **333**, 1456–61

Forrest, A.P.M. (1986) *Breast Cancer Screening: Report to the Health Ministers of England, Wales, Scotland and Northern Ireland*, HMSO, London.

Fugh-Berman, A. and Epstein, S. (1992). Tamofixen: disease prevention or disease substitution? *Lancet*, **340**, 1143–5.

Kedar, R.P., Bovine, T.H., Powles, T.J. *et al.* (1994). Effects of tamofixen on uterus and ovaries of postmenstrual women in a randomised breast cancer prevention trial. *Lancet*, **343**, 1318–21.

Miller, A.B., Howe, G.R. and Wall, C. (1981) The national study of breast cancer screening. *Clin. Invest. Med.*, **4**, 227–58.

Miller, W.R., Ellis, I.O., Sainsbury, J.R.C. and Dixon, J.M. (1994) Prognostic factors. *BMJ*, **309**, 1573–6.

Paci, E. and Duffy, S.W. (1991) Modelling the analysis of breast cancer screening programmes: sensitivity, lead time and predictive value in the Florence District programme (1975–1986). *Int. J. Epidemiol.*, **20**, 852–8.

Powles, T.J. (1992). The case for clinical trials for prevention of breast cancer. *Lancet*, **340**, 1145-7.

Shapiro, S., Strax, P. and Venet, P. (1971) Periodic breast cancer screening in reducing mortality from breast cancer. *JAMA*, **215**, 1–9.

Silverstein, M.K., Poller, P.N., Waismain, J.R. *et al.* (1995). Prognostic classification of breast ductal carcinoma-*in-situ*. *Lancet*, **345**, 1154–7.

Tabar, L., Fagerberg, C.J.G., Day, N.E. and Holmberg, L. (1987) The Swedish two-county trial: update and initial results on the screening interval. *Br. J. Cancer*, **55**, 547–51.

UK Trial of Early Detection of Breast Cancer Group (1988) First results on mortality reduction in the UK trial of early detection of breast cancer. *Lancet*, **ii**, 411–16.

Wilson, J.M.G. (1966) Some principles of early diagnosis and detection, in *Proceedings of a Colloquium, Magdalen College, Oxford, July 1965* (ed. G. Teeling-Smith), Office of Health Economics, London, 1966.

Further reading

Treatment

Bundred, N.J., Morgan, D.A.L. and Dixon, J.M. (1994) Management of regional nodes in breast cancer. *BMJ*, **309**, 1222–5.

Sacks, N.P.M. and Baum, M. (1993) Primary management of carcinoma of the breast. *Lancet*, **342**, 1402–8.

Richards, M.A., Smith, I.E. and Dixon, J.M. (1994) Role of systemic treatment for primary operable breast cancer. *BMJ*, **309**, 1363–6.

Watson, J.D., Sainsbury, J.R.C. and Dixon, J.M. (1995) Breast reconstruction after surgery. *BMJ*, **310**, 117–21.

Prognostic indicators

Neville, A.M. (1991) Prognostic factors and primary breast cancer. *Diagn. Oncol.*, **1**, 53–63.

Nicholson, S., Harris, A.L. and Farndon, J.R. (1991) Role of receptors in the management of patients with breast cancer. *Diagn. Oncol.*, **1**, 43–52.

Psychosocial factors

Meyer, L. and Aspegren, K. (1989) Long term psychological sequelae of mastectomy and breast conserving treatment for breast cancer. *Acta Oncologica*, **28**, 13–18.

Risk factors

Hulka, B.S. (1990) Hormone replacement therapy and the risk of breast cancer. *CA Cancer J. Clin.*, **40**, 289–96.

Schlesselman, J.J. (1990) Oral contraceptives and breast cancer. *Am. J. Obstet. Gynecol.*, **163**, 1379–87.

WHO Collaborative Study of Neoplasia and Steroid Contraceptives. (1990) Breast cancer and combined oral contraceptives: results from a multinational study. *Br. J. Cancer*, **61**, 110–19.

Pathology

Schnitt, S.J., Silen, W., Sadowsky, N.L. *et al.* (1988) Ductal carcinoma *in situ* (intraductal carcinoma) of the breast. *N. Engl. J. Med.*, **318**, 898–903.

Genetics

Roberts, L. (1993) Zeroing in on a breast cancer susceptibility gene. *Science*, **259**, 622–5.

Porter, D.E. and Steel, C.M. (1993) Recent advances in the genetics of heritable breast cancer. *Disease Markers*, **11**, 11–21.

16   Cervical cancer

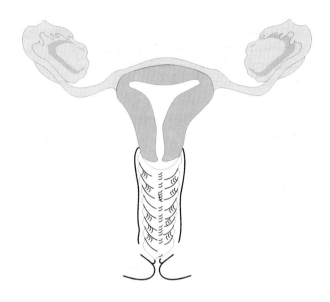

There are two types of cervical cancer, squamous carcinoma and adenocarcinoma. The most common squamous type is believed to be mediated by human papillomavirus and other tumour promoter factors. The disease mostly affects middle-aged women, survival depending on the stage of the disease at diagnosis. It can largely be prevented by regular attendance at cervical screening.

The progression of cervical cancer is characterised by a precancerous stage known as cervical intraepithelial neoplasia (CIN). The abnormalities at this stage are readily detected in cytological smears, and can be confirmed by colposcopy or histological evaluation of tissue biopsies. Treatment at this stage is relatively straightforward and generally halts the progression of the disease.

Invasive cervical cancer is usually treated by radiotherapy or surgery. Radiotherapy results in loss of ovarian function, but usually the woman is still able to have sexual intercourse after treatment. Conversely, surgery can spare the ovaries, but it may be necessary to remove at least part of the vagina.

Pre-test

- **How common is cervical cancer?**
- **Can any woman develop the disease?**
- **Can cervical cancer be prevented? If so, how?**
- **How is cervical cancer detected?**
- **What are the treatments available for cervical cancer?**

Aims of this chapter

By the end of this chapter you will have increased your knowledge of:
◆ The epidemiology of cervical cancer: who is affected and the risk factors involved in development of the disease
◆ The pathological features of precancerous and cancerous conditions of the cervix
◆ Methods for screening, diagnosis and treatment of cervical precancers and cancers

In addition, this chapter will help you to:
◆ Understand who is most at risk of developing cervical cancer and discuss how the disease can be most effectively prevented
◆ Distinguish between the pathology of precancerous and cancerous conditions and assess the likelihood of disease progression in treated and untreated women
◆ Describe a typical sequence of events following the detection of an abnormal lesion
◆ Evaluate the merits of ablation and excision methods in the treatment of non-invasive cervical cancer

Introduction

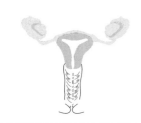

> *Cervical cancer is a significant cause of death in women, but is largely preventable by screening*

Worldwide, cervical cancer is the second most common form of cancer in women (after breast cancer). It is particularly prevalent in countries of Africa, South America, and parts of Asia. Mortality and morbidity rates in the UK are higher than in other developed countries (Figure 16.1), with about 4000 cases of invasive disease and 2000 deaths occurring each year (Figure 16.2). In North America cervical cancer kills 2000 women each year.

In many areas of the world, particularly Scandinavia and the USA, incidence and mortality from invasive cervical cancer have fallen since the introduction of cytology screening programmes. Cervical cancer tends to be a locally invasive tumour, with most patients developing symptoms before distant metastases develop. Treatments at this stage are relatively successful; hence in developed countries cervical cancer is not as prominent a cause of death as in less developed countries where medical facilities are limited.

Epidemiology

In most parts of the world the death rate from cervical cancer is declining. This trend has also been seen in the UK, although over the last few years the incidence and mortality in younger women have increased. In 1971, deaths from cervical cancer in women aged under 35 were 2.5% of all cervical cancer deaths; but by 1988 this figure had increased to 5.5%. Most deaths from the disease are in older women (Figure 16.3).

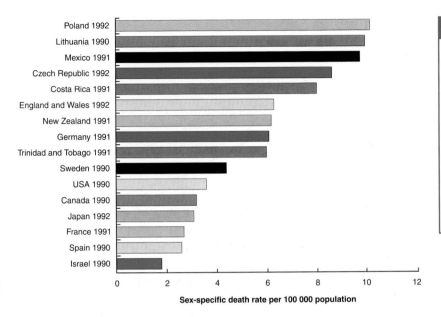

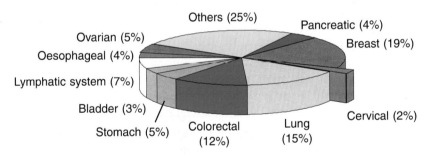 Figure is at cx 0.34, cy 0.26 — the bar chart.

Sex-specific death rate per 100 000 population

▲ Key points

Cervical cancer incidence and survival

▲ In England and Wales 4000 new cases are seen each year
▲ About 2000 women die every year
▲ The disease mostly affects women over the age of 45 years
▲ Five-year survival (all stages): 52% at age 45, 40% at age 65

Figure 16.1 Geographical differences in deaths from cervical cancer. There is wide variation in death rates from cervical cancer around the world. Some of this variation can be explained by differences in lifestyle risk factors (such as religious beliefs and moral values limiting sexual experience outside marriage). In some countries (Canada and the USA, for example) deaths from invasive cervical cancer have been limited by widespread cervical screening. (Data from WHO, 1994.)

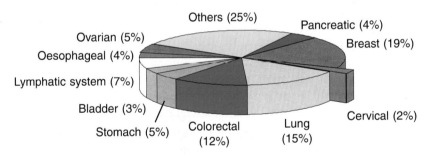

Figure 16.2 Deaths from cancer in women, England and Wales. Cervical cancer accounts for about 4% of all deaths from cancer in England and Wales and the disease is the fourth most common cause of cancer in women. Total is not 100% because of rounding. (Source: OPCS.)

Risk factors in cervical cancer

Human papillomavirus (HPV), which is thought to be transmitted by sexual activity, has been implicated as a causative agent in cervical cancer. Not all cases of cervical cancer are infected with HPV and there are many examples in which HPV-infected cells show only mildly abnormal changes and do not become malignant.

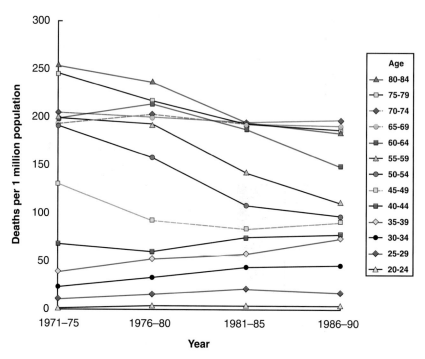

Figure 16.3 Age specific mortality rates for cervical cancer in England and Wales, 1971–1990. The number of older women dying from invasive cervical cancer is declining but the trend in women below 50 years is upwards. Most deaths still occur in middle-aged and older women. (Source: OPCS.)

> *Women who do not attend screening are at greatest risk of developing cervical cancer*

Epidemiological studies point towards sexual activity, non-attendance at cervical cytology screening, smoking and use of oral contraceptives as the main risk factors in cervical cancer. Women who have not had a smear taken for cytology in the last 10 years have a fourfold excess risk of developing carcinoma of the cervix than those who regularly attend screening. Women from lower socioeconomic groups have an increased prevalence of cervical cancer (Figure 16.4) because of generally increased exposure to lifestyle risk factors and poor attendance at cervical screening.

Sexual activity

> *The large majority of cervical cancers are in women who are, or who have been, sexually active*

Most other risk factors for the disease are associated with sexual activity. The risk relates to the number of sexual partners for either the woman or her partner, and the greater the number of sexual contacts the greater the risk. The age of first sexual intercourse is not of itself a significant risk factor, other than the possibility that earlier age allows the accumulation of more sexual partners.

The use of oral contraceptives is associated with increased risk, whereas use of barrier methods of contraception is associated with decreased risk. It has been postulated that this difference is related to the differences in exposure of the cervix to seminal fluid with barrier and non-barrier contraceptive methods.

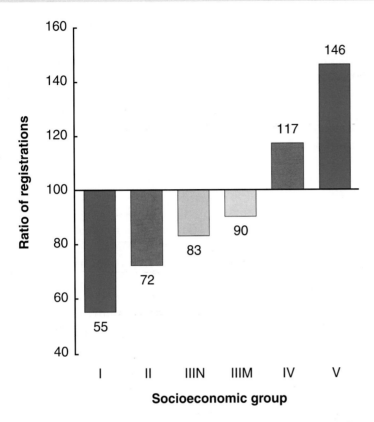

Figure 16.4 The incidence of cervical cancer is much higher in socioeconomic groups IV and V. In 1984, for every 145 registrations in women from socioeconomic group IV there were only 55 registrations in group I. (Source: OPCS.)

Viral infection

Originally, type 2 herpes simplex virus was believed to be the most likely candidate for a sexually transmitted agent in cervical cancer, but extensive studies have failed to support this. The focus has therefore shifted to an examination of the possible involvement of HPV in cancer and precancerous changes of the cervix. To date about 70 types of this virus have been identified, differing in the sequence of nucleotide bases in their DNA. Most of these are capable of infecting cells to produce benign changes, but some high-risk types are capable of inducing malignant changes. The malignant potential of this class of viruses has been shown in animal experiments with rabbit papillomavirus: the virus appears to act as a tumour initiator, and the transformation to malignancy can be completed by exposure to a chemical tumour promoter.

In humans, HPV is involved in development of genital warts, and has been identified in both precancerous and cancerous cervical lesions. However, a history of venereal warts or other venereal infection does not appear to be related to cervical cancer, which suggests that different types of the virus are

Most cases of cervical cancer are initiated by human papillomavirus

Some HPV strains are low-risk and produce only benign changes; other types have malignant potential

associated with warts and cervical cancer. Genital warts contain HPV types 6, 11, 42, 43 or 44 whereas most cases of preinvasive cervical cancer contain types 16 or 18. A minority of cervical cancers contain HPV types 31, 33 and 35. It therefore seems that there are low-risk and high-risk types of the virus; dysplasia in a warty cervical epithelium equates with low-risk, and severe dysplasia or preinvasive cancer may be synonymous with infection by high-risk HPV.

Sequences of DNA corresponding to those in HPV can be found in 80–90% of cervical cancers but the virus has also been found in 5–10% of histologically normal cervical biopsies. These findings raise the question as to how HPV is involved in the production of cervical cancers. Its absence in some cancers may simply be due to insensitivity in the method of detection, but these cases *could* have been caused by other, as yet unidentified, factors.

The presence of the virus in normal epithelium is consistent with the multistage process of neoplasia: both tumour initiators and promoters need to be present before malignant transformation occurs (see Chapter 13). HPV in normal cells could indicate a malignancy waiting to happen, through exposure to other promoting factors. These other promoting factors remain unidentified, but candidates are the metabolites of cigarette smoke or other sexually transmitted agents. Epidemiological studies indicate that there is an excess risk of cervical cancer associated with non-specific genital infections, but this may reflect an increased vulnerability of damaged cervical mucosa to viral infection.

The presence of HPV in cervical cells is readily detected in cytological smears. Infected cells have a large perinuclear halo and the cytoplasm is more darkly stained at the periphery of the cell. These distinctive cells are termed **koilocytes**. A more efficient method for detecting HPV infection is the polymerase chain reaction (see Chapter 3), in which specific nucleotide sequences corresponding to HPV are amplified and visualised with a labelled probe.

Several studies have shown an increase in both cervical lesions and HPV infection in HIV-positive women – especially those with symptomatic HIV infection (AIDS-related complex or AIDS itself), and the Centers for Disease Control (CDC) clinical categories of HIV infection include cervical neoplasia (see p. 775). The recurrence rate of CIN (see p. 515) after treatment is higher in HIV-positive women, and invasive cancers are usually more aggressive and less responsive to treatment. These differences are probably due to the immunodeficiency caused by HIV infection, rather than a direct oncogenic effect of HIV itself.

Cigarette smoking

Cigarette smoking is an independent risk factor in cervical cancer and constituents or metabolites of tobacco smoke have been demonstrated in cervical mucus. These may act directly on the cervical cells, or may offer an environment favouring infection by certain types of papillomavirus.

There is some evidence that formation of DNA adducts with some of the chemical constituents in cigarette smoke is a critical early stage in malignant

---

> *Infection with HPV alone is not enough to produce cancer – some other promoting agent must be present*

▲ **Key points**

HPV and cervical neoplasia

Low-risk HPV types producing benign lesions:
▲ HPV 6 and 11
▲ Causes genital warts (condyloma acuminata)

High-risk HPV types with malignant potential:
▲ HPV 16 and 18
▲ HPV 31, 33, 35 (intermediate risk)
▲ Initiates changes that may lead to cervical cancer

▲ **Key points**

Risk factors in cervical cancer

▲ Absence of cervical screening
▲ Sexual history of multiple partners in the woman, or in any of her partners
▲ Oral contraceptive use (non-barrier methods)
▲ Smoking
▲ HIV infection

DNA adducts: new chemical species formed by direct combination of a chemical agent with DNA.

transformation of the cell, possibly because the adducts act as tumour promoters after initiation by HPV. Also, smokers have reduced numbers of Langerhan's cells in their cervical epithelium, which means they may not be able to mount an immunological response adequate to eliminate viral infection.

> *The constituents of cigarette smoke could act as tumour promoters*

Mechanisms of HPV pathogenesis

In histologically normal tissues (and in some precancerous stages) the viral genome is present as a circular plasmid and is not integrated into host DNA. In many invasive cancers, the viral genome becomes linear and is then integrated into the host cell DNA. As the virus is incorporated into host DNA some of its own genes are lost or disrupted, particularly those responsible for controlling viral replication. The result is that more sustained growth characteristics are conferred on both the virus and the host cell.

Experimental studies have shown that HPV can induce a number of changes to host cell DNA and modulate the production or activity of gene products essential for the control of cell growth and proliferation. Most notable are co-operative effects with activated oncogenes and inactivation of the gene products arising from tumour suppressor genes, including *Rb* and *p53*.

Some effects on the host cell are caused by continued production of viral proteins in the infected cell. The virus has a number of genes, which are divided into two functional groups, described as early (*E*) and late (*L*) genes. The seven *E* genes control viral replication and transcription. Two *L* genes encode structural viral proteins. Some of the *E* genes are disrupted during viral integration into the host cell genome, but two genes (*E6* and *E7*) encode proteins that can transform cells to a malignant phenotype.

Langerhan's cells: antigen-presenting cells, responsible for initiating a local immune response.

Plasmid: circular double-stranded DNA capable of independent replication inside a bacterium.

P53 gene: a tumour suppressor gene that is mutated in about half of all cancer types. The normal protein product is involved in the induction of apoptosis following DNA damage.

Rb gene: mutations of this tumour suppressor gene were first identified as a cause of retinoblastoma. Its normal product is a nuclear phosphoprotein with DNA-binding activity. This protein inactivates tumour-causing proteins. *Rb* is important in suppressing a range of tumours in addition to retinoblastoma.

Oncogenes

In-vitro studies using human and rat cell lines of HPV interaction with host cell genes have shown that incorporation of viral *E6* and *E7* from HPV type 16 into host cells can result in their extended growth or immortalisation (this is a characteristic feature of cancer cells in culture). The viral genes appear to affect the activity of the proto-oncogenes *H-ras* and *c-fos*. In experimental studies this occurs only after the proto-oncogenes have been activated with promoters such as glucocorticoids.

There is evidence that other hormones, such as progestagens in contraceptive tablets, can also activate proto-oncogenes in animal cell lines. These virally infected cell lines are capable of producing tumours when transplanted back into the original species. Interestingly, enhanced oncogene activation is associated with infection by high- and medium-risk HPV types 16, 18, 31 and 33, but not by low-risk HPV 6.

Mutation to the *H-ras* oncogene is common in cervical cancer, especially in more advanced tumours. However, some proto-oncogene mutations (*c-myc* for example) do not appear to be influenced by HPV infection. This suggests

> *HPV acts on cancer genes only after they have been activated by other agents*

that other factors must be involved in the pathogenesis of invasive cervical cancer.

Tumour suppressor genes

> *Proteins produced by HPV can inactivate normal regulatory proteins, locking the host cell into a cycle of proliferation*

Apoptosis: programmed cell death, enabling surplus, worn or damaged cells to be removed from tissues without inflammation.

One contributory factor in the neoplastic transformation of the HPV-infected host cell is believed to be the binding of a virally encoded protein (E6 protein) to the protein product of the *p53* tumour suppressor gene. This results in degradation of p53 protein, so the cells do not undergo p53-mediated apoptosis after induction of DNA damage. Further DNA mutations will accumulate in these immortalised cells (Figure 16.5). In contrast, E6 proteins produced by low-risk HPV types do not efficiently bind p53 protein, explaining the benign clinical behaviour of cells infected by low-risk HPV.

Not all cervical cancers are HPV-positive, but nonetheless contain *p53* mutations. In these cases it is likely that p53 protein has not been produced in the first place, or is incorrectly assembled, because of defects in the encoding gene. The result is the same: the cell is unable to undergo apoptosis. However, not all HPV-negative cervical cancers contain *p53* gene mutations, indicating that inactivation of p53 protein or mutation of the gene is not a prerequisite for the development of invasive cervical cancer.

Inactivation of p53 protein also occurs in another HPV-mediated cancer: anal cancer. The HPV types are the same, and women with cervical cancer are at risk of also developing anal cancer. In one study, conducted in the UK, nearly 20% of women with CIN III (see p. 501) also had histological evidence of anal cancer or precancerous lesions. Most of the anal lesions were found in women who had multiple foci of disease, in the vulva or vagina, in addition to the cervix. Anal cancers are more likely to occur in HIV infected men and women (see Chapter 25).

Viral proteins probably modulate the activities of other host cell tumour suppressor genes. For example, E7 protein (produced by HPV types 16 and 18) binds to the protein product of the retinoblastoma (*Rb*) gene.

Does HPV infection cause cervical cancer?

Point	Counterpoint
HPV, particularly types 16 and 18, is detected in 80–90% of early cervical cancers	10% of normal cervical biopsies show evidence of HPV infection. Not all invasive cancers are infected with HPV
HPV initiates changes that may lead to cervical cancer	Not all HPV-infected CIN lesions progress to cancer
HPV E6 protein binds to p53 protein, blocking apoptosis and locking the	Some invasive cervical cancers show no evidence of alteration to either

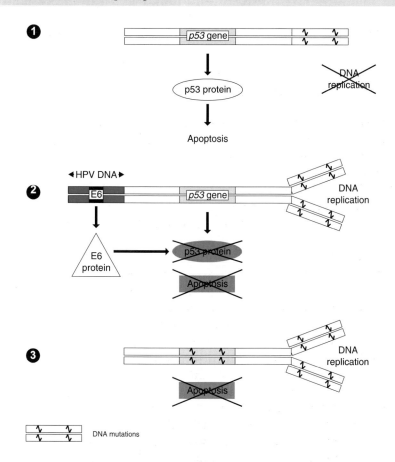

Figure 16.5 Human papillomavirus modifies *p53*, DNA replication and apoptosis. 1: The *p53* gene plays a crucial role in the 'decision' to initiate apoptosis or to repair damaged DNA by replication. Apoptosis is mediated by the p53 protein. 2: When HPV is incorporated into the host cell genome the viral E6 protein continues to be produced. This inactivates p53 protein so that apoptosis cannot take place. The cell instead 'repairs' the DNA, thereby 'fixing' the mutations. Both HPV and the mutations will be replicated whenever the cell divides. 3: Mutations to the *p53* gene itself will stop p53 protein production. The cell will instead become fixed in a growth and division cycle, replicating any mutated DNA.

cell into continued proliferation	p53 protein or its gene
HPV E7 protein binds to *Rb* tumour suppressor gene product	May not be a necessary feature of invasive cervical cancer
HPV *E6* and *E7* gene sequences induce cell immortalisation and co-operate with known oncogenes *in vitro*	Co-operation with cell oncogenes occurs only if expression promoted by other agents

Review question 1

Explain why human papillomavirus is believed to be a causative agent in most cases of cervical cancer

Author's view

In some women infection with 'high-risk' HPV types probably initiates the production of early CIN changes (see p. 501). Some HPV types are capable of inducing several 'hits' to host DNA and cellular control, by co-operating with oncogenes or inactivating tumour suppressor genes or gene products. Whether or not this occurs could depend on the persistence of infection, and this in turn will depend on the host response. Immunosuppression from any cause will encourage persistency.

Other women are able to eliminate the virus, and this presumably is largely responsible for the capacity of early precancerous lesions to regress to normal.

The progression to cancer probably requires other risk factors that would act as tumour promoters (e.g. metabolites of cigarette smoke) or would adversely affect host response (e.g. HIV infection). These factors alone, without HPV infection, are sufficient to induce invasive cervical cancer in some women but it would seem that HPV is involved in most cases of cervical cancer, probably in the early stages.

Pathology of cervical neoplasia

Precancerous lesions and cervical cancer usually occur within the transformation zone

The predominant type of cervical cancer is **squamous cell carcinoma**. The rarer **adenocarcinoma** arises from the columnar cells of the cervical canal. It makes up about 10% of primary cervical cancers and is more often found in women over 60 years of age, but is becoming increasingly common in younger women. Precancerous lesions (described as **cervical intraepithelial neoplasia**, or **CIN**) and preinvasive cervical cancers are usually asymptomatic and are discovered only by screening. By far the majority of women who die from invasive cervical cancer do not have a recent history of cervical screening.

The cervix comprises the lower third of the uterus. Cancer of the cervix usually arises in a small area at the junction of the squamous epithelium and columnar epithelium of the ectocervix, referred to as the **transformation zone** (Figure 16.6 and Plate 2). The precise location of this zone, and the types of cells within it, changes during a woman's life. Initially the epithelium comprises a single layer of mucus-secreting cells. Following hormonal changes at puberty the exposed epithelial surface becomes more acid and causes conversion (metaplasia; see Chapter 4) of the simple columnar epithelium to the thicker, more protective stratified squamous epithelium. In the adult an area of metaplastic cells will always be present, and it is in this zone that most precancerous and cancerous changes occur.

The natural history of cervical cancer in its advanced stages is unpleasant, with spread into the urinary tract and the bowel. Metastatic spread most often occurs through the lymphatic circulation. The lymph nodes usually affected are the parametrial, paracervical, obturator, hypogastric, iliac and sacral nodes within the pelvis. Lymph nodes outside the pelvis (mediastinal and supraclavicular) may also become involved.

Cervical canal: passage between the vagina and the uterine cavity. Lined with mucus-secreting columnar epithelium.

Columnar epithelium: a single layer of cells in the shape of columns or long rectangles. Often found arranged into glands.

Squamous epithelium: a layer of flattened cells lining the surface of organs such as the skin and vagina. In these sites the epithelium consists of multiple layers (stratified) of cells.

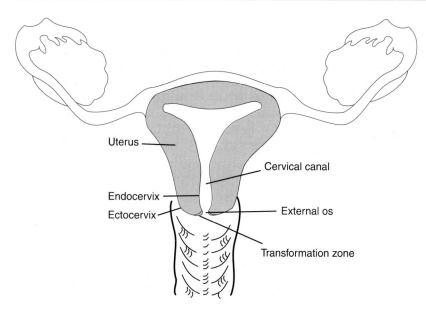

Ectocervix: usually describes tissue lying outside the external os.

Endocervix: tissue lying inside the cervical canal.

External os: the point at which the cervical canal opens into the vagina.

Figure 16.6 Cervical cancers arise in the transformation zone, a metaplastic region of the ectocervix and endocervix composed of stratified squamous epithelium.

Signs and symptoms of cervical cancer

Overt symptoms are seldom produced in the preinvasive phases of the disease and the main way these abnormalities come to attention is through regular screening.

The early symptoms of invasive cervical cancer include vaginal discharge, usually of watery bloodstained fluid: vaginal bleeding between periods, post-menopausal and post-coital bleeding are also signs. Symptoms of advanced disease include pelvic, abdominal or back pain, lack of appetite and weight loss. Involvement of the pelvic lymph nodes can obstruct venous flow and result in oedema in the legs. Tumour spread towards the bladder can cause obstruction of the ureters, urinary tract infection and uraemia.

Keratinising: the ability to form keratin, a protein found in the cornified layer of the skin.

Uraemia: excess blood in the urine.

Types of tumour

The most common malignancy of the uterine cervix is squamous cell carcinoma (about 90% of cervical cancers). These squamous cell types are subdivided into:

• Large-cell keratinising tumours
• Large-cell non-keratinising tumours
• Small-cell non-keratinising tumours

The small-cell tumours are associated with a poorer prognosis.

Malignant and premalignant changes also take place in the glandular epithelium of the cervix; malignant tumours are termed adenocarcinomas.

▲ Key points

Signs and symptoms of invasive cervical cancer

▲ Offensive vaginal discharge
▲ Unexpected vaginal bleeding
▲ Post-coital and contact bleeding
▲ Malaise, nausea and loss of appetite
▲ Lower abdominal and back pain
▲ Hard irregular ulcerated cervix
▲ Leg oedema

These can account for 10% or more of the total numbers of cancers of the cervix, but the incidence appears to be increasing. Adenocarcinomas generally have a poorer prognosis than squamous carcinomas, probably because they occur further up in the cervical canal and often remain undetected by cytology until a large tumour mass is present. Occasionally (in about 5% of cases) mixed adenosquamous tumours occur. Other malignant tumours, such as lymphomas, melanomas and sarcomas, can be encountered but are rare.

Histological stages

A range of cellular abnormalities can be detected by histological examination, corresponding to precancerous and cancerous states. Precancerous lesions have the capacity to develop to malignancy or revert to normal. In the intermediate stage (carcinoma *in situ*) these cells can persist for many years without invading the surrounding tissue. Complete removal of the lesion at a precancerous or *in-situ* stage will probably result in a complete cure.

The final stage in the process is that of invasive cancer. Treatment of this can be more problematic, and the prognosis is related to the degree of tumour spread.

Precancerous stages

The normal epithelium in the adult cervical transformation zone is a metaplastic stratified squamous epithelium. Usually three discrete cell layers are seen within this epithelium: a single layer of basal cells at the bottom, several layers of rounded polygonal cells in the middle and flattened epithelium at the surface.

Histological abnormalities

A series of morphological changes can be seen in the progression towards invasive cancer. Changes can be seen in the individual cells, and in the thickness of the abnormal epithelium. These changes are classified as grades of CIN, also referred to as **dysplastic** changes.

> *CIN classifications refer to changes in cell morphology in a progression towards invasive cancer*

Essentially, the cell changes that occur represent disorder of cell development and maturation. This is seen as:

- Atypical maturation of the different epithelial cell layers
- Abnormal keratinisation
- Nuclear and cytoplasmic changes
- Hyperactivity or expansion of the relatively undifferentiated cell population in the basal or parabasal layers, so that they constitute a major portion of the epithelium.

Precancerous conditions of the cervix are always confined to the epithelium: there is no penetration across the basement membrane into the underlying stroma. Three grades of CIN are used to describe the degree of cell differentiation and the thickness of epithelium affected (Figure 16.7). This

Basal, parabasal: the deepest layers of cells in a stratified epithelium, adjoining the basement membrane. Comprise 'reservoir' cells that frequently divide. The newly formed cells eventually reach the surface as dead cells and are removed from the surface layers.

grading is artificial in the sense that the progression towards invasive cancer is a continuum, starting with mild change and ending with undifferentiated cells, which, if not yet invasive, soon will be.

CIN I

In the early CIN I stage cells in the basal layer of the epithelium have larger nuclei than normal – there is an increase in the nuclear:cytoplasmic ratio. The nuclei are also **pleomorphic** (exhibit a variety of shapes). These cells may be several layers thick, but do not occupy more than the lower third of the epithelium. The upper two-thirds contain normal stratified squamous cells.

CIN II

The main change in CIN II is that the abnormal cells now involve the lower half of the epithelium. The upper half of the epithelium shows relatively normal stratification and maturation.

CIN III

CIN III is the most severe change possible before the development of invasive cancer. Many of the cells are already cancerous, but they are so far confined to the epithelial layer and show no sign of invasion into the underlying stroma (the CIN III classification encompasses carcinoma *in situ* but not invasive cancer). CIN III changes involve most of the epithelial cell layers, with perhaps one or two layers of normal squamous cells on the surface. The cells have large intensely stained (**hyperchromic**) nuclei and mitoses are common (the cells are actively dividing).

Cytological abnormalities

The cellular changes are reflected in cytological smears. Smears contain cells only, so that the extent of epithelial involvement cannot be ascertained. More importantly, the extent of invasion into the underlying stroma cannot be revealed by the cytological method, which is why the detection of cytological abnormalities is usually followed by biopsy.

The cytological appearances of the cells in a cervical smear are categorised according to the overall size and shape of the cells and, crucially, the size, shape and staining properties of the nucleus. Alteration in the structure of the nucleus is termed **dyskaryosis**, of which there are three grades: mild, moderate and severe (Plate 3). Invasive cancer is also detectable by cytology (Plate 4). It is possible to detect a minimal alteration to the cell structure known as **borderline change**. This is usually associated with inflammation or physical or chemical irritation.

As the cells are assessed by their microscopic appearances the classification into grades is somewhat subjective. Generally, mild, moderate and severe dyskaryosis correspond to CIN I, II and III respectively. However, cytology tends to underestimate the severity of the lesion (the histological findings often result in upgrading of CIN stage).

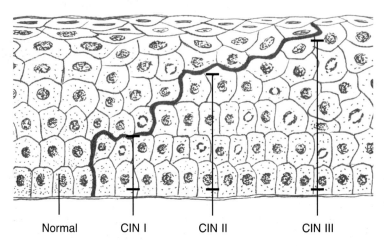

Figure 16.7 Depth of cervical epithelium involved by CIN changes. CIN I change involves only the lower third of the cervical epithelium whereas virtually the full thickness of epithelium contains abnormal cells in CIN III. Although CIN I and CIN II are apparently confined to the lower epithelium, the abnormal cells migrate to the surface and are exfoliated as part of epithelial cell turnover – this is why it is possible to detect early CIN changes by cytological examination of cells that have been scraped from the surface. The spectrum of CIN changes is not usually seen at any one time in a single lesion but represents a progression with time.

Progression to invasive cancer

> *Not all cervical abnormalities progress to invasive cancer*

> *Disease progression is more likely in the presence of HPV*

Early dysplastic (CIN) changes may persist for several years then may revert to normal or progress to invasive cancer. It is impossible to predict which lesions will progress or which regress. Regression to normal occurs in up to two-thirds of patients with CIN I and may be spontaneous, caused by anti-inflammatory therapy or the physical trauma of biopsy.

The potential for progression varies with the severity of the cervical lesion. Mild abnormalities are more likely to regress to normal (Figure 16.8). Up to 25% of untreated cases of CIN I progress to CIN III within 4–5 years. The factors influencing progression are unclear although infection with HPV (types 16 and 18 in particular) may predispose towards disease progression. Not all HPV-infected lesions progress to invasive cancer, which suggests that other cofactors may be important. Treatments are available which effectively halt disease progression but these are usually given only once CIN II or CIN III abnormalities are present. Intervention at an earlier stage is probably over-treatment.

Malignant stages

Cervical cancer is first locally invasive, spreading upwards into the corpus uteri or downwards into the vaginal wall. Fistulas can be produced by spread

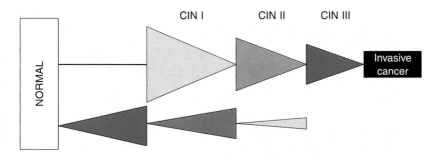

Figure 16.8 The natural history of cervical cancer. Cervical abnormalities proceed through a series of morphological changes (CIN I to CIN III) before the production of invasive cervical cancer. The further the progression, the greater the likelihood that the disease will ultimately end in invasive cancer, but there is some potential for regression. Regression to normal is much more likely in the early stages of the disease. Detection by screening and treatment at any CIN stage is effective in arresting the transition to cancer. However, in the early stages some women will be treated unnecessarily. There is no way of predicting which lesions will regress and which will progress to invasive cancer.

into the bladder or rectum. Spread towards the spine proceeds along the uterosacral ligaments, leading to involvement of the sacral plexus (Figure 16.9). This gives rise to intractable sciatica.

Lymphatic spread of the cancer is usually along the paracervical lymph tract towards the external iliac lymph nodes. Blood-borne spread in cervical cancer is unusual and occurs very late in the disease. When it does occur, metastases are usually seen in the liver, lungs and skeleton.

Invasive cervical cancer is usually staged by taking into account the degree of invasion and involvement of lymph nodes.

- **Stage 0:** carcinoma *in situ* – a localised area of cancer cells within the cervical epithelium that can persist unchanged for several years
- **Stage I:** invasion of the underlying connective tissue stroma. Tumour is confined to the cervix. There are two sub-classifications: **IA** (microinvasive carcinoma), in which cancer cells have broken through the basement membrane but have not entered blood or lymphatic systems and depth of tumour invasion is less than 3 mm; **IB**, in which cancer cells have spread more than 3 mm from the basement membrane and lymphatic vessels may be involved
- **Stage II:** tumour spread beyond the cervix into the upper vagina but not as far as the pelvic wall
- **Stage III:** tumour has reached the pelvic wall and the lower third of the vagina
- **Stage IV:** the tumour has spread into surrounding organs such as the bladder and rectum

As with all cancers the prognosis depends on the stage of the disease. Practically all cases of stage 0 cervical cancers are permanently curable but 5-year survival rates range from 94% for stage IA cancers to 30% for the more

▲   **Key points**

Staging of invasive cervical cancer

▲ Physical examination: bimanual vaginal and rectal examination, palpation of lymph nodes
▲ Radiological examination: intravenous pyelogram, barium enema, chest and skeletal radiographs, radionuclide bone scan, CT (or MRI) scans
▲ Laboratory: histology, fine-needle aspiration cytology
▲ Surgical staging

advanced stage III and IV cancers (these survival rates are based on outcomes after appropriate treatment). The surgical treatment of invasive cervical cancer is usually limited to stages I and II. More advanced cases are treated by radiotherapy.

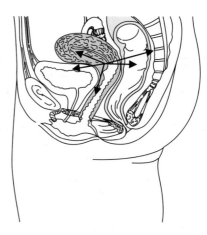

Figure 16.9 Spread of invasive cervical cancer. Cervical cancer spreads downwards along the vaginal walls, upwards into the body of the uterus, forwards into the bladder and backwards to involve the rectum and sacral plexus.

Detection and assessment of cervical lesions

Following the initial presentation of symptoms or detection of cervical abnormalities by routine cervical screening, the condition is assessed by visual inspection, bimanual pelvic examination, colposcopic examination and tissue biopsy. In the early stages there may be no obvious signs on bimanual examination or visual inspection. The appearances may remain normal for some time, particularly if the growth is within the cervical canal. The initial appearance may be of an inflamed-looking outgrowth of the external os. As the cancer infiltrates the wall of the cervix it will become harder, forming a barrel-shaped mass. Infiltration of the vaginal fornices will cause the cervix to become fixed in place. The surface of the growth is friable and bleeds when touched.

There is usually little doubt about the diagnosis once these physical signs become apparent but a biopsy is usually taken for histological confirmation. Other conditions that can give rise to similar signs are cervical inflammation (cervicitis) and infected benign mucous polyps.

Once malignancy is confirmed by histological assessment of the biopsy a number of investigations may be undertaken to assess the stage of the disease. Cystoscopy, proctosigmoidoscopy or barium enema may be performed to determine any involvement of the bladder or rectum. Other investigations might include chest radiography, intravenous pyelogram, or CT scanning of the pelvis. Any nodal involvement is best assessed by CT in combination with

Cystoscopy: visual examination of bladder wall and urethra through a cystoscope.

Intravenous pyelogram: a soluble radio-opaque substance (e.g. iodine-131) is injected. This is filtered by the kidney glomeruli, concentrated in the tubules and excreted in the urine. Its passage can be followed by timed serial X-rays. Useful for demonstrating sites of obstruction and space-occupying lesions in urinary tract.

Vaginal fornix: a recess at the upper end of the vagina where it is surrounded by the cervix.

fine-needle aspiration cytology of any suspicious nodes. Unless the condition is inoperable or the patient is to be treated with radiotherapy alone, the findings of any staging investigations should be confirmed by surgical exploration and histological evaluation of excised tissues.

Colposcopy

Colposcopy is a simple procedure carried out without anaesthesia in a hospital outpatient department, although the correct interpretation of the appearances requires skill and experience. The colposcopist must distinguish between normal and abnormal squamous epithelium and the glandular or columnar epithelium. The identification and evaluation of abnormal lesions are based on colour, surface irregularities and patterns of the underlying blood vessels.

> *Colposcopy involves visual examination of the cervical and vaginal walls with a modified microscope*

It is common practice to apply a dilute (2–3%) solution of acetic acid to the cervix. This produces a whitened appearance confined to areas of CIN, because of differences in the protein composition of the cells (Plate 5). The distribution and extent of any abnormalities can indicate the type and severity of disease. The normal columnar and glandular epithelium can be distinguished by its papillary (projections on the surface) appearance.

Biopsy procedures

Punch biopsy

When abnormal areas are seen by colposcopy the usual protocol is to take a punch biopsy of the lesion for histological assessment. Often more than one lesion will be present in the transformation zone and all of these should be sampled. Sometimes an experienced colposcopist is able to grade the lesions, in which case biopsies of only the highest-grade lesions will be necessary. It is also usual to examine the vaginal walls, which can contain HPV-infected lesions.

> *Biopsies will be taken from any abnormal areas seen by colposcopy*

Large loop excision

Large loop excision of the transformation zone (LLETZ) is becoming increasingly popular and involves the use of an electrically heated wire loop to remove a cone of tissue from the cervix, to include all of the transformation zone. Different designs of loop can be used to excise different amounts of abnormal tissue. The area excised is less extensive than that of a cone biopsy (see below) and the method offers a quick and acceptable out-patient alternative. Like the cone biopsy LLETZ serves both diagnostic and treatment purposes.

> *Occasionally sufficient tissue is taken at biopsy to serve both diagnostic and treatment purposes*

This technique is normally performed under local anaesthesia. Slight vaginal bleeding may persist for several days or even weeks after the procedure, and patients should avoid sexual intercourse or use of tampons for about 4 weeks. If the blood loss approaches that of the normal menstrual flow the patient should be re-examined: the cause is usually a small bleeding point which can be cauterised under local anaesthesia.

The amount of tissue removed by LLETZ is more extensive than that destroyed by ablation treatments, increasing the likelihood that all abnormal areas will have been included in the treatment. For this reason some gynaecologists advocate LLETZ in preference to the more common ablation methods. About 25% of specimens contain no serious abnormalities (these patients have thus been over-treated). Other gynaecologists favour the more conservative ablation treatments, particularly as the after-effects, such as vaginal discharge, are less extensive. Occasionally, LLETZ biopsy specimens are difficult to evaluate histologically because they have been damaged by heat.

Cone biopsy

In some postmenopausal women it may be difficult to visualise the transformation zone, where most of the abnormalities occur. These require cone biopsy. Cone biopsy is a surgical procedure requiring general anaesthesia. The intention is to remove a cone of tissue around and including the cervical canal with all of the transformation zone. Other indications for the procedure are cytological abnormalities repeatedly seen in successive smears and diagnosis of adenocarcinomas (these often cannot be visualised by colposcopy).

Cone biopsy yields a piece of tissue 2–3 cm in diameter at its base. This is sent for histological assessment, to confirm the nature of the abnormality and to check that the abnormal lesion has been completely excised. If it has, the biopsy has served the dual purpose of providing both diagnostic information and treatment.

The procedure is associated with a high incidence of immediate complications such as haemorrhage and infection. Cryocautery is used after cone biopsy to stop bleeding. Treatment is usually followed by a vaginal discharge for some weeks. Other complications are cervical stenosis which can affect fertility, and a tendency for spontaneous abortion in subsequent pregnancies.

Endocervical curettage

Occult lesions in the cervical canal can be sampled by curettage. This yields fragments of tissue suitable for histological evaluation of squamous cell carcinoma or adenocarcinoma. However, since this is only a superficial biopsy there is usually insufficient material to establish the depth of tumour invasion. Abnormal findings in curettings must confirmed and further evaluated in a cone biopsy.

Treatment of CIN lesions

The aim of treatment in women of reproductive age is to eliminate CIN, while retaining the cervix and its function

The results of the colposcopic examination and the histology will determine whether treatment is needed. The type of treatment used will depend on the type and extent of lesion. The age of the woman and her possible desire to remain fertile also need to be taken into account. Pregnancy alters the timing, rather than the type, of treatment because of the possibility of inducing haemorrhage or abortion. The course of CIN lesions is not affected by pregnancy and therefore treatment can be delayed until after delivery. Many of the initial diagnostic investigations, including exfoliative cytology, colposcopy and biopsy, can be performed without risk to the fetus.

Local ablative treatment

Review question 2

Explain the relative merits of punch biopsy, LLETZ treatment and cone biopsy in the diagnosis of cervical cancer

CIN II and III lesions can be easily ablated if the transformation zone is exposed in the external os. In older women the transformation zone lies further up the cervical canal and cone biopsy may be necessary. A variety of ablation methods use heat or cold to destroy the tissue: cryocautery, diathermy (electrocoagulation), cold coagulation and laser treatment.

Unfortunately the ablation methods do not yield tissue that can be used for histological confirmation of the diagnosis or to see whether the lesion has been completely removed. Follow-up examinations and cytology are very important after treatment to ensure that the disease has been eradicated.

Cryocautery

This is also known as cryosurgery or cryotherapy. It is performed without anaesthesia on an outpatient basis in about 15 minutes with little discomfort to the patient. A probe is applied to the exposed cervix and the area frozen by high-pressure nitrous oxide or carbon dioxide. Tissue is usually destroyed to a depth of 2 or 3 mm. The technique is recommended for small CIN I or CIN II lesions, for which it has a success rate of 80–90%. Follow-up smears and colposcopy should be undertaken within 6 months and the cryocautery repeated if necessary. Minor side-effects include faintness, mild abdominal cramps and a watery discharge for 2–3 weeks after treatment.

The transformation zone can be destroyed by freezing

Diathermy

This procedure is normally carried out under general anaesthesia but can be done with local anaesthesia. It involves destruction of the abnormal lesion using heat generated through needle and ball-shaped electrodes. The needle electrode is used for deeper penetration and destruction of the glands underlying the cervical surface, while the ball electrode is more effective in destroying areas on the surface.

Wide and deep destruction of the transformation zone can be achieved with needle and ball electrodes

The entire transformation zone is treated by inserting the needle electrode at approximately 2–3 mm intervals, to a depth of 7–8 mm on each occasion, in a 'pepper-pot' pattern. This is followed by application of the ball electrode systematically to the entire surface of the circumscribed area. The treatment is highly effective in eliminating all degrees of CIN and most patients require only one treatment.

Inevitably some of the surrounding normal tissue is damaged by this procedure and a bloody discharge should be expected for 2–3 weeks after treatment. Stenosis of the cervical canal may occur – this will make taking future smears difficult. It may also make menstruation painful if the flow is obstructed; dilation of the cervix may be necessary.

Cold coagulation

Despite its name, the cold coagulation method uses electrically heated probes to destroy the transformation zone by blistering. Various sizes and shapes of Teflon-coated probes are available to suit the contours of the area to be treated. The probes are heated electrically to 100–120°C and applied to small sections of the cervix for up to 30 s until the whole abnormal area is covered.

The probe temperature is lower than that used in diathermy – hence 'cold' coagulation. The treatment is usually given under local anaesthesia and has a 95% cure rate for CIN III. Side-effects can include heavy discharge due to destruction of some healthy tissue.

Laser treatment

A carbon dioxide laser can be used to vaporise tissue

Laser treatment has the advantages of precision: there is minimal destruction of surrounding normal tissue, healing is rapid and side-effects less severe. It is possible to outline the lesion and destroy it by heat vaporisation to a depth of 1 cm. The procedure produces little pain and only local anaesthesia is required. Bleeding should be minimal because the blood vessels are sealed by the laser. This is the most convenient and effective ablation treatment but the equipment is expensive and may be limited to clinics in the larger hospitals. It is more time-consuming and requires a greater degree of skill.

Excision procedures

Adequate excision of the lesion may already have been performed by LLETZ or cone biopsy used for diagnosis. Provided that histological examination of the excised tissue confirms that all abnormal cells have been removed, no further treatment is required except for follow-up cytological screening or colposcopy.

Cone biopsy

The availability of less extensive ablation and excision methods has led to a decline in the use of the cone biopsy in management of CIN. The remaining therapeutic indications for cone biopsy are for removal of extensive CIN lesions and for treatment of women in whom follow-up is likely to be a problem. Cone biopsy can be used to manage microinvasive (stage IA) cervical cancer if the woman wishes to remain fertile but in most cases the treatment of choice is simple hysterectomy.

Hysterectomy

Fibroids (leiomyoma): tumour of smooth muscle in the wall of the uterus, the most common benign tumour of the female genital tract. Usually 2–4 cm in size but can be 20 cm or larger. Causes abnormal menstrual bleeding or infertility.

Menorrhagia: abnormal premenopausal bleeding.

Total hysterectomy may be chosen for the older woman who does not wish to have more children. Other indications for hysterectomy are:

- Aberrant smears or colposcopic appearances that persist despite local ablation or cone biopsy
- Presence of associated gynaecological symptoms of menorrhagia, uterine

fibroids or uterovaginal prolapse
- The woman has early invasive cervical cancer

Review question 3

Explain why some precancerous lesions of the cervix may be left untreated

> ▲ **Key points**
>
> **Ablation and excision methods for treating CIN**
>
> | | Application | Disadvantages |
> |---|---|---|
> | **Ablation methods:** | | |
> | Laser treatment | Treatment of choice | Equipment is expensive |
> | 'Cold' coagulation | | Treatments can fail because of inadequate extent and depth of treatment |
> | Diathermy | | Large extent and depth of treatment increase the likelihood of adverse side-effects |
> | Cryocautery | | |
> | **Excision methods:** | | |
> | Cone biopsy | Diagnosis (usually in older women). Treatment of stage IA invasive cancer in women who wish to remain fertile | Can affect fertility and ability to bring pregnancy to term (risk is low) |
> | Large loop excision of transformation zone (LLETZ) | Diagnosis and treatment | Ensures any undetected microinvasion is eliminated but can be over-treatment |
> | Hysterectomy | Treatment of persistent abnormalities despite ablation or cone biopsy. Treatment of early invasive cancers | Not suitable for younger women who wish to remain fertile |

Treatment of invasive cancer

The type and degree of treatment necessary to eliminate invasive cervical cancer depend on the histological stage. In contrast to the earlier CIN changes, invasive cancer involves tumour spread beyond the epithelial basement membrane. Consequently the treatment needs to be more extensive, usually involving radiotherapy or surgery.

Early invasive cancers are usually treated by simple hysterectomy

Early invasive cervical cancer (stages I and II)

If tumour invasion has not extended beyond 1 mm of the basement membrane (early stage IA) then the condition can be managed conservatively by a wide

Hysterectomy: surgical resection of the uterus and supporting tissues. Operations vary in complexity from simple (uterus and very small cuff of vaginal wall only) to radical.

Modified Wertheim radical hysterectomy: removal of the uterus, ovaries and tubes, most of the vagina, supporting ligaments, and pelvic and iliac lymph nodes. Many surgeons carry out a block dissection, removing the pelvic nodes and fat, and then the uterus and vagina all in one piece. The end result is clearance of all pelvic structures down to the muscle fascia, leaving only vessels, nerves, rectum and bladder.

Type III hysterectomy: radical hysterectomy with removal of only the upper third of the vagina.

> *Radiotherapy can be used to treat invasive cervical cancer at any stage*

Afterloading: plastic housing for intrauterine and vaginal fornix sources are introduced first. Low-dose radioactive source introduced manually after housings are correctly placed. Local or epidural anaesthesia is usually sufficient.

'Cathetron' or 'Selectron' high-dose treatment: applicator tubes are placed in position manually. The patient is taken to a side-room and the radioactive source is introduced into the applicators by remote control.

Intracavitary radiotherapy: packs containing the radioactive source (usually caesium-137) are placed in the cervical canal and in lateral vaginal fornices.

cone biopsy or simple hysterectomy. Invasion beyond this would be treated by more radical hysterectomy or radiotherapy. In the surgical treatment of younger women the ovaries are conserved whenever possible to preserve oestrogen function. The ovaries rarely become involved by cervical cancer. It is not possible to preserve ovarian function with radiotherapy and patients undergoing radiotherapy will require HRT.

The advantage of surgery is that the disease can be accurately staged by visual examination and histological assessment of the excised tissues. Disadvantages are initial sexual dysfunction or even complete loss of coital function if the procedure has involved excision of the upper portion of the vagina. After type III hysterectomy the vagina lengthens with regular sexual intercourse.

Survival after surgery depends on lymph node involvement, the size of the tumour and depth of invasion. Patients in whom nodes are uninvolved have a 90% 5-year survival: this drops to 20–60% when lymph nodes are involved. Survival at the higher end of this range can be expected if only the pelvic lymph nodes are involved, but involvement of the common iliac nodes is associated with a worse prognosis. The number of lymph nodes involved also influences prognosis.

Radiotherapy

The goal of radiotherapy is to deliver the highest possible radiation dose to the cervix and associated lymph nodes without damaging normal tissues. The radiation dose is administered internally (intracavitary radiotherapy) or externally by beam therapy. Intracavitary radiotherapy allows a relatively high radiation dose to be delivered to the central site of the cancer, but the dose is not adequate to treat large tumour masses or the pelvic lymph nodes.

In these instances external beam therapy from a cobalt source or megavoltage linear accelerator is chosen. In practice both approaches are used in a single patient. With small tumours the practice varies as to which method is used first, but large tumours should first be treated by external beam therapy to shrink the tumour and reduce anatomic distortion. This will allow more precise positioning and dosage from the intracavitary source.

Treatment is not without complications, which may include radiation damage to the ureter, rectum, small intestine and the vagina. Very similar survival rates (about 85% 5-year survival) are associated with surgical or radiation treatments for stage IB cancer of the cervix. The 5-year survival for radiotherapy-treated stage II cancer is about 60%, 30% for stage III and 10% for stage IV. One reason for failure of radiotherapy treatment is the presence of undetected metastatic spread outside the treatment fields. This usually involves lymph nodes in the para-aortic region.

Side-effects of the external radiotherapy include fatigue, diarrhoea, cystitis and radiation-induced menopause. The internal treatment produces a vaginal discharge, dryness, soreness, inflammation and narrowing of the vagina. Resumption of sexual intercourse will therefore be painful and to help avoid this the woman should be given a dilator to insert into her vagina with a lubricating jelly for the first 6 weeks after treatment. Sexual dysfunction can persist after radiation therapy because of vaginal shortening, fibrosis or atrophy of the epithelium.

Advanced cervical cancer (stages III and IV)

There is no real hope of a cure by either surgery or radiotherapy when cervical cancer has advanced to stages III or IV, although survival may be extended – 5-year rates of 30% can be achieved for stage III cervical cancer. Treatments are designed to suit the individual, and are likely to involve radiotherapy.

Pelvic exenteration can be used as a primary treatment, but is more likely to be performed when the tumour is small and localised with no distant metastases. It is a very specialised procedure and only a dozen or so operations are carried out each year in the UK. With careful selection of patients (no lymph node or pelvic side wall involvement) there is a good chance of cure. The extent of surgical treatment depends on involvement of the bladder or rectum: these organs may need to be removed along with the genital tract and pelvic lymph nodes. Occasionally the surgeon will find that full tumour clearance is impossible or too dangerous for the patient.

Cervical cancers are poorly sensitive to chemotherapy and consequently this approach has not been commonly used. Further evaluation is under way to investigate the potential of chemotherapy for tumour debulking before other treatments. Some chemotherapy agents increase the radiosensitivity of cervical cancers and a combination of chemotherapy and radiotherapy can produce a better response and survival than radiotherapy alone. Cisplatin may be given as an adjunct to radiotherapy in poorly differentiated tumours.

Treatment in pregnancy

Treatment in patients with microinvasive disease (stage IA) can be delayed until the baby can be delivered normally. Some stage IB patients (depth of tumour invasion less than 5 mm) can be followed to term, the baby delivered by Caesarean section and a modified radical hysterectomy with pelvic lymph node dissection performed. Patients with more advanced cancers must be treated as soon as possible. This will depend on the stage of gestation and the wishes of the woman. Survival for babies delivered at a gestational age of 28 weeks is about 75%, rising to 90% for those delivered at 32 weeks. Treatment should not usually be delayed beyond 4 weeks. Surgery is performed at the time of Caesarean section, although vaginal delivery with post-partum radiotherapy would be another option.

Patients with advanced cervical cancer (stage IIB and beyond) require immediate treatment. If the fetus is viable it should be delivered by Caesarean section. In the first trimester external radiotherapy may be started but abortion is inevitable.

Pelvic exenteration: clearance of all pelvic organs. In advanced cervical cancer exenteration is usually confined to anterior or posterior pelvic organs. The anterior operation is more common because the bladder is more often a site of tumour invasion. In this case the ureters are diverted and implanted into either the colon or the ileum. Posterior exenteration involves removal of the reproductive tract, the rectum and part of the colon (to achieve tumour-free margins). This leaves the patient with a colostomy. Total exenteration is a formidable operation leaving the patient with both a colostomy and urinary tract diversion to the ileum.

▲ **Key points**

Treatment of invasive cervical cancer

- ▲ Stage IA: wide cone biopsy or simple hysterectomy
- ▲ Stage IB: radiotherapy or radical hysterectomy with pelvic lymph node dissection
- ▲ Stages II and III: radiotherapy alone or followed by surgery
- ▲ Stage IV: intracavitary and external beam radiotherapy
- ▲ Chemotherapy is used for very advanced or recurrent disease
- ▲ Exenteration in cases of recurrent disease without distant metastases

Cervical screening

The *Health of the Nation* target is to reduce the incidence of cervical cancer by at least 20% by the year 2000, from 15 per 100 000 to 12 per 100 000 women. The proposed means of doing this is through screening, although the contributory risk factors for cervical cancer are known and it may be possible to reduce incidence of the disease by primary prevention. This will require a health education approach to raise awareness of the risks associated with early intercourse, multiple partners, and non-barrier methods of contraception.

In many countries, particularly Scandinavia and the USA, incidence and death rates from cervical cancer have fallen since the introduction of cytology screening programmes. In the USA, the death rate due to cervical cancer has declined by 70% over the past 40 years. Reductions have not been so marked in the UK, despite the operation of opportunistic screening practices since the 1960s. The government therefore decided to rationalise the screening programme, mainly by introducing computerised call–recall systems and providing financial incentives for general practitioners to take cervical smears.

The call–recall programme was introduced nationally in 1988, aimed at routine screening of women aged 20–64 years at least every 5 years. In England 14.3 million women are eligible for screening, and by March 1992 11.5 million had had at least one adequate smear taken. Fewer than 700 000 women remained to be invited for screening but many women failed to take advantage of their screening invitation. Most invasive cervical cancers occur in women who have not attended routine screening (Figure 16.10).

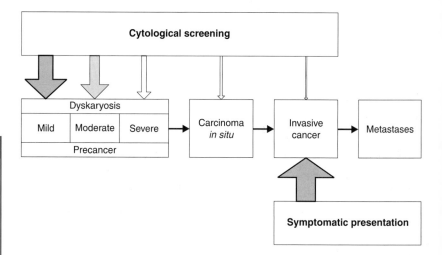

Figure 16.10 Development and detection of cervical lesions. Women who have symptoms usually already have invasive cervical cancer. Cytological screening of asymptomatic women can advance the diagnosis to a precancerous stage. With regular screening, detection is advanced to the very early mild dyskaryosis stage.

The screening method

The cervical transformation zone is relatively easily accessible for examination and treatment. Cells can be removed by inserting a speculum into the vagina and then scraping the exposed entrance to the cervical canal (the external os) using a spatula or brush. The cells are then smeared on to a glass slide. In order to see the cells under the microscope they are stained by a method developed by Papanicolaou: cytology smears are colloquially known as 'Papanicolaou smears' and the procedure known as the 'Pap test'.

Although many women find the procedure embarrassing, worrying, occasionally uncomfortable or even painful, the taking of cytology smears is a simple and rapid technique that lends itself to regular screening of large sectors of the female population. Sampling difficulties may be encountered in older women because of the relative inaccessibility of the transformation zone, which lies further up the os than in younger women (Figure 16.11). The area can be more effectively reached by using a spatula with an extended tip (Aylesbury spatula) and an endocervical brush (Plate 6).

> *The basis of the screening test is cytological examination of cells that have been scraped from the surface of the cervix*

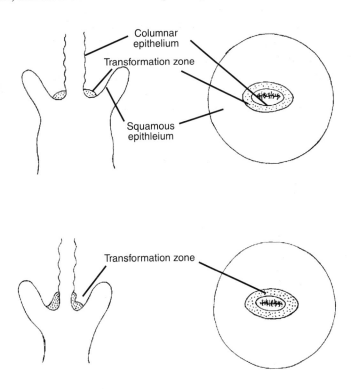

Figure 16.11 Variation in position of the transformation zone. (a) The ectocervical transformation zone. The right-hand diagram represents end-on view as would be seen by colposcopy. In younger women the transformation zone is usually easily visualised on the ectocervix. (b) Largely endocervical transformation zone. In older (postmenopausal) women the transformation zone often extends into the endocervical canal and is incompletely visible by colposcopy.

Accuracy of cytology

Estimates vary, but the frequency of false-negative results from cytology smears can be as high as 20–40%. One of the main reasons is inadequate sampling from the correct area of the cervix: ultimately the screening programme depends on the expertise and proper training of the medical practitioners and nurses who take the smears. Adequacy of the sample is determined by the numbers and types of cell removed; metaplastic squamous cells should be present, together with columnar cells from the higher endocervix. Another possible reason for failure occurs in the microscopic examination of the smears: it is possible to miss a few abnormal cells among many hundreds of normal cells.

False-positive results are extremely unlikely, although subjective interpretation can result in some misclassification within the range of possible abnormalities. Most laboratories incorporate quality control procedures, any abnormalities being re-checked and the smear throughput being randomly sampled and re-evaluated.

> *The main failing of the cytological smear test is false-negative results*

Diagnostic stage

The cytological screen does not reveal the overall tissue architecture and extent of a lesion and cannot be relied on to assess precisely how far an abnormal condition has progressed. For this reason, women with high-grade precancerous lesions detected by cytology (moderate or severe dyskaryosis) must always be referred for further colposcopic investigation and biopsy (as would women in whom there is evidence of cancer). There have been proposals to eliminate the cytology step altogether, and instead use colposcopy as the screening modality. Unfortunately, because it takes years of training and experience to recognise cervical lesions properly by colposcopy this method would not be cost-effective.

> *Abnormal findings must be further investigated by colposcopy and tissue biopsy*

Treatment stage

The treatment of screen-detected precancerous lesions is very different from that required for symptomatic cancer, in terms of both the extent and the chances of success (Figure 16.12). The goal of cervical screening is to prevent the development of invasive cancer by early treatment but this does not necessarily mean that all screen-detected abnormalities should be treated. It may be difficult to decide when such treatments should be given, because not all the abnormalities detected will ultimately progress to cancer.

There is little debate about what to do to with high-grade lesions such as CIN II and III, but the best course to take with the low-grade lesions up to CIN I is controversial. In most women any intervention would represent over-treatment because these lesions would probably return to normal, subjecting women to needless concern and increasing financial costs (about 400 000 women in the UK and 1 million in the USA have low-grade cervical abnormalities). The usual strategy is to 'watch and wait', monitoring for any disease progression by more frequent cervical smears, usually at 6-month intervals. Women who

> *Treatment of screened precancers involves local ablation or excision*

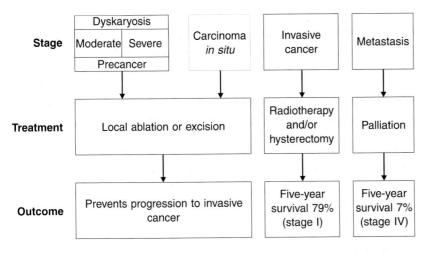

Figure 16.12 The treatment required for screen-detected cervical precancers is far less extensive than that required for invasive cancer. Moreover, with proper follow-up, treatment is virtually 100% effective in preventing progression to invasive cancer. The treatment of invasive cancer is associated with significant morbidity and does not cure all women.

have persistent low-grade abnormalities in two repeat smears (within 12 months) will usually be referred for colposcopy and possible biopsy. Given the time course usually associated with progression to cancer this is fairly safe management.

Follow-up of treated women

There is always some risk of recurrence after ablation, because the lesion was incompletely eradicated or because a further, undetected, lesion existed. Recurrence is also likely if the original lesion was severe. Overall, the recurrence rate after treatment is 5–20% and new disease may develop in up to 5% of treated cases. Generally, cytological follow-up should be started 6 months after treatment. After 1 year of follow-up, smears should be repeated yearly, and if no recurrence or new disease is detected within 5 years the woman is returned to the normal recall programme.

Effects of cervical screening

By far the majority of smears submitted for cytological examination are perfectly normal. Approximately 4–5% of smears will be classified as showing borderline changes or changes consistent with infection by HPV, and usually mild or moderate dyskaryosis will be identified in 1–2% of the smears screened. Cytological evaluation tends to underestimate the severity of the lesion: up to 30% of smears assessed as low grade are upgraded on colposcopic examination.

▲ **Key points**

Cervical screening and treatment

Screening method:
▲ Cytological examination of cells removed from the cervical surface by spatula or brush

Diagnostic stage:
▲ Colposcopy – microscopic evaluation of cervical surface and vaginal walls
▲ Tissue biopsy for histological assessment

Treatment stage:
▲ Local ablation or excision

Review question 4

Explain the fundamental differences in the approaches to treatment of precancerous and cancerous lesions of the cervix

> *The treatment of women with CIN generally prevents development of invasive cancer*

With time, screening will prevent invasive cancer and produce a general downstaging (decrease in severity) of the precancerous lesions. Data showing these trends are available from a demonstration project undertaken in the Netherlands (Boon *et al.*, 1990). The prevalence of precancerous changes is usually greater than that of the invasive cancers, because of the long time course of disease progression. With repeated screening the greatest *proportionate* decline is seen with respect to the invasive cancers; the proportion of carcinoma *in situ* (CIN III) also declines but not as markedly (Figure 16.13). Fewer cases of severe dyskaryosis are seen, although the impact on the incidence of mild and moderate dyskaryosis is less strong (Figure 16.14). This information on disease staging is another means of monitoring the effectiveness of the screening programme. The result should be the eradication of CIN III and cervical cancer in screened women.

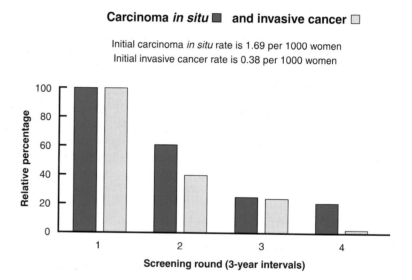

Carcinoma *in situ* ■ and invasive cancer □

Initial carcinoma *in situ* rate is 1.69 per 1000 women
Initial invasive cancer rate is 0.38 per 1000 women

Relative percentage (y-axis: 0, 20, 40, 60, 80, 100)

Screening round (3-year intervals) (x-axis: 1, 2, 3, 4)

Figure 16.13 Type and frequency of cervical abnormalities (histology) with repeat screening: carcinoma *in situ* and invasive cancer. Initial carcinoma *in situ* rate is 1.69 per 1000 women; initial invasive cancer rate is 0.38 per 1000 women. Screening has the most marked effect on severe abnormalities. By the fourth round of screening the incidence of invasive cancer in previously screened women falls to zero. For carcinoma *in situ*, the incidence in the fourth round is about 20% of that found in the initial prevalent screen. (Data from Boon *et al.*, 1990.)

The results shown by the demonstration project in the Netherlands are not as easily produced in mass screening programmes because of the population dynamics involved. Women constantly enter or leave the programme as their eligibility changes, and may not take advantage of every screening opportunity. The main problem influencing the efficiency of cervical screening programmes is that of attendance.

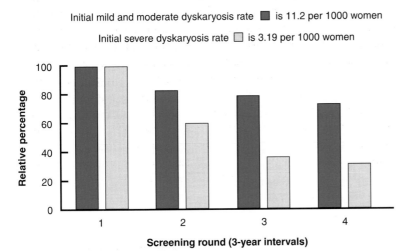

Figure 16.14 Type and frequency of cervical abnormalities (cytology) with repeat screening: premalignant (dyskaryotic) changes. Initial mild and moderate dyskaryosis rate 11.2 per 1000 women; initial severe dyskaryosis rate 3.19 per 1000 women. By the fourth round of screening the incidence of severe dyskaryosis is reduced to about 30% of that seen in the initial screening round; the effect of screening on mild and moderate dyskaryosis is less marked. It follows that in the individual woman who regularly attends screening the chances of a severe abnormality decrease as the number of negative smears increases. In established cytology screening programmes by far the greater proportion of abnormalities detected are of low grade. (Data from Boon *et al.*, 1990.)

Cervical screening in practice

Efficiency of screening

A number of factors influence the efficiency of cervical screening programmes. The programme must reach its target population. In the UK the aim is to achieve 80% attendance, and eligible women are identified and invited for screening through the Family Health Service Authority registers. These need to be maintained in an accurate condition: not an easy task in some metropolitan areas where the population is highly mobile, and it is estimated that the registers can be up to 20% inaccurate. Poor attendance is encountered in areas where there is a wide mix of ethnic groups. Some people of ethnic minorities may be reluctant to undergo the intimate examination involved in cervical screening for cultural and religious reasons, and there can be a problem of communication in women whose first language is not English.

Cervical screening must reach its target

As far as practicable the testing procedure must be tailored to women's needs and operate at suitable hours, in accessible locations, with female doctors or nurses available to take the smear. In general women in the lower socioeconomic groups are less likely to attend screening – this is particularly unfortunate as these women appear to be at greatest risk of developing cervical cancer.

> *Cervical screening is aimed at those at most risk of developing the disease*

Target population

In the UK cervical screening is offered to women aged 20–64 years. Some teenagers have cervical abnormalities but the incidence of invasive cervical cancer in this population is in the order of two per million. It is therefore considered uneconomic to screen this sector of the population, and in view of the usually slow progression of the disease it is believed safe to delay screening until the woman is in her early twenties – assuming that she attends.

Nearly half of the deaths from cervical cancer in the UK occur in women over 65 and at first glance it would seem appropriate to screen these older women. However, a substantial proportion of these cancers would have been initiated some years earlier, at a time when the women were eligible for screening (in other words, most of these cancers occur in non-attenders). Only about 10% of women of 60–64 years attend for screening, and it would seem more prudent to encourage uptake in this age group than to extend the programme beyond 65 years. There are also technical problems in screening the older woman; not only are there difficulties in sampling but the smears may also be difficult to interpret. Nevertheless, any woman over the age of 65 should be offered a smear test if she has never had one.

Screening interval

> *The interval between screens is a balance between resources, test acceptability and the incidence of interval cancers*

To some extent the repeat screening interval is determined by the number of interval cancers which appear in the screened population. More of these cases will appear with time, and hence the degree of protection afforded by screening will decline with time after the screen. In practice, the relative protection given by screening is very similar for the first 3 years, but screening once every 5 or 10 years offers considerably less protection (Figure 16.15). For this reason the screening interval is usually set at 3 years or more; there would be little extra gain in screening annually or biennially. It should be emphasised that repeat screens are necessary: a negative smear does not mean that a woman will never develop the disease.

Early recall

In some circumstances repeat testing may be necessary in advance of the usual 3-year interval – when the smear is found to be inadequate for technical reasons or when an abnormality has been detected. If the smear is inadequate the woman will be recalled immediately for a repeat. Most women with screen-detected cervical abnormalities will undergo repeat screening at more frequent intervals in order to monitor the effectiveness of treatment or, if left untreated, any further progression.

Review question 5

Why has the target age group for cervical screening in the UK been set at 20–64 years?

Is cervical screening worthwhile?

Point	Counterpoint
Cervical screening and treatment can prevent the progression of cervical	Treatment of precancerous lesions may be unnecessary because some

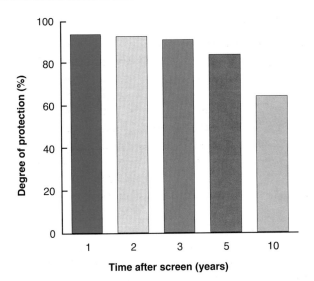

Figure 16.15 Protection from invasive cervical cancer with screening in women aged 35–64 years. In the first year after screening, protection against development of invasive cervical cancer is nearly 100%. The risks of developing the disease increase with time after screening, so that by 10 years there is only a 65% reduction in cumulative mortality from cervical cancer compared with women who had never been screened. Cancer incidence rates for the first 3 years after screening are very similar: there would be no real benefit by increasing the screening frequency to less than 3 years. (Data from IARC Working Group, 1986.)

Review question 6

With respect to cervical screening, have all of Wilson's criteria for mass screening been met?

Wilson's criteria for mass screening

▲ The disease should be common and serious
▲ The natural history of the disease should be understood
▲ The screening test should be accurate and reliable
▲ Acceptable treatment and the resources for treatment must be available
▲ The treatment should favourably influence the outcome

(After Wilson, 1966)

---

neoplastic lesions to invasive cancer	will regress to normal – there is some potential for over-treatment
Treatment of precancerous lesions is much less extensive than that required for invasive cancer, with a far greater certainty of success	Over-treatment is harmful to a woman both physically and psychologically
Call–recall cervical screening will markedly reduce incidence and mortality from cervical cancer	Routine mass screening can induce unnecessary anxieties in people who are perfectly healthy
The cervical smear test is well suited to a mass screening programme	Screening of all women aged 20–64 is expensive. The programme requires well trained staff. There is an unacceptably high rate of false-negative results

Author's view

There is no real argument over the benefits of cervical screening and all women who are offered screening should take advantage. However, the

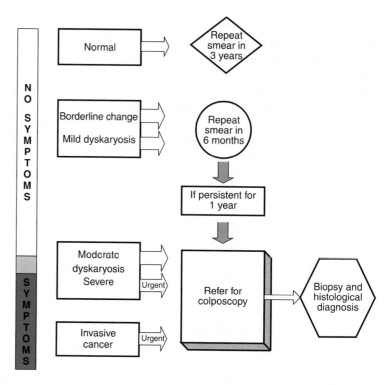

Figure 16.16 Summary of referral outcomes for normal and abnormal cytology smears

cervical smear test is far from perfect and can yield false-negative results. Much skill and experience is required to perform and evaluate the test properly. The test does not give an 'on the spot result' so that substantial anxiety can build up in the interval between attendance at screening and when the result is available. The potential for over-treatment is unfortunate, although to some extent this can be overcome by 'wait and see' referral procedures for early lesions. The problem with this is that women can easily become lost to follow-up. The 'message' to women about the purpose of the test and the implications of various test outcomes is complex, and many women do not appreciate the importance of keeping referral appointments or the need for regular screening. Laser and other ablation treatments have no long-term sequelae and their advantages over the treatment required for invasive cancer are so great that it is better to err on the side of safety.

Psychological impact of cervical precancer and cancer

Fear, anxiety, denial and depression are among the emotions felt by women who are informed of a positive smear result. There is fear of the disease itself (whether it can be treated and cured, how extensive and painful the treatment might be) and fear of recurrence after treatment. The anxieties produced can put strains on relationships. Because of the perceived associations of this disease with promiscuous behaviour the woman may blame herself for her choice of partners in the past or may blame her partner for his other relationships. Most women, even if they do not ask the questions directly, will want to know implications for herself, her partner, her sex life, her future fertility and her method of contraception. She will also want to know what the treatment involves, whether she has a sexually transmitted disease, and how frequently she will need follow-up assessment.

Many women go through specific phases in dealing with their disease. An initial phase may be one of denial. She may not listen to explanations, believing that the disease has not occurred and therefore that there is no need to listen. Later she may become emotional and will experience the need to talk and seek support. Eventually she may become ready to understand, to listen to the facts and learn about the illness. Some women adopt a 'fighting' attitude and change their lifestyle accordingly, perhaps with modifications to diet, smoking behaviour, contraceptive use and stress management.

Case study

Mrs C is a 30-year-old housewife who has been divorced and recently remarried to a textile worker. She was born in Glasgow but is now living in a rented house on an estate in Sheffield. Not long after her second marriage at the age of 28 Mrs C gave birth. She already has two children: one from her previous marriage, and one from a relationship when she was 17 (this child is now cared for by her mother). She has had one miscarriage.

Both Mrs C and her husband smoke 10–20 cigarettes a day. She has used oral contraception intermittently since the age of 17. Her previous smear, taken in early pregnancy, was reported as inflammatory. Her latest smear showed moderate dyskaryosis.

- How typical is Mrs C in respect of the age and socioeconomic group distribution of cervical cancer?
- What risk factors are usually associated with cervical cancer?
- In Mrs C's case, what would be the next stage of investigation?
- What might these investigations show?
- How would CIN III lesions be treated?
- What complications of treatment might be expected?

ANSWERS TO REVIEW QUESTIONS

Question 1

Explain why human papillomavirus is believed to be involved as a causative agent in most cases of cervical cancer

The epidemiological evidence (increase in risk associated with numbers of sexual partners, and protection from barrier methods of contraception) points towards the presence of a sexually transmitted agent. The most likely candidate would be a virus, and it is known that certain strains of HPV are involved in the production of certain benign tumours in the genital epithelium of both sexes.

It is known that certain strains of HPV (for example HPV 16 and 18) are associated with the production of precancerous (CIN) changes, although such changes can also occur in the absence of the virus. The virus may be detected (by the presence of koilocytes or using more sophisticated genetic probes) in normal cervical epithelium. Some women may be more or less resistant to the transforming potential of this virus, perhaps depending on genetic predisposition or the presence of certain additional risk factors.

Question 2

Explain the relative merits of punch biopsy, LLETZ treatment and cone biopsy in the diagnosis of cervical cancer

Punch biopsy provides a well preserved piece of tissue for histological examination but, because of the small size of the biopsy, sampling errors are possible. A further disadvantage is that the biopsy often does not completely remove the lesion, so the patient may have to attend for further treatment when the histological findings become known. However, the histology may be innocuous and no further ablative or excisional treatment might be needed.

The LLETZ procedure provides a much larger piece of tissue but much of this may be damaged because of the use of heat – not all the excised material can yield a reliable histological diagnosis. The advantage of LLETZ is that the transformation zone can be completely removed, along with any undetected lesions or areas of microinvasion. No further treatment will be necessary if the abnormality is limited to CIN.

Neither of these procedures is of any value if the transformation zone cannot be visualised (usually in the older women). In this situation a cone biopsy may be performed. No further treatment will be necessary if the abnormality is limited to CIN or stage IA cervical cancer.

Question 3

Explain why some precancerous lesions of the cervix may be left untreated

There may be no need to treat mild dyskaryotic lesions because they may disappear spontaneously. The strategy will be to increase cytological monitoring, and if abnormality persists (two consecutive abnormal smears) refer for colposcopy. It is still possible for moderate dyskaryotic lesions to regress to normal, but in view of the tendency of cytology to under-represent the severity of a lesion these cases will be referred for colposcopy and possible biopsy. Any lesion more severe than CIN I will be treated by ablation or excision.

Question 4

Explain the fundamental differences in the approaches to treatment of precancerous and cancerous lesions of the cervix

The differences are in the extent of treatment required and in survival prospects.

Treatments for precancerous (CIN) lesions are based on ablation or excision. Generally the ablation methods are reliable and are associated with only short-term side-effects such as bloodstained discharge. Excision methods usually remove more tissue than ablation methods. They can be more reliable because any undetected abnormalities will be eliminated.

Local ablative treatment is inappropriate for invasive cervical cancer. At the very least a cone biopsy will be needed (minimally invasive stage I cancers). More extensive surgical excision or radiotherapy will be required. Surgery and radiotherapy are equally effective, with 5-year survival rates of 85–90% in women with stage IB cervical cancer. The surgical procedure is usually a modified radical hysterectomy. The ovaries can be spared, which is an advantage for young women that is not possible with radiotherapy.

Why has the target age group for cervical screening in the UK been set at 20–64?

Question 5

In the UK very few women under 30 die from cervical cancer. There is therefore ample time to detect the disease process in its early stages while the woman is in her twenties. While women younger than 20 have been found to have pre-malignant cervical abnormalities, it is unlikely that these lesions will progress beyond premalignancy before she enters the screening programme. Women over the age of 65 are notorious non-attenders at screening and in the eligible 60–64 year group only about 10% of women attend. Most deaths in women over 65 years would probably have been prevented if they had attended screening when they were still eligible.

Have all of Wilson's criteria for screening been met?

Question 6

Is cervical cancer common and serious? In the UK cervical cancer is the fourth most common type of cancer in women. Premature deaths could be prevented by screening.

Is the natural history of the disease understood? A well recognised precancerous phase of the disease exists, and treatment at this stage is highly effective in arresting the disease process. There is a possibility of over-treatment, since some early lesions will regress to normal naturally.

Is the screening test accurate and reliable? Problems concern adequate sampling of cells from the correct area of the cervix, false negatives through failure to identify abnormal cells by microscopy, and misclassification within the range of possible abnormalities. A more accurate assessment can be provided by colposcopy, but in most countries this has been excluded as the initial screening modality because the examination is costly and time-consuming.

Are acceptable treatments and resources available? The treatments for precancerous lesions involve local ablation or excision. No general anaesthesia is required and, although uncomfortable, the procedures should be painless. Subsequent discomfort, abdominal cramps and vaginal discharge are usually resolved within 1 month of treatment. These treatments are far less aggressive, and the complications less severe, than those generally required for invasive cervical cancer. In the UK, the resources for treatment are allocated within the general provision for the national screening programme.

Does the treatment favourably influence the outcome? The treatments are associated with a success rate of at least 80%. Recurrence of disease after treatment does occur, but this should be picked up by adequate cytological or colposcopic follow-up, again at a preinvasive stage. That is not to say that screened and treated women do not go on to die of cervical cancer, but this is very rare. By far the majority of deaths from cervical cancer occur in unscreened women.

Case study

How typical is Mrs C in respect of the age and socioeconomic group distribution of cervical cancer?

Cervical cancer is most commonly seen in women over the age of 45 years but there is a trend towards increased mortality in younger women in the UK. Precancerous changes can occur at any age in women who are, or who have been, sexually active. Generally, the frequency of detected precancerous changes is greatest in younger women (below 45 years).

Epidemiological studies show that women from lower socioeconomic groups have a higher incidence of cervical cancer. This is likely to be related to historical differences in sexual relationships (reflected as higher rates of illegitimate births and abortions). The prevalence of cigarette smoking is higher in women in lower socioeconomic groups. It can therefore be said that Mrs C is not unusual.

What risk factors are usually associated with the disease?

The most important risk is non-attendance at cervical screening: women who have not had a smear examined in the last 10 years have a risk of developing cervical cancer that is four times as great as in regular attenders.

Other risks are associated with sexual activity: the number of partners by either the woman or the man, and absence of regular barrier contraception. These factors would maximise exposure to a sexually transmissible agent. Smoking is a further risk factor.

Infection with HIV and immunosuppression from any cause are associated with increased incidence of CIN and a worse prognosis for those who develop invasive cervical cancer.

What would be the next stage of investigation?

Mrs C was referred for colposcopy. Abnormal lesions were detected in both the cervical transformation zone and upper vaginal wall. Several punch biopsies were taken and sent for histological evaluation. The vaginal biopsies showed evidence of HPV infection but the cervical biopsy was reported as CIN III. She received laser treatment.

Any dyskaryotic change found in a cervical smear will trigger an alteration in the usual 3–5 year cycle of call–recall, even if only to repeat the smear (in cases of borderline change or mild dyskaryosis). Women whose smears show moderate or severe dyskaryosis will be referred for colposcopic examination. Any abnormal cervical or vaginal lesions seen by this examination will be biopsied for histological evaluation.

What might these investigations show?

Colposcopic examination of a woman referred as result of a moderately dyskaryotic smear would probably reveal the presence of aceto-white lesions in the transformation zone, and possibly also in the upper wall of the vagina.

Histological examination of the biopsied material allows evaluation of cellular morphological changes and the extent of epithelium affected. These changes will be classified as CIN I, II or III or invasive cancer. A moderately dyskaryotic smear will probably be either CIN II or III on subsequent histological evaluation.

How would CIN III lesions be treated?

There are a number of options for treatment based on either ablation or excision of the whole or part of the transformation zone. In Mrs C's case the vaginal lesions should also be treated, and laser therapy would be the method of choice. This would be used to ablate most of the transformation zone.

What complications of treatment might be expected?

The short-term side-effect of laser therapy will be a bloodstained discharge which may last for several weeks. The treatment is very successful (85% cure rates) and no long-term complications would be expected. Treated women will be called for repeat smears at 6-monthly intervals to monitor the effectiveness of treatment. Persistence or re-emergence of dyskaryotic changes is possible, either as recurrence of incompletely treated lesions or as development of subclinical changes that were not apparent at the time of initial treatment.

References

Boon, M.E., de Graaf Guilloud, J.C., Rietveld, W.J. *et al*. (1990) Effect of regular 3-yearly screening on the incidence of cervical smears: the Leiden experience. *Cytopathology*, **1**, 201–10.

IARC Working Group on Evaluation of Cervical Cancer Screening Programmes (1986) Screening for squamous cervical cancer: duration of low-risk after negative results of cervical cytology and its implication for screening policies. *BMJ*, **293**, 659–64.

Wilson, J.M.G. (1966) *S*ome principles of early diagnosis and detection, in *Proceedings of a Colloquium*, Magdalen College, Oxford, July 1965 (ed. G. Teeling-Smith), Office of Health Economics, London, 1966.

Further reading

Anderson, M., Jordan, J., Morse, A. and Sharp, F. (1992) *A Text and Atlas of Integrated Colposcopy*. Chapman & Hall, London.

Bridges, J. (1993) Management of advanced gynaecological malignancies. *Br. J. Hosp. Med.*, **49**, 191–9.

Campion, M.J., McDance, D.J., Cuzick, J. and Singer, A. (1986) Progressive potential of mild cervical atypia: prospective cytological, colposcopic, and virological study. *Lancet*, **ii**, 237–40.

Crook, T. and Farthing, A. (1993) Human papillomavirus and cervical cancer. *Br. J. Hosp. Med.*, **49**, 131–2.

Govan, A.D.T., Hart, D.M. and Callander, R. (1993) *Gynaecology Illustrated*, 4th edn. Churchill Livingstone, Edinburgh.

Marteau, T.M. (1990) Screening in practice; reducing the psychological costs. *BMJ*, **301**, 26–8.

Prendiville, W. (1993) Management of an abnormal smear. *Br. J. Hosp. Med.*, **48**, 595–600, **49**, 503–7.

Simons, A.M., Phillips, D.H. and Coleman, D.V. (1993) Damage to DNA in cervical epithelium related to smoking tobacco. *BMJ*, **306**, 1444–8.

Vousden, K.H. (1994) Interactions between papillomavirus proteins and tumour suppressor gene products. *Adv. Cancer Res.*, **64**, 1–19.

Wilkinson, C., Jones, J.M. and McBride, J. (1990) Anxiety caused by abnormal result of cervical smear test: a controlled trial. *BMJ*, **300**, 440.

17   Colorectal cancer

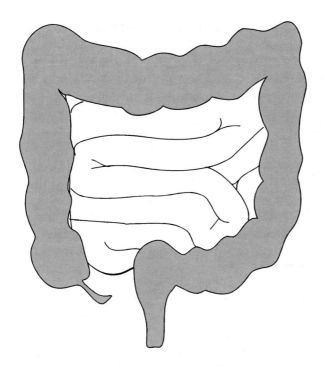

Colorectal cancer is one of the most common types of cancer in the developed countries. It is far less common in the less developed countries, which suggests that environmental factors are significant causative agents. Most notably the diet, particularly intake of fibre, fat, antioxidant vitamins and minerals, is believed to influence development of the disease. Attention to these factors could offer considerable potential for primary prevention.

Colorectal cancer is often without symptoms in its early stages, most people seeking medical attention only when the disease is advanced enough to cause symptoms. This means that survival is correspondingly poor. Surgery is the main means of treatment.

Most colorectal cancers develop from pre-existing benign tumours called adenomas. If these could be detected and treated the development of colorectal cancer would, in most cases, be prevented. A range of screening methods, designed to detect adenomas and early stage colorectal cancers are currently undergoing trials.

Pre-test

- **How common is colorectal cancer in the UK?**
- **What are the chances of dying from colorectal cancer?**
- **Are the risks of colorectal cancer the same in all parts of the world?**
- **What kind of diet should you eat to minimise the chances of getting colorectal cancer?**
- **What symptoms accompany colorectal cancer?**
- **How can colorectal cancer be treated?**
- **Can people be screened for colorectal cancer before they become aware of any symptoms?**

Aims of this chapter

By the end of this chapter you will have increased your knowledge of:

◆ The epidemiology of colorectal cancer: the age at which the disease is most likely to occur and geographical differences in incidence and mortality
◆ The genetic and possible environmental factors involved in the development of colorectal cancer
◆ The pathology of colorectal cancer and its precursor lesions
◆ Methods for screening, diagnosis and treatment of colorectal cancer and precursor lesions

In addition, this chapter will help you to:

◆ Discuss the possible role of diet in causing colorectal cancer
◆ Describe the genetic changes and sequence of events leading to benign and malignant tumours of the large intestine
◆ Evaluate the methods available for the detection of colorectal cancer and precursor lesions and their suitability for screening the asymptomatic population

> *Colorectal cancer is one of the most common cancers in affluent societies*

> *Overall survival is poor because most patients present with the disease late*

Anal cancer: anal cancers are rare, usually squamous, cancers. In women they are often associated with cancer of the cervix or vulva. Incidence is higher in male homosexuals in whom it is often (but not exclusively) associated with HIV infection. Infection with human papillomavirus is thought to play an important role in causing this type of cancer. It is curable by radiotherapy, with or without chemotherapy.

Introduction

The term 'colorectal cancer' refers to any primary cancer that occurs in the colon, rectosigmoid junction and rectum. Although the incidence and mortality statistics for cancer of the rectum often include anal cancer, this is a very different type of cancer in its causation, treatment and prognosis.

Colorectal cancer is the second most common cause of death from cancer in men in the UK; in women it is the third, after lung and breast cancer. As with most other cancers, survival is influenced by the stage of the disease at diagnosis. Other factors include the resectability of the tumour, histological grade and the degree of vascular invasion by the tumour.

The overall 5-year survival rate is about 38%, although this improves to 80% or more in patients with early stage disease (Dukes' stage A). Unfortunately, less than 10% of patients suffer from symptoms at this early stage, and consequently there is much interest in screening the asymptomatic population. However, screening trials have not demonstrably reduced mortality from the disease, possibly because of the poor sensitivity and specificity of the occult faecal blood test most commonly used for screening. More accurate methods of detection are available, such as endoscopy and barium enema radiography, but these are invasive and generally reserved as diagnostic procedures in symptomatic individuals.

Epidemiology and risk factors

The most striking feature of the epidemiology of colorectal cancer is the geographical variation in incidence and mortality. Generally, colorectal cancer is far less common in the less developed countries, although there have been some improvements in frequency in developed countries. In the USA for example, incidence and mortality from the disease have declined since the early 1970s. The trend is most apparent in whites, the rates have stabilised in black women, but in black men they are still increasing slightly (Figure 17.1).

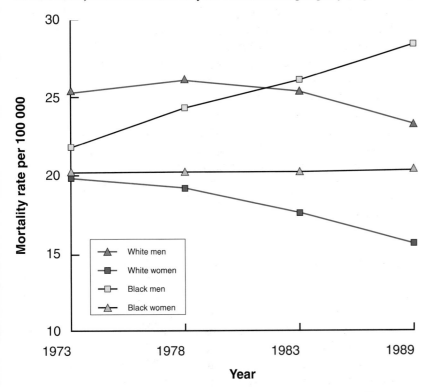

Figure 17.1 Death rates from colorectal cancer in the USA, 1973–1989. Figures are age adjusted to 1970 US standard population. (Data from Miller *et al.* (1992) *Cancer Statistics Review* 1973–89, NIH Publication No. 92-1789.)

Age

Age is a significant risk factor for colorectal cancer: 96% of deaths occur in people over the age of 50. In the USA the mean age of onset is 63 years but in less developed countries the mean age of onset is at least 15 years younger. The prognosis is usually worse when the disease occurs in people below 40 years of age. The disease is very rare in this age group but when it does occur the cancers are more frequently of the more aggressive mucinous type and are poorly differentiated.

Incidence and mortality rates for colorectal cancer increase with age

Gender

Both the sexes are vulnerable to colorectal cancer, but there is a slight excess of colonic cancers in women. In contrast, most rectal cancers are found in men.

Genetic factors

Genetic factors are evident in colorectal cancer, but most cases occur in people with no family history

Microsatellite repeats: short sequences of DNA that are repeated over and over. This repetition makes them unstable during DNA replication so that slippage, or stuttering, occurs.

Mismatch repair: mismatches of bases can occur during DNA replication, probably because of physical damage to the DNA. Sometimes a single-strand loop is formed in areas of DNA that contain repeated sequences. These are normally repaired by mismatch repair gene products.

About 15% of all patients with colorectal cancer have a family history of the disease in a first-degree relative. This may reflect a genetic susceptibility for the disease, but could equally reflect a shared environment. It follows from these figures that the large majority of colorectal cancers are sporadic.

The best characterised inherited genetic defect that confers susceptibility for colorectal cancer is in the *APC* (adenomatous polyposis coli) gene. Mutations of this gene are responsible for the rare autosomal dominant syndrome **familial adenomatous polyposis** (FAP) – more than two-thirds of patients with this syndrome have inherited germline mutations of the *APC* gene (Figure 13.9). Unless treated, all cases of FAP progress to colorectal cancer (see below); this represents about 1% of colorectal cancers.

Other patients, without polyposis but with a family history of colorectal cancer, have inherited gene mutations elsewhere in the genome. These **hereditary non-polyposis colorectal cancers** (HNPCC) account for 5–15% of colorectal cancers. The main genes responsible are located in chromosome 2 (the *hMSH2* gene) and chromosome 3 (*hMLH1*). The mutated genes differ from the normal version by the number of microsatellite repeats. The two genes are thought to act as mismatch repair genes, and their inactivation (caused by microsatellite instability) probably means that any new DNA mutations cannot be repaired. Any damage to the DNA by physical agents will become fixed in the genome, and the mutations will accumulate with each round of replication. Eventually one of these non-repairable mutations will cause the malignant transformation of the cell.

Aspirin intake

Some epidemiological reports show that regular aspirin intake can reduce the risk of colorectal cancer by up to 50%. Experiments *in vitro* indicate that aspirin induces apoptosis. Cancer cells appear to be more susceptible to aspirin than adenoma cells, suggesting that this protective effect occurs late in the adenoma–adenocarcinoma sequence (see below).

Geographic variation

Colorectal cancer is rare in less developed countries, but when people migrate to more affluent countries they take on the higher rates of the host country

The incidence of colonic cancer varies in different parts of the word by as much as 60 times, whereas the rates for rectal cancer vary by only up to 20 times. Colorectal cancer is most common in Europe and North America (Figure 17.2) but is rare in Asia and Africa, where it is seen in urban areas more than in rural areas. Migration studies indicate that environmental influences are important in the aetiology of the disease. Blacks living in the USA have much higher rates of colorectal cancer than black people in Africa.

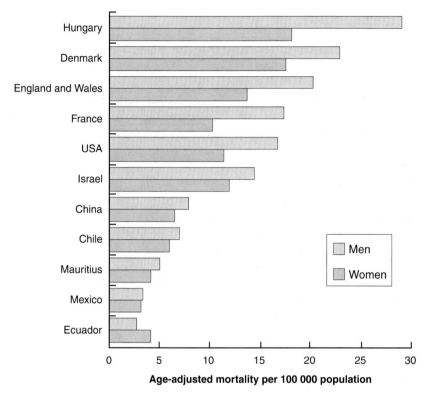

Figure 17.2 Geographical variation in mortality from colorectal cancer, 1988–1991, in men and women.

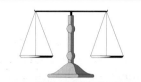

Antioxidant vitamins vs. placebo

▲ Study of 981 patients who had colonoscopic polypectomy, randomised to one of three intervention groups or placebo

▲ Interventions: 25 mg β-carotene daily, 1 g vitamin C daily with 400 mg vitamin E daily, or both

▲ End point: development of new polyps between year 1 and year 4 of follow-up

▲ Compliance confirmed by biochemical measurement of serum β-carotene and vitamin E

▲ Incidence of polyps in group receiving β-carotene 36%, in those receiving vitamins C and E 39%, all vitamins 38% and placebo 36%

Data from Greenberg et al., 1994.

Dietary factors

One of the best known and earliest examples of work on the influence of diet on the development of colorectal cancer was carried out by Professor Denis Burkitt. He observed that the mortality rate from bowel cancer was much lower in African black people, who had high intakes of dietary fibre, than in white people, who consumed much less fibre. The role of other dietary constituents such as fat, calories, trace elements, vitamins and minerals has also been evaluated.

Not all epidemiological studies have shown a relationship between fibre in the diet and colorectal cancer. It may be that the type of fibre (soluble or insoluble) is of importance. Consumption of insoluble vegetable fibre such as that in broccoli, cauliflower, cabbage and sprouts is protective whereas soluble pectin appears to be relatively ineffective. The mechanisms by which some dietary fibres may exert a protective effect include:

- Transit time in the colon is reduced, thus reducing exposure to any carcinogens
- The fibre may bind or dilute any carcinogens present in the colonic lumen
- Changes may be induced in the colonic bacterial flora which metabolise

Migration studies indicate that environmental factors, probably dietary, are important

Vegetables rich in insoluble fibre may protect against colonic cancer

carcinogenic bile acids

- Reduction in pH causes deionisation of potentially harmful free fatty acids and bile acids

Low fat consumption is associated with lower rates of colorectal cancer

Review question 1

Describe the kind of diet that could help protect against colorectal cancer. Which foods should be encouraged and which avoided?

Antioxidant vitamins are believed to be important for preventing many cancers, including colorectal cancer

Some people are genetically susceptible to the development of benign polyps, but progression to cancer may depend on environmental factors

Because dietary factors play an important role in colorectal cancer there is scope for preventing the disease

Another fundamental difference between the diets of the developed and less developed countries is fat consumption. In developed countries the higher mortality rates from colorectal cancer correlate with increased fat consumption. However, the epidemiological evidence is inconclusive and other considerations (such as the type of dietary fat and its modulation by fibre) may be important. Animal fats are thought to increase the risks, but animal studies show that vegetable oils and polyunsaturated fats are associated with higher incidences of experimentally induced tumours. Fish oils and monounsaturates (olive oil, for example) may exert a protective effect.

Epidemiological data and animal studies equate increased calorie consumption with enhanced risk for colorectal cancer. It is unclear whether this is a consequence of the excess calorie intake, or is related to the composition of the food and its influences on metabolic rate and body weight.

Other dietary components that are considered to influence colorectal carcinogenesis are minerals, vitamins and trace elements. Calcium may exert a protective effect by neutralising bile and free fatty acids, which are considered to be strong cancer promoters in the colon. Vitamins C and E, and selenium, are antioxidants and could protect against cancer by neutralising the damaging effects of free radicals. Vitamin A could also have an anti-cancer effect. Epidemiological studies have shown that depleted amounts of these micronutrients are associated with increased risks for many types of cancer.

Almost all colorectal cancers arise from benign tumours or polyps called **adenomas**. The propensity for adenoma formation is probably genetically determined, but environmental factors (gut bacteria, bile acids, and dietary factors) are probably necessary to stimulate transformation from adenoma to adenocarcinoma.

The evidence that various nutritional factors play a role in the promotion or inhibition of colorectal cancer suggests that primary prevention by manipulation of the diet may offer a way of controlling the disease. Some of the epidemiological studies designed to evaluate the effects of dietary and other dietary components are discussed in Chapter 7.

So far, the data for the inclusion of specific components in the diet as a means of prevention are not very promising. In one study (Greenberg *et al.*, 1994), the effect of antioxidant vitamins was examined in relation to the development of adenomas (generally regarded as precursor lesion for colorectal cancer, see below). Patients who had a polyp removed were randomised to antioxidant supplementation or placebo, and examined for the development of new polyps after four years. There was little or no difference in the incidence of polyps between the treatment and placebo groups. It could be argued that a protective effect of antioxidant vitamins was missed: antioxidants could help stop the transition from adenoma to adenocarcinoma, rather than the transition from normal cells to adenoma. Proving this in humans is impossible for ethical reasons.

Pathology

The typical cancer of the colon or rectum consists of a polypoid mass with central ulceration and irregular edges which easily bleed. Most tumours are adenocarcinomas. Other types exist, such as squamous carcinoma, adenosquamous carcinoma and small-cell carcinoma, but are uncommon. Most adenocarcinomas (about 85%) produce only small amounts of mucin, the remainder being mucinous or colloid adenocarcinomas.

Most colorectal cancers are adenocarcinomas, arising from mucus-producing glands

Many cases of colorectal cancer arise from adenomas, although the progression from benign tumour to malignancy is not inevitable. The risk of progression has been estimated at 2.5% in adenomas that have been present for 5 years, rising to 24% at 20 years.

Many colorectal cancers arise from benign polyps

About one in 30 patients present with more than one tumour and roughly 20% of patients with colorectal cancer will also have benign adenomas in the colon or rectum at first presentation. It is therefore important to examine the entire colon and rectum for other tumours when a single benign or malignant tumour is discovered. Patients who have had part of their bowel removed for the treatment of a cancer are at increased risk of developing further tumours and should be kept under close surveillance.

Benign polyps and cancer may be present at the same time in different areas

About 1% of patients with colorectal cancer have had previous chronic ulcerative colitis, the risk of colorectal cancer increasing with duration of the ulcerative colitis; 3% at 15 years, 5% at 20 years and 9% at 25 years. It may therefore be advisable to conduct annual colonoscopic surveillance in patients with ulcerative colitis, starting from 10 years after diagnosis. Another chronic inflammatory disease of the gastrointestinal tract, Crohn's disease, does not always involve the large intestine and consequently is associated with a lower risk of subsequent colorectal cancer, although the risk is higher than in the unaffected population.

Crohn's disease: an inflammatory bowel disease of no known cause. Inflammation affects the full thickness of the intestinal wall. It is most common in the terminal ileum but can affect any part of the gastrointestinal tract as discontinuous ('skip') lesions. Macroscopic examination of the mucosa shows a characteristic 'cobblestone' pattern, caused by oedema and deep-fissured ulcers.

Prognosis

The likelihood of survival in treated patients is determined by the assessment of tumour spread into surrounding and distant tissues (tumour staging). Another valuable indicator in colorectal cancer is histological grading. Other factors include the site of the tumour, its resectability, the degree of vascular and lymphatic infiltration, and whether the large intestine has been obstructed or perforated by the tumour.

The prognosis in colorectal cancer is largely determined by how much the tumour has spread at initial presentation

Hundreds of adenomas develop in the colon of patients with FAP. These are particularly likely to progress to malignancy, usually when the patient reaches their third or fourth decade. Adenomas first appear in late childhood or adolescence and can become cancerous without producing symptoms. Therefore the offspring of affected individuals should be monitored regularly by colonoscopy. Colectomy is carried out when adenomas are detected to stop the inevitable progression to malignancy.

Ulcerative colitis: an inflammatory disease of the large intestine with no known cause. The lesion begins in the rectum as proctitis, extending upwards to involve variable amounts of colon. Mucosal ulceration does not extend through the full thickness of the bowel wall. Patients typically have episodes of diarrhoea containing blood or mucus.

Staging of colorectal cancer

The best guide to prognosis in colorectal cancer is surgical staging. In the UK the Dukes' staging system is most commonly used.

- Stage A: cancer confined to intestinal wall (mucosa and submucosa)
- Stage B: invasion through the muscle wall, but no involvement of lymph nodes
- Stage C1: any degree of local spread, with involvement of adjacent lymph nodes
- Stage C2: any degree of local spread, with involvement of distant lymph nodes, or metastases
- Stage D: with metastases

Stage A colorectal cancers are associated with a 5-year survival rate of 95–100%, but only about 15% of cases are diagnosed at this stage. Stage B is associated with 60–80% survival, stage C1 30–50% and C2 10–25%. Most cases are diagnosed at stages C1 or C2.

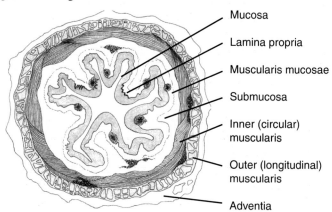

Mucosa

Lamina propria

Muscularis mucosae

Submucosa

Inner (circular) muscularis

Outer (longitudinal) muscularis

Adventia

Figure 17.3 Structure of the large intestine. The wall of the large intestine may be divided into six layers. The innermost layer, containing the epithelial cell lining, is the **mucosa**. This is supported by a layer of loose connective tissues containing many small blood vessels, the **lamina propria**. Underlying this is a thin wall of smooth muscle, referred to as **muscularis mucosae**. A further layer of loose connective tissue and blood vessels is called the **submucosa**. There are then two layers of smooth muscle, one circumferentially arranged and the other longitudinally, known as the inner circular and outer longitudinal **muscularis**. An outer layer of connective tissues and blood vessels is referred to as the **adventitia**. Finally, the exposed outermost layer is lined by a single layer of epithelial cells, known as the **serosa**.

Genetic alterations in adenoma and colorectal cancer

Progression to colorectal cancer is a multistage process involving oncogene activation and loss of tumour suppressor gene activity

Genetic alterations have been detected in both adenomas and adenocarcinomas. Invasive colorectal cancer is the result of a multistage process, starting with small adenomas which grow progressively larger and then become malignant.

These processes involve mutations in proto-oncogenes and tumour suppressor genes (see Figure 13.9).

Oncogenes and tumour suppressor genes

An early change involves the loss of a (presumed) tumour suppressor gene on the long arm of chromosome 5. The loss is detectable in both benign polyps and in malignant tumours, and in most cases arises as a sporadic event. However, this mutation can be inherited and, when both alleles are mutated, causes familial adenomatous polyposis.

Almost 50% of large adenomas and colorectal carcinomas display *ras* gene mutations. These mutations are less common in smaller (<1 cm) benign adenomas. The size differential suggests that the mutation in *ras* is a late change, perhaps initiating the transformation of the adenoma into cancer.

Further sporadic losses of tumour suppressor genes occur in other specific chromosome regions, the most common example in colorectal tumours involving chromosome 17p, which is seen in about 75% of colorectal carcinomas but only infrequently in the earlier adenomas. This area contains the *p53* tumour suppressor gene. Another common allelic loss, occurring in both large adenomas and colorectal cancers, involves chromosome 18q. The area contains a probable tumour suppressor gene, the DCC (**d**eleted in **c**olorectal **c**arcinoma) gene. Deletion of this part of chromosome 18 in patients with colorectal cancer is thought to signify poor prognosis.

The loss of genetic material in chromosome 5 is characteristic of all patients with FAP. For this reason the putative tumour suppressor gene in this site is known as the *APC* gene. The normal version of the *APC* gene is expressed in a variety of tissues, including normal colonic mucosa and white blood cells. The function of the gene and its product are not known but its expression in white blood cells means that it could be possible to devise a simple and reliable screening test for familial adenomatous polyposis. Genetic linkage analysis is now available for early identification of the mutated gene in the children of affected patients. Hitherto all the offspring had to undergo regular and uncomfortable colonic examinations, since it could not be shown which individuals had inherited the aberrant gene. Now, only children who are known by genetic testing to have inherited the condition need be regularly monitored.

Sites affected by colorectal cancer

More than half of all colorectal cancers are found in the rectum and rectosigmoid area. A further 30% of cancers are located in the caecum and ascending colon. The transverse and descending parts of the colon are relatively unaffected (Figure 17.4).

Symptoms

In its early stages colorectal cancer is generally asymptomatic. One of the earliest

The initial change, seen in benign polyps, involves loss of genetic material in chromosome 5: this can be inherited

*Transformation to cancer is probably initiated by **ras** gene mutation*

Further losses of tumour suppressor genes complete the change to invasive cancer

*Inheritance of **APC** gene mutations can be detected by genetic linkage analysis*

Review question 2

Why are benign polyps in the large intestine a cancer risk?

Review question 3

In what ways do the genetic alterations in FAP differ from those in colorectal cancer?

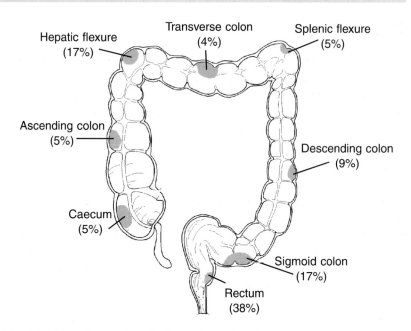

Figure 17.4 Site distribution of colorectal cancers.

abnormalities is bleeding into the stools, which can be detected by an occult blood test.

Colonic cancer

> *Constipation, diarrhoea and abdominal pain are symptoms of colon cancer*

Early colonic cancer may not cause symptoms. Symptoms of colonic cancer include altered bowel habits, constipation and diarrhoea, and colicky abdominal pains caused by obstruction. Obstruction does not usually occur when the cancer is on the right side because the bowel contents are fluid and the tumours tend to grow into the intestinal wall. Common symptoms in right-sided colonic cancer are anaemia, weight loss, abdominal pain and a palpable abdominal mass.

Outgrowing tumours in the descending or rectosigmoid colon tend to obstruct the passage of faeces. This may be evident as a history of laxative use, coupled with other signs such as thin pencil-like stools. Anaemia may be caused by bleeding.

Rectal cancer

> *Rectal bleeding is not only caused by haemorrhoids: it is also a sign of rectal cancer*

Rectal cancer is often associated with the passage of blood (usually bright red) and mucus along with loose stools. Unfortunately, diagnosis may be delayed because the bleeding may be mistaken by the patient as a sign of haemorrhoids. A feeling of urgency to defecate, or of incomplete passage of stools may also be experienced. A mass may be felt by digital rectal examination. Pain is an infrequent sign in the early stages of rectal cancer.

Diagnosis

The diagnosis is of colorectal cancer based on the results of clinical findings, endoscopy, radiography and laboratory investigations.

A clinical assessment is made by taking the patient and their family's history, visual examination of the abdomen, palpation of any masses or areas of distension and digital examination of the rectum.

Clinical evaluation is most frequently followed by endoscopy or barium enema radiography

Digital rectal examination: examination of the rectum with a gloved finger.

Endoscopy

Sigmoidoscopy is suitable for examination of the lower 60 cm of colon. About 50% of colorectal cancers occur within this range. Rigid sigmoidoscopes are cheaper to buy and easier to maintain than the flexible types, but limit examination to the distal 15–20 cm of the bowel. In recent years a trend in the site distribution of the tumours has been noted, with greater numbers of proximal tumours. These are more easily detected by the flexible sigmoidoscope than the rigid type.

Development of the flexible fibreoptic colonoscope allowed a more complete examination of the colon, and has the advantage that polyps can be removed by snare diathermy through the instrument at the time of examination. Endoscopy, particularly colonoscopy, can be highly invasive and the patient may need to be sedated.

Flexible fibreoptic instruments enable the large bowel to be visualised

Barium enema

Tumours of the large intestine can also be detected by double-contrast barium enema radiography (Figure 17.5). The entire colon can usually be examined by this method, and is comparable with colonoscopy in its ability to detect tumours. Whether endoscopy or barium enema radiography is used is a matter of preference, expertise and the facilities available.

Laboratory investigation

Laboratory tests centre on the investigation of blood haemoglobin in the faeces (faecal occult blood), any consequent anaemia, and the presence of tumour markers such as carcinoembryonic antigen (CEA).

The faecal occult blood test is based on the supposition that all colorectal cancers bleed, and that the blood becomes incorporated in the faeces. However, this is not always the case and a range of other bowel conditions might cause bleeding. The test is therefore prone to producing high numbers of false-positive and false-negative results.

Even when bleeding does occur, it may not be detectable because the haemoglobin becomes degraded as it passes down the tract, especially when the lesion is in the proximal portion of the intestine. The test may also fail to detect rectal lesions since there is less opportunity for blood to diffuse widely into the stool.

Bleeding from the cancer may be detectable in the faeces

Carcinoembryonic antigen: a cell-surface glycoprotein produced by many epithelial tumours. Also produced by normal colonic epithelium but not in amounts measurable in blood unless the patient is a heavy smoker or has inflammation or a tumour in the bowel.

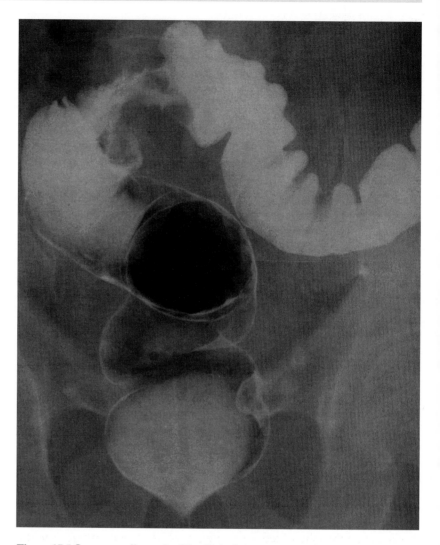

Figure 17.5 Contrast radiograph of familial adenomatous polyposis. Multiple polyps can be seen throughout the lower colon and rectum.

Loss of blood from colorectal tumours may become evident as anaemia, and estimation of blood haemoglobin and a haematocrit can be helpful. In many cases, however, the bleeding may be so minor as to be unnoticeable.

Cancers of the colon and rectum may produce CEA and its estimation in blood often has diagnostic value. However, the levels of CEA may also be raised by tumours in other sites, in some inflammatory conditions and in heavy smokers with no bowel pathology, which limits its usefulness as a diagnostic test. Measurement of blood CEA is most useful for postoperative monitoring of patients in whom the CEA levels had been raised: blood levels should rapidly fall after surgery. Any subsequent rise is likely to be a sign of recurrence of tumour.

> *Tumour recurrence can be monitored by measurement of CEA in blood*

Treatment

Provided that the tumour is resectable, surgery is the treatment of choice. Multiple tumours may require total colectomy, although single tumours of the transverse colon may be treated by more limited resection. Most patients with tumours of the upper rectum can be treated by sphincter-saving surgery that preserves the anal sphincters and hence faecal continence. In some cases it may be necessary to remove the whole rectum, with formation of a permanent colostomy. Radiotherapy and chemotherapy are of only limited value.

> *Curative treatment for colorectal cancer always involves surgery*

Surgery

The surgical procedures employed will be determined by the health of the patient and the location and extent of the cancer. A colectomy is usually performed, with removal of lymph nodes for prognostic assessment. The resection involves removal of diseased colon and its arterial supply, with end-to-end joining (anastomosis) of the remaining sections. A tumour on one side of the colon will be removed by resection of that half: a left or right **hemicolectomy**. Tumours in the transverse colon will be removed by **transverse colectomy**, and in the sigmoid colon by **sigmoid colectomy**. The length of colon to be removed is determined by the position of the tumour in relation to the main arteries and lymphatics.

Anastomosis

The objective of anastomosis is to achieve a passageway for the bowel contents, without leakage from the join. This can be done with sutures or, for a rectal anastomosis, with steel staples inserted with a stapling gun. Minor leakage from the join is fairly common but does not interfere with recovery. The waste is eliminated by inflammatory defences and very often a cuff of scar tissue forms around the join, effectively sealing it. More serious leakage, into the abdominal cavity or to the surface through the surgical wound, is relatively rare. Further surgical intervention is needed to deal with this, often by fashioning a temporary colostomy upstream of the anastomosis to allow healing.

Faecal occult blood: occult (hidden) blood in the faeces usually indicates gastrointestinal bleeding. The standard test is the guaiac method which detects peroxidase-like activity in haemoglobin. False-positive results may be recorded because peroxidase activity is present in dietary components including red meats, poultry, fish and certain raw vegetables and fruits. A new immunochemical test for human haemoglobin (HemeSelect) eliminates the specificity problem, and is thought to have a higher sensitivity for adenomas than the standard guaiac tests.

Colostomy

Radical surgery for rectal cancer may necessitate permanent colostomy, particularly if the lower rectum is involved. In these cases the entire rectum is removed and sphincter control is lost. The bowel end is stitched to the opened abdominal surface, forming a stoma to which a bag can be attached to receive the faeces and flatus. Permanent colostomy is never needed for the treatment of colonic cancer and is not always necessary for rectal cancer.

> *It may be necessary to perform a colostomy, so that waste is eliminated through the abdomen*

Local excision of the tumour with only a narrow margin of normal tissue may be an alternative to radical surgery. The adequacy of the excision, particularly at the resection margins, must be checked by histological examination. In the past this procedure was used as a palliative measure in patients who were thought to have incurable tumours, who were thought to represent a poor risk with more radical surgery or who absolutely refused a permanent colostomy. Nowadays, in carefully selected patients the procedure can be curative. The main indication that local excision might be successful is the mobility of the tumour – a mobile tumour is less likely to involve the full thickness of the intestinal wall. Further radical surgery is indicated if histological examination of the excised tumour shows that it is not confined to the bowel wall, the resection margins are involved or the tumour is poorly differentiated.

The physical complications of a stoma include prolapse or retraction of the bowel, necrosis of the stoma or stenosis (narrowing) of the opening, hernia, bleeding or infection. These complications may require further surgery to re-form the colostomy and create a new stoma.

Radiotherapy

Radiotherapy is seldom employed as a primary curative treatment but is usually used as an adjuvant therapy or for palliation in inoperable cancers of the sigmoid colon and rectum. Radiotherapy may also be given preoperatively to reduce the viability of tumour cells.

Chemotherapy

Chemotherapy is sometimes used as adjuvant therapy in patients who have resectable lesions and in those with metastases.

Chemotherapy is now commonly used as an adjuvant therapy to Dukes stage C colorectal cancer

The most commonly used drugs are 5-fluorouracil, mitomycin, folinic acid and levamisole. Initial trials with various drug regimens yielded disappointing results but more recent drug combinations and approaches to administration are encouraging. The combination of fluorouracil and levamisole has been found to reduce the relapse rate by 40% and the mortality by one-third in patients with node-positive colorectal cancer.

A new approach to administration is portal vein infusion immediately after surgery. The US National Surgical Adjuvant Breast and Bowel trial of fluorouracil infusions (Slevin, 1996) demonstrated a reduction in the incidence of liver metastases, with corresponding improvements in 5-year survival (23% mortality, compared with 29% in control patients).

Psychological effects of colorectal cancer

A stoma fundamentally changes body image and leads to both physical and psychological problems

Not surprisingly, the greatest psychological problems occur in patients in whom sphincter function could not be preserved and who have been given a permanent colostomy. Patients will require counselling before and after surgery to come to terms with a new and unwelcome body image. The practical procedures of changing the appliance are relatively easily overcome, but the psychological and social traumas are complex, and can lead to introversion and social isolation, depression, suicidal tendencies and other emotional disorders.

A variety of physical traumas affect the daily lives of people with a colostomy. These include bowel hyperactivity (with the result that many patients have to give up their job or change their working habits), changes in diet, urinary problems and sexual difficulties.

Review question 4

Why is the overall 5-year survival rate for colorectal cancer so poor?

Screening for colorectal cancer

The 5-year survival rates for patients diagnosed with Dukes' stage A colorectal cancer approaches 100%, but only about 15% of patients are diagnosed at this stage. Deaths from colorectal cancer could be reduced substantially if more cancers were detected at an early stage. Screening also offers the potential for cancer prevention because most colorectal cancers are preceded by adenomas – if these could be detected and treated the progression to invasive cancer will be prevented. Because most cases of colorectal cancer occur in people over the age of 50 screening could be limited to this sector of the population.

The aim of screening is to detect adenoma or early colorectal cancer

The screening method

A prerequisite of screening tests is that they should be relatively non-invasive, inexpensive and quick and simple to apply (see Chapter 10). Digital rectal examination fulfils these criteria but, unfortunately, is not appropriate for a mass screening programme because, at its best, it can detect only those 10–15% of cancers which occur in the lower rectum. Rigid sigmoidoscopy is limited by the range of the instrument. Flexible sigmoidoscopes reach further and are less uncomfortable for the patient, but are more expensive to use. A colonoscope can be used to examine the entire colon but colonoscopy is a time-consuming and expensive examination: the bowel must be prepared with a purgative, the patient needs to be sedated, and there is a slight risk of perforating the bowel wall. Barium enema radiography also allows the entire colon to be examined, but the procedure is lengthy and uncomfortable.

Although these methods are appropriate for investigation of symptoms, it is unlikely that any would gain acceptance for the regular screening of an asymptomatic target population.

Most of the screening trials currently under way use the faecal occult blood test because it is the least invasive. Unfortunately, the test lacks sensitivity and specificity, particularly for detection of precursor adenomas. Lack of specificity means that it is therefore necessary to refer people with consistently positive results to a diagnostic stage, normally colonoscopy or barium enema radiography. This does not solve the problem of poor sensitivity, as the false negatives will not reach the diagnostic stage until symptoms develop or they are detected at the next screening round.

Screening is limited by the methods available for detection

Annual faecal occult blood screening can reduce deaths from colorectal cancer by up to one-third

Numerous trials of faecal occult blood screening are taking place in various countries. Most are randomised trials, in which participants are stratified according to age, sex and place of residence and then assigned to either a control group or the screening group. Screening intervals vary, but the most promising results have come from annual screening. One of the largest randomised trials currently taking place in the UK is based in Nottingham, with more than 160 000 participants (Hardcastle *et al.*, 1989). The screen employs the Haemoccult guaiac test, and all positive findings are further investigated by colonoscopy or by double-contrast barium enema radiography. The trial was initiated in 1984, and yields a detection rate of 1.97 colorectal cancers per 1000 people screened.

The most recent analysis of the Nottingham trial data (Hardcastle *et al.*, 1996), after a median follow-up of nearly 8 years, showed significant improvement in the colorectal cancer mortality rate for the screened group. The cancers detected in the screened group were at an earlier stage (20% in Dukes' stage A compared with 11% in the unscreened group). This translated into a 15% cumulative reduction in colorectal mortality in the screened group. The benefits could have been even greater, but a problem was that only 38% of people in the screened group completed all the tests offered.

Comparable results were obtained in a study of 60 000 people aged 45–74 in Funen, Denmark (Kronberg *et al.*, 1996). Faecal occult blood tests were offered every 2 years for a total of 10 years in a screening group of 30 967 people. Over the course of the study the incidence of colorectal cancers in both the screened and control groups was virtually identical, but in the control group detection was at an earlier stage (22% at stage A compared with 11% in the control group). This earier detection resulted in reduction in colorectal mortality of 18%, but again the results could have been better since only 46% of the screened population completed all the screening tests. It should be emphasised that both the Nottingham and Danish studies were limited trials, designed to test the methods and the feasibility of introducing a national screening programme. It may in the future be possible to increase compliance by education and by the publicity that a well-organised national screening programme would attract.

The most promising picture has emerged from a 13-year randomised trial conducted in Minnesota (Mandel *et al.*, 1993). More than 46 000 men and women aged 50–80 years were assigned to annual screening, biennial screening and unscreened groups. All abnormalities detected by the occult blood screen were further investigated and all diagnosed polyps and cancers were treated. The screen-detected cancers were effectively downstaged: there were fewer cases of Dukes' stage D cancers than in the unscreened group (Figure 17.6). The mortality rate from colorectal cancer was 33% lower in the annually screened than in the unscreened group.

One reason for the success of this particular trial is believed to be the occult blood test protocol used. This differed from practice elsewhere by rehydrating the paper slides when they were received in the laboratory, which increased the sensitivity of the test, but at the expense of specificity. The rate of positive results from the occult blood test was nearly 10% (compared with about 2% in

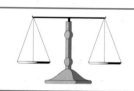

Nottingham trial

Faecal occult blood screening vs. control

▲ More than 160 000 subjects aged 50–74 years age and sex stratified. Subjects randomised into test and control groups

▲ Minimum follow-up 7 years

▲ Participants sent a faecal occult blood kit to be returned to laboratory for analysis

▲ Response rate exceeds 60%

▲ Positive test rate about 2%

▲ Initial diagnostic phase comprises clinical examination and rigid sigmoidoscopy

▲ Further referral to colonoscopy or barium enema radiography

▲ Cancer detection rate 1.97 per 1000 persons screened

Data from Hardcastle *et al.*, 1989.

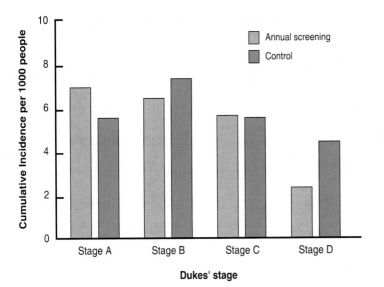

Figure 17.6 Effect of annual screening on colorectal cancer stage (Minnesota study). Screening by annual faecal occult blood testing can result in a downstaging of colorectal cancers. More early cancers (Dukes' stage A), and correspondingly fewer cases of advanced Dukes' stage D cancers, are seen in the screened group than in controls. (Data from Mandel *et al.*, 1993.)

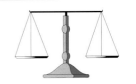

Minnesota trial

Annual faecal occult blood screening vs. biennial screening vs. control

▲ More than 46 500 subjects aged 50–80 years
▲ Randomised into annual and biennial test groups and control group
▲ Follow-up 13 years
▲ Rehydrated guaiac occult blood screening test
▲ Positive test rate about 10%
▲ Diagnostic phase usually colonoscopy
▲ Colorectal cancer mortality was 8.83 per 1000 in control group, 8.33 in biennial screened group, 5.88 in annual group.

Data from Mandel *et al.*, 1993.

the Nottingham trial). The effect was that a large number of colonoscopies were required in cases which ultimately turned out to be false positives. This increases the costs as well as subjecting people to unnecessary examinations. To be weighed against this was a reduction in deaths from colorectal cancer, from a cumulative 8.83 per thousand people to 5.88 per thousand in the 13 years of the study.

It has been calculated that most of the benefit of colorectal screening could accrue by a once-only flexible sigmoidoscopy examination when a person reaches 55–60 years of age. This examination represents one of the best ways of detecting precursor adenomas. Because it probably takes 10 years or more for an adenoma to develop into invasive cancer, and most adenomas are seen in people older than 50, the accurate detection and removal of lesions in people of this age ought to confer at least 10 years' protection.

Not all tumours would not be detected by flexible sigmoidoscopy but detection of the lower (distal) adenomas is more important because these very often serve as an indication that further adenomas are present in the proximal colon. Hence patients with distal tumours could be referred to a diagnostic stage intended to search for proximal tumours. Although sigmoidoscopy is an invasive and often uncomfortable procedure, restriction of the screening requirement to a once-only examination could be acceptable to many people. At present there exists nothing more than a proposal to set up a randomised controlled trial, but on theoretical grounds this is probably the most sensible way forward.

> ### ▲ Key points
>
> #### Screening and treatment of colorectal cancer
> ---
>
> **Screening method:**
> ▲ Digital rectal examination
> ▲ Estimation of faecal occult blood
> ▲ Sigmoidoscopy examination (proposed once-only after age 55 years)
>
> **Diagnostic stage:**
> ▲ Sigmoidoscopy
> ▲ Colonoscopy
> ▲ Barium enema radiography
>
> **Treatment stage:**
> ▲ Colonoscopic removal of precursor adenomas prevents development of most colorectal cancers
> ▲ Surgical treatment of early stage colorectal cancers associated with improved survival

ANSWERS TO REVIEW QUESTIONS

Question 1

Describe the kind of diet that could help protect against colorectal cancer. Which foods should be encouraged and which avoided?

Choose a low-fat high-fibre diet with plenty of fresh fruit and vegetables. Saturated fats should be avoided, and there is evidence that monounsaturates may be beneficial. Calcium, obtained from low-fat dairy foods, may also be beneficial.

The main dietary factors in prevention of colorectal cancer appear to be insoluble fibre, adequate vitamins and minerals, without excessive calories and fat. Insoluble fibre and most of the vitamins would be provided by plenty of fresh fruit, vegetables and cereals. The important vitamins and minerals are those with antioxidant activity: vitamins A, C and E, and selenium. Vitamin A is present as retinol in animal products such as liver, egg yolk, milk fat, butter and cheese and as carotenes in yellow and orange vegetables, particularly carrots. Vitamin C is found in a wide range of fruit and vegetables. Vitamin E is present in cereals. Selenium occurs in cereals, fish and meat.

It cannot be certain whether this regime will actually prevent colorectal cancer. A clinical trial of antioxidant vitamins in the development of adenoma was not encouraging. In this, supplementation was with pills and capsules: fresh fruits and vegetables in the diet could exert different effects by the combination of fibre and antioxidant vitamins.

Question 2

Why are benign polyps in the large intestine a cancer risk?

The answer to this is in two parts. First, there is evidence showing that over time some benign polyps will eventually become malignant. Patients with familial adenomatous polyposis invariably develop colorectal cancer because they have many hundreds of polyps, at least one of which will eventually become malignant.

Second, benign polyps have already progressed through a number of genetic changes. The initial alterations to chromosome 5q have occurred, as has activation of the *ras* oncogene. When the polyps become larger deletions of tumour suppressor genes may occur. If there are genetic influences and environmental factors sufficient to cause this kind of damage, and if exposure to these continues, then presumably it is not going to take much more to produce the further damage necessary for malignant change.

How do the genetic alterations in FAP differ from those found in colorectal cancer?

Question 3

The main differences, as far as is known, concern damage to chromosome 5q, which can be regarded as the initial event. In FAP the alteration is a mutation, which can be inherited. In most cases of colorectal cancer a deletion of part of the genetic code in chromosome 5q occurs as a sporadic event. Furthermore, there are two genes of interest in this part of the chromosome, the *APC* and *DCC* genes.

In familial adenomatous polyposis the alteration is to the *APC* gene. This alteration may also occur in sporadic colorectal cancers, but is usually accompanied by deletions in the *DCC* gene. Deletions in *DCC* are not seen in non-malignant FAP. Thereafter, progression to benign polyps, dysplasia and invasive cancer is probably similar in both polyposis and sporadic cases.

Why is the 5-year survival rate for colorectal cancer so poor?

Question 4

By the time symptoms develop the tumour may already be at an advanced stage with micrometastases in other parts of the body even if they remain undetectable. Furthermore, symptoms of colorectal cancer can easily be mistaken as signs of other, more innocuous, diseases and patients may delay seeking medical attention. Most cases of colorectal cancer are at Dukes' stage C at the time of surgery; the tumour has already spread to the lymph nodes. Lymph node involvement is always a poor prognostic sign. The overall 5-year survival in colorectal cancer is about 38%. The diagnosis can be advanced by screening, but this is not routinely performed in the UK or in most other countries.

References

Greenberg, E.R., Baron, J.A., Tosteson, T.D. *et al.* (1994) *N. Engl. J. Med.*, **331**, 141–47.

Hardcastle, J.D., Chamberlain, J., Sheffield, J. *et al.* (1989) Randomised controlled trial of faecal occult blood screening for colorectal cancer. *Lancet*, **i**, 1160–4.

Mandel *et al.* (1993) Reducing mortality from colorectal cancer by screening for foetal occult blood. *N. Engl. J. Med.*, **328**, 1365–71.

Slevin, M.L. (1996) Adjuvant treatment for colorectal cancer. *BMJ*, **312**, 392–3.

Further reading

Austoker, J. (1994) Screening for colorectal cancer. *BMJ*, **309**, 382–6.

Cawkwell, L. and Quirke, P. (1995) A new class of colorectal cancer gene. *Gut*, **36**, 641–3.

Fearon, E.R. and Vogelstein, B. (1990) A genetic model for colorectal tumorigenesis. *Cell*, **61**, 759–67.

Groden, J., Thliveris, A., Samowitz, W. *et al.* (1991) Identification and characterisation of the familial adenomatous polyposis coli gene. *Cell*, **66**, 589–600.

Hardcastle, J.K., Chamberlain, J.O., Robinson, M.H.E. *et al.* (1996) Randomised controlled trial of faecal-occult-blood screening for colorectal cancer. *Lancet*, **346**, 1472–7.

Kinsella, A.R. (1993) *Colorectal Cancer. A Scientific Perspective*, Cambridge University Press, Cambridge.

Kronberg, O., Fenger, C., Olsen, J. *et al.* (1996) Randomised study of screening for colorectal cancer with faecal occult blood test. *Lancet*, **348**, 1467–71.

Kune, G.A. (1995) The causes of colorectal cancer. *GI Cancer*, **1**, 25–31.

Norris, H.T. (1991) *Pathology of the Colon, Small Intestine and Anus*, 2nd edn, Churchill Livingstone, New York.

Northover, J.M.A. and Kettner, J.D. (1992) *Bowel Cancer: The Facts*, 2nd edn, Oxford University Press, Oxford.

Shike, M, Winawer, S.J., Greenwald, P.H. *et al.* (1990) Primary prevention of colorectal cancer. *Bull WHO*, **68**, 377–85.

18   Prostate cancer

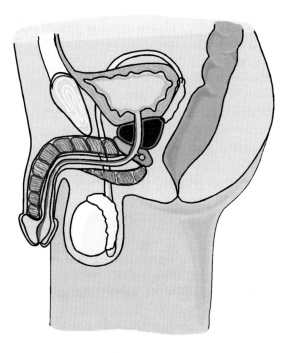

Prostate cancer mainly affects men over the age of 50 years, in whom it is a major cause of death. The disease has a very variable natural history: in some men it progresses very rapidly, in others tumour growth is so slow that the man dies from other causes without ever experiencing symptoms of prostate cancer.

The diagnosis of advanced disease is relatively straightforward, relying on clinical examination, ultrasound and the estimation of tumour markers (such as prostate-specific antigen in the blood). This last method is particularly useful in monitoring response to treatment and tumour recurrence.

Treatment of prostate cancer involves surgery, radiotherapy or, in advanced cases, hormone manipulation. Treatment is radical, even in early stages of the disease. A high proportion of patients treated by surgery or radiotherapy suffer side-effects of urinary incontinence and impotence. The chances of cure are highest when the cancer is confined within the prostatic capsule, but most symptomatic cancers have already spread beyond this.

Screening for prostate cancer is problematic because the non-invasive tests available are not very good at detecting the localised disease for which there is a high chance of cure. Technical advances have improved test sensitivity, but the risk of over-treatment remains because many localised cancers never progress to invasive disease. At present there is no means of distinguishing between the slow-growing and the life-threatening types.

Pre-test

- How common is prostate cancer?
- Who is likely to develop the disease?
- What are the symptoms of prostate cancer?
- What other conditions cause similar symptoms?
- How is prostate cancer diagnosed?
- What treatments are available for this disease?

Aims of this chapter

By the end of this chapter you will have increased your knowledge of:
♦ The frequency of prostate cancer and risks of developing the disease
♦ The pathology of prostate cancer
♦ Current methods used in diagnosis and treatment

In addition, this chapter will help you to:
♦ Compare the accuracy and reliability of non-invasive and invasive methods of diagnosis prostate cancer
♦ Discuss the potential of screening to reduce morbidity and mortality from prostate cancer
♦ Evaluate the prospects for development of more effective treatments

Introduction

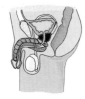

Prostate cancer is the third most common cause of deaths from cancer in men in the UK

Prostate cancer is a common cause of cancer deaths in men, ranking third in the UK after lung and colorectal cancers (Figure 18.1). It causes about 8500 deaths each year in England and Wales. The tumour can grow very slowly and is a frequent finding at post-mortem examination, even in men who had no symptoms and died from other causes. Unfortunately, in some men the cancer appears at an early age and grows rapidly for some time before symptoms appear. Nearly 60% of men with prostate cancer have metastatic disease at the time of presentation. With treatment the median survival for those with metastatic cancer is about 2.5 years; for those with locally invasive disease it is 4.5 years.

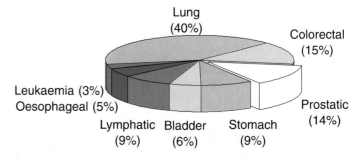

Figure 18.1 Deaths from cancer in men in England and Wales, 1989. The total adds up to more than 100% because of rounding. (Source: OPCS.)

Epidemiology

In the UK incidence and mortality rates for prostate cancer have nearly doubled over the last 30 years

Exactly why the incidence of prostate cancer is increasing (Figure 18.2) is not fully understood. It may be that the disease is diagnosed more easily by ultrasonography and CT scanning, and the increasing popularity of transurethral resection for the treatment of prostatic hyperplasia has meant that more tissue samples have become available for histological examination (prostate cancer is frequently an 'incidental' finding when these tissues are examined). Nevertheless this does not explain the near-doubling in mortality over the last 30 years. Epidemiological studies have been undertaken to assess the influence of environmental or lifestyle factors on the disease, which might also have changed over time, but none has identified any environmental factors of significance. The most important associations are unalterable factors such as age, family history and race. There is therefore little prospect of reducing the incidence of prostate cancer by primary prevention measures involving alteration of lifestyle risk factors.

Prostatic hyperplasia (benign): formation of large nodules which compress and partially obstruct the urethral canal. Probably caused by hormonal stimulation of prostate cells. Affects up to 90% of men by the eighth decade of life. Only 5–10% of men with the condition require treatment.

Transurethral resection: an endoscopic instrument is introduced through the urethra and small fragments of prostate tissue are removed with an electrical wire loop.

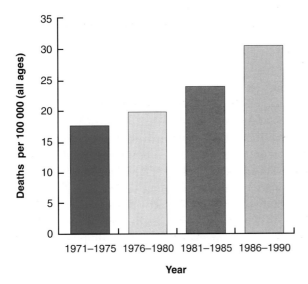

Figure 18.2 Deaths from prostate cancer, England and Wales, 1971–1990. (Source: OPCS.)

Age

Incidence and mortality from prostate cancer increase with age (see Figure 1.8). Essentially, prostate cancer is a disease of older men; more than 80% of prostate cancers are diagnosed in men over the age of 65, while only 1% are detected in men under the age of 50. In England and Wales only two deaths from prostate cancer were recorded for men under the age of 44 during 1992 but over 2000 were recorded in the 75–79 age group, who comprise a much smaller proportion of the male population.

Post-mortem studies indicate that nearly 35% of all men over the age of 50 have asymptomatic Stage A disease, and this increases to 60% or more of men over the age of 80. In the great majority of cases the cancer never progresses beyond the non-invasive stage; however, 5–10% of cases become invasive, and progression is more likely in men below the age of 60.

Prostate cancer is primarily a disease of older men

Anabolic steroids: synthetic hormones that accelerate protein synthesis and growth, used illegally by 'power' athletes to increase muscle mass. Side-effects include acne, baldness, shrunken testes, infertility, heart disease, kidney damage. In women, anabolic steroids induce masculinisation.

Follicle-stimulating hormone (FSH): produced by the anterior pituitary gland, regulates function of gonads, stimulates sperm production and maturation of ovarian follicles.

Luteinising hormone (LH): produced by the anterior pituitary gland. Promotes production of hormones by the gonads and stimulates testosterone production by interstitial cells.

Oestrogens: normally produced in small amounts by interstitial cells of the testis but is overwhelmed by the effects of testosterone. Rare testicular tumours may increase the production of oestrogens and cause feminisation.

Prolactin: produced by the anterior pituitary, structurally similar to growth hormone. Best known for stimulating milk production in mammary glands, but also affects hormone production in the ovaries and testes.

Testosterone, dihydrotestosterone: hormones secreted by interstitial cells of the testis. Responsible for initiation (in adolescence) and maintenance of spermatogenesis and the development of male secondary sexual characteristics.

Family history

There is a tendency for prostate cancers to cluster in families. Up to 40% of patients diagnosed with prostate cancer have a family history of the disease. A family history of breast cancer is also believed to increase the risk of prostate cancer.

The familial clustering of prostate cancer points either to a genetic susceptibility for the disease or to shared exposures to environmental agents. In the USA, about 1 in 5 men will develop symptomatic prostate cancer at some time in their lives. A candidate gene has been identified by genetic linkage studies in some hereditary prostate cancer cases. The gene, located on the long arm of chromosome 1 and designated *HPC1* (for hereditary prostate cancer 1), was found by testing individuals from more than 90 cancer-prone families in the USA and Sweden. It has not yet been cloned and its function is unknown but it is more likely to correspond to an oncogene rather than a tumour suppressor gene because prostate cancer cells occasionally carry extra copies of the chromosome 1 region containing the gene.

Extra copies of the gene implies that the prostate cancers are produced through increased activity rather than by the inactivation which occurs when tumour suppressor genes are mutated or deleted. It is estimated the *HPC1* gene is involved in only about a third of inherited prostate cancer cases, which in turn form about 3% of the total. None the less, it is possible that the same gene becomes mutated or abnormally activated in cases where there is no family history of the disease. Once the gene has been precisely located and cloned, it may become possible to screen for disease susceptibility in men who have a family history of prostate cancer.

Race and geography

The incidence rate of prostate cancer in American black men is one of the highest in the world. The reasons for this are unclear and more comprehensive genetic and epidemiological data are needed. Scandinavia is also an area of high incidence, whereas the incidence is low in Japan, Greece and Mexico (Figure 18.3).

Hormones

A possible role for the sex hormones in the development of prostate cancer has been postulated because the disease only very rarely develops in castrated men. Survival can be improved by manipulation of hormones produced by, or which regulate the function of, the testis: testosterone, dihydrotestosterone, prolactin, FSH, LH and oestrogens. Epidemiological studies have shown that the risk of developing prostate cancer increases with raised blood levels of LH and a high ratio of testosterone to dihydrotestosterone. Intense physical activity correlates with reduced risk, possibly because of its testosterone-lowering effect. Men who take anabolic steroids have an increased risk of prostate cancer.

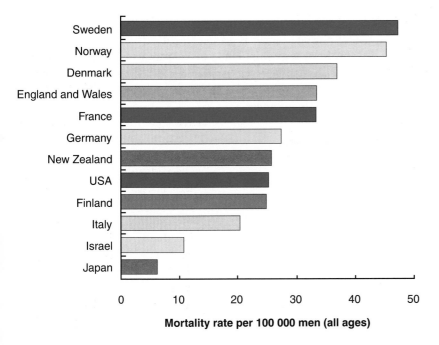

Figure 18.3 Geographical variation in deaths from prostate cancer in men between 30 and 74 years of age. (Data from *WHO World Health Statistics Annual*, 1992.)

Environmental factors and diet

Migration studies suggest that environmental factors have some influence on the disease. The low mortality rates in Japan are not seen in Japanese men who have migrated to the USA – these men take on a rate intermediate between those in Japan and the host country. The environmental factors responsible are elusive. There is an association between overall fat consumption and the prevalence of prostate cancer in different parts of the world. It is believed that dietary fats influence the production of the sex hormones, and hence their ability to act as a tumour promoter. The lower mortality rate in Japan may be influenced by the generally lower-fat diets of people in that country. When Japanese men migrate abroad more fat is probably included in their diet as they adapt to the indigenous lifestyle.

Epidemiological studies have also shown that the risk of prostate cancer is slightly increased in farmers, metal workers and mechanics. A larger increase in risk has been found in teachers, but the significance of this finding is unclear.

Previous prostatic and venereal disease

The most common pathological condition of the prostate is a nodular enlargement caused by the proliferation (hyperplasia) of non-cancerous gland cells. This condition is often referred to as benign prostatic hyperplasia, but hyperplasia is benign by definition. Some epidemiological studies indicate that the risk of prostate cancer is greater in patients who have a history of prostatic hyperplasia. Why this should be so is difficult to explain, because hyperplasia and cancer usually arise in different parts of the gland. Case-control studies also report that more men with prostate cancer have had a venereal disease than men without cancer.

Clinical features

Clinically, prostate cancer can be detected at several stages in its evolution. Initially there are no symptoms at all and the cancer is detected only as an incidental finding *post mortem*. This constitutes **latent prostate cancer**. During life, prostate cancers may be palpated by rectal examination as a hard nodule on the surface of the gland. The presenting symptoms are usually non-specific 'rheumatism' or 'arthritis', and the patient may have a short history of incontinence and pain when urinating. In advanced cases, symptoms such as pain in the back, sciatica and anaemia are caused by tumour metastases. Oedema of the legs can occur if the lymphatics are occluded, and fractures may occur at sites of skeletal involvement.

Pathology

Prostate cancer and hyperplasia arise in different parts of the gland and it is therefore unlikely that prostatic hyperplasia is a precancerous change. The common incidental finding of prostate cancer in surgical and autopsy material far exceeds the number of symptomatic cases of the disease: only about 1% of men over the age of 50 experience symptoms.

Local spread

Tumours commencing in the lateral area of the gland often spread into the prostatic urethra and in advanced cases the base of the bladder can be involved. The rectum may become stenosed by tumour growth around it, but direct infiltration into the rectum occurs only in the terminal phase of the disease (Figure 18.4).

Tumours originating in the posterior portion of the gland spread upwards to involve the seminal vesicles. Eventually one or both ureters may become obstructed.

Metastases

Prostate cancer metastases are most frequent in the bones and lungs

Malignant tumour cells from the prostate may spread into the bloodstream or lymphatic circulation. The most common site of distant metastases is bone, particularly the pelvis, lower lumbar vertebrae, femoral heads, rib cage and skull. Blood-borne spread to the lungs is also often seen at post mortem.

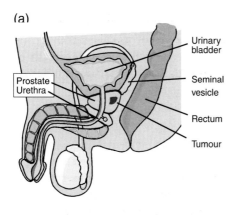

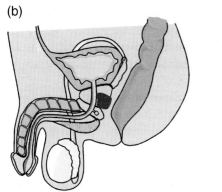
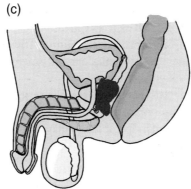

Figure 18.4 Local spread of prostate cancer. (a) Stage A tumour is confined within the prostatic capsule and cannot be felt by digital rectal examination. (b) Stage B tumour is a well defined nodule, apparently confined to the prostate. (c) Stage C tumour extends beyond the confines of the prostate, typically involving the bladder wall and seminal vesicle. There is no evidence of metastasis.

Lymphatic spread occurs along vessels at the sides of the rectum or over the seminal vesicles, depositing tumour cells in the retroperitoneal lymph nodes and eventually the mediastinal and supraclavicular lymph nodes. It is now recognised that lymph node involvement usually precedes tumour spread to the bones.

Cancer staging and grading

In common with most cancers, prostate tumours are staged according to the degree of spread:
- Stage A: cancer unsuspected and detected in tissue removed for hyperplasia
  A1: well differentiated, unifocal adenocarcinoma
  A2: diffuse or moderate to poorly differentiated
- Stage B: tumours palpable by digital rectal examination

▲ Key points

Pathology of prostate cancer

Latent cancer:
- ▲ Very common in older men who remain asymptomatic
- ▲ Only detected at post-mortem or in tissue removed for prostatic hyperplasia
- ▲ Stage A latent cancers unlikely to cause death, Stage B cancers become invasive
- ▲ Treated cancers are associated with a 10-year survival rate of 50–80%

Clinical cancer:
- ▲ Symptomatic only in the later stages (C, D) of the disease
- ▲ Lymph nodes usually involved
- ▲ Urinary problems are most common but advanced metastatic disease can cause bone pain
- ▲ Disseminated cancers have a 10-year survival rate of 10–40%

Cribriform: a perforated pattern, like a sieve.

Papillary: small projections of the tumour into surrounding tissue.

> *The expected survival depends on the stage at which the disease is diagnosed*

B1: adenocarcinoma of less than 2 cm

B2: adenocarcinoma greater than 2 cm

- Stage C: locally invasive tumours but no clinically evident metastases. Tumour extends through the prostate capsule or into the seminal vesicle
- Stage D: tumours with distant metastases

D1: lymphatic metastasis confined to pelvis

D2: metastases outside of pelvis, usually involving bone or lymph nodes

Stage A1 disease is usually an incidental finding and in most men there is no evidence of tumour progression when followed over a period of 5–10 years. The risk of progression and eventual death from prostate cancer is greater in younger men (below 60 years) because they have a longer life expectancy and possibly because of an inherited predisposition. The stage A2 lesions are more serious: 30–50% of cases progress to invasive cancer if left untreated.

Stage B cancers can also be completely asymptomatic and are detected by digital rectal examination, perhaps in routine screening or health checks. Inevitably these lesions will progress to invasive cancer if not treated by surgery or radiotherapy.

Most patients present with stage C or D cancer, usually because of urinary symptoms or bone pain arising from metastatic disease. At this stage the cancer is often inoperable and may be unsuitable for radiotherapy because of its bulk.

Histological grading

There is also a histological grading system for prostate cancer, known as the **Gleason** system. This system is based on morphological appearances corresponding to the size and pattern of the tumour:

- Grade 1: single, separate, closely packed uniform glands with a margin delineating the edge of the tumour
- Grade 2: single, separate glands that are less uniform and more loosely arranged, with a less definite margin
- Grade 3A: single, separate, but variable glands that may be widely separated and have a poorly delineated margin
- Grade 3B: microglandular tumour composed of tiny cell groups, or cords, or both
- Grade 3C: sharply circumscribed, rounded tumour with a cribriform or papillary pattern
- Grade 4A: infiltrating tumour with fused glands
- Grade 4B: similar to 4A but with large, clear cells
- Grade 5A: circumscribed masses of cribriform tumour, often with central necrosis
- Grade 5B: diffusely infiltrating anaplastic carcinoma

Prostate cancers are not always consistent in their morphology. The Gleason system takes account of this by awarding a primary grade based on the tumour type occupying the greatest area and a secondary grade for the less representative tumour. The primary and secondary grades are added together to give a value up to 10. Homogeneous tumours are given the same primary and secondary grade. Gleason values up to grade 4 are usually well differentiated, with relatively good prognosis. Higher Gleason grades are more poorly differentiated.

Background information: The prostate gland

The prostate gland is an extension of the urinary bladder and is connected to the prostatic urethra and ejaculatory ducts. Its main function is to produce secretions which form part of the seminal fluid. The secretions are produced by gland cells arranged in acini and are carried to the urethra by ducts. The glandular tissue is arranged in zones about the urethra. These zones can be seen most clearly in the young adult; parts of the prostate invariably enlarge with age and render the zonal architecture indistinct.

The area of the prostate immediately surrounding the urethra is known as the **transitional zone**: hyperplasia develops in this region. At the base of the prostate is the **central zone**, comprising 25% of the prostate gland. The remainder, the **peripheral zone**, is located on the posterior and lateral aspects of the prostate.

Most cancers are found in the peripheral zone, but some can arise in the central and transitional zones. Usually the cancer appears in a number of focal areas within the affected zone, arising from the gland cells.

Diagnosis

Enlargement and hardening of the prostate gland can be detected by digital rectal examination. Confirmation that the changes are caused by cancer relies on imaging and laboratory investigation.

Imaging

A number of suitable imaging techniques are now available, including transrectal ultrasonography, CT and MRI. These imaging techniques cannot detect microscopic deposits of cancer and it is therefore necessary to obtain tissue samples for histological examination.

Transrectal ultrasonography

Transrectal ultrasonography is usually carried out with the patient lying on his side with his knees bent. Cancers are usually hypoechoic – they appear as a darkened area on the image – although not all cancers produce changes in image density. Prostate cancer usually occurs in the periphery of the gland and several discrete foci may appear in different areas of the scan. Staging can be carried out by assessing the integrity of the fibrous capsule surrounding the prostate.

Hypoechoic areas within the scan may be caused by conditions other than cancer – prostatitis, glandular hyperplasia and prostatic infarcts. It is therefore necessary to establish the true cause by means of biopsy. Ultrasound can be used to guide the biopsy needle.

Transrectal ultrasonography is the best imaging method for diagnosis of prostate cancer

CT scanning

This is not the most effective or efficient means of diagnosing prostate cancer but it is of value for staging the disease. Transrectal ultrasonography and MRI are preferable.

MRI

This is the best technique available for staging prostate cancer. Improvements in the accuracy of MRI for staging have come through the recent development of phased array coils and endorectal surface coils.

Radionuclide imaging

Radionuclide imaging is used to detect bone metastases

Radionuclide imaging may be performed as a staging procedure. Phosphate complexes labelled with technetium-99m are given intravenously and are selectively taken up by the bones. Increased uptake on the bone scan corresponds to increased vascularity and high bone turnover, which is usually indicative of metastatic tumour deposits.

Laboratory investigation

Tumour markers

PSA is a useful tumour marker for monitoring disease activity

Two useful tumour markers produced by prostate cancer cells are detectable in blood. These are **prostate-specific antigen** (PSA) and **prostatic acid phosphatase**. The former is regarded as having the greater specificity.

The normal value for PSA in serum is less than 4 ng/ml; values up to 15 ng/ml can be found in men with prostatic hyperplasia. Levels of PSA generally reflect overall tumour mass and concentrations in excess of 80 ng/ml would reflect extensive local disease or metastases. However, PSA levels are not always raised in prostate cancer, particularly if there are no metastases. The most important application of PSA as a tumour marker is for monitoring the response to treatment: a rise after previously low levels in a treated patient is very likely to reflect recurrence of tumour.

The estimation of prostatic acid phosphatase levels is less useful because raised blood levels are usually found only in advanced disease, with metastases. Normal blood prostatic acid phosphatase levels are below 2 ng/ml.

Raised serum alkaline phosphatase can signify bone metastases

Prostatic metastases in bone stimulate osteoblastic activity. The osteoblasts, responsible for bone synthesis and mineralisation, produce alkaline phosphatase. If bone metastases are widespread the total serum alkaline phosphatase levels will rise, reflecting increased osteoblastic activity. When this occurs, it is virtually diagnostic of secondary prostate cancer. However, in common with many other cancers, secondary prostate cancer deposits are more likely to stimulate dissolution of bone by signalling the resorption process (see Chapter 22).

Histology and cytology

The diagnosis of prostate cancer can be confirmed by histological or cytological assessment of biopsy material obtained by a needle introduced through the rectum. A wide-bore needle yields a solid core of tissue, and is better than a transurethral resection which removes tissue from only the central portion of the gland. A finer-bore needle is used to aspirate cells for cytological assessment, from the prostate, or from pelvic lymph nodes which may be enlarged because of metastatic spread.

Treatment

Patients with confined non-invasive disease can be treated by radiotherapy or radical prostatectomy, giving 5-year survival rates of 75–85%. Radical prostatectomy is suitable only for younger, fitter patients. In most cases local invasion or metastases are already present and curative treatment is not possible. Nevertheless, about 80% of these advanced cancers can be controlled by means of hormonal therapy.

Radical prostatectomy

Radical prostatectomy (using either retropubic or perineal approaches) is curative in cancers confined to the prostate. The surgical approach is either retropubic or perineal. Permanent impotence occurs in up to 90% of patients (this varies with age and tumour stage), urinary incontinence in about 5%, urethral stricture in up to 25%, and about 3% of patients die during surgery. The operation is usually undertaken only in men who have a life expectancy of at least 10 years.

For many years most men were considered unsuitable for the operation, but earlier detection by digital rectal examination and PSA screening (more common in the USA) has increased the number of referrals for this procedure. In men whose cancer is confined within the prostate a nerve-sparing retropubic radical prostatectomy can be carried out to preserve erectile function by avoiding injury to the cavernosal neurovascular bundles.

Radical radiotherapy

Localised prostate cancer may be treated by radiotherapy, an approach that is more popular in the UK, and is more suitable for older men who are not fit enough to undergo radical surgery. Unlike radical surgery, invasion beyond the prostatic capsule is not a contraindication to treatment.

External beam therapy is most commonly given to the whole of the gland and the immediate area. Excessive radiation to surrounding tissues, such as the bladder, prostatic urethra or rectum can cause serious side-effects. The usual acute complications (in 30–50% of patients) are proctitis, cystitis and urinary retention. Chronic complications include proctitis (about 2%), impotence (up to 50%) and urethral stricture (about 4%).

▲ **Key points**

Prostate-specific antigen

▲ Most specific of the tumour markers for prostate cancer
▲ Upper limit in symptom-free men is 4 ng/ml
▲ Early prostate cancers are unlikely to raise levels above 20 ng/ml
▲ Blood levels are raised in prostatic hyperplasia (8–15 ng/ml)
▲ Levels above 80 ng/ml probably reflect metastatic disease
▲ Some cancers may not increase levels of PSA, particularly in early stages

▲ **Key points**

Imaging prostate cancer

Transrectal ultrasonography:
▲ Does not use ionising radiation, does not require anaesthesia or analgesia
▲ Cancer usually appears as hypoechoic areas in peripheral zone

Computed tomography:
▲ No value in diagnosis of confined prostate cancer
▲ Useful for cancer staging

Magnetic resonance imaging:
▲ Staging localised and early advanced disease

Radionuclide imaging:
▲ Staging procedure: localisation of secondary skeletal deposits

Brachytherapy: a form of radiotherapy in which radiation sources are planted directly into a malignant tumour.

Orchidectomy: surgical removal of the testes. A relatively safe procedure carried out under general or spinal anaesthesia.

Radical prostatectomy: resection of the prostate, prostatic urethra, seminal vesicles and surrounding connective tissue. Only suitable for treatment of prostate cancers confined within the prostatic capsule, without lymph node involvement.

Brachytherapy

Brachytherapy offers the theoretical advantage of delivering a high radiation dose to a confined volume of tissue while sparing adjacent normal tissue; this is particularly attractive for treating prostate cancer because of the proximity of the bladder and rectum.

Brachytherapy is not a popular treatment for prostate cancer because results of early trials were disappointing. The main problem was difficulty in correctly positioning the radioactive implants. The introduction of new radioisotopes and modern imaging methods has renewed interest in the technique. These improvements allow greater accuracy and dose distribution, and the modern after-loading devices give greater radiation protection for health care workers as well as allowing optimal placement of the implant.

The recent experience of brachytherapy, in which permanent radioisotope implants are placed in the prostate, is that cure rates for early cancer are similar to those of radical prostatectomy or conventional external beam radiotherapy. A further application of brachytherapy is as a boost to external beam radiotherapy in the treatment of locally advanced prostate cancers. The value of these approaches will become more clear over the next few years.

Hormone therapy

Inhibition or removal of the main source of androgens is used to control advanced prostate cancer

Male androgens are primarily produced by the testes but are also produced by the adrenal glands. The most effective treatment should be achieved by blocking androgens from all sources. This can be achieved directly by manipulating the hormones produced by the testes, or indirectly by inhibiting testicular stimulation by the hypothalamus–pituitary axis (Figure 18.5).

In practice, removal or blockade of the testicular source appears to be just as effective as total androgen blockade. This can be achieved with drugs or by orchidectomy. Orchidectomy is the longest-standing of these treatments and hence the efficacy of new drug treatments are compared with this standard. Over time, prostate cancers become refractory to hormonal manipulation.

Hormone treatments can give significant survival advantages for most patients, but in all cases initial remission is followed by renewed tumour growth. This is probably because prostate cancers are generally a mixture of well differentiated androgen-dependent cells and a population of poorly differentiated androgen-insensitive cells. It follows that only the androgen-dependent cells will be depleted by the treatment, while the poorly differentiated cells continue to grow. It is also likely that androgen-dependent cells lose their sensitivity over time, to grow independently of androgen stimulation.

Orchidectomy

Orchidectomy slows down the growth of prostate cancer

Orchidectomy usually produces a good response, arresting tumour growth in most patients for a median time of 50 weeks. After this, tumour cells resume growth and other methods of control or palliation must be considered. Serum

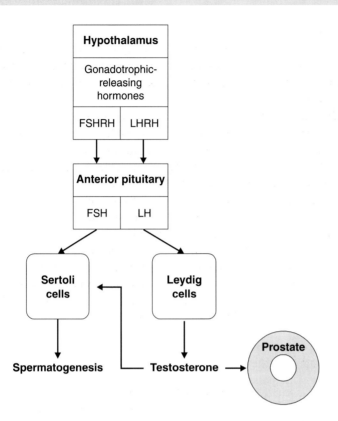

Figure 18.5 Stimulation of testosterone synthesis and spermatogenesis by the hypothalamus–pituitary axis. Most prostate cancers are stimulated by androgens produced by the testes and adrenals. Testosterone production by the testes is regulated by the hypothalamus–pituitary axis through a negative feedback mechanism. Two gonadotrophins produced by the anterior pituitary stimulate the testes – LH and FSH. The former acts on the Leydig cells in the testis to regulate testosterone secretion, the latter on the Sertoli cells of the testis, involved in spermatogenesis. Both hormones are controlled by hypothalamic gonadotrophic-releasing hormones. The growth of cells in prostate cancer may be inhibited by controlling the activity of testosterone directly or indirectly through the hypothalamus and pituitary hormones. In the prostate, testosterone is converted to a more active form, 5-alpha dihydrotestosterone, by the enzyme 5-alpha reductase. LHRH = Luteinising hormone releasing hormone; FSHRH = follicle stimulating hormone releasing hormone.

testosterone levels are rapidly reduced by orchidectomy, causing side-effects of hot flushes and impotence. Many patients are unhappy or unwilling to submit to this treatment, and those who do often experience adverse psychological effects. The advantage is that it is one of the most effective forms of intervention for advanced prostate cancer.

Anti-androgen drug therapy

One of the earliest anti-androgen drug treatments used was oestrogen (diethylstilboestrol), which blocks the production of testosterone. It is now

Surgery is not the only option for managing advanced prostate cancer

rarely used because of a risk of cardiovascular complications and stroke. Diethylstilboestrol also causes gynaecomastia and indigestion.

An alternative to diethylstilboestrol is **cyproterone acetate**, a synthetic steroid which inhibits the testicular production of testosterone and blocks androgen receptors in target tissues. The non-steroidal compound **flutamide** competitively inhibits the binding of testosterone to its cellular receptors in the hypothalamus and other target organs. Other treatments are based on suppressing pituitary–hypothalamus axis stimulation of the testes. This can be achieved using analogues of **luteinising hormone releasing hormone** (LHRH). The two most commonly used LHRH analogues, goserelin acetate and leuprorelin acetate, are usually administered as depot preparations in the subcutaneous tissue of the abdominal wall, on a monthly basis.

Ultimately, prostate cancers become refractory to these manipulations. The most effective regimen appears to be a combination of an LHRH analogue with flutamide: the median progression-free interval for advanced cancers treated in this way is 16 months, with median survival of 3 years.

> *In time prostate cancers no longer respond to hormonal manipulation*

Other treatments

Another option is chemotherapy, but men with prostate cancer are often old and debilitated by the disease and therefore most chemotherapy regimens are unsuitable. One possibility, presently under trial, is to introduce cytotoxic agents as an adjunct to hormonal therapy. Most prostate cancers contain hormone-insensitive clones of cells and it may be best to attempt early control of their growth. The chemotherapy regimen currently on trial consists of doxorubicin, mitomycin and vinblastine, but only small numbers of patients have been treated to date.

Once hormone manipulation fails to control tumour growth further treatment options are limited and the emphasis is on palliation of symptoms. Bone pain, arising from metastases, is probably best controlled by radiotherapy. Opioid drugs and bone protecting agents such as the bisphosphonates are also useful as palliative agents.

Fundamentally, we really need more effective agents to deal with hormone-refractory disease. Some new agents are being developed (such as suramin, which acts as a growth factor antagonist) but at present it is far too early to know how effective these will be.

> *A priority is to find a better way of treating hormone-refractory cancers*

Prevention

Review question 1

How do the treatments for prostate cancer differ from those available for other types of cancer?

Because no obvious alterable risk factors are involved in the development of prostate cancer, primary prevention is not a practical possibility. Most effort has focused on screening as a secondary prevention measure, but an alternative is chemoprevention (this is analogous to the tamoxifen trials currently taking place for women at high risk of developing breast cancer). Trials are currently taking place using the drug finasteride, which inhibits the conversion of testosterone to the more active dihydrotestosterone in the prostate. It is hoped

▲ **Key points**

Hormonal control of prostate cancer

▲ Cancers shrink in response to androgen deprivation but usually recur in 15–18 months

Bilateral orchidectomy:
▲ An effective treatment but has poor acceptability and adverse psychological effects

Anti-androgen drugs:
▲ Interfere with production of testosterone and its binding to target cells
▲ Single-agent therapy is effective, but usually given with LHRH analogues
▲ Cyproterone acetate used to counter initial testosterone surge produced by LHRH treatment
▲ Flutamide interferes with formation of testosterone–receptor complex without reducing testosterone levels, causing fewer side-effects

LHRH analogues:
▲ Reduce testosterone production by modifying hypothalamic–anterior pituitary stimulation of testicular Leydig cells
▲ Goserelin acetate or leuprorelin acetate used as monthly depot treatments

that the main stimulus to prostate cell growth can be blocked by this agent before malignancy develops.

Screening for prostate cancer

Prostate cancer is easily curable when the disease is confined within the prostatic capsule. There is therefore considerable potential to reduce morbidity and mortality from the disease by earlier detection and treatment.

Prostate cancer can be difficult to detect in its early stages

In practice the early detection of prostate cancer is problematic and, so far, no screening programme has produced any significant reduction in mortality. The main reasons for this are the sensitivity and specificity of the screening tests available: false-positive and false-negative results are common. Furthermore, the biology of prostate cancer is very variable; in some men it advances rapidly, in others the disease is relatively quiescent and does not spread or produce any symptoms.

It is impossible to predict the men in whom the disease will remain latent, or who will go on to produce clinically significant disease. Therefore, even if all early-stage cancers could be reliably detected, some latent cancers which would never bother the patient will be needlessly treated. In these cases the treatment could be worse than the disease; both radical prostatectomy and radiotherapy can cause permanent side-effects.

Screening methods

The methods that have been tried in prostate screening include digital rectal examination, measurement of serum PSA and transrectal ultrasonography.

Digital rectal examination

Digital rectal examination offers a quick and easy method of detecting the prostatic enlargement and surface irregularities which may be signs of prostate cancer. However, digital rectal examination is relatively insensitive and any prostate cancers detected are likely to have already advanced beyond the prostatic capsule: its capacity to detect those cancers which can most easily be cured is therefore limited. Other detection methods show that cancer can be present in up to 30% of palpably normal prostate glands.

Benign conditions can also give positive findings and therefore further investigations are necessary to ascertain the cause of the enlargement.

Transrectal ultrasonography

This technique suffers from lack of sensitivity and specificity and high cost. The method can lead to the detection of greater numbers of non-palpable tumours, but many of these prove to be benign. Its use as a screening method is also limited by acceptability: there are many men who will not undergo the embarrassment and discomfort of this test when they have no symptoms and, in most cases, have nothing wrong with them.

Prostate-specific antigen

Of the proteins produced by prostate cancers, PSA is the most sensitive tumour marker currently available. If it were accurately to reflect the presence of cancer cells, estimation of PSA would be a non-invasive test ideally suited for screening purposes. However, this is not always the case and prostatic hyperplasia and prostatitis can give results above the normal range. Additional diagnostic investigations will be required in the large numbers of men who test positive, most of whom do not have prostate cancer. A further shortcoming is that in early prostate cancer the PSA levels are often within normal limits.

Because of the limitations in the individual methods for the detection of prostate cancer current practice is to use a combination of methods for screening and confirmatory purposes. Initially both digital rectal examination and PSA estimation should be used: PSA levels can be elevated in the absence of any palpable abnormality and palpably abnormal prostate glands have been detected without any elevation in PSA.

The detection rate by digital rectal examination alone is 1–2% of men over the age of 50; this increases to 2–2.5% by combining rectal examination with PSA measurement, although the patients identified are not always the same individuals. Abnormal results with either method should therefore be further investigated by transrectal ultrasonography, and biopsies taken from any suspicious areas. If PSA levels are elevated but the ultrasonographic examination is normal, further, repeated, PSA estimations should be made and biopsy undertaken if the levels continue to increase.

It is uncertain whether prostate screening reduces mortality rates from prostate cancer. Very few controlled trials have been undertaken in which subjects are randomised into screening and control groups. Prostate screening is difficult to evaluate because of the effects of lead-time and length-time bias (lead-time bias is a particular problem). The more aggressive tumours are likely to produce symptoms and be investigated. Therefore any differences in survival between screened and unscreened populations may actually be due to inherent differences in tumour biology rather than an effect of screening.

For these reasons long-term prospective studies are needed to evaluate mortality from prostate cancer. One such study is being organised in the USA by the National Cancer Institute (Kramer *et al.*, 1993). This will randomise 150 000 men into a screened group who will receive annual digital rectal examination and PSA estimation, and an unscreened group who will receive only their normal health care. Both groups will be followed for 15 years.

> *The value of prostate cancer screening is not proved*

The diagnostic stage

Any 'positive' or suspicious findings must be confirmed in a subsequent diagnostic stage. Whatever the initial screening method, confirmation of suspected prostate cancer requires biopsy and histological examination of the tissue. Fine-needle aspiration can be used for cytological examination of cells but is less reliable for determining the tumour grade.

Treatment of screen-detected prostate cancer

It is possible to treat cancer confined to the prostate by transurethral resection, but most prostate cancers arise in the peripheral portion of the gland which cannot be removed by this means. Transurethral resection relieves symptoms, and for some slow-growing cancers may be all that is required. However, the procedure is associated with high recurrence rates and a higher rate of metastases, which are thought to arise from dissemination of tumour cells into the bloodstream at the time of resection.

For these reasons early-stage prostate cancer would usually be treated by radical prostatectomy. An alternative to surgery is radiotherapy, but this is also associated with complications because of the damage of closely situated organs such as the rectum and bladder: early reactions include diarrhoea, rectal bleeding, dysuria and cystitis. Hormonal therapy is presently reserved for the treatment of (symptomatic) advanced cancers.

> *Treatment of screen-detected prostate cancer differs very little from the treatment of symptomatic prostate cancer*

▲ Key points

Screening and treatment of prostate cancer

Screening method:
▲ Combination of digital rectal examination and serum PSA estimation

Diagnostic stage:
▲ Transrectal ultrasound
▲ Fine-needle aspiration cytology
▲ Trucut needle biopsy for histological assessment

Treatment stage:
▲ Radical prostatectomy

Is prostate cancer screening worthwhile?

Point	Counterpoint
Prostate screening can reduce mortality by detection of localised prostate cancers	Reduction in mortality from prostate cancer by screening has not been conclusively demonstrated

Review question 2

Have all of Wilson's criteria been met with respect to prostate cancer screening?

Wilson's criteria for mass screening

▲ The disease should be common and serious
▲ The natural history of the disease should be understood
▲ The screening test should be accurate and reliable
▲ Acceptable treatment and the resources for treatment must be available
▲ The treatment should favourably influence the outcome

(After Wilson, 1966)

Treatment of screen-detected lesions have a greater certainty of success	Many localised prostate cancers grow very slowly and will not become a problem during a man's lifetime – there is potential for over-treatment. Since there is no way of distinguishing between slow-growing and aggressive cancers, all must be treated aggressively. Radical prostatectomy is associated with high risk of impotence and urinary incontinence
Suitable tests are available for use in a mass screening programme	The non-invasive tests available are not very sensitive for detection of localised prostate cancers. Even if it were possible to increase the sensitivity of the test this would increase the potential for over-treatment

Author's view

Because of lack of sensitivity a negative result can provide false reassurance. Difficulties also arise with a positive test result. Treatment of a localised prostate cancer in asymptomatic men could enhance survival prospects but a prostate cancer becomes life-threatening only when it becomes symptomatic. Treatment at the asymptomatic stage will represent over-treatment for many men. In view of the short and long-term sequelae of radical prostatectomy or radiotherapy this could be unacceptable, depending on the age and life-expectancy of the man. A short period of 'watchful waiting' may be warranted, monitoring for tumour progression by PSA measurement and ultrasound. The position in the UK seems to be that improvements are needed in screening and treatment, with demonstrable improvement in mortality rate, before mass screening is introduced. Many Americans think differently.

Case study

John is a 58 year-old film producer, born and currently living in California. His older brother recently died from prostate cancer and his maternal grandmother and aunt both died from breast cancer. John presented with a recent history of difficulty in starting urination and in stopping the stream. After investigation a diagnosis of advanced prostate cancer was established.

• What are the usual presenting symptoms of prostate cancer?
• Are there any identifiable risk factors in John's history?
• What investigations would you recommend?
• What other conditions might feature in the diagnosis?
• What are the treatment options?
• What side-effects of treatment can be expected?

- What check-ups should be instigated to monitor the disease and the response to treatment?
- What investigations would be used to evaluate the presence of metastatic disease?
- What new symptoms might be related to progression of the disease?
- What is the typical survival of patients with symptomatic prostate cancer?

ANSWERS TO REVIEW QUESTIONS

How do the treatments for prostate cancer differ from those available for other types of cancer?

Question 1

Surgery, radiotherapy and chemotherapy are similar in principle to those commonly used to treat other types of cancer. The main difference in treatment of prostate cancer is control of tumour growth by hormone manipulation. In some respects this is a similar strategy to the use of tamoxifen in breast cancer. A problem is that the tumours already contain, or will contain, hormone-refractory cells. When this stage is reached, the survival prospects are poor.

Have all of Wilson's criteria for screening been met?

Question 2

Is prostate cancer common and serious? Clearly yes; prostate cancer is one of the most common causes of deaths from cancer in men, second only to lung cancer in some countries.

    Is the natural history of the disease understood? This is a problem. There are many men who had died from other causes who have been found at post-mortem examination to have prostate cancer: in many cases the disease caused no symptoms and did them no harm. At present there is no way of differentiating these slow-growing cancers from the aggressive cancers which rapidly produce symptoms.

    Is the screening test accurate and reliable? No test is capable of reliably detecting the disease in a precancerous or even preinvasive phase. The most promising screening test is a combination of digital rectal examination and PSA estimation. In many instances a considerable tumour load must be present before PSA concentrations are raised: at this stage the cancer is probably not far off producing symptoms, and therefore there is very little advance in the time of diagnosis. Prostatic enlargement detected by digital rectal examination could be caused by a variety of conditions, not just cancer.

    Are acceptable treatments and resources available? The treatments may be acceptable if the man has symptoms and knows that without treatment he will soon die. Without symptoms, it cannot be said with certainty that the screen-detected disease is of the aggressive type which could cause death, or the slow-growing type which will do no harm. Treatment offers peace of mind, but affects quality of life. The resource issue does not really apply in the UK since prostate screening is not available as a mass programme.

Does the treatment favourably influence the outcome? Because there is no way of knowing whether the screen-detected cancer is slow-growing or aggressive, it is difficult to determine whether the detection and treatment of asymptomatic prostate cancers actually influence the outcome.

Case study

John was referred for further investigation, including transrectal ultrasound and needle biopsy, estimation of prostate-specific antigen and a CT scan.

Prostatic enlargement was confirmed by the ultrasound scan, and the tumour appeared to involve the seminal vesicles and pelvic lymph nodes. Histology of the needle biopsy showed a poorly differentiated tumour. Serum PSA was elevated at 40 ng/ml. A bone scan revealed a possible 'hot spot' in one rib (upper left 6). Stage D2 prostate cancer was diagnosed.

Are there any identifiable risk factors in John's history? John's main risk factor is his family history of prostate and breast cancers. The disease becomes more common with increasing age – 58 years is a little young but not exceptional for advanced disease. He also lives in a country where the frequency of prostate cancer is high.

What are the usual presenting symptoms of prostate cancer? Symptoms of urinary obstruction are usual. Less specific features such as tiredness and 'rheumatism' could also be expected.

What investigations would you recommend? Investigations should be directed at diagnosing the cancer and estimating how far it has spread. Visualisation of the prostate itself is best achieved by transrectal ultrasonography. An enlarged prostate can also be felt by digital rectal examination. Extensive prostate cancer may be reflected as increased serum PSA. The possibility of metastatic disease is evaluated by serum PSA and alkaline phosphatase measurements, radionuclide bone scanning and CT scanning.

What other conditions might feature in a differential diagnosis? With urinary symptoms alone John's condition could be caused by prostatic hyperplasia. This can be alleviated by transurethral resection of the prostate. The operation leaves some of the prostate gland behind, in which cancer could develop in the future.

Because of the degree of spread, surgical and radiotherapy interventions were considered inappropriate. John was counselled and given the choice of bilateral orchidectomy or hormonal therapy, and elected for the latter. He was prescribed monthly depot injections of leuprorelin and flutamide.

His serum PSA levels returned to normal and the repeat ultrasound scan revealed that the tumour bulk had reduced. Consequently he was given a series of radiotherapy treatments, over 6 weeks, with a total dose of 70 Gy to the prostate. He was referred for repeat investigations in 6 months.

The repeat bone scan showed no further skeletal changes; however, the CT scan showed possible secondary deposits in the liver and one lung. The liver finding was further investigated by ultrasonography and hepatic angiography. The lesion was a small haemangioma (a benign focal proliferation of blood vessels). He was referred for a repeat CT scan of the lungs in 6 weeks (this would show enlargement of the lesion if caused by secondary tumour since these grow rapidly).

No further change was detected in the lung by CT scan, effectively ruling out the possibility of an actively growing invasive secondary tumour at this stage. However, his elevated PSA (100 ng/ml) was noted. At further review 3 months later the PSA levels had risen further to 150 ng/ml, indicating that the tumour had become refractory to the hormonal treatment.

What are the treatment options? Radical prostatectomy or radiotherapy in early stages of the disease are curative. Later, inoperable cancers are treated by bilateral orchidectomy or anti-androgen drug therapy. Combined anti-androgen treatment is probably better than single agent therapy. John could have been offered chemotherapy as he is relatively young for this sort of disease, although the radiotherapy regime he received after hormonal tumour debulking is probably just as effective.

What side-effects of treatment can be expected? John felt well throughout his treatment with the exception of some hot flushes in the initial stages of the hormonal treatment. Radiotherapy is associated with lethargy and loss of appetite.

What check-ups should be instigated to monitor the disease and response to treatment? Monthly PSA measurement, repeat imaging investigations every 6 months.

What investigations would be used to evaluate the presence of metastatic disease? In John's case a repeat CT scan showed some anomalies in the lung and liver which could correspond to secondary tumour deposits. The liver finding was further investigated by means of ultrasonography and hepatic angiography. It was concluded that this lesion was a small haemangioma (a benign focal proliferation of blood vessels of no clinical significance). It was decided to wait for 6 weeks to see if the possible secondary in the lung enlarged (lung secondaries grow rapidly).

What new symptoms might be related to the progression of the disease? The main problem in advanced cases of prostate cancer is bone pain. Secondary tumour deposits in the lungs might become evident as shortness of breath, chest infections and expectoration of mucus and blood. Liver failure or jaundice could arise from extensive secondary deposits in the liver.

What is the typical survival of patients who have symptomatic prostate cancer? The median survival time with treatment in advanced cases such as John's is about 2.5 years. Once the cancer becomes refractory to hormonal treatment the median time of survival is 15–18 months. The remaining treatment options will be aimed at making life as comfortable for John as possible.

References

Kramer, B.S., Brown, M.L., Porok, P.C. *et al.* (1993) Prostate cancer screening: what we know and what we need to know. *Ann. Intern. Med.*, **119**, 914–23.

Wilson, J.M.G. (1966) Some principles of early diagnosis and detection, in *Proceedings of a Colloquium, Magdalen College, Oxford, July 1965* (ed. G. Teeling-Smith), Office of Health Economics, London.

Further reading

Brewster, S.F. and Gillat, D.A. (1993) Advanced prostate cancer: What's new in hormonal manipulation? *Br. J. Hosp. Med.*, **49**, 710–15.

Catalona, W.J. (1994) Management of cancer of the prostate. *N. Engl. J. Med.*, **331**, 996–1004.

Clements, R. (1993) Imaging the prostate. *Br. J. Hosp. Med.*, **49**, 703–5.

Dearnaley, D.P. (1994) Cancer of the prostate. *BMJ*, **308**, 780–4.

Horwich, A. (1993) Prostate cancer. *Lancet*, **342**, 901–5.

Porter, A.T., Blasko, J.C., Grimm, P.D. *et al.* (1995) Brachytherapy for prostate cancer. *CA Cancer J. Clin.*, **45**, 165–78.

Saini, A. and Waxman, J. (1992) Recent progress in the treatment of advanced prostatic cancer. *Br. J. Hosp. Med.*, **47**, 122–6.

Slawin, K.M., Ohori, M., Dilloglugil, O. and Scardino, P.T. (1995) Screening for prostate cancer: an analysis of early experience. *CA Cancer J. Clin.*, **45**, 134–47.

19 Peptic ulcers and gastric cancer

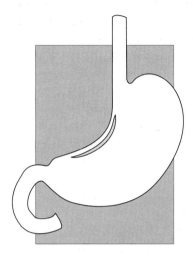

A large proportion of peptic ulcers, and possibly some gastric cancers, are initiated by infection with *Helicobacter pylori*. The natural habitat of this bacterium is the stomach, and it is ubiquitous in some populations. Its mode of transmission is unclear, but is believed to be primarily by the faecal–oral route. With improved living standards in developed countries infection rates, particularly in children, appear to be decreasing, which might explain the noticeable decline in the incidence of stomach cancers in developed countries.

Formerly, excess acid production was believed to initiate damage to the epithelial lining of the stomach and induce an inflammatory response in the underlying tissue, eventually causing a peptic ulcer. The rationale of treatment was to limit acid production or to protect the surface from damage. These treatments can be very effective, but once the treatment is stopped the damage is likely to recur.

The recognition that most peptic ulcers are initiated by *H. pylori* has resulted in new treatments designed to eradicate the organism. This can be very effective and lead to permanent cure, but problems are arising with response rates and increasing resistance by the organism.

Gastric cancers are the product of a sequence of changes, often starting with inflammation. In some cases the inflammatory changes are probably initiated by *H. pylori*. Unfortunately, the eradication of *H. pylori* will not completely remove the public health problem of either peptic ulcers or gastric cancer.

Pre-test

- **What factors are responsible for the development of peptic ulcer?**
- **What is the best treatment for an ulcer?**
- **How important is gastric cancer as a health problem in (a) the developed countries, (b) the less developed countries?**
- **What factors contribute to the development of gastric cancer?**

Aims of this chapter

By the end of this chapter you will have increased your knowledge of:
◆ The epidemiological distribution and possible risk factors involved in the production of peptic ulcers and gastric cancers
◆ The pathology of peptic ulcers, gastric cancers and precursor lesions
◆ Methods for diagnosis, prevention and treatment
In addition, this chapter will help you to:
◆ Discuss the possible reasons for changes in the incidence of gastric cancer
◆ Discuss the common features in the aetiology of peptic ulcer and gastric cancer
◆ Evaluate the potential for prevention and treatment

Introduction

*Many peptic ulcers and gastric cancers are initiated by infection with **Helicobacter pylori***

The stomach and duodenum are the sites of some very common disorders, ranging in severity from gastritis to peptic ulcer and, more ominously, to gastric cancer. About 10% of adults will at some time suffer from duodenal ulcer and gastric cancer is one of the most common causes of death from cancer. Gastric cancer is unusual in that its prevalence is falling dramatically in most Western countries, without any deliberate intervention. Almost uniquely for a cancer, a bacterial infection is believed to be involved in its development.

The most common type of gastric cancer is preceded by a range of conditions involving inflammation and atrophy (shrinkage) of the mucosal glands. These conditions are described as superficial and chronic gastritis. The lesions can resolve with or without treatment, may become metaplastic or, more rarely, dysplastic and then cancerous (Figure 19.1). Peptic ulcers may be preceded by a milder inflammatory condition or metaplasia.

In many cases a contributory factor in producing gastritis is infection with the bacterium *Helicobacter pylori*: the production and recurrence of gastric and duodenal ulcers and the development of gastric cancer may well have been influenced by this organism. Duodenal ulcers in particular have a very strong association with *H. pylori*. However, other factors are also involved in the development of these conditions, and it is not uncommon for ulcers and cancers to be found without identifiable *H. pylori* infection.

In the initial stages some gastric diseases are without symptoms. One of the main presenting features, common to gastro-oesophageal reflux, gastritis and peptic ulcer, is dyspepsia. The principal means of investigation is endoscopy. Non-invasive serological screening can be used to detect previous or current *H. pylori* infection.

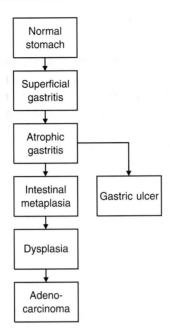

Figure 19.1 Ulcers are a very common and distressing condition of the stomach and duodenum. In the stomach the condition is preceded by an inflammatory condition called gastritis. Occasionally, persistent gastritis can lead to intestinal metaplasia and eventually cancer. There is very little risk of ulcers becoming cancerous.

Background information: Functional anatomy of the stomach

Food is passed into the stomach from the oesophagus. The **cardia** of the stomach is a small area immediately adjacent to the oesophageogastric junction (Figure 19.2). The **fundus** is an enlarged portion to the left side, above the cardiac orifice. The main portion of the stomach is known as the **body**. The **antrum** is a distal, non-acid-secreting portion of the stomach. Cells in this area are responsible for the secretion of gastrin, the hormone that stimulates secretion of hydrochloric acid. The terminal portion of the stomach, the **pylorus**, leads to the gastroduodenal sphincter.

The mucosal cells mostly have secretory functions and are therefore arranged into glands that penetrate downwards from the surface. These areas are described as the **gastric pits** or **foveolae** (Figure 19.3). In the body of the stomach, parietal cells are involved in the production of hydrochloric acid and intrinsic factor. Hydrochloric acid is necessary to activate pepsinogen into the protein-digesting enzyme pepsin. Pepsinogen is produced by **peptic cells**, present at the base of the gastric pits; its production is regulated by the hormone gastrin, which is produced by endocrine cells in the fundus.

Because of the highly acid conditions in the stomach the cell lining is

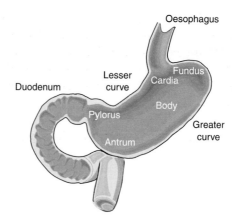

Figure 19.2 Anatomy of the stomach.

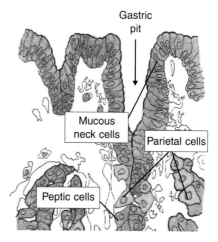

Figure 19.3 Microscopic structure of the stomach.

protected by the production of mucus from **mucous neck cells**. In addition, the epithelial cells secrete bicarbonate ions to keep the environment underneath the layer of mucus more alkaline.

Superficial and chronic gastritis

Gastritis is recognised histologically by the presence of an inflammatory cell infiltrate. In **superficial gastritis** the infiltrate is confined to the zone between the gastric pits. Deeper extension of inflammation into the pits, accompanied by loss of the glands and their replacement by fibrous tissue, is **chronic atrophic gastritis**.

Reactive gastritis is a further distinct entity. It is characterised by foveolar hyperplasia, dilation of blood vessels, oedema in the lamina propria and a lack of inflammatory cells. Reactive gastritis is often caused by use of NSAIDs.

Gastritis is now scored according to the Sydney System (named after the World Congress of Gastroenterology, held in Sydney; Price, 1991), a grading system that also takes into account aetiological features of the disease. The system calls for separate assessment of inflammation and metaplasia in biopsies from different areas of the stomach.

Chronic inflammation of the gastric mucosa is commonly found by endoscopy and biopsy in both symptomatic and asymptomatic individuals.

Peptic ulcer

Aetiology

A peptic ulcer is a full-thickness defect in the surface mucosa that is exposed to acid and pepsin in the gastric juice (any area of the stomach and upper part of the duodenum). About 80% of peptic ulcers are located in the first portion of the duodenum, the remainder being in the stomach (gastric ulcer). Most peptic ulcers heal without therapy, although they frequently recur. They usually first appear in middle to later life.

Most ulcers are thought to result from an imbalance in the gastroduodenal defensive and aggressive forces (Figure 19.4). Aggressive forces are acid secretion and pepsin enzymatic activity, infection with *H. pylori* and use of NSAIDs. The defensive forces are principally the surface layer of mucus and secretion of bicarbonate ions into the mucus layer. The extent of any damage will also be determined by the regenerative capacity of the mucosal cells, and maintenance of an adequate submucosal blood flow: the production of prostaglandins by the mucosal cells is believed to be influential in these defensive activities.

Peptic ulcers are probably caused by disturbances to acid and pepsin secretion, or to the defensive mucus–bicarbonate barrier

Alteration in any one of these factors may be sufficient to cause ulceration. In some people the ulcer may be caused by excessive production of pepsin and acid; in others, whose levels of gastric acid and pepsin are normal and who are free of *H. pylori* infection, ulceration may be caused by use of NSAIDs or by reduced prostaglandin synthesis. No specific dietary factors have been associated with peptic ulcer.

Prevalence

The prevalence of peptic ulcer appears to be falling in the UK from a peak in the 1920s. Hospital admissions and surgery for peptic ulcer have dramatically declined because of advances in drug therapies that control acid secretion or improve the protection by mucus.

Symptoms

The symptoms of peptic ulcer are usually a gnawing or burning pain that

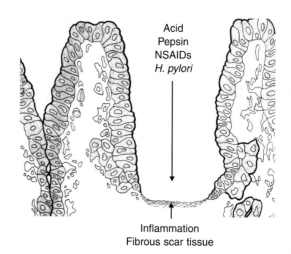

Figure 19.4 Development of peptic ulcers. In chronic peptic ulcer the epithelium is destroyed by peptic acid and pepsin stimulating an acute inflammatory response. Because the damaging agents persist there is penetration into deeper layers and formation of fibrous scar tissue. In an established ulcer the opposing forces of epithelial damage and inflammation occur at the same time, so that a 'stalemate' is reached. If the damage persistently exceeds the capacity for repair, penetration of the full thickness of the wall will lead to perforation.

occurs 1–3 hours after eating, which is often worse at night. The pain is sometimes relieved by alkali or by food. Other symptoms include nausea, vomiting, bloating, belching and significant weight loss. A minority of peptic ulcers are discovered because they haemorrhage or perforate.

Malignant transformation

Malignant transformation of duodenal ulcers is unknown, and is rare in gastric ulcers (1% or less). The complications of peptic ulcer include perforation, haemorrhage, fibrosis and stenosis. Death is usually caused by perforation of ulcer and gastric bleeding, but usually the condition impairs the quality of life rather than shortens it.

Gastric ulcer

Chronic gastritis is often a prelude to gastric ulcer, the position of the ulcer being related to the distribution of the gastritis. Most gastric ulcers appear at the boundary between the inflamed non-acid-secreting antral mucosa and the acid-secreting mucosa in the body of the stomach and are accompanied by *H. pylori*-positive chronic gastritis. About 70% of patients with gastric ulcer have, or have had, *H. pylori* infection. The remaining ulcers are mostly secondary to a reactive gastritis induced by NSAIDs.

Duodenal ulcer

Most duodenal ulcers are found in the first part of the duodenum immediately after the gastroduodenal sphincter. The vast majority of patients with duodenal ulcer also have *H. pylori*-associated gastritis. There seems to be a familial association for duodenal ulcer, a positive family history being present in up to 40% of patients. Individuals with blood group O have a 30% greater risk of duodenal ulcer than other individuals. About 40% of patients with duodenal ulcer secrete excessive amounts of acid.

Focus on H. pylori

H. pylori is a spiral bacterium with several flagellae at one end. It was first cultured and implicated as a cause of gastrointestinal disease in 1984. Initially the organism was classified as *Campylobacter pylori*. *H. pylori* colonises the stomach of a number of species including humans. Up to half of the world's population may be infected but fortunately in most individuals the organism produces no symptoms or untoward effects.

The organism is Gram-negative, microaerophilic and possesses potent urease activity. Urease activity increases the pH of the immediate environment, enabling the organism to protect itself from stomach acid.

Epidemiology of *H. pylori* infection

Individuals infected with *H. pylori* are found in all parts of the world. Generally the infection is extremely long standing, with individuals remaining infected for several decades. Estimates of the prevalence of *H. pylori* infections are usually based on serological tests. Endoscopy may be used to confirm the results of serological tests, but this is more likely in developed countries because of the resources required. Studies indicate that the great majority of cases of gastritis are accompanied by *H. pylori* infection. In the USA and Europe infection is generally much more common in adults, and increases with age from 5–20% in people below 20 to 30–60% of those over 50. In African and Asian countries infection rates are higher (60–90%), and children become infected in early life. It is estimated that in some locations virtually the entire population is infected. Generally, the poorer the population the higher the infection rate, and the younger people are when they become infected.

The likelihood of new infection is now much reduced because of improved hygiene and development of antibiotics. In the developed countries infection rates vary with socioeconomic group; infection is less common in adults of high socioeconomic status. Racial group and gender do not appear to alter the risk of infection. The age-related change in prevalence seen in Europe and the USA is probably a cohort effect: people who are now over the age of 50 were more likely to have been infected as children than present younger adults who probably acquired the infection

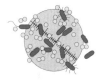

*The intestine is the natural habitat of **H. pylori***

Microaerophilic: organisms that survive only in a reduced oxygen atmosphere.

Urease: an enzyme that hydrolyses urea to ammonia.

▲ **Key points**

Features of *H. pylori*

▲ Urease activity provides protection against the acidic environment by providing an alkaline buffer around the organism
▲ Multiple flagellae allow motility in the mucus overlying the gastric epithelium
▲ Adheres to specific glycolipid receptors present on the surface of antral epithelial cells

after childhood. There appears to be no relationship with alcohol consumption or with smoking, and vegetarians appear to be just as susceptible as meat-eaters.

Transmission of *H. pylori*

The main mode of transmission of *H. pylori* is probably the faecal–oral route. The organism can be grown (with difficulty) from faecal samples and from dental plaque and its DNA has been identified by the PCR in these sources. Epidemiological data show that *H. pylori* infection follows a distribution pattern very similar to that of some viruses known to be transmitted by the faecal–oral route, such as hepatitis A. There is some evidence to suggest that water supplies may be a vehicle for *H. pylori* infection.

H. pylori in the development of peptic ulcer

H. pylori adheres to gastric-type mucosa, in the normal stomach or in metaplastic duodenum

In the stomach *H. pylori* adheres to normal gastric epithelial cells, under a layer of mucus which serves as protection against the acid environment. There is evidence that the organism actually binds to the epithelial cells, but does not normally penetrate the epithelial cell layer. From this position the organism is still able to influence events in the underlying tissue probably by releasing cytotoxins into the cells to which the organisms are bound. The tissue response to this is the production of inflammation – **gastritis**. With time the gastric mucosa becomes metaplastic, converting to an intestinal type of epithelium. *H. pylori* does not adhere to this metaplastic epithelium.

Ultimately, infection in the stomach is self-limiting as the normal mucosa is replaced by metaplasia. Total intestinal metaplasia does not occur in most people, and some people are able to eliminate the organism by immunological means before this stage is reached.

*In the duodenum **H. pylori** adheres to gastric-type metaplastic epithelium*

The production of duodenal ulcers is believed to be related to acid-induced injury. The defensive response to excess acid in the duodenum is production of a metaplastic epithelium of the gastric type (similar to that of the normal stomach). Areas of gastric metaplasia are then infected by *H. pylori*, causing further injury to the mucosa and eventual duodenal ulceration. The specific association of *H. pylori* with only normal gastric epithelium or gastric metaplasia may be related to the type of mucus produced: the mucus produced by normal duodenal epithelium and intestinal metaplasia is more acid.

The question remains whether infection by *H. pylori* is essential to the development of duodenal ulcer. The yield of the organism in duodenal biopsy is very low, but more than 90% of patients with duodenal ulcer also have *H. pylori* gastritis. One theory is that inflammatory mediators released in the stomach (as part of the gastritis) are washed down into the duodenum. The presence of these mediators in the duodenum could then initiate a local immune response and mucosal damage, leading to ulceration. Conversely, the vast majority of individuals with *H. pylori* infection are symptomless carriers. The question must therefore be asked why the organism is completely harmless in some people but in others is involved in ulcer disease or even cancer. The answer is uncertain, but probably involves both bacterial and host factors.

It appears that some strains of *H. pylori* secrete factors chemotactic for monocytes and neutrophils. These inflammatory cells probably initiate tissue damage and ulceration by the release of oxygen free radicals or proteolytic enzymes. This inflammatory response is enhanced by the secretion of interleukin-8 (IL-8) by gastric epithelial cells; IL-8 is a potent chemoattractant for neutrophils, but secretion is induced only by certain *H. pylori* strains, meaning that some strains are more pathogenic than others. People vary in their response or ability to produce IL-8 when infected by *H. pylori*.

Diagnosis of ulcer disease

In most cases peptic ulcers are diagnosed on the clinical signs alone, but the 'gold standard' investigation is endoscopy. Laboratory tests centre on the investigation of secretory function and *H. pylori* infection. Some of these investigations can help to determine the optimum treatment and to monitor the response to therapy. Methods are also available to assess changes in various protective factors, but these are currently confined to experimental studies.

Gastric acid output

Gastric output analysis is used to monitor response to antisecretory drugs that interact with parietal cell H_2 receptors. The gastric juice is aspirated and its pH determined. About 50% of patients with antral gastric or duodenal ulcer are hypersecretors and will benefit from drugs that inhibit acid secretion. However, most patients with ulcers of the body and fundus of the stomach exhibit no secretory abnormalities. Gastric aspiration is the principal method for diagnosis of Zollinger–Ellison syndrome.

Pepsin secretion

Gastric ulcers may be associated with altered secretion of pepsin. This enzyme, and its isoenzymes, can be estimated in the gastric juice or in gastric or duodenal biopsy samples. Most patients with duodenal ulcer secrete more pepsin, particularly during the active stages of the disease. However, the estimation of pepsin secretion is of little value for determining the type and site of ulcers.

Detection of *H. pylori*

H. pylori is definitively identified by microbiological culture and histological examination of biopsy samples. Culture also enables the antibiotic sensitivity of the organism to be evaluated. The organism is identified (usually with special staining procedures) in tissue sections by its spiral or curved shape, its position on the mucosal surface and its usually high population density. Detection in some precancerous lesions can be difficult: the population density decreases as the severity of the lesion increases. *H. pylori* colonisation is rare in atrophic areas and absent in intestinal metaplasia.

Pepsin: a proteolytic enzyme that breaks down proteins into large fragments.

Pepsinogen: the inactive precursor of pepsin. Activated by hydrochloric acid and by pepsin itself.

Zollinger–Ellison syndrome: caused by a tumour of the gastrin-producing cells of the pancreas. Gastric acid production is over-stimulated, resulting in peptic ulcers. Treatment involves excision of the neoplasm and control of gastric acid secretion with histamine H_2 blockers.

*This urea breath test is a quick and easy test suitable for screening purposes and confirmation of **H. pylori** eradication*

▲ **Key points**

Diagnosis of *H. pylori* infection

Biopsy-based tests:
▲ Culture on selective media: 'gold standard' method giving indisputable identification
▲ Histology: identification relatively easy, slides can be referred for a second opinion
▲ Urease test: based on pH change as ammonia is released from the urease substrate
▲ All biopsy-based methods may give false-negative results because of sampling error

Non-invasive methods:
▲ Urea breath test (^{13}C or ^{14}C), based on release of radio-labelled CO_2 from urea substrate
▲ Serology: detects antibodies to *H. pylori*, useful in epidemiological studies but also indicates past as well as current infection

A more rapid routine test for diagnosis of infection is the **biopsy urease test**. A gastric biopsy specimen is placed in a urea broth: the urease activity of the bacteria hydrolyses urea in the broth to alkaline ammonia and raises the pH of the medium, which is detected by a colour change of phenol red indicator. This is a much simpler test than culture or histology, and the results can be obtained while the patient is still present. However, the test lacks sensitivity (some positives will be missed), particularly if patients have received antimicrobial or bismuth treatment. Cultures should still be set up for serotype and sensitivity testing in order to determine the most appropriate treatment. Histological assessment of the gastric mucosa may still be desirable, particularly if the purpose of endoscopy and biopsy is to monitor response to treatment.

An alternative test, which does not rely on endoscopic biopsy, is the **urea breath test**. The test relies on the ingestion of radiolabelled (^{13}C or ^{14}C) urea, which, in individuals with *H. pylori* infection, appears in the breath as labelled CO_2. If the bacteria are not present then the urea is not hydrolysed and no labelled CO_2 is produced. The gas is collected in a respiration chamber and measured by scintillography. The radioactive dose is not (unduly) dangerous, being about 10% of that received when a single plain radiograph of the abdomen is taken. The test lacks sensitivity, particularly if treatment has reduced the number of organisms but has not eliminated the infection (i.e. it does not distinguish between suppression and eradication of the bacteria). If the test is to be used to evaluate treatment, it should be performed at least a month after the treatment has finished.

Infection with *H. pylori* results in the production of antibodies, and these can be detected by serological methods. This will indicate current infection and any previous infection that may have been successfully eradicated. It is therefore necessary to use one of the other methods to diagnose active infection. Serological tests are mainly used for evaluating the prevalence of *H. pylori* infection in epidemiological studies.

Treatment of peptic ulcer

Before the recognition of the importance of *H. pylori* in the pathogenesis of peptic ulcer, drug therapies were designed to:
• Reduce gastric acid secretion
• Increase defensive barriers against acid and enzymatic attack

Suppression of gastric acid

Antacids raise the pH of the gastric juice

The simplest approach to reducing the acidity of gastric juice is to neutralise it with alkaline agents or antacids. Unfortunately, this increases the rate of gastric emptying so that any effects are short-lived. This transient action may relieve some of the symptoms of peptic ulcer but does not promote healing. The commonly used antacids are sodium bicarbonate, magnesium hydroxide and aluminium hydroxide.

H2 histamine antagonists are currently the first-line drugs in ulcer treatment

A more reliable approach is to reduce the amount of acid secreted by the parietal cells using H_2 receptor antagonists. Normally, acid secretion is stimulated by the neurotransmitter acetylcholine and the hormone gastrin. These messengers work indirectly, by stimulating the release of histamine from nearby paracrine cells, which then binds to the parietal cell H_2 receptors, causing acid secretion.

The principal H_2 receptor antagonists are cimetidine and ranitidine. Their chemical structure is so similar to that of histamine that they block the receptor but do not stimulate the parietal cell into acid secretion. Acid production is reduced, as is pain from the ulcer and, because the mucosal cells are no longer repeatedly damaged, healing is encouraged. A dose in the evening usually inhibits about 80% of nocturnal acid production. Up to 80% of ulcers are healed within 2 months. The drugs do not generally have significant side-effects, although cimetidine is associated with a very low incidence of impotence.

Another useful agent is omeprazole, particularly for patients with Zollinger–Ellison syndrome. This drug inhibits ATPase, which is necessary for the proton pump responsible for transporting H^+ ions out of the parietal cells. Inhibition of this enzyme is irreversible and acid secretion resumes only when new enzyme is synthesised.

Antagonists: substances that bind to receptors without activating them. The bound receptors are temporarily unavailable for interaction with the physiological activating agent. Antagonist drugs compete with the natural agent for receptor binding.

Histamine H_2 receptor antagonists: block the action of histamine on parietal cells, thereby reducing acid secretion.

Parietal cells: secrete acid into the stomach lumen by means of an energy-dependent proton pump which exchanges intracellular H^+ for extracellular K^+.

Defensive barriers

The agents that increase defence against acid and enzymatic attack work either by forming a barrier on the ulcer surface or by influencing the production of prostaglandins, which may stimulate mucus secretion and bicarbonate production. Sucralfate is a complex of sulphated sucrose and aluminium hydroxide. In the acid conditions of the stomach the molecules polymerise to form a sticky gel that adheres to the base of the ulcer. Further damage is minimised, thereby encouraging the healing process.

A well established treatment is bismuth chelate. This has a strong affinity for the glycoprotein component of mucus, rendering it more resistant to breakdown by gastric acid and enzyme. It is also active against *H. pylori*, which could explain its effectiveness in promoting ulcer healing.

A synthetic analogue of prostaglandin E_1 has been found to promote ulcer healing. However, this agent, misoprostol, has unpleasant side-effects, particularly diarrhoea, and is not commonly used.

Some treatments provide physical protection by binding to the ulcer surface, giving it a chance to heal

Eradication of *H. pylori*

Eradication of *H. pylori* infection in patients with peptic ulcer alleviates the symptoms. Conversely, reinfection leads to renewal of active ulcer disease. In practice, eradication of the bacteria can prove difficult. A variety of antimicrobial agents is available, but their effectiveness depends on a host of factors including the bacterial strain, the pH of the gastric environment and the immunological status of the patient. The treatment courses can be long (6 weeks or more) and some of the drugs are unpleasant to take, producing problems with compliance. New treatment regimens are evolving, including some 1-week regimens, which should improve compliance. Standard triple therapy, and the dual use of omeprazole and amoxycillin, are now recommended for use as 2-week courses.

The effectiveness of eradication therapy increases with a combination of agents, but side-effects are more likely

Vagotomy: surgical incision of the vagus nerve.

Review question 1

How has the treatment of peptic ulcer changed over the last 20 years?

A double therapy of omeprazole and amoxycillin over 6 weeks can eradicate the organism in about 80% of patients. A triple therapy of bismuth chelate, metronidazole and tetracycline, administered for 4–6 weeks, gives eradication rates of up to 90%. Unfortunately, bismuth chelate is unpleasant to take and metronidazole increases the side-effects (usually diarrhoea and possibly allergic reactions) of the regimen. There is also a high incidence of antibiotic resistance to metronidazole. Eradication is no guarantee that the problem is forever resolved in a patient: in one evaluation of triple therapy re-infection rates of about 20% were found within a year.

Reinfection and ulcer recurrence may occur because antibiotic therapy does not immediately change the environment for *H. pylori* colonisation. *H. pylori* cannot exist in the duodenum without gastric metaplasia, and duodenal ulcers do not occur without it. Until the metaplasia disappears the patient is vulnerable to reinfection or, more likely, regrowth of organisms which were not completely eliminated by treatment.

Surgical management

Surgical treatment of peptic ulcer has markedly declined with the advent of the H_2 receptor antagonists. Before this, two types of partial gastrectomy were performed to remove the antral area of the stomach responsible for secretion of gastrin. The operations differ in how the remaining portion of the stomach is connected to the small intestine: in one procedure (Bilroth I) the lower part of the stomach is removed and the remaining portion connected to the duodenum; in the Bilroth II procedure the stomach remnant is connected to the jejunum, and the duodenum is closed off. The principal long-term complication of surgery is recurrence of peptic ulcer in the stomach remnant, duodenum or jejunum.

Another surgical approach to the management of peptic ulcer is **vagotomy**, aimed at reducing the sympathetic nervous stimulation of acid secretion. This was often carried out in addition to the Bilroth II operation but surgery is now reserved for the management of complications such as uncontrolled haemorrhage, perforation or obstruction of outflow (this can occur if a pyloric or duodenal ulcer swells with oedema, or if the healing process involves scarring).

Intestinal metaplasia

Intestinal metaplasia is regarded as a (reversible) precancerous condition of the stomach

Persistent inflammation of the stomach eventually leads to **intestinal metaplasia** (Figure 19.5).

The three types of intestinal metaplasia are referred to as Type I (complete), Type II (intermediate) and Type III (incomplete). Only Type III is strongly associated with progression to dysplasia and cancer, although small risks are attached to the other types.

In incomplete intestinal metaplasia the mucosa retains some of the features

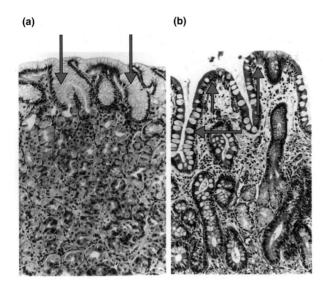

Figure 19.5 (a) Normal glandular architecture of the stomach in which the mucosa is invaginated to form gastric pits (arrows). (b) Intestinal metaplasia of the stomach showing villus projections into the lumen (arrows). The mucosa contains discrete goblet cells (horizontal arrow). Photograph provided by Dr E.J. Kuipers and reproduced by kind permission of the *Lancet*.

of the original gastric mucosa, intermixed with some characteristics of the small intestine, particularly the presence of goblet cells. This type of change occurs often in populations at high risk for gastric cancer. It is very often seen adjacent to a gastric cancer, particularly an intestinal adenocarcinoma. Intestinal metaplasia can also be associated with gastric ulcers. In the complete type the glands of the gastric mucosa are replaced by crypts lined by cells characteristic of the small intestine, notably Paneth cells, mucus-secreting goblet cells and absorptive epithelial cells.

Gastric cancer

Gastric cancer is not a single entity. The most common type, making up about 95% of gastric cancers, is adenocarcinoma. The adenocarcinomas are divided into two principal categories, **intestinal** or **diffuse**, according to histological appearance. Intestinal adenocarcinoma has a glandular structure, whereas the diffuse type comprises small clusters of cells separated from each another. The intestinal type is associated with specific precancerous lesions and is more common in older patients; diffuse adenocarcinoma is more common in populations in which the incidence of gastric cancer is low, and the patients are often younger. The remaining 5% of gastric cancers are usually lymphomas and leiomyosarcomas.

Gastric cancers also differ according to their site in the stomach, intestinal adenocarcinomas being more common in the fundus and antrum and diffuse adenocarcinomas more common in the cardia.

> *The most common type of gastric cancer involves the fundus and antrum*

Leiomyosarcoma: a malignant tumour of smooth muscle. Affects the uterus, gastrointestinal tract, abdomen, retroperitoneum and walls of blood vessels. Tumour is rare in children.

Epidemiology

Although decreasing, gastric cancer is the second most common form of cancer world-wide

The incidence of gastric adenocarcinoma varies widely, the highest incidences being in Japan and South America (Figure 19.6). In the UK it currently ranks sixth as a cause of death from cancer. Both incidence and mortality rates of gastric cancer are decreasing in developed countries. For example, in the USA the incidence in 1930 was 38 per 100 000 men and 30 per 100 000 women; by 1980 these figures had fallen to 10 per 100 000 men and 5 per 100 000 women. These trends are continuing (Figure 19.7).

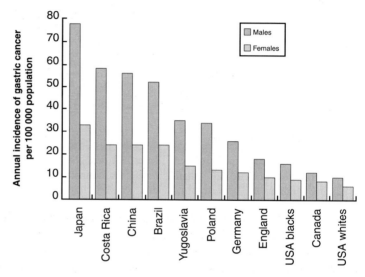

Figure 19.6 Geographical variation in gastric cancer in men and women. (Data from International Agency for Research on Cancer.)

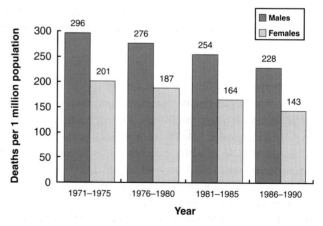

Figure 19.7 Variation in death rate from gastric cancer in men and women in England and Wales, 1971–1990. A marked decline has been observed this century. Over the past 20 years this trend has continued, although there no significant changes have been made in public health measures or treatments specifically aimed at containing the disease. In comparison with other cancers this rate of progress is remarkable. (Source: OPCS.)

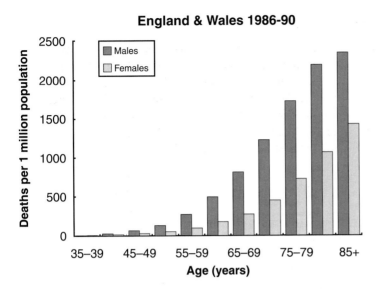

England & Wales 1986-90

Figure 19.8 Variation in deaths from gastric cancer with age in men and women, England and Wales, 1986–1990. Deaths from gastric cancers increase with age. The excess of deaths (and incidence) in men is seen in every age category. (Source: OPCS.)

The reasons for this decline are unclear. Certainly diagnostic criteria and accurate ascertainment of the disease have changed with time, but these changes would not account for such a marked reduction. Observed differences in the incidence of gastric cancer in first and second-generation Japanese who have moved to the USA point towards the involvement of environmental factors. Although the trends in the developed countries are welcome, on a global perspective the disease remains a significant public health problem. Generally, the risk of death from gastric cancer increases with age (Figure 19.8). There is also an unexplained gender imbalance, male deaths exceeding those of females.

Risk factors

Although *H. pylori* is implicated in the early stages of the most common types of gastric cancer this agent cannot be solely responsible for the disease in all individuals. The response to infection varies greatly among individuals: in most people infection is asymptomatic, but some develop gastritis, others develop peptic ulcer and a small minority develop gastric cancer. Which of these outcomes becomes apparent depends on the host's response to the infection, which in turn is genetically controlled. Other superimposing or predisposing factors in the environment probably help to stimulate progression through gastritis, atrophy, metaplasia and dysplasia (Figure 19.9).

To date no predisposing gastric cancer gene has been identified, although certain oncogene and tumour suppressor gene mutations characterise stages in the evolution of the disease. The only association with individual genetic characteristics is that the incidence of the diffuse type of gastric cancer is higher

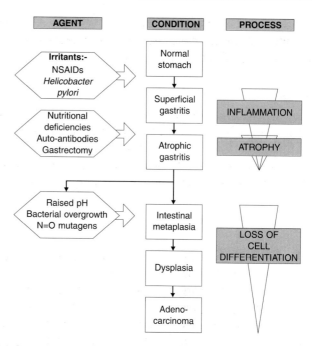

Figure 19.9 Correa's model of the chain of events leading to adenocarcinoma of the fundus and antrum (Correa, 1988). Adenocarcinoma of the fundus and antrum is preceded by inflammation and atrophy of the gastric mucosa. This may be initiated by irritants such as *H. pylori* infection and use of NSAIDs. Owing to atrophy of the mucosal glands secretion of gastric acid and pepsin are reduced and the consequent rise in pH may result in the production of mutagens from bacterial activity and dietary components. Mutagens are more likely to cause damage in the absence of antioxidant vitamins and minerals. Changes become apparent as intestinal metaplasia, leading to dysplasia and eventually to invasive adenocarcinoma. Most of the precancerous changes are reversible.

in individuals of blood group A. The role of environmental factors is uncertain and so far most attention has focused on the diet.

Dietary factors

Factors in the diet may be tumour initiators and promoters. Epidemiological studies suggest that patients with intestinal metaplasia consume fewer fruit and vegetables than unaffected individuals. Nutritional deficiencies probably impede mucosal repair and early lesions are more likely to increase in severity than regress. The antioxidant vitamins and minerals may be particularly important in this respect. For example, vitamin C is essential for wound healing, but in the stomach it is believed also to prevent the formation of carcinogenic nitroso and diazo compounds from nitrates and nitrites. Vitamin C also appears to affect the metabolic action of some carcinogens.

It has been suggested that the introduction of refrigeration and non-chemical means of preserving foods has influenced the decline in gastric cancers.

Refrigeration increases the availability of fresh fruit and vegetables, avoids the need for salting or nitrate preservation and helps to prevent contamination by bacteria and fungi (which could synthesise procarcinogens).

Salt consumption

There appears to be some correlation between infection with *H. pylori* and salt consumption. Without *H. pylori*, salt does not affect proliferation of mucosal cells, but in infected individuals gastric mucosal cell proliferation increases with salt intake. Increased cell proliferation is often regarded as a circumstance in which the active cells are more vulnerable to damage and neoplastic transformation.

H. pylori

Normally the stomach actively secretes vitamin C, so the intragastric concentration is above that of the blood. This mechanism is inhibited by *H. pylori*, but is restored after the organism is eradicated. The loss of vitamin C and the possible consequent production of carcinogens could be one of the mechanisms underlying the association of *H. pylori* with gastric cancer. The organism also generates oxygen free radicals and can induce a chronic inflammatory response, both of which can increase the tendency for cells to become damaged and undergo neoplastic transformation.

The urease activity of the bacteria generates ammonia; this is very toxic to the gastric mucosa and is probably responsible for the loss of mucosal glands in chronic atrophic gastritis. Some, but not all, *H. pylori* strains produce a toxin that could cause cell damage, although it appears that peptic ulcer disease and gastric cancer can develop independently of a toxin-producing strain.

Pernicious anaemia

Gastric cancer is about four times more common in people with pernicious anaemia than in the general population. In pernicious anaemia the production of autoantibodies to stomach parietal cells results in an atrophic gastritis (as well as reducing the production of intrinsic factor and hence the absorption of vitamin B_{12}). Risk of gastric cancer is also increased in patients with gastric stumps following partial gastrectomy for the treatment of benign gastric ulcer.

Pathology

Gastric adenocarcinoma

About 50% of gastric adenocarcinomas occur in the antral and pyloric region of the stomach, 20% involve the lesser curve, 5% the greater curve, 5% the fundus, 10% the cardia and 10% are diffuse. The incidence of adenocarcinoma of the cardia is increasing, but the reasons for this are not known. Adenocarcinoma of the cardia is believed to be unrelated to *H. pylori* infection.

Gastric cancer spreads by infiltration through the stomach wall via the lymphatics and blood circulation. Perigastric lymph nodes are often involved

---

▲ Key points

Risk factors in gastric cancer

- ▲ High salt intake
- ▲ Excessive alcohol consumption
- ▲ Foods with high nitrate/nitrite content
- ▲ Low intake of fruit and vegetables
- ▲ Infection with *H. pylori*
- ▲ Bile acid reflux
- ▲ Pernicious anaemia

Preventive measures:
- ▲ Food refrigeration
- ▲ Avoidance of highly salted and pickled foods
- ▲ Reduction of nitrates and nitrites in food and drinking water
- ▲ Supplementation with vitamins C and E

at presentation. More distant lymph nodes around the left gastric, common hepatic, coeliac, splenic, middle colic and para-aortic arteries, hepatoduodenal ligament and mesenteric roots may also be involved. Secondary deposits of gastric cancer are common in the greater omentum, peritoneum and in the ovaries. The small and large intestines may also be involved and the resultant stricture is a well recognised clinical presentation of the disease. The more common intestinal type of adenocarcinoma is associated with intestinal metaplasia – this type has a better prognosis than the diffuse type.

Pre-cancerous gastric lesions

Intestinal adenocarcinoma is preceded by a series of precancerous lesions

A hypothesis for the chain of events leading to adenocarcinoma of the fundus and antrum was proposed by Correa in 1988 (Figure 19.9). In this model adenocarcinoma is preceded by a spectrum of precursor lesions, starting with superficial gastritis. Infection by *H. pylori* is believed to play an important role by initiating inflammatory changes. Subsequently, *H. pylori* disappears from the lesion as it becomes metaplastic. The general trend is a gradual worsening of the lesions.

Hypochlorhydria: decreased hydrochloric acid production in the stomach.

At first the gastritis is superficial but if it persists it may spread more diffusely to other areas of the stomach, producing a chronic multifocal atrophic gastritis. This causes hypochlorhydria and bacterial overgrowth. These conditions may be more favourable for the conversion of nitrites in the food to carcinogenic nitrosamines, which leads to a sequence of cellular changes resulting in the morphological lesions of metaplasia, dysplasia, and finally gastric carcinoma.

In common with precancerous lesions in other sites (cervix, for example) the changes leading to intestinal adenocarcinoma may regress or ultimately progress to invasive cancer. Progression from gastritis to adenocarcinoma takes one or more decades, but occurs in only a very small proportion of patients.

Tumour stage

The prognosis for patients with gastric cancer depends on tumour stage and grade (Figure 19.10). This is based on a TNM system according to the depth of local invasion, involvement of lymph nodes and presence of metastases. The stage is determined by a combination of diagnostic procedures (for example radiography, endoscopy), by biopsy and ultimately by surgery and examination of the resection specimen.

Stage IA tumours invade only the lamina propria or submucosa, without involvement of lymph nodes and without metastases. Stage IB shows the same degree of local tumour invasion but perigastric lymph nodes within 3 cm are also involved.

Five-year survival correlates with tumour stage

Subsequent stages of gastric cancer all involve tumour invasion beyond the submucosa and all are described as 'advanced' gastric cancer. The intermediate stages (IB, II, IIIA and IIB) correspond to increasing degrees of invasion, lymph node involvement or metastases. A stage IV tumour has invaded through the serosa into adjacent structures, involves lymph nodes, and may or may not have metastasised. The 5-year survival for stage IA gastric cancer is about

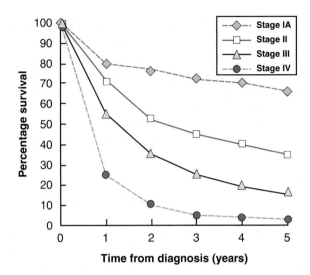

Figure 19.10 Gastric adenocarcinoma: relationship between survival and TNM stage. (Data from Thompson *et al.* (1993) *Lancet*, **342**, 713–718.)

65%, but 5% or fewer patients with stage IV gastric cancer survive beyond five years. Because of the usual late presentation of the disease, the overall 5-year survival rate for gastric cancer is only about 10%.

One important macroscopic classification, seen by endoscopy, is termed early gastric cancer (EGC). This is a cancer that is confined to the mucosa, or to the mucosa and submucosa only. These cancers have characteristic surface appearances, such as a slight elevation or depression of the mucosa or the presence of a polypoid lesion.

Before the introduction of endoscopy EGCs were fewer than 5% of gastric cancer cases. Now, with endoscopy, up to 15% of cases seen in Western countries are EGC. In Japan up to 40% of cases are EGC, the larger number of early cases seen in Japan probably being due to the much more common use of endoscopy as a screening modality. The prognosis for patients with EGC is very favourable; 5-year survival, after surgery, being about 90%.

> *An early form of gastric cancer can be distinguished by endoscopy*

> *Most cases of early gastric cancer are curable by surgery*

Histological grade

The histological grading system comprises four grades: I–IV. Grade IV is the most anaplastic tumour and carries a poorer prognosis (5-year survival about 65% for grade I, reducing to about 10% for grade IV). The DNA ploidy (a measure based on change in chromosomal number) correlates with the depth of tumour invasion and lymph node involvement.

Genetics of gastric cancer

Alterations to both proto-oncogenes and tumour suppressor genes have been found in gastric cancers. Activation of the *ras* and *c-erb-B2* oncogenes have been shown, as have mutations to the *p53* tumour suppressor gene. Frequency

Review question 2

**Why is infection with *H. pylori*
asymptomatic in some people
but associated with peptic ulcer
or even gastric cancer in others?**

of *p53* mutations correlates with tumour stage, lymph node metastasis and survival. The *p53* mutations probably play a crucial role in the conversion from dysplasia to malignancy.

Gastric lymphoma

This is a rare form of gastric malignancy with an annual incidence in the USA of about 0.6 per 100 000. In appearance the lymphoma is very similar to lymphoid tissue seen elsewhere in the gut such as the Peyer's patches (a characteristic feature of the small intestine). The normal lymphoid deposits are known as mucosa-associated lymphoid tissues (MALT). The gastric MALT lymphoma is essentially a malignancy of B cells.

The prognosis of gastric lymphoma is better than that of gastric adenocarcinoma because the tumours are amenable to chemotherapy. The recent recognition of *H. pylori* infection in the development of B-cell MALT lymphomas has transformed the treatment strategy and survival prospects for patients with this disease. Eradication of *H. pylori* by antibiotic therapy resulted in complete regression of the lymphoma in five of six patients with low-grade B-cell gastric MALT lymphoma (Wotherspoon *et al.*, 1993). The one failure suggests that there may be an optimal time for initiating antibiotic therapy in these lymphomas, but this remains to be determined.

Diagnosis

Gastric cancer usually occurs in people over 60 years of age, but can be seen from the third decade onwards. Following physical examination the usual diagnostic investigations are fibreoptic endoscopy and gastric biopsy, barium meal radiography or cytology of stomach washings. CT is increasingly used in diagnosis.

Screening for gastric cancer

At present the only formal mass screening programme for gastric cancer in existence is in Japan, in recognition of the much higher incidence of the disease in that country. Screening is aimed at detecting EGC by endoscopy with biopsy. Other screening methods less commonly employed include photofluorography and gastric washings. Detection of EGC reduces the number of cases of advanced gastric cancer and the number of deaths. The trend towards detection of EGC has also occurred in Western countries that do not have mass screening, and it is therefore difficult to evaluate just how much of the Japanese success has been because of the mass screening programme.

Treatment

Treatment depends on the extent of the disease. As with most cancers the mainstay of treatment is surgical resection of the tumour. In advanced cases surgical intervention offers no survival advantage, hence patients should be assessed preoperatively for evidence of metastases to peripheral lymph nodes, the bowel, liver and bones.

Unfortunately, gastric cancer is rarely diagnosed early. Only 10–20% of patients initially present with disease that is confined to the stomach and about 30% have distant metastases at the time of presentation. Most patients present with tumour invasion of adjacent structures and lymph node involvement.

Surgery

The most common surgical interventions are:
- Partial gastrectomy for distal tumours (in the antrum or pylorus)
- High partial resections for small lesions in the body of the stomach
- Total gastrectomy for multicentric, larger lesions in the stomach body, and proximal tumours (in the cardia or fundus)

These operations include resection of the lesser and greater omenta and the perigastric lymph nodes. As might be expected operative morbidity and mortality increase with the extent of stomach resection and removal of adjacent structures such as lymph nodes, spleen, pancreas, adrenal glands or colon.

Surgery is also employed with palliative intent. Obstructions can be bypassed by gastrojejunostomy so that the patient can continue with normal oral nutrition, but gastric resection (which means that oral nutrition is no longer possible) treats the symptoms better and improves the chances of survival.

Chemotherapy and radiotherapy

Radiotherapy can be used as a palliative treatment but administration is difficult because of the close proximity of radiosensitive organs. There is no evidence that single or combination chemotherapy prolongs survival.

Role of *H. pylori* in development of peptic ulcers and gastric cancer

There is a minority opinion that *H. pylori* infection in chronic gastritis, peptic ulcer and gastric cancer is opportunistic rather than causative. Koch's third postulate ('when a pure culture is inoculated into a susceptible animal species, the typical disease must result'; see Chapter 6) has not been fulfilled: many people are infected by the organism without suffering ill effects. This ignores the fact that ulceration and neoplasia are multifactorial diseases; *H. pylori* infection alone would not be expected to produce the condition.

There are also instances in which antibiotic therapy alone does not help the condition. However, use of acid-suppressing drugs alone is associated with very high recurrence rates. The only exception is the treatment of Zollinger–Ellison syndrome, in which worthwhile responses are produced by administration of proton pump inhibitors, despite infection in some patients by *H. pylori*. Most patients with peptic ulcer are therefore treated, either

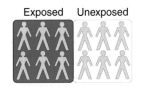

Exposed   Unexposed

Long-term sequelae of *H. pylori* gastritis

▲ Prospective study of 58 subjects with *H. pylori* infection and 49 non-infected subjects
▲ Presence of *H. pylori* infection confirmed by serology and histology of gastric biopsies
▲ Presence of infection at follow-up determined by culture and histology
▲ Mean follow-up 11.5 years
▲ Atrophic gastritis and intestinal metaplasia developed in 16 (28%) infected subjects and in 2 (4%) non-infected subjects
▲ *H. pylori* infection is a significant risk factor for development of atrophic gastritis and intestinal metaplasia

From: Kuipers *et al.*, 1995.

concurrently or sequentially, with bismuth or an acid-suppressing drug as well as the antibiotic therapy.

Undoubtedly many gastric cancers are produced in the absence of *H. pylori*, but there is evidence that the progression of precancerous lesions to invasive cancers is influenced by the organism (Kuipers *et al.*, 1995). The regression of MALT lymphomas following antibiotic therapy supports the role for *H. pylori* as a cancer-causing agent, although this condition is much more rare than gastric adenocarcinoma.

Is *H. pylori* a causative agent in peptic ulcers and gastric neoplasia?

Point (From Graham, 1995)	Counterpoint
Koch's third postulate has not been fulfilled	Koch's postulates apply only to single-agent diseases: ulceration and neoplasia involve several risk factors
Antibiotics alone are relatively ineffective at healing peptic ulcers	Acid-suppressing drugs given alone do not protect against ulcer relapse
Improvements in patients with Zollinger–Ellison syndrome obtained with proton-pump inhibitors, despite *H. pylori* infection	The fundamental defect in Zollinger–Ellison syndrome is a disturbance in gastrin secretion and acid production: it is to be expected that treatments aimed at correcting the prime defect would be most effective
Many gastric cancers, particularly adenocarcinomas of the cardia, are found in patients without *H. pylori*	Progression of precancerous lesions to adenocarcinoma is more likely in the presence of *H. pylori*. MALT lymphomas regress following eradication of *H. pylori*

From Graham (1995).

Author's view

The advantage of adding antimicrobial therapy to the treatment of peptic ulcers is inescapable: healing rates are shorter than usual and the chances of relapse are much reduced. At the very least this demonstrates that *H. pylori* exacerbates the condition and, from the perspective of treating patients, it is academic whether *H. pylori* is a causative organism or an opportunistic infection on a background of mucosal inflammation. It seems likely that in Zollinger–Ellison syndrome *H. pylori* is superimposed on a pre-existing condition, but it does not necessarily follow that this must apply to all other cases on non-NSAID-induced peptic ulcer. It is likely that most non-NSAID peptic ulcers are multifactorial in their aetiology, involving disturbances in acid and pepsin secretion as well as *H. pylori* infection. Tackling both processes gives the greatest chance of success.

The development of gastric cancer is certainly multifactorial. Even if *H. pylori* does not itself initiate changes leading to malignant transformation, its presence as an agent which causes cell damage and inflammation could increase susceptibility to other carcinogenic agents.

Prevention of peptic ulcers and gastric cancer

The involvement of *H. pylori* in the development of peptic ulcer and gastric cancer presents an opportunity to arrest these diseases at an early stage. Primary prevention could be achieved by limiting transmission of *H. pylori*. In the developed countries this has largely been achieved by improvements in sanitation and overcrowding, producing a marked decrease in the incidence of gastric cancer.

This is not so readily achievable in less developed countries. A vaccine might help matters, although effective immunisation will be difficult because of variability in the bacterial strains. Even if a vaccine is eventually developed it will not be possible to eradicate gastric cancer. With the possible exception of the rare MALT gastric lymphoma, *H. pylori* infection is not essential for the development of every case of gastric cancer. It seems likely that *H. pylori* infection is not involved in the production of adenocarcinoma of the cardia. Currently, the incidence of this type of gastric cancer is increasing. It is debatable whether some countries would be able to afford a vaccine.

It is likely that the changes in living conditions that have benefited people in the developed countries have lessened exposures to other risks, particularly dietary factors. Environmental conditions are the key to this disease. Improvement in the less developed countries would not only help to reduce the problem of gastric cancer but also to reduce the burden from a whole host of human diseases.

There is some potential for preventing gastric cancer by manipulating various other cofactors in its development. In Linxian province, China, the incidence of gastric cancer was reduced markedly by giving supplements of β-carotene and vitamin E (see Chapter 7). An intervention study has begun in Europe (Reed, 1994), in which patients with biopsy-proven intestinal metaplasia are randomised into treatment groups designed to evaluate the effect of *H. pylori* eradication and/or vitamin C supplementation (2 g daily) given over 3 years. The results are awaited with interest: primary prevention by vitamin supplementation would be cheaper to apply and would have fewer problems of transport and storage than a vaccination programme.

*Many peptic ulcers and some gastric cancers could be prevented by avoiding or eliminating **H. pylori***

Vaccination alone would not address the other risk factors involved in development of peptic ulcers and gastric cancer

Secondary prevention by antibiotic eradication of *H. pylori* might be considered suitable for developed countries but is probably impractical. Screening would be required to find out who is infected and who is not and, although screening for *H. pylori* is technically feasible, it would not discriminate between the majority of people who will remain asymptomatic and those who will develop disease. Most people will be treated unnecessarily, with the associated risk of encouraging antibiotic resistance of *H. pylori*. Progression to intestinal metaplasia might offer a suitable alternative intervention point for antibiotic therapy. Screening would not be required because patients would come to attention by their presentation of symptoms. Another aim of the European intervention study is to find out whether this approach is effective.

ANSWERS TO REVIEW QUESTIONS

Question 1

How has the treatment of peptic ulcer changed over the last 20 years?

Initial treatments were aimed at neutralising excess stomach acid by the use of antacids. In extreme cases surgery, usually consisting of a partial gastrectomy, was necessary. Later treatments attempt to reduce the production of acid at source. Although these are effective, as soon as treatment is finished, excessive acid production restarts.

New treatments are aimed at eradicating infection by *H. pylori*. It could be said that all the previous treatments were akin to preventing rain from a leaking roof reaching the floor by judicious placement of a bucket: eradication of *H. pylori* offers the opportunity to repair the leaking roof.

Question 2

Why is infection with *H. pylori* asymptomatic in some people but associated with peptic ulcer or even gastric cancer in others?

Probably because of the combination of host and bacterial factors. Strains of *H. pylori* differ in their secretion of chemoattractants (to attract monocytes and neutrophils) and probably of most importance, in their ability to induce IL-8 secretion by gastric epithelial cells. The localised inflammatory response at the site of infection probably causes most of the tissue damage and ulceration.

Why some individuals develop gastric cancer and others do not probably depends on a series of other host and environmental factors. These may include availability of antioxidants in the diet which could limit the damage caused by neutrophil-generated free radicals.

References

Correa, P. (1988) A human model of gastric carcinogenesis. *Cancer Res.*, **48**, 3554–60.

Graham, J.R. (1995) *Helicobacter pylori*: human pathogen or simply an opportunist?

BMJ, **345**, 1095–7.

Kuipers, E.J., Uyterlinde, A.M., Pena, A.S. *et al.* (1995) Long-term sequelae of *Helicobacter pylori* gastritis. *Lancet*, **345**, 1525–8.

Price, A.B. (1991) The Sydney System: a histological division. *J. Gastroenterol. Hepatol.*, **6**, 209–22.

Reed, P.I. (1994) The ECP-IM intervention study. *Eur. J. Cancer Prev.*, **3** (Suppl. 2), 99–104.

Wotherspoon, A.C., Doglionin, C., Diss, T.C. *et al.* (1993) Regression of primary low-grade B-cell gastric lymphoma of mucosa-associated lymphoid tissue after eradication of *Helicobacter pylori*. *Lancet*, **342**, 575–7.

Further reading

De Koster, E., Buset, M., Fernandes, E. and Deltenre, M. (1994) *H. pylori*: the link with gastric cancer. *Eur. J. Cancer Prev.*, **3**, 247–57.

Plebani, M., Vianello, F. and Di Mario, F. (1994) Laboratory medicine in ulcer disease. *Clin. Biochem.*, **27**, 141–50.

Rathbone, B.J. and Heatley, R.V. (1992) H. pylori *and Gastroduodenal Disease*, Blackwell Scientific Publications, Oxford.

Sinicrope, F.A. and Levin, B. (1993) Gastric cancer. *Curr. Opin. Gastroenterol.*, **9**, 930–7.

Thompson, G.B., van Heerden, J.A., Sarr, M.G. (1993) Adenocarcinoma of the stomach: are we making progress? *Lancet*, **342**, 713–18.

20 Atherosclerosis and coronary heart disease

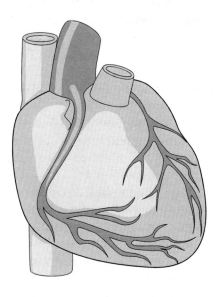

Pre-test

- **What is a heart attack?**
- **What are the symptoms of heart attack?**
- **What is angina and why does it often precede a heart attack?**
- **What can we do to reduce the risks of heart attack?**
- **What is meant by the term atherosclerosis?**
- **Why is cholesterol of importance in coronary heart disease?**
- **How is a heart attack diagnosed?**
- **What treatments are available for angina?**
- **What can be done after a heart attack to reduce the chance of further cardiac events?**

Atherosclerosis is a focal thickening in the wall of an artery caused by a fibrofatty plaque. In developed countries, most people will have some evidence of atherosclerosis by the time they reach 40 or 50 years of age. Although the plaques are focal, people often have multiple lesions, either in the same arterial tree or in different arteries. The principal complications of atherosclerosis are coronary heart disease (CHD), stroke, gangrene and aneurysm.

In developed countries coronary heart disease accounts for more deaths than any other single disease. Although there is a significant genetic component to the disease, people can do much to reduce risks by changing their lifestyle; most notably by stopping smoking, decreasing the amount of fat and calories in their diet and increasing the amount of exercise they take. Changes can favourably influence the overall quality of life and offer protection against other diseases.

Many of the risk factors in CHD appear to operate together and magnify the effects; hence paying attention to more than one risk factor will lead to greater benefits. There is also evidence that risk for atherosclerosis can to some extent be laid down very early on in life.

To some extent illness from CHD can be controlled medically, and deaths from myocardial infarction can be reduced by swift thrombolytic therapy. The 'gold standard' surgical intervention is coronary bypass surgery but costs are extremely high and waiting lists are long. Alternatively, use of a balloon catheter to widen the artery (coronary angioplasty) will provide revascularisation of heart muscle – but this procedure may cause complications of abrupt vessel closure or longer-term restenosis.

Aims of this chapter

By the end of this chapter you will have increased your knowledge of:
- Population differences in susceptibility to coronary heart disease
- How atherosclerosis and thrombosis develop and how they contribute to coronary heart disease
- The risk factors involved in atherosclerosis and thrombosis
- Means of diagnosing and treating coronary heart disease

In addition, this chapter will help you to:
- Describe the biochemistry of lipid metabolism and the importance of lipoproteins in influencing atheroma formation
- Discuss the current theories of atheroma formation and describe the role of thrombus in producing arterial occlusion
- Evaluate the role of environmental and behavioural risk factors as contributory causes of coronary heart disease
- Describe the methods available for the diagnosis and evaluation of atherosclerosis and myocardial infarction
- Describe the treatments available for persistent angina and for people who have suffered a heart attack
- Identify interventions that could be used to prevent coronary heart disease

Introduction

Coronary heart disease (CHD) is the largest cause of illness and deaths in the UK. The disease is usually caused by atherosclerosis in the coronary arteries; these become partially or completely blocked by a fibrofatty plaque.

The complications of atherosclerosis arise because blood supply to tissues supplied by the occluded artery is decreased. The artery may be occluded by the plaque itself, but because the plaques have a tendency to bleed the artery can suddenly become blocked by thrombus. Atherosclerosis in other arteries can lead to stroke, aneurysm, peripheral vascular disease or gangrene.

The incidence of CHD varies in different parts of the world, which supplies clues about the environmental factors influencing the disease. The mortality rate in the UK (particularly Scotland, Northern Ireland and the north of England) is one of the highest in the world. Similarly, regions of Finland and the USA have a high incidence of CHD. These trends correlate with high prevalence of smoking, intake of dietary saturated fats and serum cholesterol levels. In contrast, the incidence of CHD is much lower in some Mediterranean countries and Japan, where the population has correspondingly lower saturated fat intakes and serum cholesterol levels.

This is an overly simplified picture: atherosclerosis is caused by a combination of environmental influences, or risk factors, that act in a genetically susceptible individual – it is a multifactorial disease. Some of the environmental agents can be favourably altered by adjustments to lifestyle, particularly by stopping smoking, taking more exercise and controlling diet.

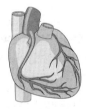

In developed countries CHD is responsible for more deaths than all types of cancer

CHD is caused by atherosclerosis and thrombosis in the coronary arteries, blocking blood supply to heart muscle

CHD is much more of a problem in developed countries, and is related to differences in lifestyles

Aneurysm: thinning and weakening of the artery causing dilatation or bulging outwards into a sac. Thrombus (blood clots) can form in the sac and lead to embolism. Aneurysms have a tendency to rupture.

Gangrene: necrosis or putrefaction of tissue.

> *CHD and strokes are the most common outcomes of atherosclerosis*

Peripheral vascular disease: any disorder of arteries, veins or lymphatics – except those of the heart. Impaired circulation to the extremities causes muscle weakness and pain, ulceration and gangrene.

Stroke: a sudden loss of brain function, lasting for more than a day, because of disruption in the blood supply. Also described as a cerebrovascular accident (CVA). Ischaemic strokes involve a decrease in the blood supply, usually because of atherosclerotic plaque. Haemorrhagic strokes are caused by rupture of a blood vessel.

CHD is usually diagnosed by the assessment of clinical symptoms (chest pain for example), ECG measurements and a variety of imaging techniques and laboratory investigations. Treatment centres on medical control of the symptoms or surgical intervention in the form of a coronary bypass operation or coronary angioplasty. The *Health of the Nation* objectives for CHD (see Chapter 12) place greater emphasis on primary prevention, by assessment of patient history (especially hypertension and family history of CHD) and the presence of lifestyle risk factors such as smoking.

Epidemiology

Atherosclerosis is responsible for nearly half of all deaths of the adult population in Western society. The most common manifestation of atherosclerosis is CHD; this alone is responsible for more than 150 000 deaths each year in England and Wales. Another condition commonly caused by atherosclerosis is stroke, which is the third most common cause of death in the UK (Figure 20.1).

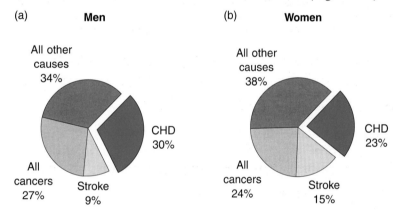

Figure 20.1 Deaths from CHD in the UK, 1990 in (a) men and (b) women. (Source: OPCS.)

Deaths from CHD increase with age; the disease accounts for about 15% of all deaths in people between 35 and 44 years, and 30% of all deaths in people over 55 years of age. For most age groups deaths from CHD are more common in men than in women (Figure 20.2). Only in people over 80 do more women die from CHD deaths than men, but by this age the proportion of women in the population is higher.

The death rate from CHD varies from country to country (Figure 20.3), and from one region to another within a country. In the UK the mortality figures rise steeply from the south-east to the north-west and Scotland (Figure 20.4).

Encouragingly, the mortality rates for CHD have declined since the mid-1980s in both the UK and the USA, particularly in men below the age of 55 years (Figure 20.5). The reasons for this are obscure but are probably attributable to a combination of primary prevention (for example by stopping smoking)

> *There are international and regional variations in deaths from CHD*

> *There is some evidence that mortality rates from CHD are in decline*

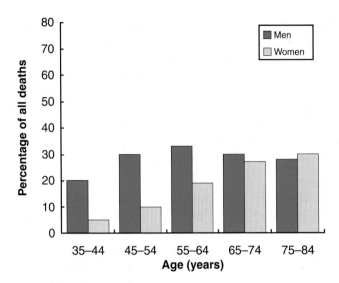

Figure 20.2 Variation in deaths from CHD with age and sex in the UK, 1990. In early and late middle age CHD is the predominant cause of death in men. In women, the disease is much more of a problem in older age groups. (Source: OPCS.)

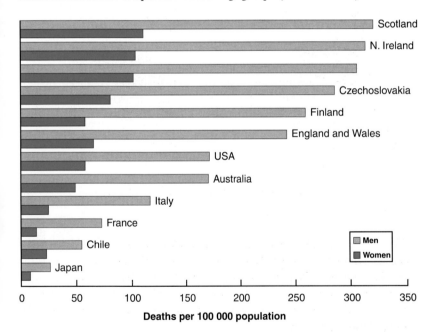

Figure 20.3 International comparison of deaths from CHD (age-specific rates in men and women, 1988). Deaths from CHD in the UK are among the highest in the world. (Source: World Health Statistics Annual, 1989.)

and improved treatment for myocardial infarction. However, this good news does not apply equally across the population. In Scotland the incidence of CHD in women has risen, which correlates with increases in smoking and alcohol consumption. There is no reason for complacency: in the UK as a

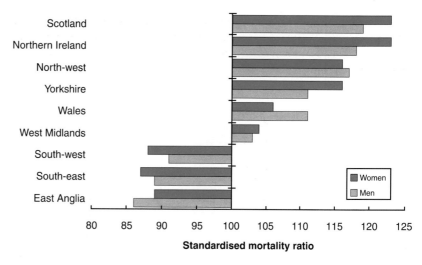

Figure 20.4 Regional variation in deaths from CHD in men and women in the UK, 1985. People living in northern regions of the UK are more likely to die from coronary heart disease compared with those living in the south. The difference is particularly marked among women. (The death rate for the UK as a whole is represented as 100; a figure above this value represents greater than average risk. (Source: OPCS, Registrar General's Offices of Scotland and Northern Ireland, 1987.)

whole the groups showing most resistance to the trends of reduced alcohol and tobacco consumption are young adults of both sexes. Unless corrected, this behaviour pattern will soon become evident as CHD.

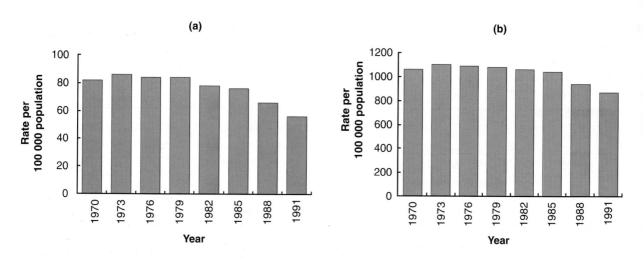

Figure 20.5 Rates of mortality from CHD in England (1970–1991) in (a) people under 65 and (b) 65–74 years. There have been some encouraging signs that mortality from coronary heart disease is decreasing, especially in people below 65 years of age (note the graph scales are different: deaths from CHD are much more common in old age). (Source: OPCS.)

The death rate from CHD also varies significantly with social class, both men and women in the lower socioeconomic groups being at increased risk (Figure 20.6). The gradient across the social classes is the opposite of that seen 60 years ago, when CHD was more common among classes I and II.

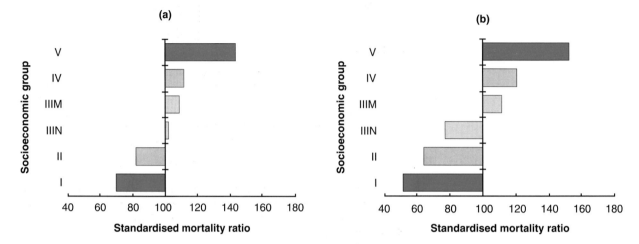

Figure 20.6 Mortality from CHD and socioeconomic group in the UK, 1979–1983 in (a) men and (b) women. Both men and women in the lower socioeconomic groups are more likely to die from coronary heart disease. (Source: OPCS.)

Biochemistry of lipid and cholesterol metabolism

Lipids are used by the body in two main forms: as fatty acids and as cholesterol. Because lipids are insoluble in blood plasma they are transported in the circulation complexed with protein. These complexes are referred to as **lipoproteins**.

The transport of lipids can be viewed in two interlinked portions. The **exogenous system** transports dietary lipids from the intestine to the liver and peripheral tissues. The vehicles for delivering triglycerides and the usually small amounts of cholesterol absorbed from the diet are the **chylomicrons**.

The **endogenous system** transports triglycerides and cholesterol that are continuously produced by the liver. These are secreted and delivered to the peripheral tissues as **very-low-density lipoprotein** (VLDL). Progressive removal of triglyceride from VLDL in the peripheral tissues gives rise to smaller **intermediate-density lipoprotein** (IDL) and **low-density lipoprotein** (LDL) particles. A consequence of triglyceride removal is that the cholesterol inside the particles becomes more concentrated, particularly in the LDL particles.

There is also a mechanism for returning excess cholesterol to the liver, where it is either processed and put back into the blood circulation or used for the production of bile salts. The vehicle for returning cholesterol to the liver is **high-density lipoprotein** (HDL).

Review question 1

Why do more people in social classes IV and V die of CHD today than those in social classes I and II whereas 60 years ago the opposite was true?

All lipids are transported in the body as complexes with specific proteins

Cholesterol: used by all cells for the production of membranes (these comprise a lipid bilayer with protein). In specialised tissues, such as the adrenal glands, gonads and liver, cholesterol is also used as precursor for the synthesis of adrenocortical hormones and the sex steroid hormones. Although physiologically important, these are of little importance in terms of cholesterol turnover. Cholesterol is also used to produce bile salts.

Fatty acids: derived from triglycerides (also called triacylglycerols). A very rich source of energy for cells.

Types of lipoprotein

The five major types of lipoprotein are classified according to their biochemical properties and, most importantly, their ratio of lipid relative to protein. Chylomicrons are synthesised only by the intestine and are mostly triglyceride. VLDL carries triglycerides and cholesterol synthesised by the liver. Most of the circulating cholesterol is present in LDL particles, although some is returned from the peripheral tissues to the liver as HDL.

The protein components of the particles are known as **apolipoproteins**, shortened to apo. The most important apolipoproteins are apo A-I, apo E, apo C and apo B – apo B-48 and apo B-100. Apo B-48 is the carrier protein in chylomicrons, apo B-100 is associated with VLDL.

Some apolipoproteins have functions other than merely acting as a carrier for lipid. The interaction of some lipoproteins with cells depends on their binding to specific receptors on the surface of the cells. It is the apolipoprotein component that acts as the binding 'glue' between the lipoprotein particle and the cell. For example, the liver can take up and process chylomicron remnants (see below) by binding with receptors for apo E. Liver cells cannot process chylomicrons because their apo E is masked by apo C. Another apolipoprotein is involved in the activation of lipoprotein lipase, an enzyme used to release triglycerides from their carrier proteins (Table 20.1).

Table 20.1 Lipoproteins and their functions in lipid metabolism

Lipoprotein	Lipid constituent	Principal apolipoprotein	Site of production	Function
Chylomicrons	Triglycerides and small amounts of cholesterol. Also contain fat-soluble vitamins	apo B-48, apo C-II	Intestine	Transport of dietary fat to liver and peripheral tissues
VLDL	Liver-synthesised triglycerides and cholesterol (derived from any source)	apo B-100, apo C-II	Liver	Transport of triglyceride to peripheral tissues
IDL	Triglyceride and cholesterol	apo B-100, apo E	Remnant, after removal of triglyceride from VLDL	Taken up by liver cells, or undergo further removal of triglyceride, resulting in LDL

LDL	Cholesterol	apo B-100		Deliver cholesterol to liver and peripheral cells
HDL	Cholesterol	apo A-I, apo A-II, apo C, apo E	Liver and intestine	Take up cholesterol from cell membranes in peripheral tissues, transporting it (after esterification) to the liver

Exogenous system transport of dietary lipids

Chylomicrons

Most of the lipids needed by the body are obtained from dietary sources. Dietary fats are broken down into fatty acids and glycerol, which are absorbed, assembled into triglycerides and combined with a protein carrier. The triglyceride–protein complexes are the chylomicrons, which serve to transport triglycerides and any absorbed cholesterol to the peripheral tissues (Figure 20.7).

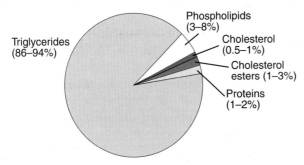

Figure 20.7 Chylomicrons mostly comprise triglycerides derived from dietary fats. They also contain small amounts of cholesterol and phospholipids. A protein component enhances solubility of the particle so that it can be transported in the lymphatics and bloodstream.

When the chylomicrons reach the peripheral tissues the triglycerides are released from their carrier protein and broken down into their constituent fatty acids and glycerol by lipoprotein lipase (Figure 20.8). This enzyme is present on the surface of capillary endothelium in muscle and adipose tissues and is activated by apo C-II on chylomicrons. The fatty acids are an extremely rich energy source and the glycerol (which is water-soluble) can also be used by the liver and muscle cells as an energy source. The triglyceride-depleted

chylomicrons, or **chylomicron remnants,** still contain a small amount of triglyceride, together with cholesterol and the carrier proteins. The remnants are circulated to the liver where they are used to manufacture VLDL.

Blood concentrations of chylomicrons are always highest shortly after a meal and gradually decrease until all are used (12–14 hours). Because chylomicrons are the only means of transporting fat from dietary sources, they also transport the lipid-soluble vitamins, dissolved within the triglyceride.

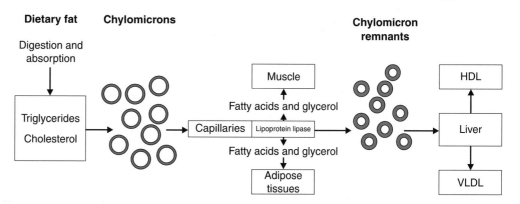

Figure 20.8 Dietary fat and cholesterol are transported to peripheral tissues in chylomicrons. In the peripheral tissues, triglycerides are separated from the protein carrier by the enzyme lipoprotein lipase. The breakdown products (fatty acids and glycerol) are absorbed by muscle and adipose tissues. The chylomicron remnants, containing protein, some triglyceride and cholesterol, are circulated to the liver.

Endogenous system transport of liver-processed triglycerides and cholesterol

To compensate for variation in the fat content of the diet, the liver produces triglycerides continuously so that cell energy requirements can always be met. Cholesterol can be produced by the liver and peripheral tissues (Figures 20.9 and 20.10).

VLDL and IDL

Triglycerides synthesised by the liver are transported as VLDL (Figure 20.11). Near the destination the triglycerides are released from their transport proteins by the action of lipoprotein lipase.

The removal of triglyceride results in IDL particles. These are either transported back to the liver or further hydrolysed in the plasma. Hydrolysis results in further loss of triglyceride and release of apo E. These are transferred to HDL. The particle remaining is LDL.

LDL

LDL is the major cholesterol-transporting lipoprotein

About 70% of plasma cholesterol is carried as LDL (Figure 20.12). Cholesterol is needed as a component of cell membranes and for the synthesis of

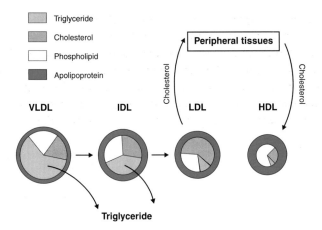

Figure 20.9 Removal of lipids from lipoproteins. Lipoprotein particles undergo sequential delipidation as triglycerides and cholesterol are removed and used by the peripheral tissues.

adrenocortical hormones, sex hormones and bile salts. Most of the cholesterol required is synthesised by the liver from fatty acids, although it can be obtained directly from foods such as eggs and liver.

When LDL particles reach the peripheral cells they bind to the cell surface at specific receptor sites. The LDL–receptor complexes are taken into the cells by endocytosis, and the LDL particle delivered to the lysosomes where cholesterol is released by enzyme activity. The receptor portion of the complex is recycled to the cell surface. The free cholesterol accumulated within the cell inhibits the synthesis of new LDL receptors, thus preventing the entry of further LDL. The activity of receptors on all cells is a major determinant of plasma LDL concentration. The free cholesterol within the cells is used for the synthesis of membranes and other components or is esterified with fatty acids to produce cholesterol esters, the storage form of cholesterol.

Lipoprotein (a)

This is a modified form of LDL containing the protein apo (a). Circulating levels of lipoprotein (a) (Lp(a)) correlate with occurrence of CHD independently of any other risk factor. Apo (a) is related to plasminogen, a protein precursor of the enzyme plasmin that dissolves blood clots. The activation of plasmin from plasminogen is induced by **tissue plasminogen activator** (t-PA). It is believed that apo (a) competitively inhibits activation of plasminogen by t-PA. The consequent inhibition of fibrinolysis could mean that small thrombi, which would otherwise be dissolved, either cause occlusion or are incorporated into a plaque, contributing to its enlargement.

HDL

Excess cholesterol is transported to the liver by a process called **reverse cholesterol transport**. The cholesterol is accepted from the cells by HDL (Figure 20.13). It is believed that HDL can transfer this to the liver directly by

Endocytosis: means by which substances are brought into cells. In receptor-mediated endocytosis the molecule to be brought inside the cell first binds to its receptor on the plasma membrane. The receptors are clustered in shallow depressions in the plasma membrane termed coated pits. The plasma membrane folds back on itself and the complex buds off, forming a vesicle.

HDL transfers cholesterol from the peripheral tissues to the liver

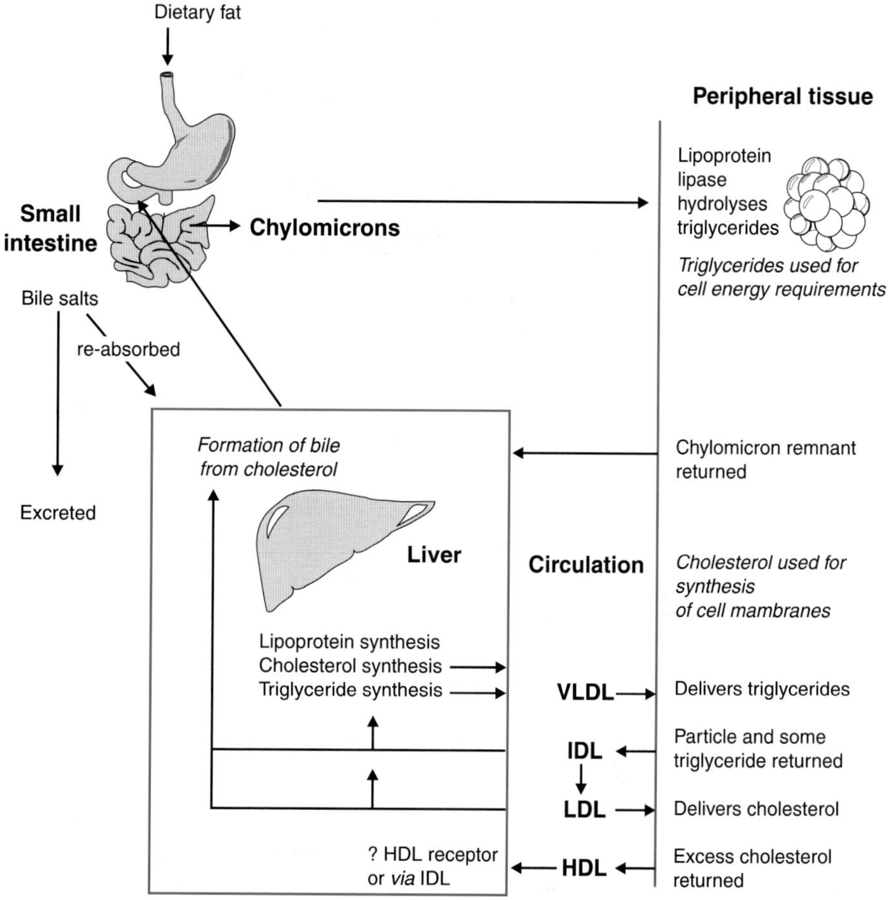

Figure 20.10 Transport and metabolism of lipids and cholesterol. Dietary fats are absorbed in the small intestine and carried to the peripheral tissues in the form of chylomicrons. Fatty acids are removed by the action of lipoprotein lipase, leaving a chylomicron remnant containing residual triglyceride and cholesterol derived from the diet. In the liver the triglycerides and cholesterol are coupled to apolipoproteins to form VLDL. Cholesterol is carried in the blood on LDL to the peripheral tissues, where it is needed to carry out essential functions such as the synthesis of cell membranes. Excess cholesterol in the peripheral tissues is carried back to the liver in the form of HDL (this is why HDL is important in inhibiting atherogenesis – excess cholesterol in the arteries can be cleared by HDL). Much of the cholesterol synthesised by the liver is used to produce bile acids. Anything that encourages the excretion of bile acids will reduce the cholesterol pool, thereby reducing blood concentrations.

binding to a HDL receptor on the cell surfaces. Alternatively, cholesterol esters taken up by HDL are transferred to IDL, which then binds to liver cell LDL receptors. The returned cholesterol is either reprocessed into VLDL particles or used in the production of bile salts.

Precursor HDL particles are mainly assembled and secreted by the liver; small amounts can also be synthesised by intestinal mucosal cells. Once in the circulation, HDL particles are completed by exchanging lipid with other lipoprotein particles.

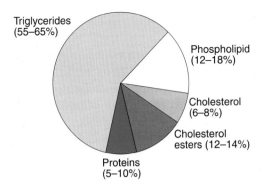

Figure 20.11 Composition of VLDL. VLDL is formed continuously in the liver. The particles mostly comprise triglycerides together with cholesterol and phospholipids. They contain more protein than the chylomicrons.

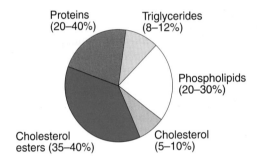

Figure 20.12 Composition of LDL. LDL results from the progressive removal of triglyceride from VLDL and IDL. It is a smaller particle, with a greater proportion of protein. About 50% of the LDL particle is cholesterol and its esters.

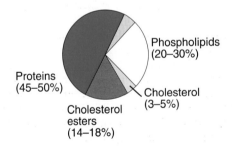

Figure 20.13 Composition of HDL. HDL is the smallest of the lipoproteins and contains the largest proportion of protein.

There are three types of HDL: HDL_1, HDL_2 and HDL_3. Phospholipids and cholesterol that remain after the depletion of triglyceride-rich particles are usually transferred to HDL, particularly the small HDL_3 particle. In turn this becomes transformed in the circulation to a larger HDL_2 particle. Plasma levels of the HDL_2 particle, carrying esterified cholesterol, are inversely related to risk of CHD.

Genetic influences in lipid metabolism

Because lipids must be transported by a carrier protein inappropriate production of these proteins can play havoc with the balance of lipids and cholesterol in the plasma and peripheral tissues. Inherited disturbances of lipid metabolism are derived from abnormalities in the apolipoproteins, lipoprotein receptors or enzymes such as lipoprotein lipase (since genes code for proteins, not lipids). The result is either an abnormal increase (**hyperlipoproteinaemia**) or decrease (**hypolipoproteinaemia**) in the concentration of specific lipoproteins.

These defects may often be diagnosed by quantifying the various lipid moieties but a more accurate assessment is obtained by estimating the amount of the relevant protein or its activity. Levels of apo A-I, apo B-100, and Lp(a) can be used to determine the risk of premature CHD. People with defects in the apo A-I gene fail to synthesise the apolipoprotein and have virtually no HDL in their plasma.

Lipid can be exchanged between carrier particles and cells only if the cells have the receptors appropriate for those particles. The elaboration of cell receptors is under genetic control, and if there are too few receptors the plasma will contain increased amounts of the particular lipoproteins.

Risk factors

There is no single cause of atherosclerosis: it is produced by a combination of genetic susceptibility and risk factors. Some of these risk factors can be altered by changes in lifestyle and behaviour, some are more difficult to alter and may require treatment with drugs, others cannot be altered.

Many epidemiological studies have attempted to identify the agents that contribute to CHD. Over the past four decades about 246 risk factors have been associated with this disease. One of the longest-running studies is the Framingham study, initiated during the early 1950s in Framingham, Massachusetts, USA.

The risk factors identified as being of importance in CHD operate at different phases in the disease process. The main processes involved in CHD are atherosclerosis and thrombosis. Some risk factors increase the tendency for the arterial wall to become damaged and infiltrated with lipid; others influence the tendency of blood to clot and produce thrombosis. Many single risk factors, such as smoking, influence both these processes (Figure 20.14).

Thrombosis

Thrombosis is influenced by three principal mechanisms, often referred to in pathology texts as **Virchow's triad**:

- Changes to the intimal surface (for example atherosclerosis or cellular injury)

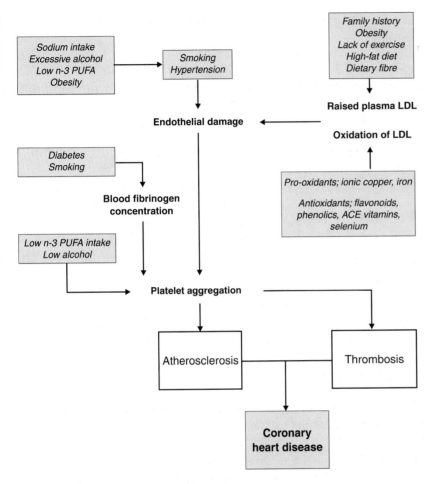

Figure 20.14 Pathological processes and risk factors in CHD. The underlying causes of CHD are atherosclerosis and thrombosis. Dietary factors influence a variety of events in the atherosclerotic process and the tendency for platelet aggregation. Other factors, such as family history and smoking, are also important.

- Blood flow (for example blood turbulence at arterial branches)
- Changes to blood constituents (for example increased platelet aggregation)

Atherosclerosis

Usually atherosclerosis is unsuspected until angina or a heart attack occurs. However, the atherosclerotic process will have been under way for many years, influenced by exposure to risk factors. The process of atherosclerosis usually begins with damage to the endothelium (the cell lining of the vessel wall).

Risk factors can influence the development of atherosclerosis by altering endothelial damage produced by inflammation or high blood pressure, and by

affecting the concentration of plasma lipoproteins and their propensity for oxidation.

Plasma cholesterol concentration

Total plasma cholesterol is a measure of cholesterol, including that in HDL and LDL

One of the most important risk factors in atherosclerosis is total plasma cholesterol concentration. The adverse effects of high plasma cholesterol concentrations hold for all the clinical outcomes of atherosclerosis such as stroke and peripheral arterial disease as well as CHD (Figure 20.15).

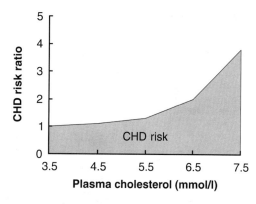

Figure 20.15 Plasma cholesterol concentration and CHD. Total plasma cholesterol levels above 5.2 mmol/l are associated with increased risks of coronary heart disease. (Source: Framingham Heart Study.)

> ### ▲ Key points
>
> **Blood cholesterol concentrations**
> ___
> ▲ Ideal below 5.2 mmol/l
> ▲ Marginal risk 5.2–6.4 mmol/l: give standard dietary advice
> ▲ Intermediate risk 6.5–7.8 mmol/l: dietary and other risk factor intervention needed
> ▲ High risk >7.8 mmol/l: dietary intervention essential and drug treatment may also be needed

There are four main tenets of the lipid hypothesis:
* A high intake of fat, especially of saturated fatty acids, leads to a high concentration of plasma LDL
* High plasma cholesterol concentrations lead to high mortality rates from CHD and stroke
* Reducing dietary intake of fat, especially saturated fatty acids, lowers the plasma concentrations of total and LDL-cholesterol
* Reducing plasma LDL leads to reductions in risk of deaths from CHD and stroke

Some alterable risk factors affect plasma cholesterol concentrations

Plasma cholesterol concentrations can be modified by lifestyle factors which include diet, smoking, stress, exercise and body weight. In addition, a number of factors cannot be changed (or at best are only partially modifiable): age, gender, race, family history, diabetes mellitus, obesity, hypertension and personality type. Some of these risk factors may also act independently of plasma lipoproteins. For example, smoking also influences atherosclerosis because chemical components of smoke in the blood irritate the endothelial lining of the arterial wall.

Up to 70% of the British population have total plasma cholesterol concentrations over the ideal limit of 5.2 mmol/l. People who have consistently raised cholesterol concentrations should modify their lifestyle risk factors or

seek treatment (see Chapter 12).

Because they function to remove and transport cholesterol from the tissues, HDL protects against atherogenesis. Epidemiological studies indicate that plasma HDL concentrations are inversely related to risk of coronary heart disease in both sexes (Figure 20.16). A 1% decrease in HDL cholesterol is associated with a 3–4% increase in the risk of coronary heart disease.

> *The ratio of HDL to LDL is probably more important in determining CHD risk than total cholesterol concentration*

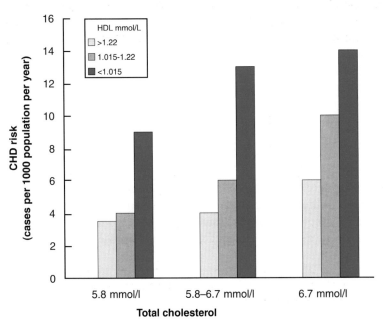

Figure 20.16 Plasma HDL, total cholesterol and CHD. Risk of CHD increases with total cholesterol concentration, particularly when HDL levels are low (<1.015 mmol/l). (Data from: Kannel, 1988.)

Although high total cholesterol concentration is an important risk factor, it should not be treated in isolation. Mortality rates will be reduced only by an overall reduction in lifestyle risk factors. At any given total cholesterol concentration there is considerable variation in the clinical expression of atherosclerosis. Hence, the current widespread promotion and adoption of cholesterol screening tests in the UK may falsely reassure many people: a complete lifestyle and risk factor profile is needed for each individual. The estimation of plasma cholesterol levels alone is a poor predictor of who will develop CHD.

> *Some risk factors operate independently and do not simply affect cholesterol levels*

Triglycerides

The role of triglycerides in coronary heart disease is controversial. They probably do not act as an independent risk factor but become relevant in conditions of insulin resistance, notably diabetes mellitus. Present recommendations are that total plasma triglyceride concentrations should not

exceed 1.5 mmol/l.

Plasma fibrinogen

High concentrations of plasma fibrinogen is an independent risk factor for CHD. One factor in the development of atherosclerotic plaques, and more importantly as a cause of sudden myocardial infarction, is thrombosis. High plasma concentrations of fibrinogen increase the propensity of the blood to clot. Fibrinogen also contributes to platelet stickiness and plasma viscosity, which in turn contributes to atheroma progression and thrombosis. Other blood coagulation components such as factor VI and factor VIII, and the haemolytic system (factors involved in dissolving blood clots) probably also affect risk of CHD.

Unmodifiable risk factors

Age and gender

CHD accounts for 36% of deaths in men aged 45–64 years, but only 10% of deaths in women of this age

The risk of developing atherosclerosis and its complications rises with age, as plasma total cholesterol levels rise with age. In men this continues until about 50 years of age; in women, cholesterol values peak at a later age and after the menopause levels greatly exceed those in men of similar age (Figure 20.17).

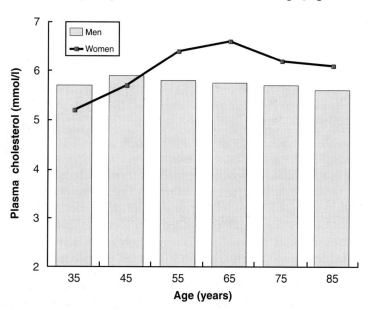

Figure 20.17 Variation in plasma total cholesterol concentration in men and women with age. In young and middle-aged men the average total blood cholesterol concentration is generally lower than in women of comparable age. After the menopause the cholesterol concentration in women is consistently higher than in men of similar age. (Source: Framingham Heart Study.)

Before the menopause, oestrogen helps to keep total cholesterol levels low,

with a relatively high level of HDL. Oestrogens raise the levels of HDL-cholesterol by increasing the synthesis of the carrier protein (apo A1) in the liver. After the menopause LDL-cholesterol and triglyceride levels increase while HDL levels remain fairly constant, or show only slight reductions (Figure 20.18). Hormone replacement therapy reverses the trend, reducing total and LDL-cholesterol and increasing HDL_2 cholesterol.

Women tend to develop heart disease later in life than men, with a lag in morbidity and mortality rates of about 10 years. After the menopause, morbidity rates in women increase and eventually match the rate for men.

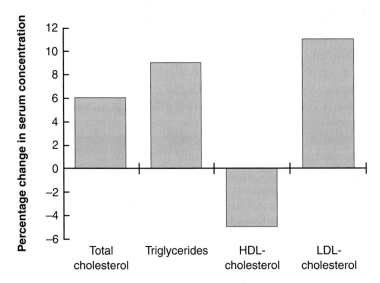

Figure 20.18 Changes in serum lipid and lipoprotein at menopause. Loss of oestrogen at the menopause causes significant changes in blood cholesterol concentration. Total and LDL cholesterol and triglycerides are generally increased, whereas there is a slight fall in HDL concentration. (Data from Jensen, J. *Baillière's Clinical Obstetrics and Gynaecology*, Vol. 5, No. 4, published by Baillière Tindall, 1991.)

Race
In the USA the death rates for coronary heart disease are higher in black people than in whites, probably because black people tend to have higher blood pressures.

The difference in both hypertension and CHD rates may be attributed to socioeconomic disadvantage and concomitant variations in diet, smoking prevalence, alcohol consumption and stress. In addition, there is a possible genetic cause related to the production of endothelin, a protein that constricts blood vessels. Healthy blacks and whites have about the same circulating levels of endothelin, but black people with hypertension have markedly raised levels compared with healthy black, healthy white and hypertensive white people.

Family history and genetic susceptibility
The risk of myocardial infarction or CHD is influenced by family history.

Children are at increased risk if either parent developed CHD before the age of 60 years. The risk does not increase if the disease occurred in a parent older than 60.

The genetic risks of developing CHD involve regulation of lipid metabolism and the propensity of platelets to stick together. Platelet aggregation is influenced by a platelet surface receptor called glycoprotein IIb/IIIa; slight alterations to this glycoprotein enhance the ability of platelets to bind with coagulation factors such as fibrinogen. About 20% of the American population carry the genetic polymorphism for this altered protein but in a study at the Johns Hopkins hospital (Weiss *et al.*, 1996) nearly 40% of patients who had been admitted for heart attack or severe angina carried the polymorphism.

Another inherited determinant of risk is the plasma concentration of Lp(a). This modified LDL particle is present in serum at 0.01–2 g/l. Much of this variation is genetically determined, although levels can be influenced to some extent by diet. Concentrations over 0.3 g/l occur in about 20% of white people; their risk of CHD increases by a factor of two. If high Lp(a) concentrations are accompanied by raised LDL levels the risk estimate increases further. The risk attached to Lp(a) is due to its property of promoting blood coagulation and, therefore, atheroma progression and thrombosis.

Hyperlipidaemia or hyperlipoproteinaemia is usually caused by a combination of environmental factors with genetic susceptibility. In some people the genetic factors are so dominant that atherosclerosis develops regardless of lifestyle. Inherited defects are referred to as the **familial** or **primary** hyperlipidaemias, of which the several types have been classified by the World Health Organization according to the lipid present in excess. Conditions caused by an excess of cholesterol are referred to as **hypercholesterolaemias**; those involving an excess of triglyceride are the **hypertriglyceridaemias**.

Familial hypercholesterolaemia

This inherited disorder is caused by a deficiency of LDL receptors. As a result markedly high plasma LDL concentrations occur from birth, and atherosclerosis arises at an early age. The heterozygous form of the gene occurs in one in 500 people, and affected individuals develop CHD about 20 years earlier than would be expected in the general population. The disorder has other signs beyond its effect on blood cholesterol concentration: cholesterol becomes deposited in the cornea (**corneal arcus**), in the tendons (**tendon xanthomata**) and eyelids as yellow plaques or nodules (**xanthelasma**).

The homozygous form of the gene is extremely rare (about one in a million people) and patients have no LDL receptors. Without drug therapy these individuals do not survive beyond their early twenties, and myocardial infarcts have been reported in children as young as 18 months.

Familial mixed hyperlipidaemia

This disorder affects about one in 200 individuals and causes excessive synthesis of VLDL. It is associated with an increased risk of atherosclerosis, and roughly 15% of deaths from CHD in people under 65 are caused by this condition.

Familial type III hyperlipoproteinaemia

This relatively rare disorder (incidence one in 5000) features accumulation of chylomicron and VLDL remnants in plasma which are not cleared by the liver at the normal rate. The uptake by the liver depends on interaction between the remnant and LDL receptors. Normally lipoprotein particles bind with LDL receptors by their apo E protein component. In type III hyperlipoproteinaemia patients have a less active form of apo E and uptake of the remnants is slower. The result is an increased concentration of plasma triglycerides and cholesterol, causing corneal arcus, xanthelasma, **tuberoeruptive xanthomata** (groups of yellow nodules in the skin over the joints) and **palmar striae** (yellow raised streaks across the palms of the hands). Patients are also predisposed to the early development of atherosclerosis.

Familial lipoprotein lipase deficiency

Deficiency of lipoprotein lipase reduces the ability to use the triglycerides carried by chylomicrons and VLDL and these components accumulate in the plasma. Affected individuals usually present in childhood with abdominal pain, enlarged spleen, eruptive xanthomata and retinal deposition of lipid (**lipaemia retinalis**). Because the defect concerns triglyceride, rather than cholesterol, metabolism there is no increase in susceptibility to atherosclerosis. The main complication is acute pancreatitis. The disorder occurs in one person per million.

Familial apo C-II deficiency

Apo C-II, one of the protein components of chylomicrons and VLDL, activates lipoprotein lipase so that triglycerides carried by these particles can be liberated. In heterozygotes lipoprotein lipase activity is 50–80% of normal, which is sufficient to maintain normal plasma lipid levels. Homozygotes cannot activate lipoprotein lipase at all, and plasma concentrations of triglyceride are extremely high. The usual complication is acute pancreatitis.

Partially modifiable risk factors

Secondary hyperlipidaemia

A number of conditions (including certain disease states or drug treatments) alter blood lipid profiles as a secondary effect. The impact of these conditions on an individual's lipid profile will also depend on other risk factors such as a person's genetic predisposition for hyperlipidaemia and dietary habits. Usually, a modification of the initiating condition, by treating the disease for example, will also correct the altered lipid profile. The most notable disease states that produce secondary hyperlipidaemia are diabetes, hypothyroidism, chronic renal failure and obesity. Some of these conditions (diabetes for one) exert additional effects on risk of CHD that are independent of the hyperlipidaemia.

Diabetes

Atherosclerosis and its related diseases are more common in patients with insulin-dependent or non-insulin-dependent diabetes: at all ages incidence of CHD in diabetics is approximately double that for non-diabetic men, and three times that for non-diabetic women. Many diabetics have other conditions, including obesity, hypertension and hyperlipidaemia which themselves increase risk. Nevertheless, diabetes is an independent risk factor: it has its own unique effect in worsening the risk.

Diabetes (see Chapter 23) is a disorder of carbohydrate, lipid and protein metabolism. Insulin lowers plasma triglyceride levels, probably by inhibiting liver synthesis of VLDL and reducing the activity of lipoprotein lipase. People with poorly controlled diabetes often have severe hypertriglyceridaemia. This is more likely in non-insulin-dependent diabetes, since insulin control is the norm in insulin-dependent diabetics.

The increased prevalence of CHD in diabetics is probably also caused by the higher blood levels of fibrinogen, which increases the likelihood of thrombus formation. The control of glucose in diabetic patients does not markedly reduce the risks of CHD. Because of the magnifying effect of risk factors when placed together, diabetics should pay particular attention to their general lifestyle risk factors that apply to the rest of the population (smoking, diet and exercise).

Lipid disturbances and a greater predisposition for thrombosis contribute to the greater prevalence of deaths from CHD in diabetics

Hypothyroidism

Altered blood lipid profiles are commonly seen in patients with untreated hypothyroidism. The usual outcome is hypercholesterolaemia, but severe hypertriglyceridaemia is also found in some patients. These abnormalities are usually resolved by thyroid hormone replacement therapy.

Hypothyroidism: functional disorder caused by deficiency of circulating thyroid hormones. Primary hypothyroidism is congenital (cretinism) or acquired. Secondary hypothyroidism is caused by deficiency of hypothalamic or pituitary thyroid-stimulating hormones. Classic symptoms are mental slowness, dry thin hair, slow heart action (bradycardia) and pericardial effusion.

Chronic renal failure

This is one condition in which the commonly available treatments do not resolve the secondary hyperlipidaemia. Patients with chronic renal failure usually have hypertriglyceridaemia in the pretreatment phase, or after undergoing haemodialysis or peritoneal dialysis. The hypertriglyceridaemia is caused by reduction in lipoprotein lipase activity.

Obesity

Obesity is associated with a number of deleterious health effects including glucose intolerance, hypertension and altered blood lipid profiles. All of these will themselves influence the risk of developing atherosclerosis. Controlling for these and other variables such as smoking still shows obesity to be an independent risk factor, with a twofold increase in CHD risk for those who are 20% or more above their ideal body weight. Even mild or moderately overweight people display an increased risk.

There is some correlation between body fat distribution and CHD; abdominal fat appears to be associated with increased risk of myocardial

Obesity and overweight cause a number of health problems, including CHD

infarction.

It is not clear whether losing weight has any impact on risk of deaths from CHD. The problem is that most people sustain their weight loss for only a short period relative to the timescales that operate in the pathogenesis of CHD.

Hypertension

The risk of CHD is increased in hypertensive people: the higher the blood pressure the greater the risk. Hypertension can influence the process of atherosclerosis in the cerebral arteries (or example by causing endothelial damage), which in turn can lead to ischaemic stroke. Hypertension is also a major risk factor for haemorrhagic stroke (see Chapter 12).

Hypertension increases the risk of CHD at any plasma cholesterol level, but there is little evidence that drug treatment of hypertension reduces the risks. A possible reason for this is that many of the drugs employed, such as the thiazide diuretics and β-blockers, adversely affect blood lipid profiles and may counteract any advantages obtained by reducing blood pressure. Other strategies to reduce hypertension, such as the control of diet, smoking and stress, undoubtedly also affect risk of CHD.

Blood pressure increases with age – one in five adults become hypertensive

Diastolic pressure: blood pressure at the moment the heart relaxes between contractions.

Hypertension: consistent elevation of blood pressure. Defined as a systolic blood pressure equal to or greater than 160 mmHg, and/or diastolic blood pressure equal to or greater than 95 mmHg.

Systolic pressure: peak pressure at the moment the ventricles contract.

Personality type and behaviour

Type A behaviour (chronic sense of urgency) is believed to carry a greater risk of CHD than the more placid Type B behaviour, although the evidence is inconclusive. Although there is little potential for altering personality, the risk could be lowered by avoiding stressful situations. Socioeconomic circumstances, however, make it impossible for some people to avoid stress. Other effects which may be contingent on personality type, such as social isolation and expression of hostility, are also believed to influence risk of CHD.

Modifiable risk factors

A number of CHD risk factors are controllable although in practice this is often easier said than done, particularly when it concerns giving up smoking or cutting down on alcohol consumption.

Cigarette smoking

The risk of atherosclerosis rises in proportion to the number of cigarettes a person smokes. Overall epidemiological data for the UK show that the risk of a fatal heart attack is three times greater in smokers than in non-smokers. This risk improves on cessation of smoking and 3–5 years after ceasing the risks are similar to those for people who have never smoked. Smoking is in decline in some groups of the population; this may explain why mortality rates from CHD are decreasing for middle-aged men in the UK. Unfortunately the prevalence of smoking in females, particularly teenage girls, has not decreased.

There is a dose–response relationship between risk of CHD, duration of smoking and number of cigarettes smoked

▲ **Key points**

Benefits of exercise

▲ Increased cardiac strength
▲ Weight reduction
▲ Increased muscle mass, reduces fat
▲ Regression of atheroma
▲ Improved blood clotting profile
▲ Improved blood lipid profile
▲ Lower mean blood pressure
▲ Results in a sexy look!

Smoking influences a number of mechanisms involved in the production of CHD, most notably damage to the arterial walls by carbon monoxide and metabolites carried in the bloodstream, reducing plasma HDL and increasing plasma triglycerides. Smoking may also affect platelet aggregation by increasing plasma fibrinogen levels.

A further effect is depletion of antioxidant vitamins, particularly vitamin C, which contributes to free radical damage of the vascular endothelium and oxidation of LDL. Unfortunately for smokers, studies indicate (Chapter 7) that vitamin supplementation does not negate the adverse health effects of smoking. It is interesting to note that although cigarette smoking is common in Japan coronary artery disease is relatively rare because the concentrations of plasma cholesterol are generally low in the Japanese population. In other populations where blood cholesterol levels are generally higher, probably the most influential effect of smoking is toxic damage to the arterial wall, allowing excessive amounts of cholesterol and other agents across.

Active people are less likely to suffer heart attacks than people who lead sedentary lives

Physical activity

The classic study relating activity levels to risk of heart disease was undertaken among drivers and conductors of London double-decker buses (Morris, 1989). The drivers were far more likely to suffer heart attacks than the conductors.

Exercise increases general physical fitness, with benefits to the heart in lowering blood pressure and pulse rate and in increasing collateral circulation. It also reduces body weight and adrenergic stress. Exercise can also alter blood parameters; lower triglyceride levels increase HDL concentrations and decrease platelet adhesiveness. Exercise also improves general physical and mental well-being and improves self-esteem (Chapter 1). It can help to sustain motivation and adherence to other lifestyle modifications. For example, ex-smokers often find that participation in exercise can help combat their urge to return to smoking.

The precise amount and type of exercise required to achieve these benefits is not known. There is much individual variation and most epidemiological studies have simply compared self-reports of sedentary individuals and highly active people. Overall, moderate-to-high activity levels, at least 30 minutes three times a week (or the equivalent of running 10 miles a week) are required. Recent activity is more important than past activity, but this needs to be carried out for 6–12 months before any real improvement in blood lipoprotein levels is seen.

▲ **Key points**

Influence of smoking on CHD

▲ Reduces plasma HDL levels and increases triglycerides
▲ Increases blood fibrinogen levels, enhances platelet aggregation, rendering blood more likely to clot
▲ Nicotine and carbon monoxide injure endothelial cells, enhancing deposition of fibrin and lipids within artery walls

Diet and CHD

In the past the focus of dietary advice for reducing the risk of CHD was to modify fat intakes: plasma concentrations of total and LDL-cholesterol can be influenced by dietary cholesterol, polyunsaturated fatty acids and saturated fatty acids. Other dietary factors, such as antioxidants and fish oils, are also important in influencing atherosclerosis and thrombosis. These are discussed in Chapter 7.

Pro-oxidants

Epidemiological studies have revealed that consumption of large quantities of antioxidants may be protective against CHD. However, antioxidants can be neutralised by excessive generation of free radicals. Some chemical agents, or **pro-oxidants**, are efficient inducers of free radicals.

The most important of these are the chemicals found in the blood of smokers, although pro-oxidants are also present in the diet, most notably as the ionic forms of copper or iron. Both these ions have the capacity to oxidise LDL but are usually prevented from initiating free radical generation because they are bound to the plasma proteins transferrin and ceruloplasmin. Nevertheless, the atherogenic effect of high plasma LDL-cholesterol may be enhanced in the presence of high concentrations of copper. Men with high serum ferritin concentrations (this indicates a large iron store) are more likely to suffer a heart attack, particularly if their LDL-cholesterol levels are also high.

Salt

Consumption of salt (sodium chloride) is a major determinant of the age-related increase in blood pressure found in some populations and hypertension is a well recognised risk factor for atherosclerosis, stroke and CHD. There is, however, great variation in blood pressure among individuals with similar salt intake, because of other influential factors such as genetics, age and obesity. A daily salt intake of about 1.6 mg will meet the needs of most people. In susceptible adults, more than 3.2 g per day may raise blood pressure. Reducing salt intake can decrease blood pressure, although the effects may be only minor in some hypertensives, and there is often no effect whatever in normotensive people. Generally, weight loss has a far greater effect on reducing blood pressure than salt restriction. Systolic blood pressure increases by about 0.8 mmHg for each unit increase in BMI. An obese person with a BMI of 40 could have a systolic blood pressure 16 mmHg higher than someone whose BMI is 20.

Alcohol

Moderate alcohol consumption is believed to have a beneficial effect on risk of CHD. Recent attention has focused on what has become known as the 'French paradox' – deaths from CHD are much fewer in France than in other developed countries, despite the fact that risk factors such as consumption of saturated fats, blood pressure, BMI and cigarette smoking are broadly similar (Figures 20.19 and 20.20). Early studies indicated that alcohol raises HDL concentrations and thus limits atherogenesis. Alcohol also affects platelet aggregation. However, blood concentrations of HDL are no higher in France than in other countries.

The protective effect appears to be associated mainly with the consumption of red wine; other alcoholic beverages such as white wine or beer do not offer the same advantage. This suggests that the alcohol content is not the only important factor. What differentiates red wine from other alcoholic drinks is the presence of phenolic compounds and flavonoids, which have antioxidant

In moderation, consumption of some alcohol can reduce the risk of CHD

The benefit may not be solely because of the alcohol content: red wine contains phenolic compounds which have antioxidant properties

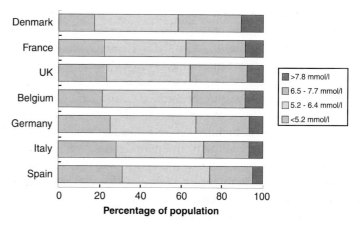

Figure 20.19 MONICA study: age-standardised cholesterol concentrations in men aged 36–64 years. The plasma cholesterol concentrations in the populations of France and the UK are broadly similar. (Source: *WHO World Health Statistics Annual*, 1989.)

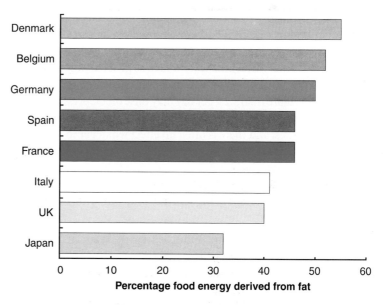

Figure 20.20 Food energy derived from fat. Despite their relatively higher fat consumption and blood cholesterol concentrations, CHD mortality rates are lower in French people than in British.

properties. The benefit is believed to be by inhibiting the oxidation of LDL and blood clotting.

The French paradox may have other explanations: differences in fruit and vegetable consumption, higher intakes of olive oil and reduced intake of *trans* fatty acids, and exposure to sunlight (vitamin D production in the skin uses a metabolite of cholesterol as a precursor).

Excessive alcohol consumption is not so benign, and increases the risk of cardiovascular disease (see Figure 2.12). Ethanol and its metabolite, acetaldehyde, has deleterious effects on both the circulatory system and the heart itself. Even moderate quantities of alcohol increase heart rate and dysrhythmias, which can be dangerous in people with heart disease.

Chronic excessive consumption of alcohol increases systolic and diastolic blood pressure. The precise mechanisms for this are unclear, but include alterations in vascular membrane permeability and vascular tissue responsiveness to constrictor agents. **Alcoholic heart muscle disease** is characterised by enlargement of the heart, dilation of the left ventricle and contractile abnormalities and, eventually, leads to heart failure. These effects reflect damage to the heart muscle by acetaldehyde, causing structural alterations and changes in cardiac enzymes.

▲ **Key points**

Principal risk factors for atherosclerosis and their mode of action

Risk factors	Action
Unmodifiable:	
Genetics	Lipid transport: production of apolipoproteins
Age: Men	Total cholesterol levels rise until middle age
Age: Women	Total cholesterol rises until menopause, then rises above the levels for men
Partially modifiable:	
Diabetes	High blood fibrinogen levels increase thrombosis risk
Hypertension	Endothelial damage
Obesity	Associated with increased total and LDL-cholesterol
Modifiable:	
Tobacco smoking	Endothelial damage, platelet aggregation, reduction of HDL-cholesterol
Diet	Influences blood lipid profiles and platelet aggregation
Physical activity	Reduces total and LDL-cholesterol
Alcohol consumption (moderate)	Increases HDL-cholesterol

Early risk factors

Some of the environmental risk factors for atherosclerosis exert their effects very early on in life. There is a north–south divide for CHD rates in the UK and, although there are some regional differences in the smoking and eating habits of adults, these do not fully account for the different CHD rates. It is logical, therefore, to look for differences that may be present in the earlier stages of life. Of interest is that past neonatal mortality and present mortality

▲ **Key points**

Possible explanations for 'French paradox'

▲ Phenolics and flavonoids inhibit LDL oxidation
▲ Alcohol increases plasma HDL concentration
▲ Higher intake of olive oil – reduces susceptibility of LDL to oxidation and contains antioxidants
▲ Higher intake of fruit and vegetables
▲ 'Sunshine factor'

Review question 2

Why is it important to control more than one modifiable CHD risk factor?

▲ **Key points**

CHD risk factors in early life

▲ Past neonatal mortality rates correlate with present CHD rates
▲ Association with low birthweight, maternal nutritional state and general health
▲ Deprivation and retarded growth in early phases of development may have long-term physiological effects
▲ The type of milk given as a baby and the age of weaning may influence blood lipid profiles
▲ Blood lipid profiles established in early life track through into adulthood

from CHD and stroke in the elderly population appear to be correlated. The characteristics of the high neonatal mortality rates in the past were low birthweight, and mothers with poor physique, nutritional state and general health. The observed association may not be causal, but retarded growth in early life due to an adverse environment during a critical period of development may cause long-term effects on physiology and metabolism and influence the risk of disease in adulthood.

Saturated fats given at an early age can determine blood lipid profiles for many years

Susceptibility for CHD may also be linked to how a baby is fed and to the age of weaning: the amount of cholesterol and saturated fat fed to infants can influence lipid metabolism throughout life. In a retrospective study of the breast and bottle feeding histories of men born between 1928 and 1930, those who had been weaned before they were 1 year old had lower mean serum total cholesterol levels than men who had been weaned later, and fewer men in the earlier-weaned group died from CHD. The type of milk may also be influential as there were fewer deaths from CHD in the men who were breast fed.

Risk factors in fetal and neonatal life may influence risk of developing CHD in the adult

Plasma cholesterol level in infancy appears to be a predictor of the cholesterol level in adult life. As high total cholesterol levels correlate with risk for CHD it may be beneficial to attempt to modify lifestyle risk factors before adulthood. With respect to dietary modifications concerns have been expressed that giving high-fibre low-energy foods to young children could lead to undernutrition and deficiencies of fat-soluble vitamins. The indications are that while normal growth and development should not be affected there can be adverse affects such as diarrhoea in younger children.

Pathogenesis

Plaques contain lipid and fibrous connective tissue

The typical lesion of atherosclerosis is a fibrofatty plaque (atheroma) in the intimal layer of the arterial wall. The plaque is a raised structure containing lipid, most notably cholesterol and its esters, and phospholipids, with a proliferation of collagenous and elastic connective tissues. The relative content of lipid and fibrous material varies depending on the artery affected (plaques in coronary arteries tend to be more fibrous) and the evolutionary stage of the plaque. This plaque narrows the artery, predisposes to thrombosis and weakens the artery wall so that an aneurysm may form.

The first histologically recognisable change in the intima and inner media is development of the **fatty streak**, a yellowed area containing lipid-laden foam cells (macrophages that have become engorged with lipid). In the aorta fatty streaks begin to appear during the first few years of life; in the coronary arteries they can be seen from about the second decade.

Plaques may develop from precursor fatty streaks, but this is controversial

There is controversy over whether fatty streaks truly represent an initial change in the atherogenic process because the location of the fatty streaks is not always the same as that of the fibrous plaques. For example, fatty streaks are more numerous in the thoracic aorta in children but fibrous plaques of adults are more common in the abdominal aorta. In certain locations fatty streaks might develop and then disappear or remain harmless, but in some predisposed individuals evolve into fibrofatty plaques. Epidemiological studies

show that the frequency of fatty streaks and fibrofatty plaques differ. Fatty streaks have been found in people throughout the world, but the prevalence of atherosclerosis has a more distinctive geographical distribution.

The appearance of both fatty streaks and fibrofatty plaques has been incorporated into a **response to injury** hypothesis of atherosclerosis. A further hypothesis is known as the **lipid infiltration** hypothesis. Both of these correlate well with the pathological and clinical findings in atherosclerosis and the known risk factors for the disease.

The response to injury hypothesis suggests that the arterial surface (endothelium) is injured, by local disturbance in blood flow at certain points near to bends and branches (which correspond to areas known to be susceptible to plaque development), by irritants in tobacco smoke or by a variety of other infectious, immunological or chemical agents. Hypercholesterolaemia may itself make endothelial injury more likely by altering the properties of the endothelial cell membrane. Injury to endothelial cells alters the permeability of the vessel wall, so that excessive amounts of lipids accumulate in the intima. Normally these are taken up by macrophages and other cells, giving the foam cells characteristic of fatty streaks. Much of the lipid that is taken up by these cells, or at least that which is most potentially damaging, originates from plasma LDL.

As LDL crosses the endothelium it is oxidised to a highly toxic form. In normal circumstances its uptake by macrophages serves a protective function but if the endothelium is injured the macrophages may become overloaded, cease to function or even die, releasing their cytotoxic LDL. This can further damage the surface-lining endothelial cells, exacerbating the excess load of LDL entering the intima.

Injury to the endothelial surface causes the adherence and aggregation of platelets. **Platelet-derived growth factor** (PDGF), which stimulates the migration and proliferation of smooth muscle cells at the injured site, is released. The smooth muscle cells lay down fibrous connective tissues, ultimately leading to thickening of the intima wall and formation of the fibrofatty plaque.

Even in the absence of endothelial injury some LDL will cross into the intima. If plasma LDL concentration is high excessive amounts of LDL are likely to cross into the intima and overload the normal uptake and metabolism by macrophages. In this situation the extracellular LDL in the intima can be oxidised by oxygen free radicals; endothelial damage could then occur and facilitate the entry of more LDL (Figures 20.21–20.23).

Further developments in the fibrofatty plaques take place over time. The most sinister of these is the tendency of the plaque to become disrupted by a fissure at its junction with the normal arterial wall. The result is an **intraluminal thrombosis**, which may completely occlude the artery. This is a prime cause of acute myocardial infarction and sudden death. Even if complete occlusion does not occur parts of the thrombus can break away, forming an **embolus**, which will travel through the arterial tree until it becomes lodged in a narrower segment (Figure 20.24).

> *Plaques may arise because of large amounts of plasma lipids crossing injured endothelium*

> *Excessive entry of LDL cholesterol can overwhelm the capacity of macrophages to metabolise it*

> *Free LDL in tissues is rapidly oxidised – when this happens the oxidised LDL itself causes cell damage*

> *The aggregation of platelets at the site of endothelial injury can initiate plaque formation*

> *Even without endothelial injury, LDL will enter the arterial wall and cause damage if its plasma concentration is high*

> *Atherosclerotic plaques have a tendency to bleed – the resulting thrombus can completely block the artery*

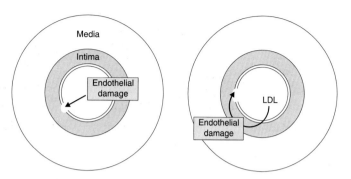

Figure 20.21 Mechanisms of endothelial injury. (a) The endothelium can be damaged from the luminal side by toxic agents carried in the blood or by high blood pressure. (b) Endothelial damage can arise from the intimal side by the cytotoxic action of oxidised LDL

Figure 20.22 Formation of fatty streaks and fibrofatty plaques. Lipid infiltration occurs in circumstances of endothelial injury or when blood concentrations are high. Fibrofatty plaques are likely to occur when there is endothelial injury, causing platelet aggregation and the release of PDGF and other growth factors. Fatty streaks accumulate as a response to lipid infiltration, without significant endothelial injury. (Adapted from Stokes J, Mancini M, eds. *Hypercholesterolaemia: Clinical and Therapeutic Implications*, published by Raven Press, New York, 1988.)

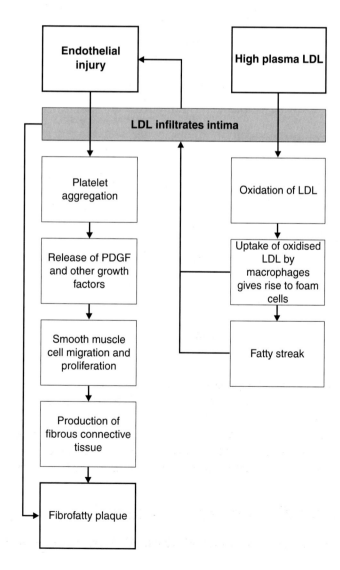

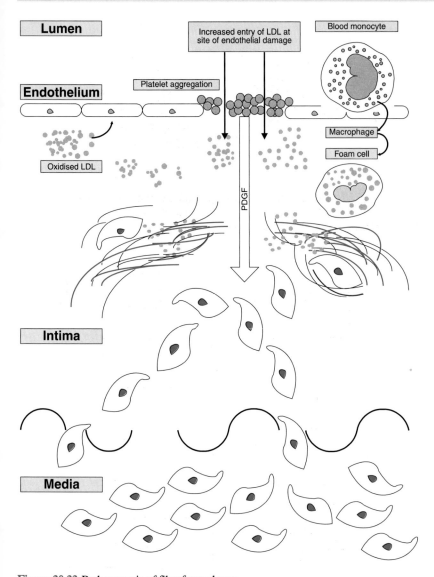

Endothelial damage causes platelet aggregation and the diffusion of PDGF into the media. Plasma LDL infiltrates into the intima. Blood monocytes cross the endothelial layer and differentiate into macrophages

Infiltrated LDL is phagocytosed by macrophages and proliferated smooth muscle cells to produce foam cells. Much of the LDL remains free in the intima and is oxidised. Oxidised LDL is cytotoxic and damages endothelial cells.

Smooth muscle cells migrate from the media and proliferate in response to PDGF. The new cells in the intima secrete connective tissues to form the fibrous component of the plaque

Figure 20.23 Pathogenesis of fibrofatty plaque.

Alternatively, the artery may not be completely occluded and the thrombus remains fixed to the arterial wall. It is then subjected to progressive fibrotic organisation and eventually becomes incorporated into the atherosclerotic plaque. By this means the plaque enlarges so that ultimately it may completely occlude the lumen (also called **stenosis**). These large plaques become necrotic and calcified at their centres, and are referred to as a **complicated lesion**.

> *Plaques can grow by incorporation of thrombotic material*

Complications of atherosclerosis

The complications of atherosclerosis (Table 20.2) arise from the gradual or

> *Atherosclerosis leads to the starvation or death of cells*

Review question 3

Explain the role of antioxidants in lipid metabolism and why they can be of importance in inhibiting atherosclerosis

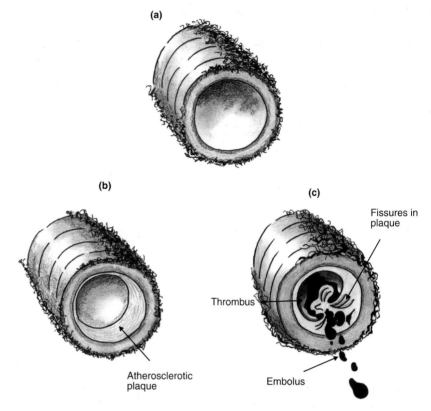

(a)

(b)

(c)

Fissures in plaque

Thrombus

Atherosclerotic plaque

Embolus

Figure 20.24 Plaque formation, arterial stenosis and thrombus. (a) The lumen of a normal artery is completely patent, allowing the free flow of blood to its destination. (b) In atherosclerosis the lumen of the artery is narrowed as a result of thickening in the intimal layer of the arterial wall. If a coronary artery is affected the reduced blood supply leads to angina. (c) The atherosclerotic plaque has a tendency to become partially detached by the pressure of blood. It will then bleed, forming a clot or thrombus, that either further blocks the lumen or is carried to a further point in the arterial network as an embolus.

Intermittent claudication: limping or lameness caused by occlusive arterial disease of the limbs. Pain and weakness commence with walking. Walking becomes impossible unless symptoms are relieved by rest.

sudden occlusion of the affected artery and from haemorrhage. The main effect of gradual occlusion of an artery is **ischaemia** (temporary lack of blood supply, depleting nutrients and oxygen) to those cells supplied by that arterial branch. In the coronary arteries the outcome would be angina pectoris, in other arteries hypertension (renal artery), intermittent muscle claudication (femoral artery for example) or dementia (cerebral artery).

An artery may become occluded suddenly as a result of thrombosis or embolism. If the occlusion is more than transient, or if metabolic requirements cannot at least partially be met by a collateral circulation, the outcome will be **infarction** (cell death). In the coronary arteries the result could be heart failure, or cardiac arrhythmia and sudden death (Figure 20.24). In some arteries the arterial wall is weakened by the atherosclerotic plaque and is susceptible to leakage or rupture; the consequent haemorrhaging is life-threatening, such as

Table 20.2 Complications of atherosclerosis

Affected artery	Gradual occlusion	Sudden occlusion (thrombosis, embolism)	Haemorrhage
Coronary	Angina, heart failure	Myocardial infarction, heart failure	
Cerebral	Dementia	Stroke	Stroke
Aorta			Aneurysm
Peripheral	Intermittent claudication, gangrene		
Renal	Hypertension	Renal infarction	

in stroke or when an aortic aneurysm bursts. For more information on peripheral vascular disease, see Chapter 23.

Angina

The main presenting symptom of coronary atheroma is angina. **Classical** or **exertional** angina becomes apparent as a gripping chest pain and tightness lasting up to 15 minutes. Pain radiates from the chest and may spread to the left arm and be referred to the neck and jaw, abdomen and back. The pain is brought about by exertion or emotional stress and is usually relieved by rest or administration of nitrates. Usually, pain is more readily provoked in the early morning. Other symptoms which may accompany angina include ashen colour, nausea and vomiting, cold and clamminess and light-headedness.

Unstable angina is of sudden (or recent) onset and is more easily provoked or lasts longer than classical angina or fails to respond to treatment. It requires vigorous treatment because many patients develop myocardial infarction within weeks. Unstable angina is probably caused by fissuring of an atherosclerotic plaque with thrombus formation. Other types of angina (decubitus angina, nocturnal angina) have other patterns of onset, usually corresponding to more severe coronary artery disease.

Angina is caused by myocardial ischaemia, a temporary insufficiency of blood supply

Acute myocardial infarction

Acute myocardial infarction is usually caused by sudden occlusion of a coronary artery by thrombus. This can cause death (infarction) of the heart muscle cells in the portion of the heart supplied by that arterial branch. The amount of heart muscle affected depends on the distribution of the artery, the degree of spontaneous recanalisation and the presence of a collateral circulation. It can take some time for the damage to spread to the full thickness of ventricular

When the blood supply to heart muscle is cut off the cells die; this is a heart attack (myocardial infarction)

> *Myocardial infarction is more serious than ischaemia – dead heart muscle cannot be replaced*

Dyspnoea: laboured or difficult breathing. Indicates inadequate ventilation of the lungs or insufficient oxygen in the circulating blood.

wall and if recanalisation occurs early enough the damage may be limited.

The chest pain caused by a myocardial infarction is more intense and prolonged than that of angina and is not relieved by resting. Other symptoms include **dyspnoea** caused by pulmonary congestion, nausea and vomiting (which can last from several minutes to days) and shock, which may lead to loss of consciousness. Blood pressure may be lowered because of damage to the left ventricle, or raised because of anxiety. Cardiac arrest is likely if the patient is not treated quickly. If a wide area of the heart is affected the normal pattern of electrical activity is disrupted, causing the heart to go into spasm (**arrhythmia**). This is a prime cause of sudden cardiac death.

▲ Key points

Correlation of arterial pathology with cardiac complications and symptoms

Event	Complications or symptoms
Fatty streak	Asymptomatic
Partial occlusion by plaque	Angina, fissure of plaque at edges leads to bleeding – thrombosis
Complete occlusion by thrombus	Myocardial infarction, sudden death
Incorporation of thrombus into enlarged plaque	Angina, myocardial infarction, heart failure
Necrosis in centre of plaque and calcification	Angina, myocardial infarction, heart failure

---

Heart failure

> *Heart failure occurs when the heart has difficulty in pumping out sufficient blood to meet all metabolic requirements of the body*

Most cases of heart failure occur because of progressive deterioration in the contractile functions of the heart, usually as a result of ischaemic injury. The outcome is reduced cardiac output, while the blood in the veins is dammed back, causing oedema in the tissues. As a response to the loss of function of injured or dead heart muscle cells, the surrounding cells increase in size (hypertrophy). Ultimately the heart becomes grossly enlarged. The enlarged heart will itself have increased metabolic requirements, becoming an added burden. The overall effect is a downward slide in the stroke volume and output of the heart, terminating in death.

As cardiac output is lost it becomes more difficult to return the blood to the heart and the veins become congested. Pressure in the veins is relieved by passage of plasma into the tissues – this causes the oedema. In the pulmonary circulation the fluid eventually finds its way into the alveolar spaces of the lung, causing decreased lung function and breathlessness.

> *Breathlessness is often seen in patients with heart failure*

The presence and increasing severity of heart failure is a predictor of poor outcome. The degree of ventricular dysfunction that accompanies heart failure may be assessed clinically by tachycardia and a third heart sound. The size of the heart can be estimated from a chest radiograph, and the lung fields may

reveal pulmonary congestion or oedema. The ejection fraction can be measured by radionuclide ventriculography – the risk of death increases as the ejection fraction falls. Echocardiography can also be used to assess left ventricular function.

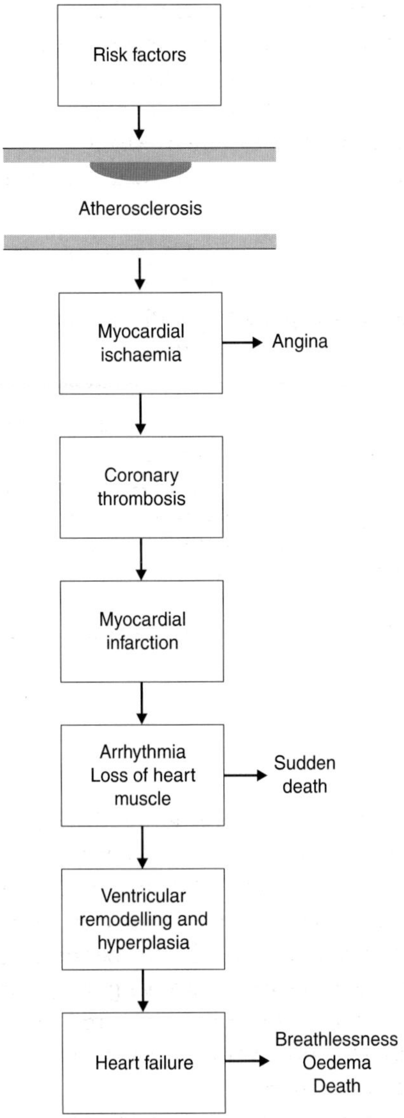

Heart sounds: best heard with a stethoscope. The first heart sound is caused by closure of the mitral and tricuspid valves. The second heart sound is caused by closure of the aortic and pulmonary valves. Additional heart sounds can be heard on filling of the ventricles. The presence of third or fourth heart sounds causes a triple or 'gallop' rhythm.

Tachycardia: rapid beating of the heart, over 100 beats per minute.

Figure 20.25 Outcomes of coronary artery atherosclerosis.

Diagnosis of coronary atherosclerosis and its complications

A variety of imaging methods can be employed to detect an atheroma, but

Electrocardiogram (ECG): a recording of the electrical activity of the heart. Electrodes are placed on the legs, arms and chest. The change in electrical polarity of the heart muscle is recorded in the form of waves and complexes. The first wave, or P wave, represents electrical changes in the atria of the heart. The second (QRS) complex represents depolarisation during ventricular contraction. The third, T, wave represents ventricular repolarisation as the ventricles relax.

diagnosis is usually based on the investigation of symptoms such as angina. The most readily available technique, conventional radiography, can be used to demonstrate advanced calcified atheromas. More complex and time-consuming examinations are needed to evaluate the extent of atheromatous deposits and their effect on the heart. Some of these techniques are highly invasive and not without risk.

Investigation of angina

Electrocardiography

Very often the ECG examination will yield normal results between heart attacks, in which case an exercise test will be required to show exertional angina. This should reveal significant ST segment depression, which is characteristic of myocardial ischaemia. The severity of the ECG changes indicates the extent of the disease.

Angiography

The internal diameter of an artery can be assessed by angiography

Angiography is a radiographic method in which a contrast agent is injected into an artery and its passage through the vessel recorded on film or as a computer-generated digital image to give an indication of the ability of the vessel to transport blood and of its internal diameter. The method has limitations in that subtle atheromatous changes may be missed. It is also highly invasive and employs iodine-based contrast agents which may be toxic.

The coronary arteries and the heart can be examined by injecting the contrast medium through a catheter which is threaded directly into the heart, usually via the femoral artery. Continuous images of the moving heart and blood flow are displayed by X-ray fluoroscopy.

Other techniques for imaging atheroma

Intravascular ultrasonography can be used only to examine large arteries

Ultrasound may be used to assess the presence of atheroma but the transducer must be introduced into the artery itself. This technique, intravascular ultrasonography, can provide fairly accurate images of the vessel wall but is not commonly used. Because of limitations on probe size the technique is used only in the examination of large vessels such as the aorta and femoral arteries, although transducers small enough to be passed into the coronary arteries are now available. It is particularly suitable for assessment of residual disease or damage after angioplasty or atherectomy.

In the future, imaging by laser and MRI may be used for the diagnosis of atheroma

Other imaging techniques currently being developed use optical lasers and MRI. The optical laser is a bundle of optical fibres with an outer diameter of about 2.5 mm which can be inserted into vessels and used to discriminate between atheromatous tissue and the normal arterial wall by differences in their fluorescence spectra on excitation by laser energy.

MRI is a means of assessing the site, size, shape and lipid content of atheromatous plaques, but the technique is yet to be established in routine clinical practice since images of small arteries such as the coronaries are difficult to interpret.

Ultrasound imaging of the heart

Echocardiography

The echocardiogram also uses sound waves to produce images of the heart. A transducer, which emits sound waves and detects those waves that are echoed back, is applied to the chest. The detected sound waves are converted into electrical signals which are displayed on an oscilloscope. There are two main types of echocardiography: transthoracic and transoesophageal.

The former can be used to evaluate structural changes in the heart and its valves, the size of the heart chambers and to differentiate between enlarged heart muscle and cardiac tamponade. Enlarged heart muscle (hypertrophy) may be produced as a consequence of earlier infarctions as surrounding cells increase in size in order to compensate for the loss of work capacity.

Transoesophageal electrocardiography works on a similar principle except that the transducer is placed down the oesophagus so that it is closer to the heart. This is a more sensitive method and valve defects and aortic aneurysms can also be identified.

> *Heart disease consequent on atherosclerosis can be detected by ultrasound*

Cardiac tamponade: compression of heart by accumulation of excess fluid in the pericardium. Can be caused by advanced lung cancer or a tumour that has metastasised to the pericardium.

Acute myocardial infarct

The diagnosis of acute myocardial infarct is obtained through evaluation of the physical symptoms, ECG measurements, the estimation of enzymes released from heart muscle cells and by radionuclide imaging.

Electrocardiography

This can detect changes within seconds of coronary occlusion. The most typical abnormality in the acute stage is regional ST elevation. This is followed by Q and T wave abnormalities. A significant proportion of patients with myocardial infarction do not produce the characteristic ST elevation on their ECG trace. Alternative methods of diagnosis are necessary for these patients.

> *One of the most convenient and reliable methods of diagnosis of myocardial infarct is ECG*

Biochemical markers

Myocardial infarction can be confirmed by the measurement of enzymes released from dying heart muscle into the blood circulation. The enzymes released include creatine kinase, lactate dehydrogenase and aspartate transaminase (previously known as serum oxaloacetic transaminase). There are two main difficulties with measurement of enzymes:

1. Some of these enzymes are also released by other cells as they die or are stressed. Examples are injury to skeletal muscle, such as that produced during resuscitation with chest compression, electrical defibrillation or intramuscular injection. Raised enzyme levels can also be observed following extreme exercise

2. Concentrations of enzymes do not peak in the blood until several hours after the event. The first 6 hours after myocardial infarction are crucial for intervention so an early diagnosis based on ECG abnormalities must be

relied on, even though ECG does not always provide conclusive evidence of an infarct.

The biochemical markers of infarction are not evident until some hours after the event

The commonly employed biochemical markers, creatine kinase and its more specific MB isoenzyme (CK-MB), increase within 4–8 hours of the infarction and peak at 12–24 hours. Lactate dehydrogenase levels begin to rise in 8–12 hours and peak at 3–6 days. Aspartate transaminase peaks at 1–2 days and falls to normal after about 3 days. As far as peak concentrations are concerned, all these markers fall outside the timescale required for optimal intervention.

Much work has been done in improving the specificity and sensitivity of the tests for biochemical markers of myocardial infarction. The first improvement relates to the measurement of CK-MB subforms. It is released from myocardial cells as $CK\text{-}MB_2$, which is converted to $CK\text{-}MB_1$ in the blood. Serum levels of $CK\text{-}MB_2$ greater than 1.0 U/l, together with a ratio of $CK\text{-}MB_2$ to $CK\text{-}MB_1$ greater than 1.5 indicate myocardial infarction. A simple and rapid test is now available for these subforms, meaning that a diagnosis of myocardial infarction can be confirmed within 2 hours of the onset of chest pains.

Other recently introduced assays are for myoglobin and the troponins. Myoglobin is a haem-containing protein which becomes raised in the blood within 2 hours of myocardial infarct. Its assay is more sensitive than that of CK-MB in the early post-infarct stage, but the marker is rapidly removed from the blood by the kidneys. The troponins are proteins present in cardiac and skeletal muscle that regulate the interaction of actin and myosin (involved in muscle contraction). The several different forms, troponin I, C and T, form a complex. In addition, several isoforms of each these proteins, encoded by different genes, are unique to cardiac or skeletal muscle. The estimation of troponin T isoforms enables the detection of the minor myocardial cell injury that accompanies unstable angina. The current assay for troponin T takes 90 minutes to complete, but it might be possible to modify the assay to considerably shorten this time. There is little advantage in using these new tests if the ECG measurement provides unequivocal evidence of myocardial infarction, or if more than 6 hours has elapsed since the onset of chest pain.

Radionuclide imaging

Radionuclide imaging is rarely employed and usually only when results of ECG and estimation of biochemical markers are equivocal

This technique can be used to diagnose coronary artery disease, cardiomyopathy and disease of the heart valves. The procedure involves intravenous injection of a radioisotope (thallium-201 or technetium-99m) followed by a scintigraphic scan to locate and measure the distribution of the radioisotope in the body. These tests may be undertaken under conditions of stress induced by exercise or drug stimulation, so that cardiac arrhythmias and ischaemic responses can be induced and monitored.

Thallium-201 accumulates in healthy well-perfused myocardium but not in infarcted areas. An initial scan is made soon after radioisotope injection to assess its uptake. Less thallium will be delivered to areas of the heart supplied by coronary arteries which are narrowed by atherosclerosis. A second scan is performed some 2–4 hours later to assess thallium clearance which will be slower in diseased areas of the myocardium. This radionuclide will not

distinguish between acute and old infarction.

In contrast, technetium-99m stannous pyrophosphate accumulates in acutely infarcted myocardium, allowing the location and size of a suspected infarct to be assessed. A disadvantage is that uptake cannot be detected until 12–24 hours after the onset of chest pain, long after any intervention to limit the size of the infarct should be implemented. Even so, the subsequent measurement of infarct size may prove to be a useful prognostic indicator.

Thallium scanning is also used to assess the operative risk in patients with evidence of cardiovascular disease who need major non-cardiovascular surgery. These patients are at risk of perioperative death, myocardial infarction or other cardiac event. An abnormal scan can be followed by therapeutic interventions (anti-ischaemic medication, revascularisation) before surgery, to reduce cardiac mortality and morbidity.

Assessment of myocardial ischaemia

Exercise stress tests

Exercise stress tests are used to identify myocardial ischaemia in all patients who might be considered for coronary angioplasty or bypass grafting. It can be used to monitor patients after therapy, providing information on the degree of residual ischaemia, ventricular dysfunction and the tendency to produce arrhythmia. Treated patients with these signs have a relatively poor prognosis.

Progressive exercise tests are used to assess the response of the heart to physical stress

A treadmill is most commonly used, but a bicycle ergometer may be used instead and an arm ergometer may be used for patients who cannot walk. In the treadmill stress test the work rate is changed every 3 minutes, in a total test time of 15 minutes, by slightly increasing the speed and the degree of incline. This will induce marked ST segment depression in patients with CHD. The exercise test may be combined with the thallium perfusion test.

Treatment of atheroma and its consequences

The accumulation of atheromatous plaques can be slowed by modification to risk factors. The main aim is to lower plasma lipid levels, if possible by dietary control. If this fails then lipid-lowering drugs are needed.

The objective in treating atheroma is to relieve symptoms and to slow down accumulation of plaque

Lipid-lowering drugs

A number of drugs reduce blood cholesterol and triglyceride concentrations (see Chapter 12). The type of drug employed depends on whether the abnormality is related to raised plasma cholesterol or triglycerides. With most of the agents available, reductions of 5–30% in lipid concentrations are achievable. Greater reductions can be realised but the side-effects, which usually include gastrointestinal irritation, limit the dose that can be used. In all cases lipid-lowering drugs are reserved for use when all else has failed: weight reduction and dietary control must be tried first.

▲   **Key points**

Diagnostic investigation of atherosclerosis and its complications

Atheroma:
▲ Angiography – Cardiac catheterisation and injection of radio-opaque contrast agent into coronary arteries
▲ Intravascular ultrasound – Small transducer introduced into arteries. More suitable for large arteries (not coronaries)
▲ Optical lasers – Can discriminate between normal and atheromatous tissue (not routine)
▲ MRI - Can detect atheroma (not routine)

Myocardial infarct:
▲ ECG - Relatively simple and rapid but some patients produce no significant changes
▲ Biochemical markers – Measure enzymes released from dying heart muscle. Changes usually follow some hours after infarct
▲ Radionuclide imaging – Thallium-201 accumulates in healthy well perfused myocardium. Technetium-99m accumulates in infarcted areas, but this may be 24 hours after infarction

Myocardial ischaemia:
▲ Exercise stress test – Identifies developing ischaemia by monitoring heart response to progressive physical stress

Heart failure:
▲ Chest radiography – Measurement of heart size, estimation of pulmonary congestion and oedema
▲ Echocardiography – Externally applied: transthoracic; internally applied: transoesophageal

The lipid-lowering drugs undoubtedly improve blood lipid profiles, but not all reduce mortality from CHD. Some of the newer agents, such as simvastatin, do produce beneficial changes in blood lipid profiles that are reflected by improved survival.

Angina

The medical control of angina is principally aimed at reducing the workload on the heart

Angina can be controlled by drug therapies but, in advanced cases, surgical intervention such as coronary bypass or coronary artery angioplasty may be necessary. The first-line medical treatment is administration of nitrates. These work by causing peripheral venous vasodilation, reducing the volume of blood returning to the heart. Distension of the heart wall is rapidly relieved, as is the pain. Acute anginal attacks are treated by dissolving a glyceryl trinitrate tablet under the tongue. The effect lasts for only about 30 minutes but more stable longer-acting nitrates are available and more suitable for the acute treatment of unstable angina. The main side-effect of glyceryl trinitrate is severe headache,

and to help avoid this the patient should spit the tablet out as soon as pain relief is obtained. **Glyceryl trinitrate** is best used as a preventive measure, immediately before exertion, rather than to relieve angina.

β-**Adrenoreceptor antagonists** (β-blockers) produce a fall in blood pressure through a reduction in cardiac output so that the oxygen demand of the heart is lower. They can also aid perfusion of blood in the ischaemic area because the reduction in heart rate extends the duration of diastole, allowing more time for blood to flow to the heart muscle. The β-blockers are unsuitable for people with asthma and bronchitis because they promote bronchospasm (by blocking β2 receptors, see Chapter 24). They also produce vasoconstriction and therefore should not be used by patients with peripheral vascular disease. Other serious side-effects include provocation of heart failure and conductance block. The β-blockers are used prophylactically to reduce the likelihood or severity of further angina attacks. The conventional therapy is with propranolol, but the more cardioselective β-blockers atenolol or metoprolol may be preferred because they have fewer side-effects.

Calcium-channel blockers are replacing β-blockers as an adjunct to short-acting nitrates because they have fewer side-effects. They relieve the workload and oxygen consumption of the heart by causing peripheral arteriolar dilation and reducing afterload. Examples of calcium channel blockers are diltiazem, nifedipine and verapamil.

β-Blockers: block β1 receptors in the heart which, when stimulated, increase the rate and force of cardiac contraction. Used to reduce blood pressure and prevent angina.

Bronchospasm: spasmodic and prolonged contraction of the bronchial airways.

Conductance block: disruption of the cardiac conductance system. The conductance system comprises neuromuscular tissue, specialised for the conduction of electric impulses. Impulses pass from the sinoatrial (SA) node through both atria, stimulating them to contract. This activates the atrioventricular (AV) node, from which the impulse travels along the atrioventricular bundle. The bundle terminates in Purkinje fibres. These deliver the impulses to the ventricular myocardium, causing contraction of both ventricles

Bypass surgery for angina

Surgical intervention is employed mainly in the treatment of selected patients with angina, and its application in acute or evolving myocardial infarction is becoming less common as the availability of thrombolytic treatment increases. Complete relief from angina can be achieved in 80% of patients who undergo coronary bypass surgery. There is, however, an operative mortality rate of about 2%, with a perioperative infarction rate of 4–5%. Overall the 5-year survival following bypass surgery is 90–95%.

The occluded segments of artery are bypassed by grafting in sections of the patient's saphenous vein or internal mammary artery. The new graft is subject to the same kind of changes that produced the atherosclerosis in the first place, but is even more susceptible. Initially the graft may be subject to acute occlusion by thrombus. Over the longer term the grafted vessel wall becomes hyperplastic, followed by a phase of atherosclerosis which partially or completely occludes the lumen. There is evidence that internal mammary artery grafts are more resistant to the development of atheroma than saphenous vein and for this reason are the conduit of choice.

One surgical treatment for angina is to bypass the area of obstruction

Some patients may require a further bypass operation because the grafts themselves become blocked by thrombus or plaque

Coronary artery angioplasty

An alternative to coronary bypass surgery for some patients is **percutaneous transluminal coronary angioplasty**. This technique was introduced by Andreas Gruentzig in 1977 for the treatment of small focal lesions in the proximal coronary arteries. The technique is now also broadly applied to patients with multiple lesions. Some patients with multivessel disease are not

In coronary artery angioplasty a balloon catheter is used to compress the atherosclerotic plaque

Afterload, outflow resistance: the resistance against which the ventricle contracts. Influenced by pulmonary and systemic resistance, physical characteristics of vessel walls and the volume of blood that is ejected. An increase in after-load decreases the cardiac output.

suited for this type of treatment, including patients who have had a recent infarct, previous revascularisation, or in whom the left main coronary artery is narrowed. Bypass grafting is preferable for these people. The technique has an initial success rate of about 90% (defined as achieving at least a 50% reduction in radiologically confirmed stenosis).

A catheter system is introduced into the coronary artery via the femoral artery under local anaesthesia. The guiding catheter carries a narrow-bore (diameter 0.5–1.25 mm) dilatational catheter with a sausage-shaped distensible segment. The position of the catheter is monitored using X-ray fluoroscopy. When it has been inserted through the obstruction and positioned against the atheroma, the balloon segment is inflated with contrast fluid to an outer diameter up to 4 mm, dilating the lumen of the artery and compressing the plaque. Multiple inflation and deflation of the balloon is usually necessary (Figure 20.26).

> ### ▲   Key points
>
> #### Coronary angioplasty
>
> ▲ Suitable for patients with normal left ventricular function and single-vessel coronary artery disease or multivessel disease that does not involve the proximal left anterior descending artery
> ▲ Less expensive than bypass surgery and hospital stay shorter
> ▲ Lower initial morbidity rate than bypass grafting
> ▲ Greater likelihood of recurrent angina, and need for subsequent revascularisation

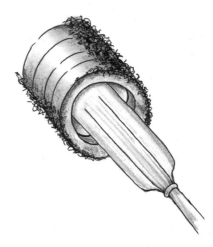

Figure 20.26 Balloon angioplasty. A balloon catheter inserted into the atherosclerotic artery is inflated to increase its external diameter and compress the atherosclerotic plaque.

> *Occlusion of an artery may be so extensive that a catheter cannot be passed through; in this case the blockage can be vaporised by laser energy*

In circumstances of severe stenosis or complete occlusion, balloon angioplasty may fail because of resistance to the passage of the catheter. This problem can be overcome by using a laser to vaporise the obstruction and produce a 'pilot hole' for subsequent balloon angioplasty. The instrument consists of a laser-power source coupled to an optical fibre and a catheter delivery system. More controlled energy can be obtained by placing a metal tip on the optical fibre so that some of the laser energy is converted into heat. Other developments include sapphire or quartz shields to attenuate the laser light and protect the optical fibres.

> *High-energy lasers can be used to punch holes in the heart wall*

A new approach to ensuring adequate perfusion of the myocardium when coronary arteries are blocked is to channel in a blood supply from the opposite direction. High-energy lasers can be used to create new vascular channels in the wall of the ventricle, which are supplied from the lumen of the ventricle.

Further clinical trials are needed to evaluate the potential of this technique.

The main complications of the procedure are myocardial infarction, arising from abrupt closure of the coronary artery, and restenosis of the vessel, which takes some months. Abrupt closure, which affects 3–5% of patients, is caused by dissection of the plaque and is the main reason for death during or after attempted coronary angioplasty. Acute vessel closure after angioplasty is treated by stenting or emergency bypass grafting. Restenosis is a less urgent problem since this occurs over several months and can be detected and further treated. Nevertheless, 25–50% of patients may require further revascularisation following coronary angioplasty.

Coronary angioplasty compared with bypass grafting

There is much interest in establishing whether angioplasty is as effective as coronary bypass surgery in terms of deaths and other outcomes such as angina and exercise tolerance. Randomised trials of the two procedures were set up in the late 1980s and it is still too early to make long-term comparisons. Initial results from the RITA (Randomised Intervention Treatment of Angina) trial of patients with multivessel coronary artery disease show that the treatments differ little in the rates of subsequent myocardial infarction or death (see page 636). However, patients undergoing angioplasty are more likely to experience further cardiac events and require repeat treatment. It is best to regard bypass surgery and angioplasty as complementary procedures; angioplasty may be used initially to treat younger patients with fairly localised disease followed, as the disease progresses, by bypass surgery.

> *Angioplasty is a cheaper treatment than coronary bypass surgery and recovery is faster, but complications and repeat treatments are more common*

Coronary stenting

The use of coronary stents was introduced in an attempt to overcome the problems of restenosis after coronary angioplasty. Stents are stainless steel slotted tubes which can be collapsed and mounted on a deflated balloon catheter. Once inserted into the stenosis the balloon is inflated so that the mesh becomes embedded within the vessel wall. The balloon is then deflated and withdrawn, leaving the stent behind (Figure 20.27). An alternative stent is an expandable mesh that is restrained by a sheath. Once put in place by a guiding catheter, the sheath is withdrawn and the stent expands into the vessel wall.

Stenting is used for acute vessel closure after percutaneous transluminal coronary angioplasty, but also has a role in the initial management of coronary stenosis. The main complication is that blood clots tend to form around the stent and very aggressive anticoagulant therapy is required, usually within 14 days of the implantation. The anticoagulant therapy can produce local haematoma at the femoral puncture site that requires blood transfusion or surgery, and abdominal or intracranial bleeding.

Results from randomised trials (BENESTENT: Serruys *et al.*, 1994 (see page 636); STRESS: Fischman *et al.*, 1994) show that coronary stenting in patients with stable and unstable angina reduces the restenosis rate by up to 40%. There were no differences in mortality rates, myocardial infarction, or need for bypass grafting. However, higher rates of bleeding and peripheral

> *Expandable metal stents can be implanted at the site of coronary stenosis*

▲ Key points

Coronary stents

- ▲ Stents consist of a wire mesh inserted by catheter, and embedded into vessel wall
- ▲ Used to prevent restenosis after coronary angioplasty
- ▲ Treatment of acute vessel closure after angioplasty
- ▲ Complications of blood clotting require aggressive anticoagulant therapy

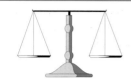

RITA

Coronary angioplasty vs. bypass graft

▲ Total 1011 patients, randomised to receive angioplasty (510) or bypass grafting (501)
▲ Similar incidences of death or myocardial infarction
▲ Similar improvements in exercise capacity over 2.5 years
▲ At 2 years, 38% of angioplasty group needed further revascularisation procedures compared with 11% of bypass group
▲ Prevalence of angina and need for drugs greater in group receiving angioplasty

Data from: RITA, 1993

BENESTENT

Coronary stent vs. balloon angioplasty

▲ Studied 520 patients with stable angina, randomised to receive stent (262) or angioplasty (258)
▲ Clinical end-points: death, stroke, myocardial infarction, need for bypass, need for second reperfusion
▲ At 7 months 20% of patients in stent group reached a clinical end-point compared with 30% in angioplasty group

Data from: Serruys et al., 1994.

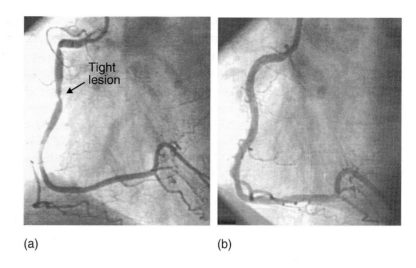

(a)   (b)

Figure 20.27 Coronary stenting. Angiographs of coronary artery before (a) and after (b) stenting. The patency of the artery is restored by the stent. Photographs provided by Dr U.M. Sivananthan.

vascular complications were associated with the stent group. The intense anticoagulation therapy required increases the rate of early complications, which so far has inhibited uptake of this procedure as a routine treatment.

A number of devices can be introduced through catheters to remove the atherosclerotic plaque. In theory, this approach should bring about fewer complications and more long-term benefits than the simple compression techniques of balloon angioplasty or stenting. One device, the Simpson Coronary AtheroCath, consists of a metal housing with an elongated window on one side. The housing contains a cutting device that can rotate at 2000 r.p.m. This is used to shave off strips of plaque which are then collected into a nose cone and removed. A similar device, the transluminal endarterectomy catheter, cuts the atheroma and removes the fragments by suction. To date, these devices are limited by their relatively large size, requiring a 4 mm catheter, so that stenosis in small or tortuous vessels cannot be reached. Results with the AtheroCath (CAVEAT randomised trial; Topol I., et al, 1993 see p.638) indicate that the method carries a higher abrupt closure rate than balloon angioplasty alone (7% vs. 3%), with similar restenosis rates.

Acute myocardial infarction

A number of alternatives are available for the treatment of myocardial infarction, all of which aim to restore myocardial perfusion. Most patients with large anterior infarctions should undergo immediate coronary angioplasty if this is available. The main alternative is thrombolytic therapy, possibly in combination with aspirin or anticoagulant therapy, depending on the course of events and contraindications. This combination may be followed by longer-term aspirin, ACE inhibitors or β-blocker treatments. Patients who have had

a recent stroke, significant trauma, recent surgery, active internal bleeding or poorly controlled high blood pressure are unsuitable for thrombolytic treatment. Significant survival benefits are associated with all types of reperfusion therapies, although many patients will still die, some from **reperfusion injury**, evident as arrhythmia, myocardial stunning and further injury to ischaemic and immediately surrounding muscle cells.

Arrhythmias are more likely when the period of ischaemia has been short or when reperfusion therapy has been completed rapidly. However, an increased vulnerability to arrhythmias arising from early thrombolytic therapy, with reperfusion after 20–30 minutes, does not appear to be associated with any increase in mortality.

Myocardial stunning is a delay in functional improvement. Usually the systolic performance of the reperfused region shows only modest improvement in the first 3 days, but recovery is faster thereafter. The clinical relevance of myocardial stunning is a possible delay in recovery from cardiogenic shock. Poor ventricular function may be mistaken for permanent damage and treated with inotropic drugs (e.g. digoxin), which will delay recovery by increasing myocardial oxygen demand and could induce further arrhythmia.

There is some controversy about the effect of reperfusion in causing further myocardial injury. It is likely that reperfusion accelerates the death of cells that were irretrievably damaged but causes minimal destruction of previously uninjured cells. Cells subjected to prolonged ischaemia will have a disturbed ionic balance because of reduced production of ATP, which drives the sodium pump (Chapter 4). The restoration of blood supply results in an influx of calcium into the injured cells. This overloads the mitochondria, which stop ATP production and eventually lyse. Calcium also activates cellular proteases and phospholipases which could disrupt the cell membrane and kill the cells, releasing free radical species which could injure surrounding cells.

Animal studies suggest that magnesium could protect against reperfusion injury, helping to restore the ionic balance between the cell and its extracellular environment by inhibiting the passage of potassium out of the cell and the ingress of sodium and calcium. Clinical trials of treatment with magnesium sulphate have produced variable results. The Leicester Intravenous Magnesium Intervention Trial (LIMIT-2; Woods and Fletcher, 1994) showed that CHD mortality could be reduced by 20% in 3 years of follow up by intravenous injection of magnesium sulphate immediately before thrombolytic therapy. In contrast, the much larger ISIS-4 trial (1995) showed no benefit, although a crucial difference might be that in this most patients were given intravenous magnesium after completion of thrombolytic therapy rather than before.

Thrombolytic treatment

Most cases of myocardial infarction are caused by obstruction of a coronary artery by thrombus. Because infarction throughout the thickness of the heart muscle wall is not instantaneous it is possible to intervene and minimise the damage by removing the obstruction. Thrombolytic treatment is aimed at dissolving the clot by enzymes. Agents currently available include

Rapid reperfusion is the only way of limiting the size of a myocardial infarct

Reperfusion could itself cause myocardial injury

Speed in initiating treatment, and selecting a treatment that acts quickly, are important prognostic factors

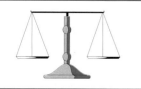

Directional atherectomy vs. coronary angioplasty

▲ Study of 1012 patients at 35 centres in the USA: 512 received atherectomy, 510 angioplasty

▲ Greater immediate reduction in stenosis in atherectomy group

▲ Reduction in stenosis to less than 50% achieved in 89% of atherectomy group and 80% in those receiving angioplasty

▲ Restenosis occurred in 50% of subjects receiving atherectomy compared with 57% of angioplasty group at 6 months

▲ Higher rate of early complications in group undergoing atherectomy (11% vs. 5%)

▲ Probability of death or myocardial infarction at 6 months 8.6% in atherectomy group, 4.6% in angioplasty group

▲ Atherectomy has no apparent clinical benefit over angioplasty

Data from: Topol et al., 1993.

streptokinase, anistreplase (a plasminogen-streptokinase activator complex), urokinase and variants of tissue plasminogen activator (alteplase, reteplase). Streptokinase treatment is much cheaper than t-PA treatments (see below): about US$500 compared with $2200 for t-PA (1993 prices).

Streptokinase is a polypeptide derived from cultured β-haemolytic streptococci. Streptokinase binds to plasminogen, forming an active complex which then splits peptide bonds on other plasminogen molecules to produce the active agent (plasmin) that disintegrates the thrombus. The plasminogen complex can also be produced *in vitro*, and is available as anistreplase. Because these agents are not human proteins their administration causes problems with allergic reactions.

Urokinase is an enzyme with thrombus-dissolving properties normally present in human tissues. It can be extracted from urine or cultures of kidney cells and can also be manufactured using recombinant DNA technology.

Tissue plasminogen activator (t-PA) is an enzyme produced naturally by vascular endothelial cells. The theoretical advantage of t-PA is that it has a binding site for fibrin in the clot, and so its action is more localised. This is in contrast to the other agents which activate to plasminogen in the general circulation. The drug is now produced by recombinant DNA techniques.

Clinical trials (FTT Collaborative Group, 1994; see p.639) have conclusively shown that early deaths (within 6 weeks of treatment) can be reduced by up to 40% by administering thrombolytic treatment within 6 hours of the onset of a myocardial infarction. The sooner treatment is initiated the better. Treatment within 7–12 hours does have some survival benefit (LATE trial, 1993; see p.639), but there is little survival advantage after 12 hours. There are some negative aspects of thrombolytic therapy: it is associated with an excess of strokes (four per 1000) that occur within 48 hours of acute myocardial infarction, but this is offset by the more substantial benefit of reduced mortality from myocardial infarction. In about 20% of cases the treatment fails to clear the blockage, and in about 15% of cases the cleared artery closes again within days of the treatment.

Clinical trials have also been used to find out whether there is any advantage in combining thrombolytic therapy with other agents such as anticoagulants or aspirin. Virtually every combination of therapies, route of administration and dose has been (or is being) tried. In general, and provided that there are no contraindications, combined therapies appear to be more effective than single therapies.

Aspirin therapy

The main effect of aspirin is inhibition of thrombus formation. It suppresses the enzyme cyclo-oxygenase that is necessary for the synthesis of certain prostacyclins. These substances stimulate the aggregation of platelets which is the initial event in thrombus formation. Very often a new thrombus is formed after successful thrombolytic therapy, probably because of the liberation of thrombin which is a potent platelet activator. As a result aspirin is thought to have the greatest potential therapeutic use immediately following thrombolytic therapy. This has been shown in clinical trials comparing combined and single therapies (ISIS-2, 1988 Figure 20.28 and p.640).

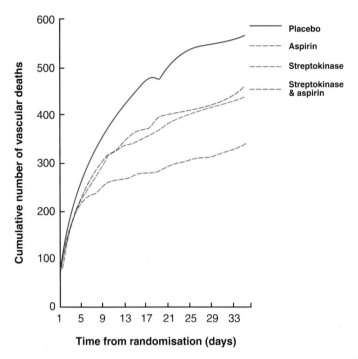

Figure 20.28 ISIS-2 comparison of aspirin and streptokinase treatments. The ISIS-2 study demonstrated the superior benefits of combined streptokinase and aspirin therapies. After 35 days, 468 (out of 4300) patients who had received oral or infusion placebo died, 461 of 4295 receiving aspirin only, 448 of 4300 receiving streptokinase only, but only 343 out of 4294 patients who had been treated with both streptokinase and aspirin died. (Data from ISIS-2, 1988.)

Anticoagulant therapy

Anticoagulants such as heparin were widely used in the management of acute myocardial infarction before the availability of thrombolytic agents. Heparin use was associated with reductions in mortality, reinfarction, deep-vein thrombosis, pulmonary embolus and stroke. None of these benefits was as impressive as those now gained with thrombolytic therapy, but the question now is whether anticoagulants have a role as an adjunct to thrombolytic therapy. Heparin is required to maintain vessel patency when t-PA is used, and this regimen appears to have some survival benefit over streptokinase and heparin (GUSTO trial, 1993; see p. 642). One important observation from the GUSTO trial is that the thrombolytic agent used is of less importance than delay in the onset of treatment.

One of the possible complications of using anticoagulant therapy is bleeding, especially the possibility of intracranial haemorrhage. An increased incidence of bleeding was borne out by both the GUSTO and ISIS-3 (1992) trials, although the problem concerned peripheral bleeding which was not related to significant mortality or major morbidity.

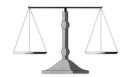

FTT Collaborative Group

Intravenous thrombolytic treatment vs. control

▲ Meta-analysis of all clinical trials of thrombolytic therapy with control with more than 1000 patients with acute myocardial infarction

▲ Excess of deaths in days 0–1 in thrombolytic groups, usually in patients treated after 12 hours

▲ Much larger benefit during days 2–35

▲ Avoidance of 20–30 deaths per 1000 infarcts

Data from: FTT, 1994.

LATE

Late thrombolysis vs. placebo

▲ Trial involving 5711 patients with symptoms or ECG consistent with myocardial infarction

▲ Patients randomised within 6–24 hours of onset to receive t-PA thrombolysis or placebo

▲ All received aspirin

▲ Overall 35-day mortality in treated group 8.86% (compared with 10.31% in those receiving placebo)

▲ In those treated within 12 hours mortality was 8.9%; this was 11.97 in patients for whom treatment was delayed

▲ Thrombolysis worthwhile up to 12 hours after infarction

Data from: LATE, 1993.

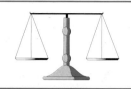

ISIS-2

Intravenous streptokinase vs. oral aspirin vs. streptokinase plus aspirin vs. control

▲ 7187 patients randomised to intervention and control groups within 24 hours of onset of myocardial infarction
▲ Intervention: 160 mg aspirin daily for 1 month, a single 1-hour streptokinase infusion, or both
▲ Reduction in vascular deaths in aspirin group at 5 weeks 23%
▲ Reduction in mortality 25% in intravenous streptokinase group
▲ Aspirin plus streptokinase reduced mortality by 42%

Data from: ISIS-2, 1988.

▲ Key points

Treatment strategies for acute myocardial infarction

Agent	Effect	Contraindication
Aspirin	Anti-thrombus	Gastric ulceration and mucosal bleeding
Heparin	Anticoagulant	Known intracranial tumour, previous neurosurgery, recent stroke, recent head trauma
Tissue plasminogen activator or streptokinase	Anti-thrombus	Recent major surgery or trauma, major trauma, recent history of bleeding (e.g. gastrointestinal bleed)
Magnesium	May limit reperfusion injury and ischaemic arrhythmia	Hypotension, bradycardia, atrioventricular block or high magnesium concentration because of antacid use, chronic renal failure
Captopril	ACE inhibitor	Renal artery stenosis
Nitrates and morphine	Control of chest pain, ischaemic ST changes	Hypotension and respiratory depression
β-Blockers	Control of residual tachycardia and hypertension	Heart block, asthma, peripheral vascular disease

Tertiary prevention of reinfarction

Most texts do not use the term tertiary prevention (Chapter 2), referring to the prevention of further episodes of myocardial infarction as secondary prevention, presumably to distinguish it from primary prevention. The main prophylactic agents are b-blockers and aspirin. b-Blockers reduce early and late mortality after infarction and may be taken by patients for years. A further strategy is the use of oral anticoagulation (acenocoumarol or phenprocoumon). A clinical trial (ASPECT, 1994; see p.643) against placebo has demonstrated that this intervention can halve the risk of recurrent myocardial infarction and also reduce the overall risk of stroke. Unfortunately, risks of cerebral haemorrhage and major extracerebral bleeding are increased.

Aspirin has also been shown to be beneficial in preventing further infarcts, although the optimal duration of treatment is not clear. A daily dose of 160–325 mg is favoured. In the absence of clear contraindications (active duodenal ulcer, gastric mucosal bleeding and anticoagulant therapy) this dose should be started as soon as possible after the diagnosis of acute myocardial infarction, and continued indefinitely. The aspirin reduces further platelet aggregation and therefore the potential for thrombus to produce plaque enlargement or

sudden arterial occlusion, probably by modulating prostaglandin-producing pathways. Clinical trials of aspirin versus anticoagulant therapy indicate no substantial differences in mortality between the two modes, but the higher risk of non-fatal major haemorrhage attached to anticoagulants, together with cost considerations, favours the use of aspirin.

Some patients will show clinical evidence of heart failure after myocardial infarction, despite treatment with thrombolytic therapy and aspirin. These patients often have a poor outcome, because of ventricular damage, myocardial ischaemia, and a tendency for arrhythmia. Recent clinical trials (AIRE, 1993; see p.643) have shown that survival in this group can be enhanced by oral administration of ramipril, an ACE inhibitor (see below).

Afterload: resistance of the arterial system to ventricular emptying. Determined by blood viscosity and the tension of arterioles and precapillary sphincters.

Preload: degree to which the cardiac muscle is stretched before it contracts. Venous dilation reduces the filling pressure in the heart and hence the preload.

Heart failure

The principal approaches to the treatment of heart failure are with diuretics and vasodilators. Diuretics increase the urinary excretion of sodium and water, thereby reducing the volume of fluid in the circulation and the workload (preload) on the heart. The main diuretics are the thiazides, and loop diuretics (frusemide and bumetanide).

The sympathetic nervous response to heart failure is to maintain blood pressure by increasing the vascular resistance. This creates a vicious circle because the resulting increased afterload further depresses the cardiac output. Reduced blood flow in the kidneys stimulates the secretion of renin. This activates the angiotensin aldosterone system to constrict peripheral blood vessels, decrease urinary excretion, and hence increase blood pressure (Figure 20.29). This decreases coronary artery perfusion and can cause infarct expansion. The ACE inhibitors (such as captopril, enalapril, ramipril) are designed to break this circle (they are vasodilators) by blocking the conversion of angiotensin I into angiotensin II (a powerful vasoconstrictor) and thereby lowering both arterial and venous resistance and decreasing preload and afterload.

A well known former treatment for heart failure was digoxin, a glycoside extracted from foxgloves, but this is not extensively used today. Digoxin increases the force of cardiac contraction and reduces oxygen consumption by the failing heart. It can cause serious toxicity, giving rise to anorexia, nausea and vomiting, and is unsuitable for older patients with impaired renal function.

The first-line treatment for heart failure is a combination of diuretics with an ACE inhibitor

Review question 4

A 53-year-old man complains of severe chest pain and a tingling sensation in the left arm. Over the previous 3 weeks he had experienced discomfort in the chest after exertion, which disappeared by resting.
- **Explain the previous and present symptoms**
- **What diagnostic investigations might be employed?**
- **What initial treatment is likely?**

Ethical concerns in the treatment of CHD

Smokers are more likely to experience further problems after coronary bypass surgery and may require reoperation: there is a higher incidence of occlusion by thrombus and vein graft atherosclerosis in smokers. At present it is not possible to carry out all the bypass operations that are required and mortality rates are high while people are on the waiting list. Treatment of smokers may

When health care resources are in short supply treatments will be aimed at the patients most likely to benefit

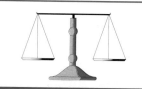

GUSTO

t-PA plus intravenous heparin vs. streptokinase plus subcutaneous heparin vs. streptokinase plus intravenous heparin vs. t-PA plus streptokinase plus intravenous heparin (all with aspirin)

▲ 2431 patients randomised to one of four reperfusion treatments

▲ Clinical end-points: coronary artery patency at 90 and 180 min, death at 30 days

▲ Patency restored soonest with t-PA and heparin (81% of patients within 90 min)

▲ By 180 min patency was the same in all treatment groups

▲ Deaths related to speed of reperfusion: 4.4% of those reperfused within 90 min died compared with 8.9 % in whom there was no flow at 90 min

▲ Mortality lowest when t-PA was given with intravenous heparin

▲ No difference in mortality rate for streptokinase with intravenous or subcutaneous heparin

Data from: GUSTO, 1993.

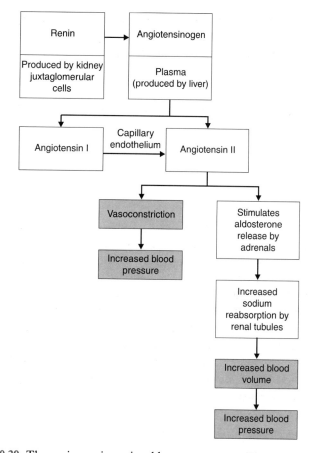

Figure 20.29. The renin–angiotensin–aldosterone system. The hormone renin is secreted by the kidneys in response to a fall in arterial blood pressure. Renin activates angiotensinogen, a plasma protein produced by the liver, to form angiotensin I, which is converted into angiotensin II by the action of angiotensin-converting enzyme present in the endothelium of pulmonary capillaries. Angiotensin II stimulates the adrenals to produce the hormone aldosterone, which stimulates sodium reabsorption by the kidney tubules. This promotes Na^+ and Cl^- retention and, by the osmotic effect, the amount of water in the extracellular fluid and arterial blood, thereby correcting the original stimulus that activated the renin–angiotensin–aldosterone system. Besides stimulating aldosterone secretion, angiotensin II is a potent vasoconstrictor, increasing blood pressure by increasing peripheral resistance. ACE inhibitors block the action of the angiotensin-converting enzyme necessary for the generation of angiotensin II, thus halting the renin–angiotensin–aldosterone system and its capacity for increasing blood pressure.

deprive non-smokers of more efficient and effective surgery – so should non-smokers be given priority? Smokers might well argue that through taxes they have contributed sufficiently to pay for their operations. There are also other risks and degrees of culpability involved – what of the overweight non-smokers who do not take exercise and refuse to alter their diet?

Whatever the viewpoint, the message is clear: smoking is becoming increasingly unpopular and smokers can expect to be asked to curb their habit,

particularly when seeking medical attention. From the viewpoint of preventing CHD, smoking is a crucial factor, but other lifestyle factors should also be given attention because they interact and even multiply the risks.

ANSWERS TO REVIEW QUESTIONS

Question 1

Why do more people in social classes IV and V die of CHD today than those in social classes I and II whereas 60 years ago, the opposite was true?

The current gradient in favour of people with greater socioeconomic status is probably due to the relative effects of the health education message: professionals tend to be more 'health aware'. There are also differences in the ability to afford and prepare fresh non-convenience foods such as fish, fruit and vegetables. The current strategy of the food manufacturing industry is to charge a premium price for 'healthy' convenience foods. There are also differences in the prevalence of cigarette smoking, which, for a variety of reasons (see Chapter 2) is higher in the lower socioeconomic groups.

The reversed trend 60 years ago was probably because of a combination of ignorance regarding the health effects of the diet, and the ability to pay for food. 'Rich' foods (that is with high fat, but low fibre content) were more expensive and people in the lower social groups often relied on their own labours to produce fresh fruit and vegetables.

Question 2

Why is it important to control more than one modifiable CHD risk factor?

CHD is a multifactorial disease and risk factors operate in different ways. Some of them, such as diet and exercise, directly influence total plasma cholesterol levels and the ratio of HDL to LDL. Others act independently of plasma cholesterol, for example, diabetes. Some factors both influence plasma cholesterol and damage the endothelium: an example of this is smoking. There is also an effect on the tendency for thrombosis. All of these factors can be controlled, albeit some more successfully than others. There is evidence that risks of CHD are multiplied by the combination of risk factors: it is therefore advisable to think carefully about diet, exercise levels and smoking habits.

Question 3

Explain the role of antioxidants in lipid metabolism and why these can be of importance in inhibiting atherosclerosis

The most damaging aspect of lipid infiltration into the arterial intima is

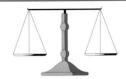

ASPECT

Oral anticoagulation vs. placebo

- ▲ Study of 3404 hospital survivors of myocardial infarction
- ▲ Randomised within 6 weeks of discharge to receive oral anticoagulation or placebo
- ▲ Mean follow-up 37 months
- ▲ Slightly fewer deaths seen in treatment group (170 of 1700 compared with 189 of 1704)
- ▲ Recurrent myocardial infarction reduced by treatment (114 compared with 242 receiving placebo

Data from: ASPECT, 1994.

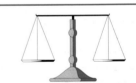

AIRE

ACE inhibitor (ramipril) vs. placebo

- ▲ 2006 patients with clinical evidence of heart failure randomised 3–10 days after infarction to receive ramipril or placebo in addition to conventional treatment
- ▲ Mean follow-up 15 months
- ▲ Mortality in group receiving ramipril 17% compared with 23% in placebo group

Data from: AIRE, 1993.

Prevention and treatment of atheroma

All subjects:
▲ Modify risk factors such as diet, exercise, smoking

Hyperlipidaemic subjects:
▲ Lower blood lipid concentration by diet control and weight reduction
▲ Use lipid-lowering drugs, for example bile acid binding resins, fibrates, nicotinic acid derivatives, statins

Patients with angina:
▲ Reduce cardiac workload with nitrates or β-blockers

Unstable angina:
▲ Coronary angioplasty to compress atherosclerotic plaque
▲ Coronary bypass surgery; avoid blockage by grafting saphenous vein or internal mammary artery

After myocardial infarction:
▲ Thrombolytic therapy, for example streptokinase
▲ Long-term aspirin to reduce the propensity for platelet aggregation

▲ β-Blockers

oxidation of LDL. Oxidation can take place as the LDL crosses the endothelium or wherever LDL is present as an extracellular tissue component, and is usually mediated by oxygen free radicals. Free radicals are normally neutralised by enzyme systems and antioxidant vitamins and minerals. When cells and tissues are damaged the excessive generation of free radicals might outstrip the defensive capacity of the enzymes and anti-oxidants. The excess free radicals can cause further cell and tissue damage. In addition, the oxidised form of LDL will cause cell damage and death. Even when there is no injury to endothelial cells from agents in the arterial lumen, injury could be caused from inside the arterial wall by oxidised LDL in the intima.

Question 4

Explain the previous and present symptoms

The patient's previous symptoms of chest discomfort are consistent with angina. He suffers cardiac ischaemia because part of the myocardium does not receive enough oxygen and nutrients to carry out the increased workload demanded by exertion. On resting the balance between the energy available to the myocardium and the required work output is restored. His present symptoms are consistent with a mild myocardial infarct. The previous angina was caused by atherosclerosis in the coronary arteries. The plaque may have been disrupted and started to bleed, producing a thrombus which could be responsible for the present symptoms.

What diagnostic investigations might be employed? The initial investigation will be ECG, where regional ST elevation would be expected. Some patients with myocardial infarction do not produce significant ECG abnormalities and other investigations might be necessary. The next step would be to monitor blood levels of creatine kinase and lactate dehydrogenase as these enzymes are released from myocardium as muscle cells die. There is some delay before the enzymes diffuse out of the heart muscle cells and reach the bloodstream and it may be necessary to start thrombolytic therapy before the outcome of these laboratory tests is known. An alternative diagnostic procedure is radionuclide imaging, but this is more rarely employed and is usually used to assess old infarcts and monitor drug treatments.

What initial treatment is likely? Initial treatment would consist of rest, drug therapy with nitrates or β-blockers to relieve the workload on the heart, and possibly thrombolytic therapy with aspirin.

References

AIRE (1993) The Acute Infarction Ramipril Efficacy (AIRE) Study Investigators. Effect of ramipril on mortality and morbidity of survivors of acute myocardial infarction with clinical evidence of heart failure. *Lancet*, **342**, 821–8.

ASPECT (1994) Anticoagulants in the Secondary Prevention of Events in

Coronary Thrombosis (ASPECT) Research Group. Effect of long-term oral anticoagulant treatment on mortality and cardiovascular morbidity after myocardial infarction. *Lancet*, **343**, 499–503.

Fibrinolytic Therapy Trialists' Collaborative Group (1994) Indications for fibrinolytic therapy in suspected acute myocardial infarction: collaborative overview of early mortality and major morbidity results from all randomised trials of more than 1000 patients. *Lancet*, **343**, 311–22.

Fischman, D.L., Leon, M.B., Baim, D.S. *et al.* (1994) A randomised comparison of coronary-stent placement and balloon angioplasty in treatment of coronary artery disease. *N. Engl. J. Med.*, **331**, 496–501.

GUSTO Angiographic Investigators (1993) The effects of tissue plasminogen activator, streptokinase, or both on coronary artery patency, ventricular function, and survival after acute myocardial infarction. *N. Engl. J. Med.*, **329**, 1615–22.

ISIS-2 (1988) Second International Study of Infarct Survival. *Lancet*, **ii**, 349–60.

ISIS-3 (Third International Study of Infarct Survival) Collaboration Group (1992) ISIS-3: a randomised trial of streptokinase vs tissue plasminogen activator vs anistreplase and of aspirin plus heparin vs aspirin alone among 41,299 cases of suspected acute myocardial infarction. *Lancet*, **339**, 759–70.

ISIS-4 Collaborative Group (1995) ISIS-4: a randomised factorial trial assessing early oral captopril, oral mononitrate and intravenous magnesium in 58,050 patients with suspected acute myocardial infarction. *Lancet*, **345**, 669–85.

Kannel, W.B. (1988) Cholesterol and risk of coronary heart disease and mortality in men. *Clin. Chem.*, **34(B)**, B53–9.

LATE Study Group (1993) Late Assessment of Thrombolytic Efficiency (LATE) study with alteplase 6–24 hours after onset of acute myocardial infarction. *Lancet*, **342**, 759–66.

Morris, J.N. (1989) Exercise versus heart attack. *MRC News*, **45**, 24–5.

RITA Trial Participants (1993) Coronary angioplasty versus coronary artery bypass surgery: the Randomised Intervention Treatment of Angina (RITA) trial. *Lancet*, **341**, 573–80.

Serruys, P.W., Jaegere, P., Kieneneij, F. *et al.* (1994) A comparison of balloon-expandable stent implantation with balloon angioplasty in patients with coronary artery disease. *N. Engl. J. Med.*, **331**, 489–95.

Topol, E.J., Leya, F., Pinkerton, C.A. *et al.*, (1993) A comparison of directional atherectomy with coronary angioplasty in patients with coronary artery disease. *N. Engl. J. Med.*, **329**, 221–7.

Weiss, E.J., Bray, B.F., Tayback, M. *et al.* (1996) A polymorphism of a platelet glycoprotein receptor as an inherited risk factor for coronary thrombosis. *N. Engl. J. Med.*, **334**, 1090–4.

Woods, K.L. and Fletcher, S. (1994) Long-term outcome after magnesium sulphate in suspected acute myocardial infarction: second Leicester Intravenous Magnesium Intervention Trial (LIMIT-2). *Lancet*, **343**, 816–9.

Further reading

Epidemiology

Elford, J., Phillips, A.N., Thomson, A.G. *et al*. (1989) Migration and geographic variations in ischaemic heart disease in Great Britain. *Lancet*, **i**, 343–6.

Keys, A. (1970) Coronary heart disease in seven countries. *Circulation*, **41** (Suppl. 1), 1–199.

Causes and risk factors

Doll, R. and Peto, R. (1976) Mortality in relation to smoking: 20 years observation on male British doctors. *BMJ*, **2**, 1525–36.

Evans, G.R. and Taylor, K.G. (1988) The paediatric origins of atherosclerosis. *Br. J. Hosp. Med.*, **39**, 132–7.

Fall, C.H.D., Barker, D.J.P., Osmond, C. *et al*. (1992) Relation of infant feeding to adult cholesterol concentration and death from ischaemic heart disease. *BMJ*, **304**, 801–5.

Ruderman, N., Williamson, J. and Brownlee, M. (eds) (1992) *Hyperglycaemia, Diabetes, and Vascular Disease*. Oxford University Press, Oxford.

Renaud, S. and De Lorgeril, M. (1992) Wine, alcohol, platelets, and the French paradox for coronary heart disease. *Lancet*, **339**, 1523–6.

Rose, G. and Shipley, M. (1990) Effects of coronary risk reduction on the pattern of mortality. *Lancet*, **335**, 275–7.

Ulbricht, T.L.V. and Southgate, D.A.T. (1991) Coronary heart disease: seven dietary factors. *Lancet*, **338**, 985–92.

Prevention and treatment

Anderson, H.V. and Willerton, J.T. (1993) Thrombolysis in acute myocardial infarction. *N. Engl. J. Med.*, **329**, 703–9.

Corr, L. (1994) New methods of making blocked coronary arteries patent again. *BMJ*, **309**, 579–83.

Esterbauer, H., Dieber-Roptheneder, M., Striegl, G. *et al*. (1991) Role of vitamin E in preventing the oxidation of low-density lipoproteins. *Am. J. Clin. Nutr.*, **53**, 314S–21S.

Isner, J.M., Lucas, A.R. and Fields, C.D. (1988) Laser therapy in the treatment of cardiovascular disease. *Br. J. Hosp. Med.*, **40**, 172–8.

Leaf, A. (1989) Management of hypercholesterolaemia: are preventive interventions advisable? *N. Engl. J. Med.*, **321**, 680–4.

Manson, J., Tosteson, H., Satterfield, S. *et al*. (1992) The primary prevention of myocardial infarction. *N. Engl. J. Med.*, **326**, 1406–16.

McMurray, J. and Rankin, A. (1994) Cardiology I. Treatment of myocardial infarction, unstable angina, and angina pectoris. *BMJ*, **309**, 1343–50.

O'Connor, P., Feely, J. and Shepherd, J. (1990) Lipid lowering drugs. *BMJ*, **300**, 667–72.

Ornish, D., Brown, S.E., Scherwitz, L.W. *et al*. (1990) Can lifestyle changes reverse

coronary heart disease? The Lifestyle heart trial. *Lancet*, **336**, 129–33.

Pepper, J. (1988) Changing controversies in surgery for angina. *Br. J. Hosp. Med.*, **39**, 16–20.

Willard, J.E., Lange, R.A. and Hillis, L.D. (1992) The use of aspirin in ischaemic heart disease. *N. Engl. J. Med.*, **327**, 175–81.

Pathology

Fuster, V., Badiamon, L., Badimon, J.J. *et al.* (1992) The pathogenesis of coronary artery disease and the acute coronary syndromes. *N. Engl. J. Med.*, **326**, 242–50.

McGill, H.C. (1988) The pathogenesis of atherosclerosis. *Clin. Chem.*, **34(B)**, B33–8.

Munro, J.M. and Cotran, R.S. (1988) The pathogenesis of atherosclerosis: atherogenesis and inflammation. *Lab. Invest.*, **58**, 249–61.

Ross, R. (1986) The pathogenesis of atherosclerosis – an update. *N. Engl. J. Med.*, **314**, 488–500.

Steinberg, D., Parthasarathy, S., Carew, T.E. *et al.* (1989) Beyond cholesterol. Modifications of low-density lipoprotein that increase its atherogenicity. *N. Engl. J. Med.*, **320**, 915–24.

Diagnosis

Hochreim, M.A. and Sohl, L. (1992) Heart smart: a guide to cardiac tests. *Am. J. Nurs.*, **92**, 22–5.

Timmis, A. (1990) Early diagnosis of acute myocardial infarction. *BMJ*, **301**, 941–2.

Walton, S. (1987) Early imaging of the myocardial infarct. *Br. J. Hosp. Med.*, **38**, 326–32.

21   Cystic fibrosis

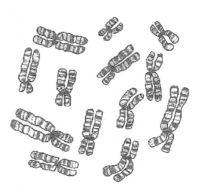

Cystic fibrosis is an inherited disorder characterised by an abnormality of mucus production. The mucus is very thick and sticky and tends to clog up small ducts such as bronchioles in the lung and the pancreatic ducts, causing infection, inflammation and tissue damage. Death often occurs from respiratory failure.

The underlying defect in cystic fibrosis is a mutation in a gene on chromosome 7, inherited as a recessive trait. The gene codes for the cystic fibrosis transmembrane conductance regulator, which acts as a chloride channel, controlling the cellular transport of water, chloride and sodium ions. In the respiratory tract of sufferers of cystic fibrosis, relative impermeability of epithelial cell membranes to chloride ions causes reduced secretion of sodium ions and water. In the sweat ducts, chloride impermeability inhibits the reabsorption of chloride and sodium ions. As a result, the mucus is very thick and the sweat is excessively salty.

The genetic abnormality can be detected by direct analysis of the gene. There are probably several hundred different mutations of the gene that can cause cystic fibrosis, some of which are unique to particular families, but testing for four or five of the most common mutations will reveal about 85% of carriers. Because it is not practicable to test for all possible mutations some negative results will actually be false negatives. In families who already have a child with cystic fibrosis a greater range of gene probes can be used to determine the precise mutation. Prenatal genetic testing can then be used in subsequent pregnancies to determine the status of the fetus reliably.

There is no cure for the disease, but over the past two decades survival has improved greatly, mainly owing to the use of replacement digestive enzymes and antibiotic treatment for respiratory infections. Some patients have also been given lung transplants. Gene therapies are being developed to replace the abnormal gene in cells of the respiratory tract by a normal version, but are unlikely to be available for some time.

Pre-test

- **What is cystic fibrosis and what systems of the body are affected?**
- **At what age does the disease become apparent?**
- **What is the average survival of patients with cystic fibrosis?**
- **How is cystic fibrosis caused?**
- **How is the disease diagnosed?**
- **Is there any way in which cystic fibrosis can be prevented?**
- **What treatments are available for cystic fibrosis?**

Aims of this chapter

By the end of this chapter you will have increased your knowledge of:
◆ The genetic and molecular defects in cystic fibrosis
◆ The pathological features of cystic fibrosis
◆ Current and future prospects for treatment

In addition, this chapter will help you to:
◆ Discuss the way in which cystic fibrosis is inherited and how the genetic changes contribute to biochemical alterations
◆ Describe the pathological changes in various organs and relate how these contribute to the symptoms and complications of the disease
◆ Evaluate the possibilities for genetic screening of carriers and affected individuals
◆ Describe the treatments currently available and evaluate the prospects that gene therapy might have for reducing the impact of the disease

Introduction

Cystic fibrosis principally affects the respiratory and digestive systems. The disease derives its name from the changes that take place in the pancreas: the glands (called acini) that would normally produce digestive enzymes are replaced by fluid-filled **cysts** and fibrous connective tissue (**fibrosis**). These changes occur together as a consequence of inflammation. The inflammatory changes are caused by secretion of abnormal mucus, which becomes lodged in the ducts or passages of various organs, leading to obstruction and infection. Another name for the disease is **mucoviscidosis**, because of the thick and sticky (viscid) mucus produced, sometimes in copious quantities.

Cystic fibrosis is an inherited defect that causes the production of abnormally thick mucus

The clinical features of cystic fibrosis are chronic pulmonary disease, pancreatic insufficiency, steatorrhoea, malnutrition, liver cirrhosis, male infertility and, less frequently, intestinal obstruction. In the sweat glands the disease causes high levels of sodium chloride in the sweat: unless the weather is particularly hot (when it causes heat prostration) this is not detrimental but it is a useful diagnostic sign.

At one time most patients with cystic fibrosis did not survive beyond early childhood, but the prognosis has improved markedly because of improvements in paediatric care, physiotherapy and antibiotic treatments (Figure 21.1). Nonetheless, only about 40% of affected individuals survive beyond 30 years. The disease is debilitating, and has no known cure. The main cause of death is respiratory failure following recurrent bacterial infections. Individuals vary greatly in the degree and severity of the illness. New treatments on the horizon, such as heart–lung transplants, are technologically complex and for the foreseeable future only available to a small proportion of patients. The prospect of gene therapy has received much publicity, but so far trials have taken place only to determine whether the theoretical possibility of gene transfer can be undertaken efficiently and safely. It is not available as a treatment and is unlikely to be so for many years, if at all.

Most people with cystic fibrosis do not live beyond 30 years of age

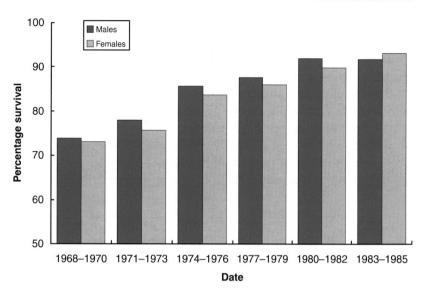

Figure 21.1 Survival to 5 years in boys and girls with cystic fibrosis in the UK. Children born with cystic fibrosis after 1980 are much more likely to survive beyond 5 years of age than those born in 1968–1970. (Data from Dodge, J.A.,*et al.* (1993)*Paediatr. Perinatol. Epidemiol.*, **7**, 157–66.)

> *The disease is inherited: it is the most common single gene disorder*

The cystic fibrosis gene was discovered in 1989, and involves mutations in the long arm (q) of chromosome 7. Until that time, no one knew what the gene did, but it is now known that its protein product, called the **cystic fibrosis transmembrane conductance regulator** (CFTR), behaves as a cellular pump to transfer chloride ions across cell membranes. The defective gene is inherited in a recessive fashion. This means that both parents of affected individuals must carry the genetic mutation, but unless they have been genetically tested they are unaware of this because they also possess a dominant normal gene (see Chapter 3).

Epidemiology

> *About 5200 people in England and Wales have cystic fibrosis*

About 50% of patients can expect to survive to 25 years of age (Figure 21.2), although 65% of the cystic fibrosis population is under 16 years of age. Estimates vary, but the maximum frequency of cystic fibrosis in large white populations is one in 2500: blacks and Orientals are rarely affected. In the UK cystic fibrosis is seen in children of Pakistani and Arab descent, but the figures for disease frequency in the originating countries are difficult to obtain. In countries in which infant mortality rates remain high a diagnosis of cystic fibrosis may often be missed. The frequency of gene carriers in whites is about one in 25 individuals.

Populations vary in the type of genetic mutation responsible for cystic fibrosis. The most common mutation, delta (Δ) F508 (see below) is responsible for nearly 70% of cases in the UK, north America and most of northern Europe.

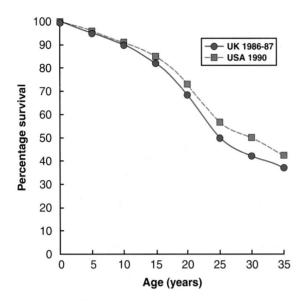

Figure 21.2 Survival of male sufferers of cystic fibrosis in the UK (1986–1987) and the USA (1990). About 40% survive to 35 years of age. Survival prospects are slightly better in the USA. (Adapted from Hodson, M.E. and Geddes, D.M. (eds.), *Cystic Fibrosis*, published by Chapman & Hall, London, 1994.)

Other mutations are more common in southern Europe. Notably, the ΔF508 mutation is found in only 22% of Ashkenazi Jews carriers living in Jerusalem, while the frequency of the W1282X mutation (which is uncommon in the UK) is about 60% (Table 21.1).

Genetics of cystic fibrosis

The normal version of the cystic fibrosis gene spans 250 000 base pairs and codes for a protein of 1480 amino acids. Much of the sequence is non-coding (introns), interspersed by 27 smaller coding areas (exons). With a gene this large the number of possible mutations that could alter the functional properties of the final protein is enormous. More than 400 different mutations of the gene locus that causes cystic fibrosis have been described, but some exist in only one or two families.

Most cases of cystic fibrosis arise from the loss of a single amino acid in a protein responsible for cell transport mechanisms

A collaborative study between 90 laboratories in 26 centres (Emery and Malcolm, 1995) has demonstrated that the ΔF508 mutation is by far the most common. A further five mutation types together account for only about 10% of cystic fibrosis cases (Table 21.1).

Table 21.1 Common mutations in cystic fibrosis

Mutation	Frequency (%)	Gene alteration	Protein alteration
ΔF508	67.2	Deletion of 3 bp at 1652–1655 in exon 10	Deletion of phenylalanine at amino acid position 508

G542X	3.4	Substitution of guanine for thymine at 1756 in exon 11	Truncated protein: glycine at position 542 replaced by stop signal
G551D	2.4	Substitution of adenine for guanine at 1784 in exon 11	Substitution of aspartic acid for glycine at position 551
W1282X	2.1	Substitution of adenine for guanine at 3878 in exon 20	Truncated protein: tryptophan at position 1282 replaced by stop signal
3905	Insertion 2.1	Insertion of extra thymine after 3905 in exon 20	Frameshift

Adapted from: Emery and Malcolm, 1995.

The ΔF508 mutation involves a deletion of three base pairs, causing the loss of phenylalanine at amino acid position 508 in the final protein. The effect of this loss is that the protein is incorrectly assembled and processed within the cell, so that it is not correctly positioned in the cell membrane. It cannot then carry out its normal function of allowing chloride ions across the cell membrane.

Substitution mutations cause the wrong amino acid to be inserted into the sequence. The mutated CFTR appears to reach the cell membrane and be correctly inserted but functions incorrectly, possibly because of changes to its three-dimensional shape. Stop mutations produce a truncated protein which is unstable and non-functional. For more on types of mutation, see Chapter 3.

Role of CFTR

The fundamental defect in cystic fibrosis concerns the operation of CFTR and its ability to allow the transport of chloride anions. The result of this defect is that epithelial cell membranes are less permeable to chloride ions. In the respiratory tract this influences the hydration of mucus; in the sweat glands chloride transport operates in the other direction and there is failure in reabsorption of salt from the sweat.

Respiratory tract
The normal function of respiratory tract epithelial cells is to transport chloride ions into the lumen, thereby maintaining adequate hydration of mucus. In cystic fibrosis chloride transport from the cell into the lumen is impaired and absorption of sodium ions from the lumen into the cell is increased (Figure 21.3).

Sweat glands
Normally, chloride and sodium ions in sweat are reabsorbed by epithelial cells

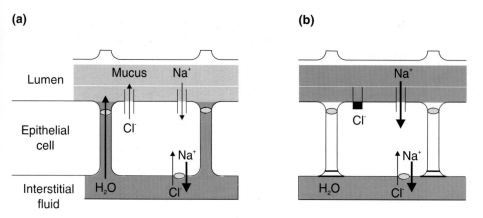

Figure 21.3 Effect of cystic fibrosis on respiratory epithelial cells. (a) Normal respiratory tract epithelial cells transport chloride ions into the lumen, maintaining adequate hydration of mucus. (b) In cystic fibrosis transport of chloride ions out of the cell is blocked and sodium ion resorption from mucus increased. Diffusion of water from interstitial fluid is reduced, causing under-hydration of the respiratory mucus. (Adapted from Elborn, J.S. (1994) *Hosp. Update*, January, 13–20.)

in the sweat duct as the sweat moves towards the surface. Failure of reabsorption leads to the characteristic excess of sodium chloride in the sweat of people with cystic fibrosis (Figure 21.4).

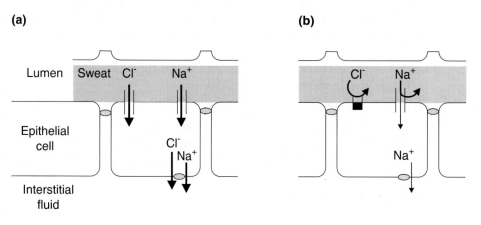

Figure 21.4 Effect of cystic fibrosis on the sweat glands. (a) Normal epithelial cells in the sweat ducts reabsorb chloride and, concomitantly, sodium ions. (b) In cystic fibrosis inability to reabsorb chloride ion results in sweat that is excessively salty.

Detection of cystic fibrosis

Before the identification of the cystic fibrosis gene, gene tracking could be undertaken only in those families with a living affected individual. The method, restriction fragment length polymorphism (RFLP) analysis, by identifying

portions of 'fingerprint' DNA that are usually inherited with the gene, works rather than probing for the cystic fibrosis gene itself. It is now possible to test any individual for defective gene status by probing for the gene mutation itself.

Neonatal screening

The early diagnosis and treatment of cystic fibrosis made possible by neonatal screening reduce short-term morbidity. In the longer term it is unclear whether screening markedly alters the outlook and prolongs survival.

Cystic fibrosis can be difficult to diagnose in the very young because it presents with a range of symptoms of varying severity. Screening therefore offers a more accurate and earlier diagnosis. The tests available are limited in terms of acceptability, sensitivity and specificity. High costs (several thousand pounds per case detected) make it difficult to justify routine screening of all neonates.

Antenatal screening

Antenatal diagnosis of cystic fibrosis has been available for some years, based on estimation of fetal membrane enzymes in amniotic fluid (see Chapter 11). Now that the gene and its common mutations have been identified fetal cells are evaluated by direct gene analysis of a chorionic villus sample. Antenatal screening is currently carried out only if a risk is known to exist – that is, if the parents already have a child with the disease. The possibility that a first-born child has cystic fibrosis (about 80% of cases) can be estimated by carrier screening.

The test is usually carried out at 10 weeks, allowing sufficient time for termination (if necessary) by 12 or 13 weeks.

The availability of gene probes for some of the common mutations has transformed the situation. Because there are so many possible mutations in cystic fibrosis cost and time limitations make it impracticable to test for them all. The usual practice is to screen for ΔF508 and five or six of the other most common mutations: in most European and American populations this would identify about 85% of cases. For any mutations that are identified the test is completely accurate. The advantage of screening for the gene itself over RFLP linkage studies is that it is not necessary to take blood from an existing family member with the disease. The method can be extended to carrier screening of unaffected families. Although not yet commonly employed, it can also be combined with *in vitro* fertilisation: the individual fertilised cells are screened for cystic fibrosis, any affected embryos are discarded and the normal embryos used for implantation.

Carrier screening

By probing for the gene mutation itself it is possible to test any individual for

defective gene carrier status. The test is simple, involving a mouthwash sample, and is quite cheap. For the reasons stated above the test detects only 85% of carriers, although a positive result is unequivocal. The main rationale for carrier screening is that pregnancy is emotionally not the best time to undertake genetic testing: a positive result necessitates the uncomfortable decision between termination or producing an affected child. Carrier screening could allow more considered decisions (although these are still not easy): whether or not to have children, to use artificial insemination or to find a new partner (the information alone could place an intolerable strain on the relationship).

Couples will be placed in three risk categories: (1) both partners are carriers; (2) one partner is a carrier; (3) neither partner is a carrier. The first group, comprising about 0.1% of couples, have a one in four risk of having a child with cystic fibrosis. In the second category there is a small residual risk because of the possibility that the other partner may carry one of the less common, untested mutations. In the third the risk is negligible. In the first category, antenatal screening can be offered, but in the first pregnancy there is still a risk of false-negatives. Clearly no further action needs to be taken when neither partner is a carrier, but in the intermediate category anxieties may become so great that they can be allayed only by antenatal testing.

Another approach to carrier screening is to apply it to the general population, perhaps in children of school age, but until the genetic status of a reproductive partner is known the information obtained by this means is of little value. There are additional problems, such as how to record the information (will the child remember the result of the test, will the information be recorded somewhere, and who will have access to the information?) and possible stigmatisation (not everyone will understand that carrier status *per se* is completely harmless.

For carrier screening to have any real value the genetic status of both partners must be known

Review question 1

Do you think it possible that you carry the cystic fibrosis gene?

Review question 2

What are the chances of a couple producing children with cystic fibrosis if both partners carry the gene?

Review question 3

Why is the risk of having a child with cystic fibrosis so much greater for a mother who already has the disease?

Pathology

Lungs

The underlying abnormality of sodium and chloride ion transport causes respiratory mucus to become abnormally thick. This impairs the mucociliary clearance of micro-organisms and irritants from the lungs. The following series of events occurs in the lungs:

- Abnormally thick mucus is produced by respiratory epithelial cells
- Small-diameter airways (bronchioles) become blocked, leading to bacterial infection and inflammation
- Normal bronchial epithelium is destroyed by inflammation
- Fibrous scar tissue forms (fibrosis)
- Abscesses form and emphysema develops
- Respiratory failure
- Heart failure

The mucus obstruction and subsequent infections lead to an inflammatory

The lungs become blocked by mucus; this leads to infection, inflammation and scarring

Atelectasis: collapse of lung tissue.

Bronchiectasis: dilatation of the bronchioles with fibrosis.

Emphysema: breakdown of the walls of individual alveoli, reducing the surface area available for gaseous exchange.

Haemoptysis: coughing up of blood.

Kyphosis: curvature of the spine.

Pneumothorax: leakage of air from the lungs into the pleural cavity.

reaction. Persistent inflammation causes further tissue damage evident as bronchiectasis (Figure 21.5). Eventually erosion of the bronchial walls by inflammation results in an abscess. The combination of blockage by mucus, infection and inflammation also leads to localised atelectasis alternating with areas of emphysema.

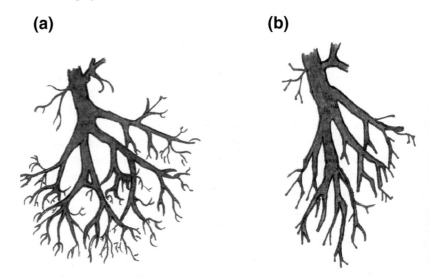

(a) **(b)**

Figure 21.5 Bronchiectasis. (a) Normal tapered branching network. (b) Bronchiectasis. The persistent inflammation in the lungs that accompanies cystic fibrosis damages the bronchial tree, causing dilation and loss of tapered ends and smaller terminal branches.

> *Sufferers of cystic fibrosis usually die from respiratory or heart failure*

The first symptoms of progressive obstructive airways disease are cough and increasing sputum production. By the age of 15 most patients produce sputum daily, often with haemoptysis. Patients suffer increasing breathing difficulties which in turn lead to chest deformity and kyphosis. Pneumothorax, haemoptysis and right-sided heart failure follow because of the pulmonary insufficiency. Precautions should be taken to minimise exposure to common respiratory infections, and patients should be immunised against whooping cough, measles and influenza. The principal bacterial organisms associated with pulmonary infections in cystic fibrosis are *Staphylococcus aureus*, *Haemophilus influenzae* and *Pseudomonas aeruginosa* (see below).

Digestive system

> *Pancreatic glands are destroyed by inflammation, resulting in fluid-filled cysts and fibrous scar tissue*

Pathological changes occur throughout the alimentary tract. In particular, the ducts of exocrine glands in the pancreas, liver and salivary glands become blocked by excessively viscous mucus. This leads to secondary tissue damage by inflammation and fibrosis.

Blockage of the pancreatic ducts prevents the digestive enzymes from reaching the duodenum. Activation of pancreatic enzymes by inflammation

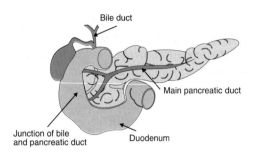

Figure 21.6 Pancreas and duodenum. The exocrine secretions of the pancreas are carried in ducts and transferred to the duodenum.

and the inflammatory process itself causes autodigestion and destruction of the glands, with formation of cystic spaces and fibrous scar tissue. As the exocrine glands are in direct connection with the ducts these are destroyed first. Ultimately the insulin-producing endocrine glands become affected as the damage spreads and diabetes may develop.

Without pancreatic enzymes, intestinal malabsorption occurs. The malabsorption gives rise to offensive and abnormally bulky stools containing undigested fat and protein; this is referred to as **steatorrhoea**. The impaction of undigested bowel contents can cause abdominal pain, distension of the bowel and vomiting. The patient may also be susceptible to malnutrition, poor growth and specific deficiencies of fat-soluble vitamins.

In about 15% of cases gastrointestinal symptoms are present at birth. These babies present with gastrointestinal obstruction or **meconium ileus**: the small intestine is blocked by viscous plugs of mucus. This may even occur *in utero* and lead to perforation of the intestine. The prospects for survival beyond infancy are poor for babies with these early manifestations of the disease. Other patients readily survive into adolescence and adulthood, and a small minority develop no significant pancreatic involvement. Homozygotes for the ΔF508 deletion invariably suffer pancreatic insufficiency.

Initially the endocrine glands of the pancreas are spared, and diabetes is more likely to be seen in older patients. The incidence of diabetes in cystic fibrosis is 8–15%, but about 50% of all patients have impaired glucose tolerance, indicating that there has been some damage to the endocrine pancreas.

Some patients also have liver problems, because of blockage of the bile duct which leads to cirrhosis. The reduced cell function in the damaged liver increases pressure in the portal circulation (portal hypertension) and can lead to oesophageal varices. Some 5% of cystic fibrosis patients have obvious liver disease and a further 20% have minor liver abnormalities.

Fertility

The vast majority of young men with cystic fibrosis are infertile because of a congenital bilateral absence or atrophy of the vas deferens (CBAVD). Semen analysis reveals azoospermia in almost all men with the disease, although

Azoospermia: semen contains no living spermatozoa, causing infertility.

Endocrine gland: a ductless gland, the secretions of which are absorbed directly into the bloodstream.

Exocrine gland: a gland that passes its secretions into ducts.

Meconium: the first dark-coloured stools passed by a newborn baby.

Meconium ileus: obstruction of the small intestine at birth.

> *The most common gastrointestinal complication is obstruction*

Oesophageal varices: portal hypertension causes blood flow in the coronary veins of the stomach to divert into the submucosa of the lower oesophagus. These veins dilate and protrude directly beneath the mucosa. There is a chance that they will rupture, causing catastrophic blood loss.

> *Patients with cystic fibrosis can become diabetic*

> *A minority of adult patients develop liver disease*

> *Men with cystic fibrosis are infertile*

Immunoreactive trypsin:
radioimmunoassay for serum trypsin
which is elevated in neonates with cystic
fibrosis. The test is limited to the
neonatal period because the antigen
falls to normal levels within a few weeks
of birth.

▲ Key points

Clinical features of cystic fibrosis

▲ Triad of obstructive lung disease, loose stools and failure to thrive

Meconium ileus:
▲ Uncommon presentation of cystic fibrosis in neonates
▲ Intestinal tract obstructed by thick mucus plug
▲ Can cause perforation and peritonitis

Pancreas and liver:
▲ Exocrine pancreas insufficiency develops in childhood and adolescence
▲ Obstruction leads to gland destruction with cystic spaces and fibrosis
▲ Enzyme deficiency causes fat and vitamin malabsorption, steatorrhoea, wasting and stunting of growth
▲ Liver fatty change and cirrhosis caused by mucus blockage of bile canaliculi: affects 5–10% of patients

Lung disease:
▲ Lung tissue progressively destroyed by infection, bronchiectasis and fibrosis

Infertility:
▲ Obstruction of epididymis and vas deferens causes male infertility

---

erectile function is unaffected. Men with CBAVD can become fathers by means of microsurgical aspiration of sperm from the epididymis, followed by *in vitro* fertilisation. The high frequency of mutations in their sperm, together with the possibility that their partner could be a carrier, makes it essential that genetic screening is carried out. Couples will also have to be counselled in view of the reduced life expectancy of the potential father: the woman may well have to cope with a dependent partner as well as a young child.

The fertility of women with cystic fibrosis is impaired because of changes in cervical mucus secretions. Female patients are often underweight and may have amenorrhoea. Nevertheless many women with the disease have undergone normal pregnancy. There is no increase in the incidence of abortions or malformations, although the baby is more likely to be born prematurely and small.

Women in sexual relationships should be counselled carefully because of the increased risk of producing a child with the disease. Because of her own short life expectancy her child might have to be cared for by someone else. If there is no history of cystic fibrosis in her partner's family the risk of producing an affected child is approximately one in 50 (assuming the partner is white and the carrier gene frequency is one in 25). This risk can be substantially reduced, but not eliminated, by genetic screening of the partner.

Diagnosis

Most patients are diagnosed within the first 2–3 years of life, usually after presenting with recurrent infections, diarrhoea, stunted growth and a generalised failure to thrive. Neonatal screening would allow patients to be identified in the first weeks of life, but this is not routinely carried out in the UK.

Most cases of cystic fibrosis can be detected by measuring **immunoreactive trypsin** in blood and confirmed by a **sweat test**. Direct **gene analysis** using a gene probe for the more common ΔF508 mutation can also be carried out. The pancreatic and liver involvement in the disease gives rise to abnormal pancreatic secretions and to altered liver function test results.

At present, prediction of the eventual severity of the disease is unreliable, although the minority of patients who have pancreatic sufficiency tend to have less severe lung disease.

Treatment

Treatment strategies are based on combating respiratory infections, improving bronchial drainage by physiotherapy and improving nutrition. This approach has served patients well, many now surviving into their fourth decade. Treatments designed to correct the fundamental defect are in early stages of development but it is unlikely that they will become available to help adult sufferers who are alive today.

Respiratory changes

The main treatment is physiotherapy combined with appropriate bronchodilator and antibiotic therapy. Adolescents and young adults may be able to manage their own physiotherapy by breathing exercises and by inhaling salbutamol and saline. The most successful form of physiotherapy in the growing child and young adult is a combination of postural drainage and forced expiration. Exercises such as jogging, weight training and even swimming should not be discouraged. Usually at least an hour a day is devoted to physiotherapy: this puts a strain on both sufferer and carers. The constant possibility of recurrent infections and the need for rapid hospital treatment make it very difficult for families to fulfil work commitments and to plan for the future.

A common complication in adolescents is haemoptysis which often accompanies episodes of infection. In most cases this bleeding is not severe or life-threatening and will stop spontaneously but occasionally the bleeding is continuous. It may be necessary to consider bronchial artery embolisation, which involves catheterisation of the bronchial arteries.

Some patients with cystic fibrosis also have asthma. This is usually treated with oral or inhaled steroids and β-agonists. Pneumothorax may present in advanced cases during adolescence or adulthood, associated with symptoms of breathlessness and chest pain. Treatment may involve oxygen therapy and antibiotics, but a large pneumothorax may require intercostal drainage and surgical intervention could be necessary to repair a persistent air leak.

A new treatment is a product of recombinant DNA technology: recombinant human DNAase (rhDNAase). The respiratory symptoms of cystic fibrosis are exacerbated by release of DNA (arising from tissue damage and inflammation) into the airways. The DNA renders respiratory mucus even more viscous and liable to block the airways. The recombinant DNAase can be introduced into the respiratory tract in aerosol form, to split the DNA into smaller fragments and hence reduce mucus viscosity.

> *Patients with cystic fibrosis need daily physiotherapy*

Breathing exercises: lung function can be improved by a cycle of exercises combining breathing control, chest expansion and huffing (forced expiration). Breathing control is breathing normally at the patient's own rate (a resting phase to avoid over-exertion), followed by chest expansion with slow, deep inspirations as far as possible and ordinary expiration. Forced expiration consists of a 'huff', which narrows the airways and forces mucus upwards. The exercises usually take 20 minutes or so to complete.

> *Recombinant DNAase aerosols can thin respiratory mucus and help clear infections*

Microbiology of cystic fibrosis

Respiratory infections often cause respiratory distress and progressive lung damage in cystic fibrosis. Infections are frequent, usually involving the bronchi and bronchioles rather than lung alveoli. The infections are typically caused by bacteria, although acute viral, fungal or mycoplasma infections also occur. There is no detectable immune deficiency in cystic fibrosis and, outside the respiratory tract, infections are no more common than in other people of similar age.

Most antibiotic therapies effective against the common infective organisms of the respiratory tract are given intravenously. Because of the frequency of respiratory infections some patients are given an implant to allow intravenous antibiotics to be given quickly and conveniently. Generally, most patients require antibiotics in higher doses over longer periods of time than unaffected

Postural drainage: drainage of mucus from the lungs is aided by placing patients with their head below their shoulders. The trunk is raised by placing pillows or a foam block under the hips. The patient lies face down, or on the left or right side to aid clearance from the different lobes of the lungs. In the face-down position the therapist claps the lower ribs, close to the spine on each side. In lateral positions the therapist claps between the collar bone and nipple on each side.

Staphylococcus aureus: this organism probably accounts for more frequent and varied human diseases than any other. It colonises the skin and mucosal surfaces and is a cause of abscesses, septicaemia, osteomyelitis, postoperative wound sepsis, CNS infections, food poisoning and toxic shock syndrome.

Sweat test: sweat production is stimulated by low-current electrodes and the pharmaceutically active agent pilocarpine placed on the skin. Sodium ion concentration in the sweat is measured by flame photometry or with an ion-selective electrode. Chloride ions are measured by titration. Concentrations of both ions are elevated in cystic fibrosis.

P. aeruginosa is the most significant pathogen of lung disease in patients with cystic fibrosis

---

Pseudomonas aeruginosa: a Gram-negative motile rod-shaped bacterium found in the general environment, especially in fresh water and soil contaminated by animals or humans. Important cause of nosocomial infections in burns victims, cancer patients and children with cystic fibrosis

people. An antibiotic is chosen on the basis of the organism identified in a sputum sample and its sensitivity to the drug.

Staphylococcus aureus

This is one of the first respiratory pathogens encountered by young patients with cystic fibrosis. It causes respiratory distress and may be responsible for some of the early lung damage but is usually well-controlled by antibiotic therapy. Before antibiotics were available few patients with cystic fibrosis survived beyond infancy: *Staph. aureus* was the main cause of death.

Some people believe that *Staph. aureus* infections can pave the way for subsequent *Pseudomonas aeruginosa* infection, which probably relies on a breakdown of local defensive barriers in the lungs. For this reason prophylactic antibiotic therapy (see below) has been widely used and is responsible for the comparative rarity of *Staph. aureus* infections.

Pseudomonas aeruginosa

P. aeruginosa is much more of a problem than *Staph. aureus*. It colonises the lungs of almost all patients by the age of 15–20 years and is almost impossible to eradicate. This organism has an innate resistance to most antibiotics and disinfectants. It does not infect healthy individuals unless some tissue damage has already occurred, such as to the skin in burns victims. In cystic fibrosis previous damage and loss of respiratory epithelium by other infections and inflammation set up the conditions for opportunistic infection.

Early in the course of infection, normal colony types are found in sputum samples but with time the organism mutates to a **mucoid** form, which in culture resembles the mucus secretions of the patient. The mucoid form adheres to the abnormal respiratory mucus, which probably accounts for its persistence in cystic fibrosis. The slimy mucoid appearance of the colonies is caused by the organism producing copious amounts of the polysaccharide **alginate**. This substance probably helps the organism to adhere to tissue and protects it against immune clearance. Most of the lung damage is caused by the inflammatory response to the organism and the mucoid material (Figure 21.7). The organism rarely invades beyond the lungs.

P. aeruginosa is ubiquitous and it is unrealistic to attempt to protect patients with cystic fibrosis from infection throughout their lives. Attempts have been made to institute treatment early or prophylactically, to eliminate infection before the organism mutates into the more resistant mucoid form. Work is continuing to develop a vaccine that will prevent colonisation.

Haemophilus influenzae

Children and young adults with cystic fibrosis are very prone to lower respiratory tract infections by the non-capsulated form of *H. influenzae*. This organism is probably responsible for some of the acute exacerbations of chronic lung disease in cystic fibrosis patients.

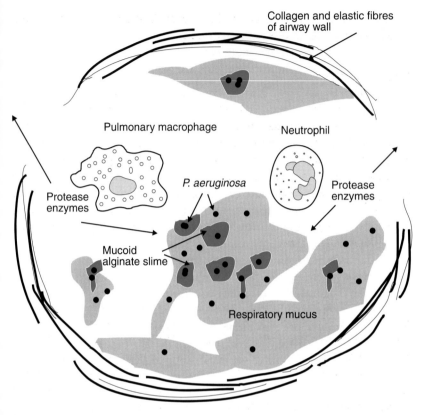

Figure 21.7 Colonisation of the small airways by *P. aeruginosa*. *P. aeruginosa* attaches itself to respiratory mucus. In time the organism mutates to the mucoid form, surrounding itself with a mucoid alginate slime. Macrophages and neutrophils, as part of the inflammatory response, release proteases in an attempt to destroy the organism. This is largely unsuccessful because of the mucoid barrier, and instead the enzymes attack collagen and elastic fibres in the airway wall, causing chronic lung disease.

Burkholderia cepacia: widely distributed in soil, water and plants. It is inherently resistant to many antibiotics and survives disinfectants. In most individuals it is not pathogenic, but can cause infections of endocardium, blood, peritoneum, bones, joints, meninges and lungs in susceptible individuals.

Haemophilus influenzae: a small Gram-negative rod-shaped bacterium with capsulated and non-capsulated forms. In the absence of cystic fibrosis non-capsulated forms are present asymptomatically in the nasopharynx and throat of most people. The capsule is the main virulence factor and the type b form is a main cause of meningitis in young children. *H. influenzae* type b is also an important cause of bacterial pneumonia, which occurs mostly in adults.

Chronic *H. influenzae* infections become established in a minority of patients. The infection is usually treated with oral ampicillin or amoxycillin but this may cause more resistant strains to produce β-lactamase. In these cases therapy is combined with β-lactamase inhibitors or other drugs (such as fluoroquinolones).

Burkholderia cepacia

A relatively new risk for patients with cystic fibrosis is infection by *B. cepacia* (formerly known as *Pseudomonas cepacia*). This Gram-negative bacillus was first described as a cause of rot in onions but it is now recognised as an important human pathogen, and infection carries a real risk of deterioration or premature death in cystic fibrosis. Infection leads to rapidly progressive lung damage and is very difficult to treat because of multiple antibiotic resistance.

Infection with *B. cepacia* in patients with cystic fibrosis was first noted in the late 1970s and infection rates have increased steadily since then. Infection seems to be transmitted by patient-to-patient contact. Many clinics now operate a strict segregation policy and patients are advised to keep social contact between themselves and infected patients to a minimum.

Prophylactic antibiotic therapy

There is controversy surrounding the prophylactic use of antibiotics. Proponents claim that it prolongs the interval before inevitable bacterial colonisation of the respiratory system and could increase life expectancy by delaying the onset of chronic lung disease. Opponents argue that anti-staphylococcal therapy increases the incidence of *H. influenzae* and *P. aeruginosa* infections. They also express concern that treatment without overt infection would contribute to emergence of antibiotic-resistant strains.

Routine administration of intravenous antibiotics to prevent infection with *P. aeruginosa* has been advocated by physicians in Denmark. A regimen comprising 3-monthly intravenous courses of tobramicyn and β-lactam antibiotics combined with inhalation of colistin (Jensen *et al.*, 1989) has yielded encouraging results: decline in lung function was slowed and survival better than in historical controls. The combination therapy protects most patients from onset of infection with *P. aeruginosa* for up to 2 years.

Digestive system

The nutritional goals for a patient with cystic fibrosis are to normalise body weight, promote growth and development, improve the immune system (thereby optimising pulmonary function and tissue repair), improve muscle strength and enhance the quality of life. The diet is modified to provide a nutritional intake high in energy and protein, with moderate-to-high fat intake.

Pancreatic enzyme replacement is essential for most patients with cystic fibrosis

In most cases the pancreas fails to produce sufficient amounts of the enzymes needed for digestion: this can be helped by replacement enzymes. Various enzyme preparations are available in the form of acid-resistant microspheres (Creon and Nutrizym GR, for example) and are to be taken just before, during, and at the end of every meal. The amount of enzyme needed varies with the amount of food and the proportion of fat in it. The dose should reduce the size and frequency of the stools and alter their consistency, with the result that the child will gain weight and grow. These drugs have side-effects, such as colicky abdominal pain, flatulence and severe constipation, particularly in large doses.

The healthy diets recommended for the general population are not suitable for patients with cystic fibrosis

Most people with cystic fibrosis need 20–50% greater energy and protein intakes than unaffected individuals of the same age because intestinal absorption is less efficient than normal, even with pancreatic enzyme replacement. An adequate calorie intake is unlikely on a low-fat high-fibre diet. Patients with cystic fibrosis are liable to become vitamin-deficient, particularly in the fat-soluble vitamins A, D and E. Their daily requirements for these vitamins are double those for unaffected people (about 8000 IU vitamin

A, 800 IU vitamin D and 100–200 mg vitamin E). Well nourished patients have a better outlook. Where possible, normal meals and nutritious snacks should be taken, together with appropriate enzyme replacement therapy but, if this is insufficient, supplemental feeds (Table 21.2) or tube feeding (usually nasogastric or nasojejunal feeds) can be given. These may be necessary where there are severe chest problems and infections.

Table 21.2 Food supplements suitable for patients with cystic fibrosis

Supplement	Product	Application
Glucose polymers	Maxijul, Polycal, Caloreen	Add to drinks, soups, sauces and puddings
Fat emulsions	Liquigen, Calogen	Add to milk, drinks and sauces
Drinks	Fresubin, Fortisip, Liquiscrib, Build-up	Add to milk, soups, sauces and puddings

Several strategies can be used to optimise nutritional intake:
- Use energy-dense foods
- Fortification of foods with extra protein (by adding grated cheese or milk powder to foods)
- Take regular snacks and meals
- Use full-cream milk
- Use food supplements, but guard against the supplement becoming a replacement for normal foods

Diabetes

Older sufferers of cystic fibrosis may become diabetic because of progressive pancreatic damage. Unlike other people with diabetes, cystic fibrosis patients do not need dietary restrictions because they need to maintain a high energy intake. Food intake should be distributed in regular small amounts throughout the day. Insulin injections are needed to control blood sugar levels.

Diabetes in patients with cystic fibrosis should be managed with insulin

Transplantation

All the treatments so far described are aimed at ameliorating the symptoms of cystic fibrosis. One approach aimed at correcting the fundamental genetic defect is to replace the principal organs involved in the disease through heart–lung or double lung transplantation. These treatments can be offered to the adolescent or adult with end-stage lung disease but the demand for these procedures far outweighs the number of organs available. In the UK this procedure was first undertaken in 1985 and some patients are still alive 8 years later. In some centres the 2-year survival rate is about 65%.

Review question 4

What diet would you recommend for children with cystic fibrosis?

Gene therapy

The aim of gene therapy is to insert a normal working gene into cells containing a defective gene

Any attempt at gene therapy relies on incorporating normal copies of a defective gene into somatic cells. The first targets for gene therapy were diseases affecting the haematopoietic system because the placement of a normal gene in bone marrow stem cells offers the possibility of providing a continuous supply of corrected cells. For example, bone marrow cells can be taken from a patient, the defective gene replaced, and the cells put back. Other genetic disorders present more of a problem because the affected cells may be widespread and relatively inaccessible.

Gene therapy presents a host of technical problems:

- The gene and associated regulatory DNA must be isolated
- Sufficient DNA for treatment must be generated
- The gene must be incorporated into a carrier which can transport it to the target cells
- The gene has to be delivered to the nucleus of the cell and incorporated into the host cell genetic material in such a way that it will be active
- Once in the cell's nucleus the gene should remain there
- Incorporation of the gene should produce no undesirable effects (such as activation of an oncogene that could initiate malignant transformation)

Genes can be introduced into cells using virus or liposome carriers

A normal gene can be placed by incorporating the normal gene into a virus and allowing the virus to infect the target cells. Many viruses are pathogenic in humans, and the goal of molecular biologists is to 'snip out' that viral DNA with pathogenic properties and replace it with desired human DNA.

The next problem is to get the virus and its human DNA into the target cell, so that it is incorporated into the genetic material and the cell makes the desired normal protein. The most efficient way is to use retroviruses, which in tissue culture have the potential to infect 100% of dividing cells and become fully integrated within the host cell's genetic material. Unfortunately, the retrovirus will infect only dividing cells, and in the respiratory tract only a few cells may be dividing at any one time. There are fears that in the long term the continued presence of extra human and viral DNA in cell clones could activate oncogenes and initiate malignancy.

An alternative strategy is to use adenoviruses as the carrier (the viruses that cause the common cold). They are able to infect non-dividing cells and are not incorporated directly into the host cell's genetic material but their genetic information does alter the function of the cell. The adenovirus and the beneficial gene it carries will, with time, be shed from the cell. Therefore any benefits are temporary and treatments must be repeated.

The possibility of using non-viral carriers (such as **liposomes**) for gene transfer is now being explored because the vector itself is less likely to elicit a pathogenic response. Liposomes are normally taken up by cell receptor mechanisms and used for a variety of metabolic tasks. A problem with this approach is that the material may not reach the desired destination – the cell might transport the liposome and its incorporated DNA to the lysosomes, where it will be degraded.

Gene therapy has the potential to treat a wide range of genetically determined conditions, including cancer as well as monogenetic diseases such as cystic fibrosis. To date about 100 clinical protocols are approved for gene therapy, involving more than 300 patients, including some with cystic fibrosis. So far there is little evidence of clinical efficacy, although most of the trials are in a very early phase and have been more concerned with establishing the procedure and matters of safety.

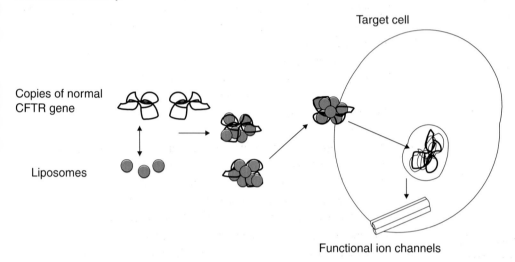

Figure 21.8 Delivery of normal CFTR gene using liposome carrier. Copies of the normal CFTR gene are made using recombinant DNA technology and the negatively charged DNA copies combined with cationic liposomes to produce DNA–liposome complexes. These will be taken up by target cells via surface receptors. The newly introduced DNA should reach the nucleus and express the normal transmembrane receptor protein.

Recent research has focused on the possibility of inserting a normal version of the CFTR gene into cells. The principal target cells are those lining the respiratory tract because, theoretically, they are relatively easily accessible by means of aerosol inhalation of modified genetic material and it is the lung manifestations of fibrosis that are the main causes of illness and death. Correction of the pancreatic deficiency would be much more difficult – and for many patients these are adequately corrected with oral pancreatic enzyme supplements.

Gene therapy may eventually become an option for treating cystic fibrosis

One approach is to incorporate the normal gene into an adenovirus which is then used to infect cells of the respiratory tract. As the adenovirus naturally infects the respiratory tract the normal gene should be incorporated into the respiratory epithelial cells. The technique has already been demonstrated in rats, and clinical trials are now under way with human volunteers in the USA and the UK. A possible disadvantage of using adenovirus is that the adenovirus itself is an infectious agent; it could elicit an inflammatory response and worsen the respiratory damage.

An alternative approach, using DNA–liposomes as the carrier, has been shown to be capable of gene delivery to mouse and rat lungs, and a human study has recently been completed (Caplen *et al.*, 1995). The results show that there is still a long way to go before gene therapy becomes an effective treatment of cystic fibrosis – in fact, no lung changes or improvement in clinical symptoms were demonstrated and the transferred material exerted only temporary effects.

Joan and Stuart Smith live in London. Both are white. Joan works part-time as a secretary for a local business and Stuart is an underwriter for an insurance company. Their son, Anthony, is now 6 years old. He weighed 6 lb 2 oz at birth and in his first few months was apparently healthy. He suffered minor colds and coughs, which resolved satisfactorily.

After his third birthday Anthony developed a persistent daily cough. He also complained on several occasions of 'tummy-ache' and appeared to have suffered episodes of diarrhoea. The family health visitor expressed concern about his weight. On the basis of the clinical history, the family doctor decided to refer Anthony for further investigation, with a provisional diagnosis of cystic fibrosis.

- Is Anthony's case typical of the age, gender and socioeconomic distribution of cystic fibrosis?
- What risk factors are usually associated with the disease?
- What laboratory tests or imaging techniques would be helpful in confirming the diagnosis?
- What are the usual symptoms of cystic fibrosis?
- What further problems can be expected?
- What is the expected survival of patients with cystic fibrosis?

ANSWERS TO REVIEW QUESTIONS

Question 1

Do you think it possible that you carry the cystic fibrosis gene?

Most people will be entirely unaware that they carry the cystic fibrosis gene because carrier status is asymptomatic. A person's carrier status becomes apparent only after they have produced a child with the disease or they have undergone genetic screening. The probability of a white person having one copy of the gene is one in 25; the gene is therefore present in 8% of couples. The problem of cystic fibrosis arises only if both partners carry the gene.

Question 2

What are the chances of a couple producing children with cystic fibrosis if both partners carry the gene?

It is possible for both partners to carry the defective gene and yet produce normal children: this is purely a matter of chance. The probability of inheriting both copies of the gene, one from each parent, is 25%.

Case study

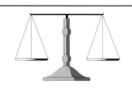

DNA-liposome complex vs. liposome alone

▲ Double-blind placebo controlled trial: nine patients received liposomes with normal CFTR gene, six received liposome alone

▲ Agent topically applied to nasal epithelium

▲ Outcome measure: electrical potential difference in nasal epithelium (elevated in cystic fibrosis because of hyper-absorption of sodium ions)

▲ 20% improvement towards normal values observed in group treated with DNA–liposome

▲ Reversion to pretreatment values by day 7

From: Caplen *et al.*, 1995.

Review question 5

What are the probable limitations of gene therapy in treating cystic fibrosis?

Question 3

Why is the risk of having a child with cystic fibrosis so much greater for a mother who already has the disease?

In a mother with cystic fibrosis both versions of the CFTR gene will be defective. If the father has two normal genes all the offspring will receive one copy of the defective gene from their mother and will therefore be carriers. If the father is himself a carrier, the probability of producing a child with cystic fibrosis is 50%.

Question 4

What diet would you recommend for children with cystic fibrosis?

Children with cystic fibrosis should be given the kind of diet that ought to horrify mothers of unaffected children, because of their need to maintain body weight in the face of the digestive enzyme deficiency: these children *never* become obese. Unfortunately, because of their short life expectancy they need not worry about the risks of high saturated fats in producing coronary heart disease.

A diet high in energy and protein (full-cream milk, full-fat cheeses and creamy yoghurts) should be encouraged. Children should be encouraged to eat generous portions of butter or margarine on bread, potatoes and other vegetables. Foods should be fried rather than grilled: this both increases the taste of the food and adds to the calorie intake.

Question 5

What are the probable limitations of gene therapy in treating cystic fibrosis?

At present it is not known whether the use of adenoviruses in humans will infect sufficient cells, or that they will express the correct gene product. As the adenovirus and its inserted gene will ultimately be shed from the respiratory tract cells treatments must be repeated. Although the start-up costs are high in terms of isolating the normal version of the gene and inserting this into the virus, the virus can be replicated in this form so that eventually the cost of individual treatments should be acceptable.

The long-term effects on the host cells are unknown and it is possible that oncogenes might be abnormally stimulated to induce malignant change. The treatment is aimed only at the cells in the respiratory tract, where the effects of the disease are most apparent, but the fundamental defect in the digestive tract will remain unaltered. Therefore, unless gene therapy can also be targeted at this area, patients will still die from gastrointestinal and liver complications.

Case study

In Anthony's case a diagnosis of cystic fibrosis was confirmed by sweat and

immunoreactive trypsin tests. Tests of liver function and pancreatic function were conducted to evaluate the severity of the disease and chest and abdominal radiographs taken. The chest radiograph revealed a slightly flattened diaphragm but no other abnormality. The abdominal radiograph revealed an obstruction in the lower bowel.

Anthony was managed by a multidisciplinary team. He was started on the anti-staphylococcal agent flucloxacillin, 250 mg intravenously four times a day. Throat swab and sputum analysis showed the presence of *Staph. aureus*. The small obstruction of his lower bowel seen was resolved by a mild laxative and rehydration with intravenous fluid. Anthony was referred for chest physiotherapy including coughing, breathing exercises, forced expiration and postural drainage.

Anthony and his parents were also referred to a dietician for assessment. He was started on a high-protein, high-calorie diet with vitamin and other dietary supplements. Pancreatic enzymes were prescribed in the form of enteric-coated Creon capsules, 10–12 capsules to be taken before and with each meal.

Is Anthony's case typical of the age, gender and socioeconomic distribution of cystic fibrosis? Yes. Cystic fibrosis is a disease of childhood and young adults. Diagnosis is usually made in the first 2–3 years of life. The incidence of the disease is roughly the same in both sexes, with slightly increased incidence in males. Males are usually infertile. There are no direct socioeconomic differences in disease frequency but there are racial differences.

What risk factors are usually associated with the disease? Other than having white parents, there are none. The disease is purely genetic in origin.

What laboratory tests or imaging techniques would be helpful in confirming the diagnosis? Sweat test: measurement of sweat electrolytes; stool microscopy and estimation of faecal fat and chymotrypsin; estimation of serum immunoreactive trypsin; chest and abdominal radiography; throat swab and sputum analysis.

What are the usual symptoms of cystic fibrosis? Poor growth; respiratory symptoms, usually recurrent or persistent bronchitis; gastrointestinal symptoms (abdominal distension/gastrointestinal obstruction, meconium ileus (in neonates), diarrhoea, offensive stools caused by pancreatic insufficiency and diabetes mellitus, usually in adults).

What further problems can be expected? A variety of medical, psychological and social problems can be anticipated. There is no cure for cystic fibrosis, and the aims of treatment are to counter infection, limit tissue damage by inflammation and to provide nutritional support. This undoubtedly prolongs both the quality and length of life for sufferers. The symptoms can become more difficult to control as the disease progresses. Fibrosis may occur at many sites (usually in the lungs, pancreas, liver and bowel) as a result of infection and chronic inflammation. Pain may be associated with the sites of inflammation, tissue damage and organ enlargement. Diabetes mellitus is likely to develop as pancreatic tissue is progressively destroyed.

Therapy may also have side-effects: pancreatic enzymes can produce abdominal pain and an allergic reaction; antibiotics can cause allergic reactions.

The course of events for many patients will include numerous admissions to hospital or clinics to deal with recurrent chest infections. This will have a disruptive effect on the sufferer and the family. The requirement for daily physiotherapy and enzyme therapy will also be disruptive: cystic fibrosis is not a disease that can be forgotten, even for a day. This weighs heavily on the lives of patients and their families, and is often accompanied by feelings of guilt, fear, anger, pain and helplessness. Psychological problems can develop as the child matures and begins to understand the true nature and prognosis of the illness. Both child and carers may require counselling and the opportunity to share experiences through contacts with other sufferers.

What is the expected survival of patients with cystic fibrosis? This depends on the respiratory and gastrointestinal features of the disease. There are approximately 6000 cystic fibrosis sufferers in the UK. In 1980 20% of patients were over 16 years of age; this figure had risen to 36% by 1990, and is expected to increase further. About 40% of patients can expect to survive beyond 30 years, but few live past 35 years. Most patients die of respiratory failure.

References

Caplen, N.J., Alton, E.W.F.W., Middleton, P.G. *et al.* (1995) Liposome-mediated CFTR gene transfer to the nasal epithelium in patients with cystic fibrosis. *Nature Med.*, **1**, 39–46.

Emery, A.E. and Malcolm, S. (1995) *An Introduction to Recombinant DNA in Medicine*, 2nd edn, Wiley, Chichester.

Jensen, T., Pedersen, S.S., Hoiby, N. *et al.* (1989) Use of antibiotics in cystic fibrosis: the Danish approach. *Antibiot. Chemother.*, **42**, 237–46.

Further reading

Goodchild, M.C. and Dodge, J.A. (1989) *Cystic Fibrosis - A Manual of Diagnosis and Management*, 2nd edn. Baillière Tindall, London.

Harris, A. and Super, M. (1995) *Cystic Fibrosis - The Facts*, 3rd edn, Oxford University Press, Oxford.

Helms, P.J. (1993) Growing up with cystic fibrosis. *Br. J. Hosp. Med.*, **50**, 326–32.

Hodson, M.E. and Geddes, D.M. (1994) *Cystic Fibrosis*, Chapman & Hall, London.

Koch, C. and Hoiby, N. (1993) Pathogenesis of cystic fibrosis. *Lancet*, **341**, 1065–9.

Littlewood, J.M. and Macdonald, A. (1987) Rationale of modern dietary recommendations in CF. *J. R. Soc. Med.*, Suppl 15, 16–24.

Ramsey, B.W. (1996) Management of pulmonary disease in patients with cystic fibrosis. *N. Engl. J. Med.*, **335**, 179–88.

Smith, D.L. and Stableforth, D.E. (1992) Management of patients with cystic fibrosis. *Br. J. Hosp. Med.*, **48**, 713–23.

Warner, J.O. (ed.) (1992) Cystic fibrosis. *Br. Med. Bull.*, **48**, 717–978.

22   Osteoporosis

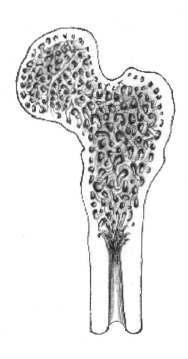

Osteoporosis often results in bone fracture and is a significant cause of disability and mortality. Women more commonly suffer from bone fractures than men because they generally have lower peak bone mass and bone loss accelerates after the menopause, although osteoporosis can be a problem in older men.

The risk of bone fracture depends on bone strength and the likelihood of trauma, usually in the form of a fall. Bone strength depends on the initial bone mass as well as subsequent bone loss. A variety of measures (mostly exercise and a diet adequate in protein, calcium and vitamin D) can be taken to reduce the risk of osteoporosis. These should be initiated early in life to maximise bone mass, and maintained throughout life to minimise bone loss.

The sex hormones oestrogen and testosterone protect against bone loss and so the administration of oestrogen (as HRT) in menopausal women effectively slows or prevents osteoporosis. Other drugs can slow bone loss, but once the bone trabeculae are separated the template for bone formation is lost and cannot be restored.

Aims of this chapter

By the end of this chapter you will have increased your knowledge of:
- The processes of bone loss and why the risk of bone fracture increases in older age
- How common osteoporosis and its consequences are
- How osteoporosis can be detected before bone fractures develop
- The measures that can be taken to prevent or treat bone loss.

In addition, this chapter will help you to:
- Suggest why osteoporosis and fracture rates are different in men and women
- Evaluate factors that may increase the risk of bone fracture
- Assess the potential for preventing osteoporosis and bone fracture
- Assess the suitability and effectiveness of methods for screening people at risk

Introduction

Osteoporosis literally means 'porous bones'. In simple terms it is described as 'brittle bone disease' or 'thinning' of the bones. Up to 40% of the original bone volume can be lost, with the result that the bone is easily fractured by very little trauma. In older people bone fractures can lead to loss of mobility and to other complications such as infection. Consequently, fractures are a leading cause of illness and death, particularly in older women. The most common sites of osteoporotic fractures are the spine (crush fractures), forearm (Colles' fracture), the hip and the pelvis. A further consequence of bone loss in the spinal vertebrae is chronic pain caused by compression of nerves, loss of height and curvature of the spine (kyphosis).

Osteoporosis results from an imbalance of the normal bone remodelling that keeps our bones healthy. In children and adolescents more bone is laid down than is removed and bone mass increases. There then follows a period when the processes of bone resorption and formation are roughly in balance. As we age bone mass reduces as more bone is resorbed than is replaced, resulting in osteoporosis.

Osteoporosis is defined in terms of bone mineral density, by comparison with the mean bone density in a population of young adults. A difference of one standard deviation (SD) below this mean corresponds to low bone mass, or **osteopenia**. An individual with a bone mass that is 2.5 SD below the mean is regarded as having osteoporosis.

In the UK about 60 000 hip, 50 000 wrist and 40 000 vertebral fractures are diagnosed clinically each year. Most of these fractures occur in women, but about 15% of vertebral fractures and 20% of hip fractures occur in men. The health service resources spent in the UK on osteoporosis are in the region of £750 million annually (1994 figures).

Bone loss is most marked in women, particularly during the first few years after the menopause. The rate of bone loss can exceed 10% per decade, and

Osteoporosis is a prime cause of illness and death in older people

Bone loss takes place over many years before it becomes apparent as fractures or kyphosis

Osteoporosis: a disease characterised by low bone mass and micro-architectural deterioration of bone tissues, leading to enhanced bone fragility and a consequent increase in fracture risk.

Osteomalacia: failure of bone to calcify because of a deficiency of vitamin D. The condition is reversible by adequate intake of vitamin D. The childhood form, rickets, can cause permanent bone deformity.

Paget's disease: characterised by progressive deformity and thickening of bones caused by acceleration of bone resorption and formation. Believed to be caused by viral infection of osteoclasts, it can lead to bone cancer.

starts before the cessation of menstruation: the median age for initial bone loss in women is 34 years. The rate of loss is not constant and is maximal during the menopause, with a slowing down in elderly women. Individuals vary in the rate of loss and also in the type of bone affected, trabecular bone being more susceptible to rapid bone loss than cortical bone.

Osteoporosis also affects men, but the bone loss is usually limited to 1–3% per decade from middle age onwards and so men are usually older when fractures occur (Figure 22.1). In addition, men usually have a higher peak bone mass to begin with.

Osteoporosis is the most common metabolic disease of bone, but becomes clinically apparent only when the complications of bone fracture and kyphosis arise. Many of the published incidence rates for osteoporosis are based on fracture rates, which does not fully reflect the true extent of the condition – before the fracture occurs, bone loss would have been under way for many years without symptoms. Other metabolic diseases of bone which can result in osteopenia or fracture include **osteomalacia** and **Paget's disease**.

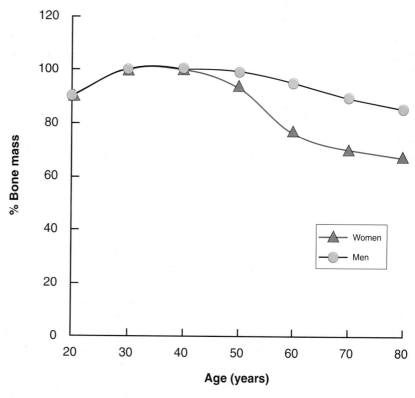

Figure 22.1 Change in bone mass with age in women and men. Most people achieve peak bone mass between 30 and 40 years of age. Thereafter bone mass decreases, but there is great variation between individuals. Women experience a greater degree of bone resorption than men because the protective effects of oestrogen are lost following the menopause. Osteoporosis can become a problem in men, particularly if they are not active or have other dietary and lifestyle risk factors. (Adapted from Cummings *et al.*, 1985.)

Because of the long time course involved it is possible to prevent or treat osteoporosis before serious consequences arise by modifying the risk factors or using drug therapy. This depends on recognising individuals most at risk of sustaining fractures by measuring their bone density or by assessing the risk factors involved. The measurement of bone mass is not without problems, usually because there is so much individual variation and low bone mass does not necessarily translate into increased risk of fracture. It may be necessary to monitor a person at intervals throughout life.

There is little evidence that the evaluation of risk factors alone can be used to predict bone density and susceptibility to fracture. Not all fractures are caused by osteopenia: perfectly healthy individuals with dense bones sustain fractures if the trauma is severe enough. In contrast, osteoporotic fractures can be sustained with little or no obvious trauma.

The likelihood of a bone fracturing is a function of several factors:

- The peak bone mass
- Degree and distribution of subsequent bone resorption
- The force applied, and the position of that force

Bone strength depends on peak bone mass and the rate of subsequent bone resorption. White men and black people of both sexes have a greater initial peak bone mass than white women and therefore have a greater 'reserve' before bone loss becomes a problem. The propensity of bone to fracture is not solely determined by its size and the degree of calcification; the integrity of the internal trabecular bone, which acts as supporting struts, is also of importance. Osteoporosis often follows an unpredictable course; sometimes very little force is required to produce a fracture, on other occasions a heavy fall results in no serious injury. This may be because of differences in the orientation of the impact.

> *Action may be taken to minimise bone loss before fractures occur*

> ▲ **Key points**
>
> **Features of osteoporosis**
>
> ▲ Most common metabolic disease of bone
> ▲ Asymptomatic until bone fractures or kyphosis develops
> ▲ Predisposes bone to fracture with little or no trauma
> ▲ Protracted natural history and an unpredictable course
> ▲ Recurrent and unexpected episodes of fractures which can cause severe pain and require hospitalisation
> ▲ Intervals free from fracture, but progressive collapse of vertebrae leads to kyphosis

Physiology of bone

Bones are not static structures; as well as providing support, protection and enabling body movement, they are active metabolically. The basic metabolic function of bone is to provide a store of calcium, which is required for a wide range of metabolic purposes (blood clotting, muscle contraction, nerve impulses and the activities of many enzymes). We cannot survive without calcium, but we cannot rely on the daily vagaries of the diet to provide a consistent supply.

There is therefore a requirement to store calcium when supplies are plentiful, and to remove it from bone when blood levels fall. Bone synthesis by **osteoblasts** depends on the activity of vitamin D (1,25 dihydroxy cholecalciferol), which influences intestinal calcium absorption. Bone resorption is carried out by **osteoclasts**, which are responsive to the activities of osteoblasts. Blood calcium levels are controlled by a feedback mechanism involving production of **parathyroid hormone** (PTH; increases plasma calcium) and the thyroid hormone **calcitonin** (reduces plasma calcium).

Bones undergo a continuous process of remodelling, with an annual turnover rate of about 25% for trabecular bone and 2–3% for cortical bone. This process

> *Bones provide an essential reservoir of calcium*

Osteoblasts: members of a family of cells that also includes osteocytes and bone lining cells, collectively involved in the formation and maintenance of bone. A major role of osteoblasts is synthesis of bone matrix. Osteoblasts are derived from mesenchymal precursors in the bone marrow.

Osteoclasts: large multinucleated cells derived from haematopoietic precursor cells in the bone marrow. Responsible for bone resorption by acid secretion and proteolytic digestion.

Calcitonin: hormone produced by the thyroid in response to a rise in plasma calcium levels. Depresses osteoclast activity. Has opposite effects to parathyroid hormone.

Cytokines: proteins involved in immune system and inflammation, described as 'hormones of the immune system'. Some regulate the growth of other cell types, including osteoblasts and osteoclasts.

Parathyroid hormone: hormone produced by the parathyroid gland in response to a fall in plasma calcium levels. Restores plasma calcium by indirectly stimulating osteoclastic resorption of bone.

Vitamin D: active form (1,25 dihydroxycholecalciferol) is produced by the kidney. Increases intestinal calcium absorption and promotes bone mineralisation.

proceeds in the **bone remodelling units** on the bone surfaces. About 1 million bone remodelling units are present throughout the skeleton, made up of osteoclasts and osteoblasts working in concert.

First, the osteoclasts resorb an area of the bone over a period of 1–2 weeks. This activity is followed by a reversal phase in which osteoblasts form new bone matrix, or **osteoid,** in the cavity left by osteoclastic resorption. Eventually this area becomes calcified and the bone is effectively renewed. Without this process the bone would become very fragile because microscopic fractures produced during normal wear and tear would not be repaired. Osteoid is mainly Type I collagen together with a variety of non-fibrous proteins. The hardness and most of the weight of bones is due to calcium hydroxyapatite (a crystalline mineral of calcium, phosphate and water), which is deposited within the osteoid matrix.

A large number of growth factors and hormones influence the activities of osteoblasts and osteoclasts. Normally bone formation is coupled to bone resorption, so that there is excess of neither removal nor formation. The activity of the osteoblasts and osteoclasts is influenced by oestrogen and testosterone. The loss of production of these (at the menopause, for example) results in

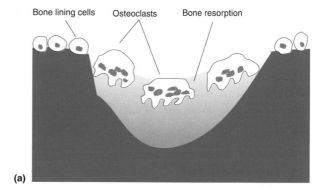

(a)

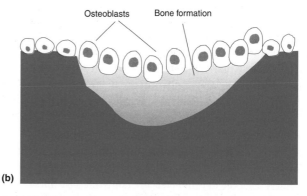

(b)

Figure 22.2 Bone resorption and formation take place at the surface in bone remodelling units. The process is cyclical, starting with resorption of old bone by multinucleated osteoclasts (a). Osteoblasts appear at the resorption site, filling the cavity with osteoid, which then becomes calcified (b).

increased production of osteoblasts and osteoclasts. These changes are mediated by altered production of cytokines such as IL-6 and IL-1, which stimulate the bone marrow progenitor cells. However, the production of osteoclasts is favoured, so that bone formation and resorption become unbalanced, eventually resulting in osteoporosis. In men, the production of testosterone is more constant and they suffer a smaller effect on bone mass.

Bone adapts to the functional forces placed on it: osteoblasts are stimulated by mechanical stress to maintain and increase bone mass. Consequently bone mass can be maintained by weight bearing and muscle contraction, but conversely disuse (such as by placing a limb in a plaster cast, or complete bed rest) leads to loss of bone.

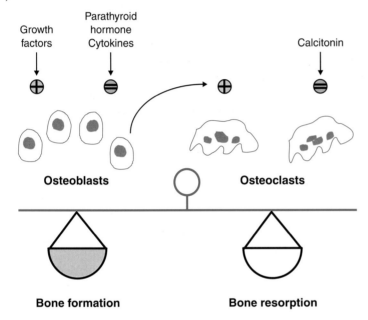

Figure 22.3 The metabolism of bone is very tightly coupled, so that when a certain amount is resorbed the same amount is formed to replace it. A principal function of osteoblasts is to synthesise bone matrix. Although osteoclasts are the only cells capable of resorbing bone, their recruitment and activity are mediated by osteoblasts. The proliferation of osteoblasts, and bone formation, is stimulated by growth factors such as TGF-β. Parathyroid hormone and some cytokines (IL-1, IL-6 and TNF-α, for example) arrest osteoblast proliferation and, indirectly, promote bone resorption. The precise nature of the 'signal' between osteoblasts and osteoclasts has not been fully elucidated. The activity of osteoclasts is also directly inhibited by calcitonin.

The structure of bone

There are two types of bone: **cortical** (sometimes referred to as compact) and **trabecular** (also called cancellous or spongy) bone. Most bones of the body are made up of both these types, although there is variation within the bone and in different bone sites.

Most calcium is removed from trabecular bone

The long bones, such as in the forearm (radius and ulna), contain about 90% cortical bone. The shaft, or **diaphysis**, of the bone is a hollow cylinder of cortical bone which encloses the bone marrow. The wider ends of the bone, or **epiphyses**, are reinforced internally by a honeycomb-like meshwork of trabecular bone (Figure 22.4).

The flatter bones, such as the vertebrae and the hip (Figure 22.5), have a much higher proportion of trabecular bone. Both the cortical and trabecular bone structures contribute to the overall strength of a bone. However, trabecular bone, because of its much greater surface area, is more metabolically active and therefore is more susceptible to hormonal influences.

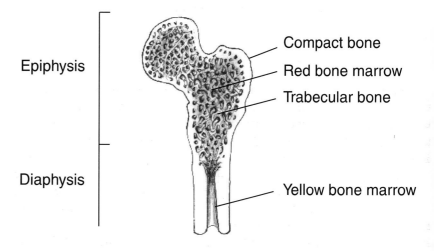

Figure 22.4 A long bone (the femur). The ends of the bone (epiphyses) are composed of trabecular bone surrounded by cortical bone. The shaft of the bone (diaphysis) is composed of cortical bone which encloses yellow bone marrow.

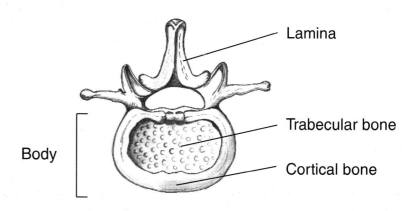

Figure 22.5 Lumbar vertebra (superior view). The body of the vertebra is principally composed of trabecular bone.

Table 22.1 Proportion of cortical and trabecular bone in different sites

Site	Cortical bone (%)	Trabecular bone (%)
Hip (trochanteric)	50	50
Neck	75	25
Vertebrae	<33	>66
Forearm:		
Distal	30–50	50–70
Middle	95	5

Data from Cummings *et al.*, 1985; Riggs et al. (1982) *J. Clin. Invest.*, **70**, 716–23; Schlenker and Von Seggan (1976) *Calcif. Tissue Res.*, **20**, 41–52.

Epidemiology

More than one in three postmenopausal women and one in 20 men can expect to sustain bone fractures because of osteoporosis. These fractures are not only painful, they can produce deformity and even contribute to premature death.

In the UK the incidence of fractures has steadily increased over the past few decades. Much of this can be explained by the larger proportion of older people in the population, but the underlying trend is still increasing. Rates are very much lower in the less developed countries, although modest increases have been reported in Africa, particularly in urban areas. These trends might reflect an increasingly sedentary lifestyle.

> *Osteoporosis is an increasing problem because people are living longer*

The main epidemiological risk factors are age, gender and race. Other risk factors include a family history, a small-boned frame, smoking, alcohol consumption and inadequate intakes of calcium and vitamin D. Because of the much more substantial loss of sex hormones at the menopause the fracture rate in postmenopausal women is much higher than in men of the same age.

The most reliable epidemiological data relate to the incidence of hip fractures because of the need for hospitalisation and operation: these account for about 20% of the occupancy of all orthopaedic beds in England and Wales. The most serious consequence of osteoporosis is hip fractures, the incidence of which has doubled over the last 30 years.

Hip fractures

Hip fracture accounts for most of the deaths, disability and economic costs associated with osteoporosis. In the UK osteoporosis is responsible for about 60 000 cases of hip fracture a year, mostly in women over the age of 65 years. In the USA the annual incidence is about 210 000 cases. Generally, incidence rises dramatically after the age of 70 years, about 50% of all hip fractures occurring in people who are over 80 years of age (Figure 22.6).

> *Most hip fractures occur in older people who are already frail: there is a high risk of disability or death*

A loss of bone mineral density may not be the only reason for this pattern. Other risk factors are likely to be the increased rate of falls in older people

Review question 1

Why are wrist fractures more common in middle-aged people and hip fractures much more common in older people?

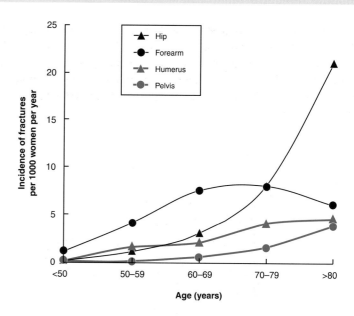

Figure 22.6 Age-specific incidence of bone fracture. The incidence of fractures of the forearm and humerus increases soon after the menopause. In older women the most frequent complication of osteoporosis is hip fracture. (Data from Cummings *et al.*, 1985.)

(who may have poor balance and eyesight) or use of drug therapies that affect motor co-ordination.

A white woman living in the USA, with a life expectancy of 80 years, has a 15% lifetime risk of suffering a hip fracture. A patient with hip fracture is 10–20% more likely to die in the 8 months following the fracture than age-matched counterparts, the highest risk being present in the first 4 months after fracture. The reasons for this are varied: many patients will be older, perhaps with pre-existing illness, not very mobile and more prone to infections such as pneumonia. Long-term nursing care may be necessary and many patients lose their ability to walk independently.

Forearm (Colles') fractures

Forearm fractures are far less serious than hip fractures

This is the most common form of fracture in white women below the age of 75 (Figure 22.6). A 50-year old woman has a 15% risk of fracturing her forearm in her remaining lifetime. Forearm fractures generally cause far less disability than hip fractures, and are rarely fatal. Fewer than 20% require hospitalisation. Some people experience persistent pain, loss of function, neuropathy and post-traumatic arthritis after forearm fracture.

Vertebral fractures

Osteoporosis in the spine initially leads to compression of the vertebrae, causing

loss of height. This is followed by multiple crush fractures and collapse of the vertebrae, giving rise to curvature of the spine (kyphosis; Figure 22.7). A substantial proportion of vertebral fractures are asymptomatic and thus the true prevalence of this condition is unknown. Initial symptoms of vertebral fracture are back pain. Some women can lose up to 23 cm in height because of spinal osteoporosis.

> *Vertebral fractures are responsible for back pain and curvature of the spine*

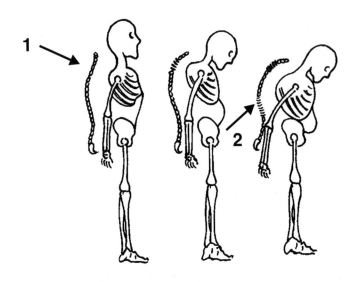

Figure 22.7 The natural history of kyphosis. The early stages of kyphosis are characterised by an asymptomatic loss of height caused by thinning of the upper thoracic vertebrae (1). Loss of bone mineral from the lower thoracic and lumbar vertebrae (2) causes crush fractures and collapse. This results in further loss of height and a stooped appearance. It can be very painful.

Crush fractures typically involve the lumbar vertebrae and can occur spontaneously during normal activities such as getting up from a bed or chair. Clinical or radiological evidence of spinal osteoporosis is seen in 25% of white women over the age of 65.

Review question 2

Why is osteoporosis a health problem?

Pathology

Osteoporosis is caused by an imbalance in the dynamic equilibrium of bone formation and resorption. As a consequence the total volume of bone is reduced, particularly in the trabecular bone (Figure 22.8). The ratio of osteoid to calcified matrix is normal. The most common type of osteoporosis, **primary osteoporosis**, occurs with age and in women is exacerbated by the menopause without any identifiable secondary cause. **Secondary osteoporosis** is a consequence of some other disease or extraneous influence.

> *Osteoporosis is caused by an imbalance in the remodelling process of bone resorption and formation*

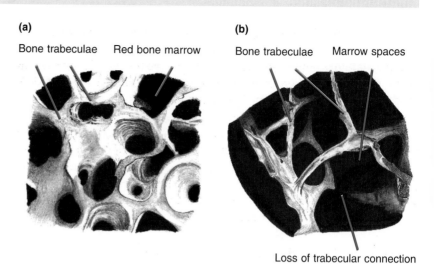

(a)

Bone trabeculae   Red bone marrow

(b)

Bone trabeculae   Marrow spaces

Loss of trabecular connection

Figure 22.8 Normal trabecular bone (a) consists of a dense honeycomb meshwork of interconnected bone trabeculae. The spaces are filled by red bone marrow. In osteoporotic bone (b) the marrow spaces are much larger and the bone trabeculae are thin, giving a much more open structure with loss of connectivity between the trabeculae.

Primary osteoporosis

Age-related osteoporosis affects both men and women

Primary osteoporosis appears to proceed in two phases, starting around the fourth or fifth decades of life. **Age-related osteoporosis** (sometimes termed **senile osteoporosis**) involves fairly modest bone losses of 0.3–0.5% a year in both trabecular and cortical bone types. Age-related osteoporosis begins after the attainment of peak bone mass in early middle age and continues for the remainder of a person's life (Plate 7). It is probably responsible for many of the hip, humeral and pelvic and some of the vertebral fractures associated with old age.

Postmenopausal osteoporosis often causes loss of height and kyphosis

Postmenopausal osteoporosis occurs in women around the menopause and usually continues for 6–7 years thereafter, but can persist for up to 20 years. It is related to gonadal hormone deficiency and is characterised by a loss of trabecular bone. During the postmenopausal period a woman can lose 1–3% of her bone mass per year, and in some cases the loss is as high as 5–6%. Postmenopausal osteoporosis is believed to be responsible for multiple crush fractures of the vertebrae. It can also occur in men with hypogonadism. The postmenopausal pattern of osteoporosis is superimposed on age-related osteoporosis. By the time she reaches 80 years of age a woman not taking HRT could lose up to 40% of the mass of vulnerable bones such as the vertebral body and femoral neck (Plate 8).

Up to half of the bone loss in an older woman is attributable to the menopause

The underlying processes in postmenopausal and age-related osteoporosis are probably different. Postmenopausal osteoporosis is believed to arise from increased osteoclast activity at the resorption sites as a consequence of lost gonadal function. The effects are most apparent in the trabecular bone, which

initially becomes thinner, with greater separation between the trabeculae until they eventually become perforated. When this happens the template for restoring bone structure is lost, and there is no known therapeutic intervention or risk factor modification capable of restoring it. Age-related osteoporosis is probably caused by decreased activity of the osteoblasts, which are unable to completely fill the spaces created by the osteoclasts. This may be related to a functional decline with age in the ability of the bone marrow to produce osteoblast precursors. Vitamin D metabolism and calcium absorption also alter with age. An age-related decrease in renal function may mean that the production of active vitamin D is reduced: hence the intestinal absorption of calcium falls, and to maintain adequate plasma levels proportionally more calcium is removed from the bones.

Table 22.2 Characteristics of primary osteoporosis

	Postmenopausal osteoporosis	Age-related osteoporosis
Age of onset (years)	50–60 approx.	40
Gender	Mainly women	Both men and women
Bone type	Trabecular	Cortical and trabecular
Rate of loss	Typically 1–3% a year, declining about 7 years after menopause	0.3–0.5% a year
Process	Increased osteoclastic activity, depends on gonadal function	Decreased bone formation by osteoblasts, possibly caused by senescence changes in bone marrow
Fracture site	Vertebrae (crush fractures)	Hip, humerus, pelvis, some vertebrae

Secondary osteoporosis

The medical conditions that cause secondary osteoporosis include chronic kidney disease, endocrine disorders such as Cushing's syndrome and primary hyperparathyroidism, multiple myeloma, chronic inflammatory diseases and conditions resulting in malabsorption, all of which affect both men and women. However, secondary osteoporosis is more likely to be a cause of fracture in men because of the relative infrequency of primary osteoporosis. The most common cause of secondary osteoporosis is corticosteroid use.

Secondary osteoporosis is caused by another medical condition or by drug therapy

Endocrine disorders

Corticosteroids produce an uncoupling of bone resorption and formation, leading to depletion of bone mass. They also inhibit gonadal production of

Corticosteroid therapy: primarily used to reduce inflammation in conditions such as rheumatoid arthritis or asthma.

Crohn's disease: an inflammatory disease of the gastrointestinal tract. Can involve the whole tract from mouth to anus, but is usually confined to the terminal ileum and colon. The usual course is slow and non-aggressive. Symptoms include diarrhoea with mucus and rectal bleeding, intermittent pain around the umbilicus or referred pain in the lower back. Arthritis or joint pain may occur.

Cushing's syndrome: arises from an excess of cortisol, either by excessive production in the adrenal cortex or by administration of exogenous synthetic steroids. The usual effects are obesity, hypertension, excessive hair growth and osteoporosis. The most common cause of the syndrome is use of synthetic steroids; more rarely tumours of the adrenal glands or the pituitary cause increased corticosteroid production.

Multiple myeloma: a malignancy of B lymphocytes characterised by continuous synthesis of immunoglobulins; may be detectable in the urine as Bence–Jones protein. Most cases occur in people over 60.

Primary hyperparathyroidism: tumour or hyperplasia of the parathyroid glands causes excessive production of parathyroid hormone and hypercalcaemia.

Rheumatoid arthritis: a chronic systemic inflammatory disease predominantly affecting the joints. Pathological process involves formation of pannus tissue derived from the synovial membrane. This inflammatory tissue destroys cartilage and erodes bone.

Ulcerative colitis: inflammation and ulceration of the wall of the large intestine (the small intestine is never involved). Main symptoms are rectal bleeding, diarrhoea, nausea, vomiting and weight loss. Symptoms can be controlled but cure is rare. Associated with increased risk of colorectal cancer.

the sex hormones, further adding to adverse effects on bone. Trabecular bone appears to be particularly vulnerable to the adverse effects of corticosteroids.

Treatment is by reversing the cause of the syndrome (for example, surgical excision of a cortisol-producing tumour or withdrawal of or dose adjustment of corticosteroids).

Add-on therapies to minimise the bone loss associated with corticosteroids are being evaluated. These include prescription of HRT in recently postmenopausal women, and supplementation with calcium and vitamin D. Bisphosphonates (see below) also seem to offer a successful prevention therapy.

Osteoporosis can also be secondary to primary hyperparathyroidism. Parathyroid hormone increases bone turnover and the concentration of calcium in the blood by directly stimulating osteoblasts, which in turn signal increased osteoclastic activity. Excess production of PTH means that osteoclastic bone resorption exceeds new bone formation, resulting in a net depletion of bone. The imbalance is abolished by surgical removal of the parathyroid glands.

Other endocrine disorders that affect bone metabolism are those which affect gonadal function, including hypogonadism associated with Klinefelter's and Turner's syndromes (Chapter 3). The effects on bone may be ameliorated by the appropriate hormone replacement therapy.

Multiple myeloma

The bone destruction in multiple myeloma is believed to be caused by the action of cytokines (produced by the tumour) on osteoclasts, mediating osteoclastic resorption.

Inflammatory conditions

The likelihood of osteoporosis is increased in patients with rheumatoid arthritis, with ulcerative colitis or with Crohn's disease. Bone loss around the inflamed joint is characteristic of rheumatoid arthritis, but this can extend to a generalised osteoporosis involving the lumbar spine, femoral neck or even the whole skeleton. Some of these changes may be ascribed to corticosteroid therapy, but there is probably also a direct effect of the inflammatory disease process itself involving the localised secretion of cytokines by inflammatory cells, affecting the activity of osteoblasts and osteoclasts.

Inflammatory bowel disease is often accompanied by arthritis which can cause local bone loss. About 3–5% of patients with inflammatory bowel disease have osteoporosis as a direct complication, probably because of malabsorption of calcium and vitamin D. These patients are also likely to be treated at some stage with corticosteroids, which would have a negative effect on bone.

Liver disease

Liver insufficiency is associated with osteoporosis. Many of the causes of liver insufficiency (excessive alcohol consumption, hypogonadism, malnutrition) are independent risk factors for osteoporosis and so the liver pathology may

simply exacerbate the condition. However, liver failure from other causes (primary biliary cirrhosis for example) is also associated with osteoporosis, possibly due to calcium malabsorption (the liver is involved in the metabolism of vitamin D).

Prevention of osteoporosis

The best strategy for dealing with osteoporosis is prevention. This can be achieved in two ways: (1) by modifying risk factors and (2) using drug therapy. Modification of risk factors entails ensuring adequate calcium in the diet and sufficient exercise to keep the bones stimulated. Behaviour that is detrimental to the maintenance of bone mass, such as smoking and excessive drinking, should be avoided. The earlier the age at which these actions are taken the better. For example, it makes sense to take up exercise before bone mass peaks in the mid-thirties so that there is a larger bone base to draw on. Thereafter, continued avoidance of risk factors will slow down osteopenia. However, only so much can be achieved in this way: to a large extent our bone mass is under genetic control. In some people, therefore, more aggressive intervention is necessary. For the menopausal woman this would usually mean HRT.

Prevention is based on realising the full potential for peak bone mass and then slowing down the inevitable loss that starts in middle age

Risk factors for osteoporosis

Risks for osteoporosis can be divided into two categories:
1. Those that influence bone density
2. Those that influence the propensity for fracture through trauma

The most important risks predisposing to fracturing osteoporosis are:
- Increasing age, white race and female gender
- Anyone who has already had a fracture with minimal trauma
- A woman whose menopause was early or who has had her ovaries removed and is not taking HRT
- A woman who has had prolonged amenorrhoea (usually because of excessive exercise or anorexia nervosa)
- Low BMI

Amenorrhoea: absence of menstrual periods.

Anorexia nervosa: a complex psychological disorder causing loss of appetite, fear of gaining weight, distorted body image.

Primary biliary cirrhosis: a chronic progressive inflammatory disease of the liver, causing impaired bile secretion.

Age
Age-related bone loss occurs throughout the skeleton, in all people regardless of race, culture and gender. This is brought about by a decline in the activity of osteoblasts and an overall slowing down of bone remodelling. Trabecular bone is most susceptible to this process, but cortical bone is also vulnerable.

Gender
The risk of osteoporosis is much greater in women (Table 22.3) for several reasons:
- They have a smaller bone mass to begin with

- There is a pronounced acceleration of bone loss in the menopausal years
- Women generally live longer than men

> *Osteoporosis is more of a problem in women, but older men also suffer bone fractures*

This is not to say that men do not suffer from osteoporosis. As facilities for measuring bone density become more widely available the condition is increasingly recognised, and is believed to be a major cause of back pain in older men and women. The incidence of fracturing osteoporosis is also increasing in men, possibly because life expectancy is increasing and lifestyles becoming more sedentary.

The gender differences are directly related to availability of the sex hormones which play a role in the maintenance of bone mass in both sexes. In women, an important predictive factor for subsequent osteoporosis is early menopause (average age of the menopause is 50 years; see Chapter 8). The role of the sex hormones is dramatically illustrated by removal of the gonads in either sex. When this occurs, for example in cancer treatment, hormone replacement should be given unless contraindicated by risks of cancer recurrence.

Table 22.3   Risk of fracture in remaining lifetime

Age (years)	Average life expectancy (years)	Risk of fracture (%)	
		Hip	Forearm
White women:			
50	31	14.7	14.7
65	19	14.7	9.7
80	9	15.2	4.7
White men:			
50	25	4.5	2.3
65	18	4.7	1.2
80	7	7.8	0.5

Data from Cummings *et al.*, 1985.

Inherited factors

Family history

A woman is more likely to develop osteoporosis if her mother had the condition. Inherited factors appear to have most influence on peak bone mass and to the degree of bone loss around the menopause. Family studies indicate that osteoporosis is a polygenic condition, but only few candidate genes have so far been implicated.

A gene for the vitamin D receptor has now been identified, and variation in this may in part explain population variations in bone density. Several combinations of the gene can be inherited: the two possible alleles b and B give the three possible genotypes BB, Bb and bb. The B allele is associated with low bone density. People with the BB genotype tend to have low bone density, bb high density and those with the Bb genotype tend to have intermediate bone density.

The association between the genotype for the vitamin D receptor and bone density is also reflected in the mean age of fracture. For people with the BB genotype the mean age of fracture is about 65 years; this rises to 69 years for the Bb genotype and to 76 years for people with the bb genotype. The b allele is believed to be protective against osteoporosis and bone fracture. The discovery of the vitamin D receptor alleles is relatively recent and it remains to be confirmed whether the results are applicable to all populations.

Another candidate genetic marker for osteoporosis is the oestrogen receptor gene. Oestrogen plays a crucial role in bone turnover as evidenced by accelerated bone loss in postmenopausal women and by the effectiveness of hormone replacement therapy. It is known that the oestrogen receptor gene exhibits polymorphism and it is possible that some polymorphisms influence the efficiency of the receptor for inducing cellular changes after binding oestrogen which, in turn, influences bone mass. In a study of Japanese women (Kobayashi et al., 1996), one particular type of oestrogen receptor gene polymorphism affecting 7.6% of the study population was associated with significantly lower bone mineral density (as determined by DXA scanning).

It is known that mutations in the genes for type 1 collagen (the major protein of bone) give rise to another bone disease called osteogenesis imperfecta. Although these genes are not abnormal in osteoporosis, it is still possible that gene polymorphisms could influence bone mass. In a case-control study (Grant et al., 1996) it was found that heterozygotes for a polymorphism in a regulatory region of the COLIA1 gene were significantly related to lower bone mass and osteoporotic fracture.

Race

Black Americans have a higher bone mass and density than their white counterparts and this is reflected in the incidence of hip fractures, which are about half those for white women. Risk for hip fracture also appears to be reduced in black men.

Dietary factors

The most important dietary factors are calcium and vitamin D. Some protein-rich diets can be detrimental because their high phosphate content increases the urinary excretion of calcium.

Calcium

Calcium intake in childhood and adolescence influences peak bone mass in adults. Later bone loss also correlates with calcium intake. See Chapter 7 for more information on calcium homeostasis.

The relationship between calcium balance and bone loss in older people has been difficult to determine because dietary changes take years to become measurable as changes in bone density. It is important to ensure adequate supply of vitamin D with calcium because absorption of calcium from the gut is less efficient if levels of vitamin D are insufficient.

> Osteogenesis imperfecta: inherited bone disorder caused by mutations in the COLIA1 and COLIA2 genes coding for type 1 collagen. The collagen in bone osteoid is abnormal, causing weakness of the bone, multiple fractures and often severe deformity.

> Calcium supplementation can reduce the rate of bone loss in some menopausal women

The rate of bone loss can be slowed (by up to 50%) in postmenopausal women 3–10 years after menopause by supplementation with elemental calcium (1000 mg daily). The type of calcium supplementation appears to be important, soluble calcium salts or dairy products being apparently more effective than calcium carbonate. To date, most studies of calcium supplementation in postmenopausal women have been conducted over only 1–2 years and it remains to be seen whether the effects can be maintained and whether a real impact can be made on fracture rates.

Vitamin D

The recommended daily intake of vitamin D is based on the amount necessary to prevent osteomalacia (the failure of bone to calcify): about 10 µg. Older housebound people may not receive enough sunlight to manufacture sufficient amounts of their own vitamin D, and so should consider taking dietary supplements of vitamin D, in tablet form or as a 6-monthly depot injection. A recent French study in a nursing home setting (Chapuy *et al.*, 1994) showed that 3 years of vitamin D supplementation can reduce hip fracture rates in older women by 20% or more.

Protein

The non-mineralised matrix of bone (osteoid) is composed of proteins and therefore adequate dietary protein is essential for bone growth and maintenance. However, too much animal protein in the diet increases the urinary excretion of calcium.

Alcohol

It is really only excessive alcohol consumption which represents a significant risk factor for osteoporosis. The mechanism of action is uncertain but a metabolite of ethanol, acetaldehyde, is believed to have a direct toxic effect on osteoblasts. Acetaldehyde also appears to suppress the activator of precursor cells in the bone marrow.

Individuals who consume large quantities of alcohol often also neglect their diet and are deficient in protein, calcium and vitamin D. Liver disease in the alcoholic will interfere with the metabolism of vitamin D and therefore with calcium absorption. Inebriated individuals are also more likely to fall and sustain a fracture. In contrast, there are indications that more moderate consumption of alcohol is protective. A prospective study found that bone mineral density tended to increase with alcohol intake at levels corresponding to social drinking (Felson *et al.*, 1995). Why this should be so is unclear. In women the effect may be related to alcohol increasing the availability of oestrogens, but this does not explain the effect on bone density in men.

Caffeine

Excessive caffeine intake promotes the loss of calcium through the urine and faeces. Products rich in caffeine include coffee, tea, cola and chocolate. However,

the calcium loss caused by the drinks can be offset by adding milk.

Medical factors

Amenorrhoea

The protection to the skeleton afforded by oestrogen is of major importance; women whose menopause comes early are more susceptible to osteoporosis. Even a hysterectomy without removal of the ovaries could represent a risk, as it is associated with early ovarian failure. Although exercise is beneficial in stimulating bone growth, a woman who takes excessive exercise can undo this advantage if she becomes amenorrhoeic – amenorrhoea from any cause is a substantial risk factor for osteoporosis. The women most at risk are professional athletes who take intense exercise (e.g. track athletes), ballet dancers and young women with anorexia nervosa.

Excessive exercise can reduce bone mass in women

As well as increasing the risk of osteoporosis a history of amenorrhoea increases the likelihood that osteoporosis will develop at an earlier age. Any non-pregnant woman under the age of 45 who has had amenorrhoea for 6 months should be referred for bone density measurement.

Underweight and obesity

The risk of osteoporosis is higher in underweight people because of the relative lack of stimulatory stresses on the bones. Conversely, the risk in overweight individuals is reduced. The role of weight and the everyday stresses and strains on the bones in maintaining their mass is succinctly demonstrated by immobilisation – the bone density in a limb immobilised in a plaster cast becomes reduced compared with the contralateral mobile limb. A further often-quoted example is that of astronauts who, after spending some time in the reduced gravity of their space station, return to earth with reduced bone mass. This is a situation that will not worry most people because when mechanical stresses on the bones are resumed the bone density increases.

Underweight women are also at risk because of their relative lack of fat stores. Adipose cells play a role in the conversion of adrenal androgens to oestrogens. Obese women have a more plentiful supply of oestrogen that will protect against excessive bone resorption.

Exercise

One of the least appreciated forms of prevention and treatment for osteoporosis is physical exercise – it can increase, not just maintain, the bone mineral content, as is often the case with other forms of therapy. Men with a history of strenuous physical exercise have a greater trabecular bone mineral density than physically inactive men. Such active individuals would therefore have more bone mineral resources to draw on.

Exercise can build strength in bone and muscle

Combined weight-loading and aerobic exercises are considered most beneficial. The duration of exercise training is also important, several years usually being necessary for any significant benefit to accrue. For example, no increases in bone densities are detectable when sedentary men are put through a 3-month training regime.

A person with thin bones may sustain a fracture in the course of vigorous exercise

---

▲   Key points

Risk factors in primary osteoporosis

- ▲ Age
- ▲ Female gender
- ▲ White race
- ▲ Excessive alcohol consumption
- ▲ Amenorrhoea
- ▲ Pregnancy and lactation
- ▲ Low calcium intake
- ▲ Poor vitamin D availability
- ▲ Smoking
- ▲ Family history
- ▲ Excessive protein in diet
- ▲ Excess caffeine consumption
- ▲ Low BMI

Fractures in older people are most often produced through the combination of weak bones and falling

The risk of falling increases with age and is compounded by some medical conditions and drug therapies

---

Exercise training is also useful to treat bone loss. Postmenopausal women can increase their bone mineral density by following a programme of light or moderate physical activity (30 minutes three times a week) for at least a year. Even women in their eighties can benefit, although it should be remembered that care is required to avoid injury and older patients may have cardiovascular limitations on the amount of exercise they can take with safety. A conservative approach should be adopted, comprising walking and extension exercises rather than vigorous jumping, stretching and sit-ups. Exercise also improves general mobility, balance and stability, which, together, would reduce the risk of a fall as well as helping to maintain bone mass.

Excessive exercise in younger women can increase the likelihood of osteoporosis rather than prevent it. This problem is encountered in long-distance runners and ballet dancers, who often become amenorrhoeic because of their intense training schedules and therefore lose some of the protection afforded by oestrogen.

Drugs

Corticosteroid therapy causes dose-related progressive bone loss. A dose more than the equivalent of 7.5 mg prednisolone daily is likely to induce bone loss. The effect is more marked in the trabecular bone. Patients at risk are those who have received steroid treatment for rheumatoid arthritis or asthma.

Smoking

Heavy smoking can accelerate the menopause by up to 5 years. The earlier loss of oestrogen is more likely to cause bone loss. Metabolites of cigarette smoke are also believed to suppress osteoblast activity.

Risk factors for trauma

A person with osteoporosis is most likely to sustain a fracture by falling, although not all falls result in injury even in an older person. This probably depends on mechanical factors and the precise point of impact in relation to the bone. The incidence of forearm fractures is higher than hip fractures in those of 50–70 years (Figure 22.6), but older people are much more likely to sustain hip fractures.

Generally, the risk of falling increases with age. Stairs are a particular hazard. It might be thought that most falls and fractures will occur at night when lighting is poor, but most incidents occur during the day.

The risk of falling is increased by some medical conditions, such as Parkinson's disease, stroke, arthritis and pneumonia. All these conditions are more prevalent in older people. Some drugs can contribute to the risk of falling: sedatives, barbiturates, tranquillisers, antidepressants, antihypertensives and diuretics may decrease alertness, affect judgement, balance or cause dizziness. All of these drugs are commonly taken by older people.

Treatment

It is possible to slow down or even reverse bone loss; however, if the loss is of such an extent that the pattern of trabecular bone has become disrupted, then the bone will never regain its strength. Various drug therapies are considered below. Risk factor modification, particularly exercise, has a role to play in treatment just as it does in primary prevention. Some therapies (HRT for example) can be used to prevent as well as treat osteoporosis.

Drug interventions for osteoporosis work either by blocking bone resorption or by stimulating bone formation. Anti-resorptive agents include oestrogen, calcitonin and bisphosphonates. Agents that stimulate bone formation include sodium fluoride, growth hormone and parathyroid hormone fragments.

> *The major aim of treatment is to reduce fracture risk by preventing further bone loss*

Review question 3

What factors have influenced the total bone mass in a 60-year-old woman?

Oestrogen-replacement therapy (HRT)

Oestrogen increases calcium absorption and decreases bone resorption. The risk of bone fractures can be reduced by 50–75% after 5 years of oestrogen treatment. However, once therapy is stopped the decline in bone mass will begin again: protection of bone mass and lowering of fracture risk may persist for some years after HRT is discontinued, but does not persist indefinitely.

Peak bone mass is declining before the menopause because oestrogen production by the ovaries is reduced for some time before menstruation ceases. It is believed that HRT is most effective as a preventive measure when started during the menopause, although HRT is still of value in the older woman and as a treatment for those with established osteoporosis.

Opposition of oestrogen by progestogen in HRT appears to have little effect on the effectiveness of therapy. The route of administration (orally as tablets or parenterally as subcutaneous implants, skin patches or creams) is not critical. The parenteral route has the advantage of achieving higher blood and tissue hormone levels through a smaller dose by avoiding first passage metabolism and elimination by the liver.

The protection of bone mass afforded by HRT continues for as long as it is taken, but currently most women are treated only for 5–10 years (see Chapter 8). There are some potential hazards attached to HRT, including increased risk of endometrial cancer and possibly breast cancer. The risk of endometrial cancer is abolished by addition of progestogen to the therapy.

Continuing HRT for 10 years carries a small risk of serious complications (see Chapter 15), and these are easily outweighed by the benefits in prevention of osteoporosis and cardiovascular disease. The risks and benefits of longer-term therapy are still being evaluated. Only about 15–20% of eligible women take HRT, and most use it short-term. Most women discontinue HRT because of continued menstrual bleeding, but exaggerated fears of cancer risks may be another factor. A newer continuous combined oestrogen and progestogen therapy overcomes withdrawal bleeding, but it appears to be associated with a high incidence of irregular bleeding. In the UK costs may also be a disincentive because the oestrogen and progestogen components of the HRT prescription

> *HRT reduces the risk of fracture by 50% or more*

Parenteral: bypassing the gastrointestinal tract, for example by subcutaneous, intramuscular or intravenous injection.

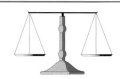

**The Fracture
Intervention Trial**

Alendronate vs placebo

▲ 2027 women aged 55–81 (mainly white) in USA with vertebral fractures

▲ Randomly assigned to 5–10 mg daily alendronate (1022) or placebo (1005)

▲ Lateral spine radiography conducted at outset and at 24 and 36 months

▲ New vertebral fractures defined as a decrease in one vertebral height of more than 20%

▲ 78 (8%) of women in alendronate group had one or more new fractures vs 145 (15%) in placebo group

▲ Alendronate can reduce the frequency of new bone fracture by about 50% in women with low bone mass

Cyclical etidronate is used to treat spinal fractures in men and women who cannot take HRT

are charged for separately.

A synthetic steroid, tibolone, has both oestrogenic and progestogenic effects and thus offers the potential for avoiding withdrawal bleeding in much the same way as continuous combined HRT. High doses of tibolone can cause irregular vaginal bleeding in some women. Preliminary data indicate that the agent is effective in reducing postmenopausal bone loss (compared with placebo), but whether it is as good as conventional HRT remains to be determined.

Anti-oestrogen drugs

The anti-oestrogen drug tamoxifen is one the most effective adjuvant treatments for breast cancer in postmenopausal women. Because the drug competes with oestrogen for receptors in breast cells, oestrogen is conserved and is available to exert its effects elsewhere in the body. Hence tamoxifen helps to maintain bone mass in postmenopausal women with breast cancer. Unfortunately, it has side-effects, including endometrial cancer in women who have not had a hysterectomy, which preclude its sole use for prevention of osteoporosis.

Several new anti-oestrogen drugs are being developed to treat advanced breast cancer (droloxifene and raloxifene for example): these appear to have a more selective action on the oestrogen receptors in cells of different tissues. This selectivity may reduce the risk of endometrial cancer yet at the same time act as an oestrogen agonist in preventing bone loss. Clinical trials of these agents for the prevention of osteoporosis are in progress.

Calcitonin

Calcitonin was first introduced as a treatment for Paget's disease. In high concentrations it inhibits bone resorption by reducing the recruitment and activity of osteoclasts. Several preparations are available but synthetic salmon calcitonin seems to be the most potent. In women with established postmenopausal osteoporosis its use appears to stabilise bone mass and reduce the incidence of vertebral and hip fractures. The hormone must be used parenterally but may now be administered as an intranasal spray. Salmon calcitonin has a short-term analgesic effect which is useful for patients with acute osteoporotic vertebral fractures.

Bisphosphonates

The first bisphosphonate drug available, etidronate, was used for treating Paget's disease. At high doses it can completely inhibit the bone remodelling process, affecting both osteoclastic resorption and bone mineralisation. At lower doses bisphosphonates can preferentially inhibit osteoclast activity and allow unopposed bone formation, hence their indication for use in osteoporosis. Etidronate is usually administered in intermittent cycles, along with calcium, to help avoid inhibition of bone mineralisation.

The bisphosphonates accumulate in the area of the bone remodelling units and bind to the calcium hydroxyapatite crystals, forming a coating. This prevents access of osteoclasts to the bone thereby inhibiting bone resorption. Several newer bisphosphonates (alendronate, tiludronate, clodronate, resedronate) are at various stages of clinical trial. These can be used at lower doses and on a daily basis. Evidence from the Fracture Intervention Trial (Black *et al.*, 1996; see p. 690) shows that alendronate is capable of increasing bone mass and reducing fracture rates by about 50% in women who have already experienced vertebral fracture. Another arm of the trial aims to evaluate the effect of alendronate on fracture risk in women without existing vertebral fractures.

However, the long-term effects of biophosphonates are uncertain because they can remain in the skeleton for 10 years or more, inhibiting bone resorption. This could have untoward effects on the quality of bone because the process of remodelling is essential to the maintenance of bone and elimination of microfractures.

Fluoride

Fluoride is familiar to most people as a means of strengthening teeth. High doses (75 mg daily) of sodium fluoride can stimulate new bone formation and clinical trials have demonstrated that substantial gains in spinal bone mass can be achieved. However, this does not seem to reduce the incidence of fracture, possibly because the new bone is abnormal in composition and strength. Lower doses of fluoride (50 mg daily) combined with calcium and vitamin D supplementation can help to maintain correct mineralisation of new bone.

Interventions that increase bone mass do not always reduce fractures

Parathyroid hormone fragments

Paradoxically, fragments of the parathyroid hormone protein can stimulate bone formation when given intermittently. Bone resorption takes place at higher doses or when the intact hormone is administered. At present the potential of this therapy for preventing fractures is uncertain and further work is required before clinical trials and licensing can take place.

New approaches to therapy

The advent of recombinant DNA technology has meant that it is possible to produce a variety of human peptides in commercial quantities. Although there is still much to understand about how osteoblasts and osteoclasts regulate bone resorption and formation, it is clear that they respond to a variety of growth hormones and signalling peptides. One factor influencing age-related osteoporosis is the availability of growth hormone. The synthesis of this hormone by the pituitary declines with age, and it may be possible to compensate for this change by stimulating the pituitary with recombinant human growth hormone releasing factor. Studies are awaited.

The activity of both osteoblasts and osteoclasts is stimulated by cytokines. Animal studies have shown that over-expression of IL-4 induces osteoporosis. Other potent inducers of bone resorption are IL-1 and TNF-α. There is therefore some potential for modulating bone metabolism by use of agents that inhibit the synthesis of these cytokines. Appropriate inhibitors are now available but have yet to be evaluated clinically.

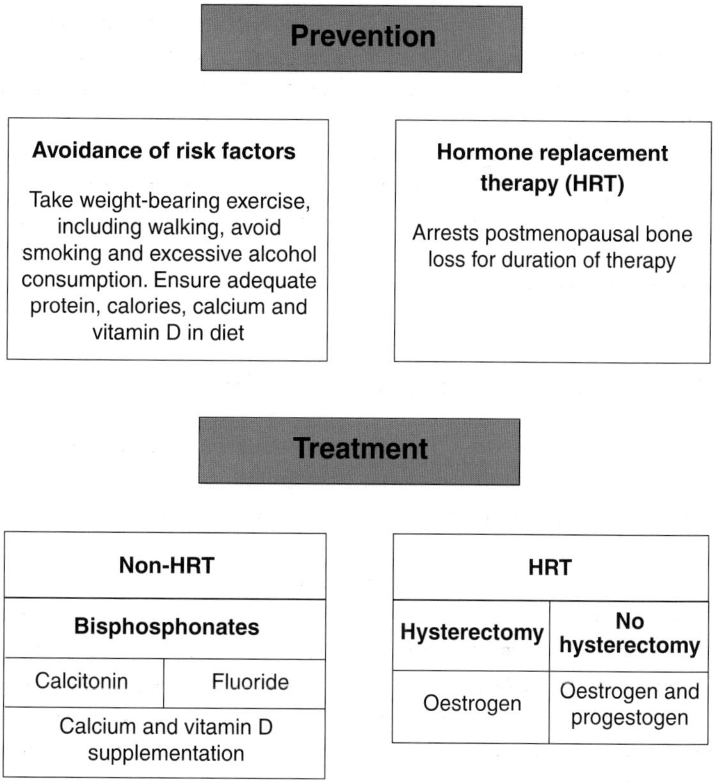

Prevention	
Avoidance of risk factors Take weight-bearing exercise, including walking, avoid smoking and excessive alcohol consumption. Ensure adequate protein, calories, calcium and vitamin D in diet	**Hormone replacement therapy (HRT)** Arrests postmenopausal bone loss for duration of therapy

Treatment	

Non-HRT		HRT	
Bisphosphonates		Hysterectomy	**No hysterectomy**
Calcitonin	Fluoride	Oestrogen	Oestrogen and progestogen
Calcium and vitamin D supplementation			

Figure 22.9 Approaches to prevention and treatment of osteoporosis.

Treatment of fractures

Review question 4

What would be the most appropriate way of helping a 60-year-old woman who recently fractured her wrist in a slight fall?

Hip fractures

Fracture of the hip is a break in the upper end of the femur. There are two kinds: femoral neck fracture, which involves the neck of the femur; trochanteric fracture, where the bone is broken below or around the greater or lesser trochanters (bony prominences of the femur below the femoral neck). Hip fractures are treatable by surgery.

Trochanteric fractures can be stabilised by the insertion of a hip nail through the femoral neck and into the head of the femur. A side plate is fitted to the

shaft with screws. Fractures of the femoral neck may require more extensive surgery, involving excision of the femoral head and the insertion of a hip prosthesis. They can also be fixed internally by inserting a three-flanged nail (Smith-Petersen type) through the femoral head and neck.

Spinal fractures

Kyphosis produces muscular and ligamentous pain which may require analgesia, ultrasound therapy or acupuncture. Recent crush fractures of the spine are particularly painful and calcitonin can be useful as an analgesic. Although the patient will need to rest it is imperative that this is not prolonged because movement encourages stimulation of the bone through mechanical stress. In some cases physiotherapy or hydrotherapy may help to restore mobility by increasing muscle strength and improving spinal movement. Someone who has lost several centimetres in height through spinal osteoporosis must not be stretched or have their vertebrae rebuilt.

Measurement of bone density

Bone density measurements are the best means of predicting bone fractures. The methods available are usually quick (often 10 minutes or less), non-invasive and involve low radiation dosage. They are used mainly for diagnosis and monitoring response to treatment, but there is great interest in using bone scanning as a means of mass screening for osteoporosis.

There are two approaches to measuring bone loss. The most accurate are **densitometric** methods that rely on measurement of the attenuation of X-rays or other radiation sources as they pass through bone (a further method relies on the measurement of ultrasound echoes reflected from bone). The second approach is to assess the rate of bone turnover by measurement of **biochemical markers**.

Densitometric methods

A variety of densitometric techniques is available for evaluating bone. Standard radiography is of little value in assessing bone density and is best used for the evaluation of bone fractures. The most accurate and widely used methods are dual photon and dual X-ray absorptiometry (DXA).

Ideally, bone density should be assessed in the bones most at risk: the spine and femoral neck

Dual photon absorptiometry
This technique can be used to estimate bone mineral density in the hips and spine. It is based on the estimation of photons absorbed by bone, which is roughly proportional to the quantity of mineral present. A radiation source (consisting of the isotope gadolinium-153) is used to emit photons with peaks in the energy spectrum at 44 and 100 keV (hence 'dual photon').

The high-energy and low-energy photons are differentially absorbed by bone and soft tissue. Subtraction of the lower energy peak allows compensation for the soft-tissue components in the examined region by comparison with the higher energy peak. The body part is scanned in a rectilinear fashion and the emerging photons continuously measured by a scintillation detector. The data is processed and analysed by computer and an image generated. In parallel with this the mineral content of the skeletal region covered is calculated. The results are displayed as a histogram showing the bone mineral density (expressed in g/cm^2).

Dual X-ray absorptiometry

> *DXA is a quick and non-invasive method of assessing bone density*

This works on a similar principle to dual photon absorptiometry, with the exception that the dual photon beams are generated by an X-ray tube instead of a radioactive isotope. This is a more efficient generator of photons and produces images of greater resolution. It also improves scan time, radiation dose and the costs of renewing the source. Measurements can be made of the spine and femoral neck to an accuracy of 1%. This is currently the method of choice for measurement of bone mineral density (Figure 22.10).

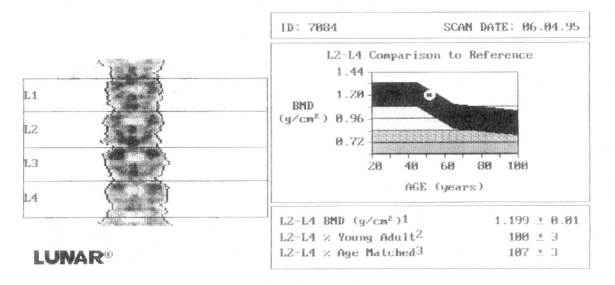

Figure 22.10 The DXA bone scan generates an image of the spine and allows measurement of bone density. This can be compared with the typical bone density from the age-matched population. In this example (a 50-year-old woman) the spinal bone density is 1.2 g/cm^2, which is at the upper end of the normal range for a woman of that age.

Computed tomography

The big advantage of CT over other densitometric methods is its ability to distinguish trabecular bone from cortical bone. Trabecular bone is the high-turnover bone that is most easily eroded and therefore its measurement is a

much more sensitive way of assessing osteopenia and predicting fracture risk. There can be problems with the accuracy of the measurement because of the variable amounts of fat and bone marrow in different parts of the bone and in different individuals. While the equipment is widely available it is costly and involves a fairly high radiation dose.

Quantitative ultrasound

Quantitative ultrasound is a newer technique that is quick to perform and free of radiation (Plate 9). Ultrasound echoes reflected by bone can provide information about bone density and quality. The preliminary indications are that ultrasound measurement is useful but whether it is as effective as DXA in predicting risk of fracture remains unclear.

Biochemical markers of bone turnover

Biochemical markers have provided insights into the bone remodelling process and its alterations in metabolic bone diseases. Markers are available that reflect bone formation and resorption. The various biochemical markers can be used in experimental studies to evaluate the mechanism of action of new therapies, and to monitor the effects of existing therapies.

The most reliable markers of bone formation are serum alkaline phosphatase and osteocalcin. Degradation products of the bone collagenous matrix, such as pyridinoline, deoxypyridinoline (derived from collagen cross-links) and hydroxyproline (collagen contains a large proportion of this amino acid), serve as biochemical markers of bone resorption.

Screening for osteopenia and osteoporosis

To date the usefulness of measuring bone density as a screening procedure is uncertain because of the large individual variation in bone mass. The problem can largely be overcome by measuring the rate of bone loss, by repeated densitometric measurements in an individual, to pick up the 'fast-losers'.

At present bone density screening is recommended for women at high risk of osteoporosis because of:
- Oestrogen deficiency caused by early (<45 years) menopause or prolonged amenorrhoea
- Long-term corticosteroid use
- Presence of disorders that can cause secondary osteoporosis (anorexia nervosa, alcohol abuse, hyperparathyroidism, hypogonadism, malabsorption syndrome, gastrectomy, myeloma)

Many people have argued that bone density screening should be extended to the broader population and a number of research projects are under way to evaluate the feasibility of screening perimenopausal women. In the past concerns were expressed about the ability of bone scans to predict future fracture risk with reasonable accuracy but there is now ample evidence that bone density

Collagen: the principal fibrous component of connective tissues. Consists of cross-linked protein chains which form insoluble fibres.

Osteocalcin: a non-collagenous protein component of osteoid, secreted by osteoblasts and present in the blood.

The rationale behind screening for osteopenia is to identify people at risk of fractures so that preventive measures can be taken

is a good predictor of fracture, although this may only relate to the particular bone sites scanned. In other words, a DXA scan of the hip is a reliable indicator of future hip fracture risk but a scan of the spine is of little use in predicting future hip fracture. Generally, the risk of fracture is at least doubled for each standard deviation fall in bone density (Figure 22.11).

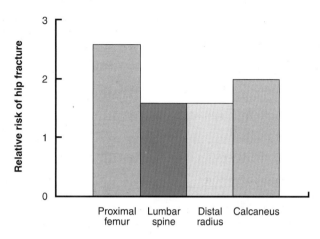

Site of bone mineral density measurement

Figure 22.11 Bone density measurement of the femoral neck is a better predictor of hip fracture than measurements of the spine or radius and is marginally better than the calcaneus (heel bone). Baseline measurements were made on 8134 American white women of at least 65 years of age, 65 of whom sustained hip fractures during 1.8 years of follow-up. Each SD decrease in femoral neck bone density increases the age-adjusted risk of hip fracture by 2.6 times. (Data from Cummings, S.R., Black, D.M., Nevitt, M.C. *et al.* (1993) *Lancet*, **341**, 72–5.)

Although there is no significant problem with attendance at screening, there is a problem with treatment compliance in women found to have low bone density because the treatment intervention (HRT) is poorly tolerated by some women. For many women the restoration of monthly bleeds is unacceptable, particularly over the long term. Even so, the proportion of women who discontinue HRT within 6 months is lower in women who have undergone bone density scanning than in women who have not been scanned. Attendance at screening increases awareness of osteoporosis, can provide a further indication for HRT for women in whom the decision was marginal, and increase compliance because the woman has more reasons for taking it.

Better intervention is needed for the women found to be at increased fracture risk. Although risk factor modification is helpful it should have been initiated some years before the menopause and even well motivated people find it difficult to change habits that have been established for many years. Therapies, like HRT, that can continue the oestrogenic effects on bone without stimulating endometrial and breast epithelium could provide a better solution. Such therapies are being developed (oestrogen agonists/antagonists, for example) but it will be some years before full clinical trials have been completed.

Should a mass screening programme be initiated for osteoporosis?

Point	Counterpoint
Reliable non-invasive methods are available for estimating bone density	Bone density estimation may not reliably predict risk of fracture
Reliability is increased by repeat screening to measure rates of bone loss	Interval screening would require enormous resources, requiring regular screening of every post-menopausal woman and older man
Women with low bone density can be identified and given HRT	There is no need to measure bone density before starting HRT
HRT is a powerful drug regimen and, without other indications, should not be given without proper evaluation of bone density	HRT is poorly tolerated by some women. Avoidance of lifestyle risk factors is good advice for everybody, regardless of their current bone density

Author's view

In one sense screening for osteoporosis provides a remedy for people who do not wish to take exercise or pay attention to other important risk factors. Risk factor intervention for the prevention of osteoporotic fractures is desirable for the general population anyway, and does not need to be preceded by screening. However, there will remain a significant number of people who will develop osteoporosis despite leading 'healthy' lifestyles. Screening would be of positive benefit for these people.

Compliance with treatment poses a problem. In most other screening programmes the intervention comprises a treatment in which the patient plays a relatively passive role but intervention for people at risk of osteoporosis requires long-term compliance in maintaining HRT. Until more satisfactory drug therapies become available, a one-off bone scan may be enough to convince some people of the need for HRT or lifestyle modification. Conversely, a person declared to have good bone density may see no need to maintain the healthy behaviour.

Case study

Mrs B is a 58-year-old part-time home help for her local council. She is white, of British nationality, and lives with her husband in an industrial town in the North of England.

Mrs B has had a history of lower back pain over the past 12 months. She is finding it increasingly difficult to sleep and sitting can be quite painful. The pain does not radiate to the legs or other parts of her back. She was initially

prescribed pain killers, but visited her doctor again 3 months later with sharp pain in the lumbar region of her back.

Mrs B has a fairly sedentary lifestyle, although her job involves some activity. She has not participated in any sport or taken regular exercise since she left school at the age of 16. She had a simple hysterectomy at the age of 43 and does not take any regular medication except self-prescribed aspirin to relieve 'rheumatism'.

She has been a smoker for 35 years and currently smokes about 15 cigarettes a day. She visits the pub on two evenings a week and usually consumes three measures of gin and tonic on each visit. This is her total weekly alcohol intake.

- Does Mrs B have any risk factors for osteoporosis?
- Are the presenting symptoms characteristic of osteoporosis? What other signs or symptoms could indicate osteoporosis?
- What other conditions might feature in a differential diagnosis?
- What useful laboratory tests are there?
- What imaging techniques are useful for detecting bone loss and bone fractures?
- What treatment options are available?
- What future problems could Mrs B expect given the treatment she received?

ANSWERS TO REVIEW QUESTIONS

Question 1

Why are wrist fractures more common in middle-aged people and hip fractures much more common in older people?

This could be related to general mobility and slowing down of the reflexes; older people are less able to break a fall with their arms and therefore fall more heavily on the hip.

Question 2

Why is osteoporosis a health problem?

Reduced bone mass increases the risk of fracture. Bone fractures are associated with pain, disability and can result in premature death. Some bone fractures are more serious than others, with hip fractures causing the most serious problems: about 50% of all people suffering hip fracture will not be able to walk unaided thereafter. The costs of treatment run into hundreds of millions of pounds a year, patients with hip fractures alone taking up about 20% of orthopaedic beds. For many people the condition is preventable.

Question 3

What factors have influenced the total bone mass in a 60-year-old woman?

The amount of bone at its peak (usually in the fourth decade), the time at which bone loss begins (in a woman this will commence with age-related loss before the menopause) and postmenopausal osteoporosis. The postmenopausal

loss is superimposed on the age-related osteoporosis. In time (usually 6–7 years after the menopause), postmenopausal loss will not be so obvious and any further losses will be caused by age-related changes.

The resultant bone loss will also be influenced by the rate at which these losses occur, which varies among individuals. Postmenopausal osteoporosis is far more detrimental to bone than age-related loss. Medical conditions, such as amenorrhoea, or drug use can also influence bone mass.

What would be the most appropriate way of helping a 60-year-old woman who recently fractured her wrist in a slight fall?

Question 4

The question suggests that the fracture was produced with only slight or moderate trauma and it is therefore likely that she has osteoporosis. If so, she will be at risk of sustaining further fractures. First, it is necessary to exclude other medical conditions or drug therapies that could be responsible for secondary osteoporosis.

Given her age, and presuming she had a normal menopause, the first-line treatment would be HRT, supplemented with calcium. She should be encouraged to take moderate exercise such as walking, to avoid excessive alcohol consumption or heavy smoking. If she cannot tolerate the initial HRT, other oestrogen preparations or routes of administration should be tried. If she remains unsuited to oestrogen therapy she should be considered for cyclical etidronate treatment.

Does Mrs B have any risk factors for osteoporosis? The woman in the case study has had a hysterectomy: this is associated with early ovarian failure and thus could have initiated osteoporosis earlier than would otherwise have been the case. She also has a fairly long history of cigarette smoking. The menopause often comes earlier in smokers than in non-smokers, and could also contribute to early ovarian failure. Alcohol is a risk factor, but Mrs B's consumption is unlikely to cause liver damage and affect calcium metabolism. Mrs B could have reduced her risk of osteoporosis through taking regular exercise. A strong risk factor is prolonged amenorrhoea, which is not applicable here.

Case study

Other osteoporosis risks are related to the likelihood of falling. Spinal fractures can be produced during quite normal activities such as getting out of bed or a chair: activities which we can hardly avoid. The risk of falling is much more important in the production of wrist and hip fractures than spinal fractures.

Are the presenting symptoms characteristic of osteoporosis? What other signs or symptoms could indicate osteoporosis? Mrs B's back pain could be a symptom of kyphosis, although there are many other possible causes ranging from muscle strain to malignancy. Osteoporosis may be completely asymptomatic even when severe, for example with collapsed vertebrae. The only sign of this may be a reduction in height but eventually the woman will complain of back pain, breathlessness, reflux indigestion and neck pain. The other early common manifestation of osteoporosis is wrist fracture, usually

with only minor trauma.

Mrs B was sent for X-ray of her thoracic and lumbar spine which showed evidence of vertebral deformity and fracture. No other conditions were identified by clinical examination and laboratory tests and she was therefore diagnosed as having primary osteoporosis.

What other conditions might feature in a differential diagnosis? Secondary causes of osteoporosis (e.g. long-term corticosteroid use, hyperparathyroidism, Cushing's syndrome) must be excluded. Osteomalacia will also result in reduced bone strength, increasing the likelihood of fracture. Metastatic tumour deposits can also erode bone.

What useful laboratory tests are there? Laboratory tests are of limited value in diagnosing osteoporosis itself. Some markers of bone turnover may be helpful: these include alkaline phosphatase and osteocalcin measurement in serum. A range of other tests are used to exclude other conditions such as multiple myeloma, Cushing's syndrome, osteomalacia and hyperparathyroidism.

What imaging techniques are useful for detecting bone loss and fractures? Plain X-rays are adequate for detecting deformity and fractures of the vertebra. Bone loss itself is better estimated using DXA.

Mrs B was advised to undertake a course of HRT but refused because a close friend had done so and suffered adverse symptoms without trying alternative preparations. She was prescribed calcium supplementation (400 mg three times daily), advised to undertake a programme of light exercise and urged to give up smoking.

A year later she still experienced back pain, but this had improved. She had decided to visit a keep fit class twice weekly but had given up after 3 or 4 months as this was too time-consuming. She also decided to walk to work instead of going by bus, except in bad weather. She was monitored by her doctor on a 3-monthly basis.

What treatment options are available? The treatment of choice in this case is HRT. In its absence, calcium therapy, exercise and attention to other risk factors such as smoking are appropriate. However, this may not be enough to arrest bone loss and prevent problems in the future. Cyclical etidronate therapy may be considered.

What future problems could Mrs B expect given the treatment she received? Kyphosis and fracture of other bones – probably initially the wrist; if this is avoided she could suffer a hip fracture when she gets older. No adverse side-effects would be anticipated with her current treatment regimen, the problem is that it is not the most effective. More aggressive treatments, such as HRT or etidronate therapy, are associated with adverse side-effects in some people.

References

Black, D.M., Cummings, S.R., Karpf, D.B. *et al.* (1996) Randomised trial of effect of alendronate on risk of fracture in women with existing fractures. *Lancet*,

348, 1535–41.

Chapuy, M.C., Arlot, M.E., Delmas, P.D. and Meunier, P.J. (1994) Effect of calcium and cholecalciferol treatment for three years on hip fractures in elderly women. *BMJ*, **308**, 1081–2.

Cummings, S.R., Kelsey, J.L., Nevitt, M.C. and O'Dowd, K.J. (1985) Epidemiology of osteoporosis and osteoporotic fractures. *Epidemiol. Rev.*, **7**, 179–208.

Felson, D.T., Zhang, Y., Hannan, M.T. *et al.* (1995) Alcohol intake and bone mineral intake in elderly men and women. The Framingham Study. *Am. J. Epidemiol.*, **142**, 485–92.

Grant, S.F.A., Reid, D.M., Blake, G. *et al.* (1996) Reduced bone density and osteoporosis associated with a polymorphic Sp1 binding site in the collagen type 1a1 gene. *Nature Genet.* **14**, 203–5.

Kobayashi, S., Inoue, S., Hosoi, T. *et al.* (1996) Association of bone mineral density with polymorphism of the estrogen receptor gene. *J. Bone Miner. Res.* **11**, 306–11.

Further reading

Aaron, J.E., Makins, N.B. and Sagreiya, K. (1987) The microanatomy of trabecular bone loss in normal ageing men and women. *Clin. Orthop.*, **215**, 260–71.

Avioli, L.V. (1993) *The Osteoporotic Syndrome (Detection, Prevention and Treatment)*. John Wiley, Chichester.

Christiansen, C. (1991) *Hormone Replacement and its Impact on Osteoporosis*. Baillière Tindall, London.

Compston, J.E. (1992) HRT and osteoporosis. *Br. Med Bull.*, **48**, 309–44.

Compston, J.E. (1994) The therapeutic use of bisphosphonates. *BMJ*, **309**, 711–15.

Dempster, D.W. and Lindsay, R. (1983) Pathogenesis of osteoporosis. *Lancet*, **341**, 797–805.

Lindsay, R. (1993) Prevention and treatment of osteoporosis. *Lancet*, **341**, 801–5.

Manolagas, S.C. and Jilka, R.L. (1995) Bone marrow, cytokines, and bone remodelling. *N. Engl. J. Med.*, **332**, 305–11.

Morrison, N.A., Qui, J.C., Tokita, A. *et al.* (1994) Prediction of bone density from vitamin D receptor alleles. *Nature*, **367**, 284–7.

Purdie, D.W. (1992) Screening for osteoporosis. *Br. J. Hosp. Med.*, **47**, 605–8.

Reid, D.M. (ed.) (1993) *Baillière's Clinical Rheumatology, Osteoporosis*. Baillière Tindall, London.

Reid, I.R., Ames, R.W., Evans, M.C. *et al.* (1993) Effect of calcium supplementation on bone loss in postmenopausal women. *N. Engl. J. Med.*, **328**, 460–4.

Stacey, T.A. (1989) Osteoporosis: Exercise therapy, pre- and post-diagnosis. *J. Manipulative Physiol. Ther.*, **12**, 211–19.

Riggs, B.L. and Melton, L.J. (1992) The prevention and treatment of osteoporosis. *N. Engl. J. Med.*, **327**, 620–7.

Valimaki, M.J., Karkkainen, M., Lamberg-Allardt, C. *et al.* (1994) Exercise, smoking, and calcium intake during adolescence and early adulthood as determinants of peak bone mass. *BMJ*, **309**, 230–5.

23 Diabetes mellitus

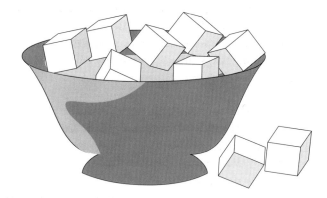

People can become diabetic at any age. The condition arises through a lack of glycaemic control, either because insufficient insulin is produced, or because it has a reduced effect. Insulin-dependent, or type I, diabetes usually becomes apparent by the age of 40; this type of diabetes can be managed only by insulin injection. The more common type of diabetes (non-insulin-dependent; type II) is more likely to become apparent from middle age onwards. It is often managed by dietary control, although some patients may need pharmacological intervention or insulin injection.

The acute symptoms of diabetes are thirst, frequent urination, tiredness and blurred vision, although many patients, especially those with type II diabetes, are asymptomatic at diagnosis. Both types of diabetes are associated with serious long-term complications: damage to the nerves, kidneys and eyes. They are also at increased risk of stroke, CHD and peripheral vascular disease. The risk of developing these complications can be reduced by good glycaemic control, but it is also important to control hypertension and hyperlipidaemia. For these reasons, people with diabetes need to pay particular attention to the lifestyle risk factors of diet, salt and alcohol intake, exercise and smoking.

Regular screening and monitoring of diabetics forms an important role in reducing the impact of complications. Early treatment can prevent early deaths from complications such as nephropathy.

Pre-test

- **What is the difference between insulin-dependent (type I) and non-insulin-dependent (type II) diabetes?**
- **What are the symptoms of diabetes?**
- **Who is likely to suffer from diabetes? Is it possible that you could develop diabetes?**
- **What are the long-term complications of diabetes?**
- **How is diabetes controlled?**
- **How is diabetes diagnosed?**
- **What can be done to treat the long-term complications of diabetes?**

Aims of this chapter

By the end of this chapter you will have increased your knowledge of:
◆ The epidemiology of diabetes: the age at which the disease is most likely to occur and geographical differences in prevalence
◆ The metabolic causes and effects of diabetes mellitus
◆ The acute and chronic consequences of diabetes

In addition, this chapter will help you to:
◆ Discuss the genetic and possible environmental factors involved in the development of diabetes
◆ Understand why good glycaemic control is necessary
◆ Distinguish between the two types of diabetes and discuss the differences in the ways they are controlled
◆ Understand how diabetes can cause damage to other body systems
◆ Understand why the objectives of the St Vincent declaration have been set and discuss how they can be met

Introduction

Diabetes mellitus is a chronic metabolic disease characterised either by insufficient secretion of insulin or by insufficient effect of insulin on peripheral tissues. This causes dangerous fluctuations in blood glucose levels, and a variety of short and long-term complications.

Most people associate diabetes with the need to inject insulin, but this is necessary only in **insulin-dependent**, or **type I**, diabetes. Before the discovery of insulin in 1921, a diagnosis of this type of diabetes was tantamount to a death sentence. Today, relatively few treated diabetic subjects die although their life expectancy is still lower because of the emergence of complications such as kidney disease and CHD: insulin replacement does not prevent the development of these conditions.

Non-insulin-dependent, or **type II**, diabetes is much more common. This has a much more insidious onset, often starting in middle age, but is sometimes not diagnosed until irreversible complications have occurred. In most cases patients retain some capacity to manufacture insulin and injections are not required: the condition is caused by a lack of response to insulin. This type of diabetes is usually controlled by careful attention to diet.

The complications of both types of diabetes can be devastating: some patients may go blind, develop renal failure or peripheral vascular disease that may require amputation of a limb. People with diabetes are more likely to die prematurely from stroke or CHD (Figure 23.1).

The disturbance of glucose metabolism in diabetes leads to changes in proteins and lipid metabolism. Glucose binds to certain amino acids within a protein: the protein is said to have become **glycosylated** or **glycated**. Glycosylated proteins cause structural changes in connective tissues and damage to the cells of blood vessels and nerves.

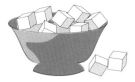

Diabetes is characterised by persistently high blood sugar levels

Diabetes can be controlled but not cured

Insulin: a hormone produced by the pancreas, essential for the metabolism of carbohydrates and fats.

Both types of diabetes mellitus have serious medical complications

Glycosylation, glycation: the non-enzymatic binding of glucose (in blood and body fluids) to proteins, particularly when glucose concentrations are high, as in diabetes mellitus. Glycosylation can have serious consequences if the proteins of the blood vessel walls and cornea of the eye are altered, contributing to atherosclerosis and blindness. Some consequences are minor, such as glycosylation of protein in hair or haemoglobin: these glycosylated proteins are measured to monitor the disease.

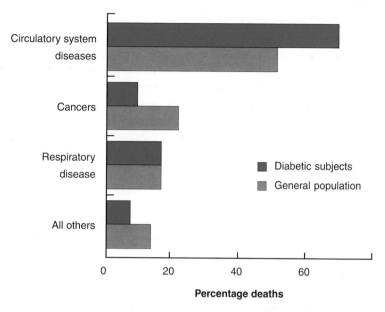

Figure 23.1 Causes of death in diabetic subjects (UK data). People with diabetes are much more likely to suffer from diseases of the circulatory system, particularly CHD, than the general population. The average life expectancy of diabetic subjects is significantly shorter than that of the general population.

Targets for treatment of diabetes

Attempts to define objectives for improving diabetes care were discussed at a meeting organised by the World Health Organization in 1989, and are set out in the **St Vincent Declaration**. These objectives (to be met within 5 years) included:

- Reduce the incidence of blindness caused by diabetes by at least one-third
- Reduce the rate of limb amputation as a result of diabetic gangrene by at least 50%
- Achieve a pregnancy outcome for diabetic women comparable to that of non-diabetic women (there is a risk of fetal death and congenital malformations)
- Reduce the numbers of people reaching end-stage diabetic renal failure by at least one-third
- Reduce the morbidity and mortality from CHD in people who have diabetes by vigorous attention to lifestyle risk factors.

At the time of writing the St Vincent declaration has not been formally adopted by all nations and in the UK the government has invited comments on the feasibility of adopting the targets. One problem is that the baseline figures (for example the numbers of diabetic patients who go blind, develop end-stage renal failure or have amputations) are not currently available and so it is not possible to monitor the targets. These data can be collected prospectively but this will require organisation of a district diabetes register,

proper measurement and assessment of outcomes, recording and audit, all of which will consume resources (although in the long term there will be savings).

Although type I diabetes is strongly influenced by environmental factors these have yet to be firmly identified, and so there is currently little potential for primary prevention. The development of the more common type II diabetes is strongly influenced by a genetic predisposition. Nonetheless identifiable environmental factors can be altered. There is, therefore, some potential for delaying onset, mainly by avoiding obesity and increasing the amount of exercise taken. Secondary prevention is of importance for avoiding the acute complications of diabetes, and there is evidence from the Diabetes Control and Complication Trial (1993) that good control of type I diabetes can minimise the long-term risks of retinopathy, nephropathy and neuropathy (see below). Attention to other risk factors such as smoking, hypertension and blood cholesterol can minimise the risk of stroke and CHD in diabetic patients.

Person-years: used in epidemiology to describe disease frequency, derived from the number of people in a study multiplied by its duration. For example, 100 000 person-years could describe 25 000 people studied for 4 years or 10 000 people studied for 10 years.

Epidemiology

Type II diabetes is three times more common than type I. At present about 500 000 people in the UK are diagnosed as having diabetes, and a further 500 000 may be undiagnosed. Both forms of diabetes have increased in incidence. Between 1973 and 1988 the incidence of type I diabetes in children in the UK increased from eight to nearly 14 per 100 000. The overall word-wide prevalence of type II diabetes is estimated at 2%. The lowest incidence is seen in Japan (1-2 per 100 000 person-years), the highest in some parts of Finland (40 per 100 000 person-years).

Type I diabetes occurs most frequently in people of northern European descent (Figure 23.2), being less common in blacks, native Americans and Asians. The prevalence of both types of diabetes is similar in both men and women. Type II diabetes becomes more common with age; 7–10% of people in the UK over 70 years have the condition.

Background information: The HLA system and disease

All cells of the body carry a complex set of proteins as part of their membrane structure. These proteins are products of the genes in the **major histocompatibility complex** (MHC), also known as the **human leukocyte antigen** (HLA) system. Among other things, these membrane proteins play a major role in cell recognition.

There is considerable individual variation in HLA genes and their products: it is very unusual to find two people with exactly the same set of HLA proteins. These proteins play a role in recognising self from non-self, an essential feature of the normal immunological defence system. The HLA proteins are recognised by the immune system when tissues or organs are transplanted from one person to another: the body will reject the newly transplanted tissue (graft versus host reaction) if they differ. Exact matches

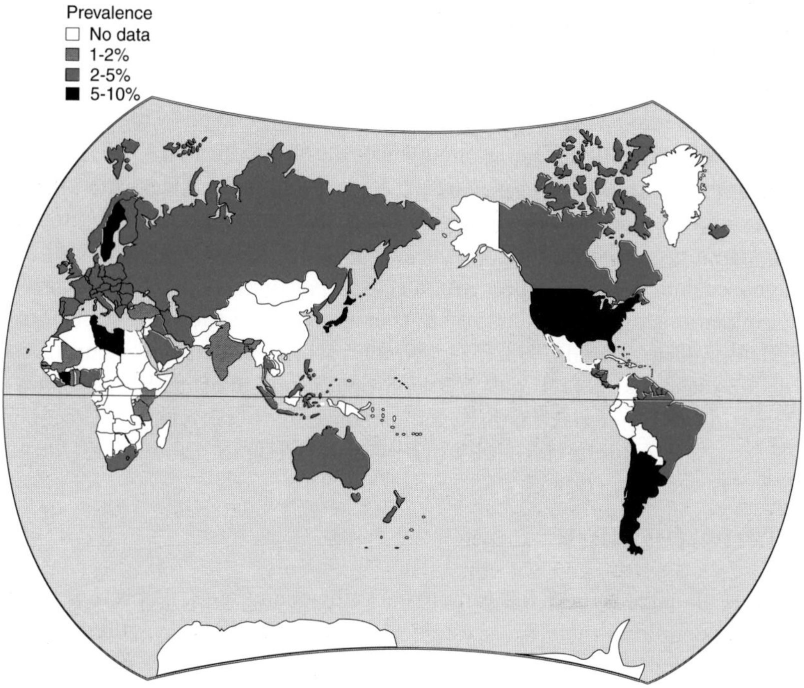

Prevalence
☐ No data
◼ 1-2%
◼ 2-5%
◼ 5-10%

Figure 23.2 Geographical variation in the prevalence of diabetes. Type I and type II diabetes are most common in the USA and South America. Most African and Asian countries currently have relatively low rates but this is increasing in populations that are changing towards a 'Western' diet. (Source: WHO, 1985.)

▲ Key points

HLA genes

Class I:

▲ HLA-A, HLA-B and HLA-C

▲ Part of the body's system of cell and tissue recognition which allows distinction between self and non-self (foreign antigens)

Class II:

▲ HLA-DP, HLA-DQ and HLA-DR

▲ Part of the body's immune response and recognition system

Class III:

▲ Includes genes coding for various components of the complement system, heat shock proteins and tumour necrosis factor

Systemic lupus erythematosus: a multisystem autoimmune disease primarily involving the joints, vascular system and serous membranes. Causes fever, anorexia, rash, malaise, weight loss, conjunctivitis and arthritis. Characteristic butterfly-shaped rash is produced on the bridge of the nose and cheeks.

are rare (from an identical twin, for example), which is why most transplant patients require immunosuppression for the rest of their lives.

The specific array of HLA proteins in an individual may be detected in the laboratory by immunological methods. The proteins are also referred to as **HLA antigens** and the detection and matching of the main types forms the basis of tissue typing. This aims to achieve a close match between donor and recipient so that the chances of transplant rejection are minimised.

The genes that code for HLA antigens are located on the short arm of chromosome 6. The entire system is divided into three classes (I, II and III) and into various gene groups (class II genes are of the HLA-DP, HLA-DQ and HLA-DR groups). The class I and II genes are primarily concerned with producing the specific proteins involved in cell recognition.

The HLA genes of all the classes are associated with predispositions for particular diseases. Class I genes are associated with ankylosing spondylitis and the class II genes with autoimmune disorders including systemic lupus erythematosus and type I diabetes.

Risk factors in diabetes

Type I diabetes

Insulin-dependent diabetes is thought to be caused by a combination of environmental factors and genetic susceptibility acting from early childhood and initiating the destruction of insulin-producing cells. Adults (usually those under 40 years) can also develop the condition.

> *Type I diabetes is caused by inflammatory destruction of pancreatic islet cells*

Genetics of type I diabetes

The genetic predisposition for diabetes is related to inheritance of genes in the HLA system. Two genes within the HLA-DQ group of class II antigens have been identified as determining susceptibility for type I diabetes. These control the way in which antigens are presented to cells and prompt an immune response. People inherit different kinds of HLA genes. Certain HLA-DQ genes confer protection against diabetes in some people but not in others, while HLA-DR3 and HLA-DR4 genes appear to confer an increased risk for development of diabetes. Some genes outside the HLA family, particularly the insulin gene on chromosome 11, may also influence the predisposition for diabetes.

Environmental factors

The environmental factors that might predispose to type I diabetes are not known. Viruses have long been suspected as causes of the disease and there is some association between infections with Coxsackie, mumps and rubella and later onset of type I diabetes; however, the large majority of people with diabetes have had no previous infection. Animal experimental studies have demonstrated that pancreatic islet cells can be destroyed and diabetes induced by infection with a range of viruses. Certain chemicals (alloxan for example) will induce diabetes in animals but no association has been conclusively shown in humans.

It is possible that an autoimmune reaction is induced by **molecular mimicry** to produce diabetes. The body mounts an immune response to a foreign antigen; if the structure of the antigen is very similar to that of a normal tissue component the antibodies generated may recognise and destroy the normal component as well as the foreign antigen. A fragment of albumin in cows' milk which bears structural similarities to a cell-surface protein (p69) is produced by pancreatic β-cells when they are infected by a virus. In some genetically susceptible individuals the environmental trigger for the destruction of pancreatic islet cells may be exposure to cows' milk during the first few months of life. This view remains controversial.

Type II diabetes

Both lifestyle risk factors and genetic predisposition contribute to the

development of type II diabetes. The known risk factors are high sugar consumption, obesity, and a lack of exercise.

Genetic factors

Identical twins are likely to be concordant for type II diabetes

Concordance: both twins of a pair have the same trait.

Studies of identical twins have established an underlying contribution of inherited genetic factors in the pathogenesis of type II diabetes. When one twin has type II diabetes there is a 60% chance that the other twin will develop the disease. The degree of concordance may be close to 100% – concordance in non-identical twins is less than 20%.

The prevalence of diabetes in people living in the same general environment also varies with ethnic group. For example, the general prevalence of type II diabetes in the USA is 7%, but in Pima Indians this rises to about 34% and similar high rates are found in the Nauru Pacific islanders. Both the Pima Indian and Nauru populations have experienced a very rapid transition to a 'Western' lifestyle and many have become obese. Diabetes is up to ten times more likely to develop in an obese person with a family history of the disease than in someone who is not obese. Over thousands of years the Nauruans and Pima Indians have inherited a metabolism that is best able to cope with food shortages. In times of plenty this causes obesity and diabetes.

The genetics of type II diabetes is less well understood than that of type I disease because its heterogeneous nature and tendency for presentation later in life make the collection of family groups for genetic analysis more difficult. The application of recombinant DNA technology to the study of well-defined clinical groups may allow identification of genes which predispose for type II diabetes.

Environmental factors

Epidemiological studies show that the prevalence of type II diabetes is very different in developed and less developed countries. Moreover, an immigrant population tends to take on the rate of the host community. This strongly suggests that environmental factors are important in the development of the disease.

Nutrition

The incidence of type II diabetes decreases in food shortages. One theory links large intakes of sugar from childhood onwards with the development of type II diabetes, possibly because large amounts of insulin are produced to deal with the sugar. This ultimately causes an early decline in the capacity of the pancreatic islet cells to produce it.

Obesity

Type II diabetes is often associated with obesity. However, not all diabetic patients are obese and not all obese people are diabetic. In obese people who are diabetic, dietary restriction is often a good way to control the disease.

Exercise

Prospective epidemiological studies suggest that regular exercise prevents or delays the onset of type II diabetes. Exercise can also be used to assist glycaemic control, reduce obesity and minimise the risks of macrovascular complications.

Low birthweight

The development of type II diabetes appears to be related to birthweight: the larger the baby at birth the less likely they are to develop type II diabetes. The reason for this is not entirely clear but it is thought that physiological 'priming' takes place in the womb. If the mother has a habitual low-calorie diet (one reason for low birthweight), the baby will also be able to deal with an austere diet later in life. A small baby will also have a smaller pancreas, with fewer insulin-producing cells to start with. The combination of 'priming' factors and a small pancreas would mean that the adult is ill equipped to cope with a diet rich in sugary and fatty foods and will more likely develop diabetes.

Low-birthweight babies who become obese as adults are particularly prone to type II diabetes

▲ Key points

Comparison of type I and type II diabetes	
Type I	**Type II**
Insulin dependent	Non-insulin dependent
Virtually no insulin produced because pancreatic islet cells are destroyed	Production of insulin inappropriate or peripheral cells do not respond to insulin
Autoimmune response evident by antibodies to insulin and islet cell proteins	No evidence of autoantibodies
Diagnosis commonly develops at 10–13 years but can occur in adults, usually below 40 years of age	Onset usually after age 40 years, incidence increasing with age
Patients are usually lean	Patients are often obese
Patients of northern European descent	All racial groups
Family history positive in about 10% of cases; 30–35% concordance in identical twins (HLA-DQ genes)	Concordance of 60–100% in identical twins indicates importance of genetic factors but susceptibility genes as yet unidentified
May be triggered by environmental factors such as viral infection	Environmental factors, obesity, lack of exercise
Patients always need insulin	May be controlled by diet, with or without hypoglycaemic agents

Background information: Insulin

Insulin is produced in the pancreas by the β-**cells** present in the **islets of Langerhans**. The insulin produced is packaged as granules within the β-cells and released in response to raised glucose concentration in the blood. Glucose stimulates not only the release of the stored insulin but also its further production by the β-cells in a **biphasic response**: an initial surge of insulin corresponding to the release of stored hormone is followed by a smaller, more sustained, response reflecting the secretion of newly synthesised insulin. The intake of food causes a fivefold to tenfold increase in the basal secretion rate of about 1 unit of insulin per hour.

The insulin is released from the islet cells directly into the bloodstream. Most insulin is degraded by the liver, only about 50% reaching the peripheral circulation. Many cells in the peripheral tissues carry receptors for insulin. The reversible binding of the hormone to these specific receptors stimulates transport and utilisation processes involving glucose, amino acids and electrolytes.

Glucose is stored as **glycogen**, a glucose polymer that forms a reserve in most body cells, particularly those of the liver and muscle. Glucose is converted to glycogen by insulin. The reverse of this process, the conversion of glycogen to glucose (in a process called **glycogenolysis**), is mediated by the hormone **glucagon**. This is also produced in the pancreatic islets, by the α-cells. These cells are unaffected in diabetes.

Acute deficiency of insulin stimulates the release of glucose from the glycogen stores in the liver. The secretion of glucagon, cortisol, catecholamine and growth factor hormones is also stimulated, all of which further increase the production of glucose by the liver. The result is a massive increase in blood glucose concentration, a condition known as **hyperglycaemia**.

Insulin also has a restraining effect on **lipolysis**, the conversion of triglycerides in adipose tissue into their constituent fatty acids and glycerol. These are transported to the liver, which produces acetyl CoA, a compound normally metabolised by the tricarboxylic acid (TCA) cycle. The TCA cycle rapidly becomes overloaded in diabetes with the result that ketones, acetoacetate and hydroxybutyrate are formed in excessive amounts and released into the blood (Figure 23.3). The glycerol liberated from the triglycerides is used by the liver to form glucose in a process termed **gluconeogenesis**.

Insulin stimulates the uptake of glucose from blood

Insulin stimulates glycogen formation

Pathology and complications of diabetes

Type I (insulin-dependent) diabetes

Histological examination of the pancreas in type I diabetes demonstrates an almost total absence of the insulin-secreting β-cells, which leaves the patient

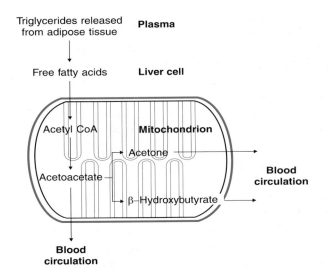

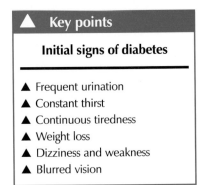

Figure 23.3 Generation of ketones from fatty acids. When insulin is in short supply triglyceride stores in the adipose tissues are mobilised and taken up by liver cells. The fatty acids released form a substrate for the mitochondrial production of acetoacetate, acetone and β-hydroxybutyrate. These ketones are released into the blood.

with no natural way of controlling blood glucose, although the types of islet cells that secrete other hormones are unaffected. The damage to the pancreatic islet cells starts some years before the onset of symptoms.

Type II (non-insulin-dependent) diabetes

Type II diabetes develops in one of two ways: either the amount of insulin produced is insufficient to prevent high blood sugar concentrations (in people who had previously produced normal amounts of insulin) or the cells in the peripheral tissues become less responsive to insulin and the patient becomes insulin-resistant. Sometimes both processes occur together, probably because of ageing processes in which the pancreatic and peripheral cells become inefficient. Occasionally lack of cellular response to insulin, even when the pancreas is still working reasonably well, causes raised blood insulin levels.

Type II diabetes is caused by insulin insufficiency or an inability to respond to insulin

Type II diabetes may be controlled by diet alone or by diet and an oral hypoglycaemic agent. Some patients are unresponsive to these forms of therapy, and need insulin to achieve control. This type of diabetes may start in early adulthood; the condition, described as **maturity onset type diabetes of the young** (MODY) was originally defined as diabetes in people under the age of 25 who could be controlled without insulin for more than 2 years. Many patients with MODY probably actually have type I diabetes; it simply takes longer than usual for the pancreatic damage to become extensive enough to warrant insulin treatment. Genuine cases of MODY usually have a family history of the condition. It is relatively rare in whites but more common in blacks.

Acute symptoms

The classic symptoms of diabetes are **polydipsia** (excessive thirst), **polyuria** (frequent urination), blurred vision and extreme fatigue. These acute symptoms are a direct result of the lack of glycaemic control. Insulin deficiency leads to **hyperglycaemia** (excessive blood sugar) and **ketosis** (excess of ketone bodies in body fluids). Hyperglycaemia is a consequence of decreased glucose uptake and utilisation by the liver and peripheral tissues, glycogenolysis, and breakdown of protein. These processes cause fatigue and weight loss. Ketosis is caused by the incomplete metabolism of fatty acids.

Polydipsia and polyuria

The accumulation of excessive glucose in the blood creates a condition called **hyperosmosis**, in which body fluids with a high sugar content are diluted by water from low-sugar fluids in other body compartments. The effect is dehydration of the body tissues and increased fluid excretion by the kidneys (polyuria). This must be compensated by increased fluid intake (polydipsia).

Blurred vision

The changes in blood glucose concentrations during the course of the disease cause changes to occur in the lens of the eye. The first sign of this is the fluctuation between normal and blurred vision that some patients experience, when blood glucose levels are either too high or too low. The lens of the eye is made up of cells and collagenous connective tissue. The cells obtain their nutrients from tissue fluid, the composition of which reflects the glucose concentration of the blood. Large variations in glucose concentration cause the lens to take up or expel water, altering its curvature. This is experienced as blurred vision.

Hyperglycaemia

Marked dehydration and salt depletion is reflected in low blood pressure and rapid pulse. Symptoms begin gradually, starting with polyuria, polydipsia, fever, nausea, vomiting and extreme fatigue.

In type II diabetes hyperglycaemia is likely to have an insidious onset, particularly in obese people. They often suffer no symptoms, the condition being detected during routine blood or urine tests.

When insulin deficiency is severe and of acute onset, as occurs in type I diabetes, the symptoms above are followed by increasing mental confusion and rapid, deep breathing. The breath takes on a characteristic 'fruity' odour.

Ketoacidosis is an acute life-threatening condition in people with type I diabetes

Ketoacidosis

Ketoacidosis is caused by a build up of the ketoacids β-hydroxybutyrate and acetoacetate in the body, leading to **acidosis** and **ketonuria**. An immediate

consequence is that the patient starts to breathe very rapidly and deeply because the nervous system response attempts to increase blood pH by expelling carbon dioxide.

Ketoacidosis is much more rare in older people with type II diabetes and is more likely to be confined to periods of acute stress, myocardial infarction or infection. In children with controlled type I diabetes ketoacidosis can be precipitated by infection. Ketoacidosis also develops if a patient does not comply with treatment and in newly diagnosed diabetes.

Ketoacidosis is less of a problem in type II diabetes but can occur in certain circumstances

Severe ketoacidosis is life threatening and is a significant cause of death in diabetics. If untreated it disrupts virtually all physiological processes, including heart activity and oxygen transport. The nervous system is depressed and eventually the patient lapses into a coma and dies. About 2% of patients admitted to hospital with a primary diagnosis of ketoacidosis die. In the EURODIAB complications trial (EURODIAM IDDM Complications Study Group, 1994) about 9% of insulin-dependent diabetics had been admitted to hospital for treatment of ketoacidosis in the previous 12 months.

Acidosis: state of abnormal acidity (high hydrogen ion concentration) in extracellular fluid.

Treatment is aimed at rehydration, re-establishment of insulin therapy and correction of the acidosis and depleted potassium. Morbidity and mortality arising from diabetic ketoacidosis are related to the time between onset of the condition and treatment, the age of the patient and presence of sepsis. The complications of ketoacidosis are usually due to the marked dehydration, which promotes blood coagulation and causes myocardial, bowel and brain infarction. The key to reducing complications of ketoacidosis is early detection and prevention by tight glycaemic control.

Hypoglycaemia

In hypoglycaemia blood sugar levels are too low. If allowed to continue the brain is starved of glucose, resulting in coma or even death. The initial symptoms are hunger and light-headedness. These symptoms should prompt the patient to take some glucose. As blood sugar levels drop even further adrenaline is released in an attempt to mobilise body glucose stores. This gives rise to sweating, palpitations and tremor. The condition may arise because insulin doses are too high or, in type II diabetes, with the use of sulphonylurea drugs.

The key to treating hypoglycaemia is to act as soon as the warning signs are noticed – a problem is the rapidly developing confusion which makes patients less able to take appropriate action. Short-acting carbohydrates such as sugar lumps or a can of (non-diet) fizzy drink should be taken. These immediately raise blood sugar, but this should be sustained by consumption of complex carbohydrates such as those present in bread or biscuits.

Hypoglycaemia can cause damage to the brain, producing alterations in behaviour or reduced consciousness. In the older person these symptoms can be misdiagnosed as TIA, stroke or dementia.

▲ **Key points**

Hypoglycaemia

▲ Potential complication arising from insulin administration

▲ Results from too little blood sugar, because of too much insulin or insufficient dietary carbohydrate

▲ Symptoms are hunger, light-headedness, sweating, tremor, confusion

▲ If untreated, leads to loss of consciousness

Chronic complications of diabetes

Long-term complications of diabetes are caused by damage to large and small blood vessels and to peripheral nerves

The chronic complications of diabetes are caused by long-term exposure to glucose, which damages large and small blood vessels and peripheral nerves (Figure 23.4). **Macrovascular disease** arises when large blood vessels are involved (as in CHD, cerebrovascular disease and peripheral vascular disease) and **microvascular disease** comprises disorders of the small blood vessels such as **retinopathy** and **nephropathy**. Separate metabolic processes cause damage to the nerve sheath (**neuropathy**). These chronic complications are all related to the duration of diabetes and the effectiveness of diabetes control. Nephropathy represents the leading cause of premature death in people with type I diabetes, while type II diabetic subjects are most likely to die from macrovascular complications.

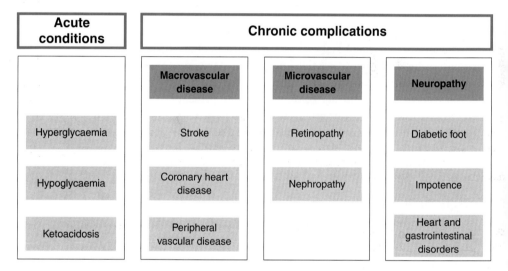

Figure 23.4 Complications of diabetes. Diabetes leads to both acute and chronic complications. The microvascular and macrovascular complications are the principal causes of disability and death in people who have diabetes mellitus.

Long-term metabolic consequences of hyperglycaemia

The long-term toxic effects of excessive glucose in the blood are probably produced by three main pathways. In one pathway (Figure 23.5; see also Figure 23.10) the body's attempts to dispose of glucose by increasing aldose reductase activity cause accumulation of sorbitol and fructose. This causes nerve damage.

In another pathway the non-enzymatic glycosylation of macromolecules leads to altered membrane and matrix proteins (Figure 23.5). These changes probably contribute to cataract and nephropathy.

There is some evidence that excess glucose activates a protein kinase in vascular tissue. Activity of this enzyme influences smooth muscle contractility and responsiveness to cell signalling factors, and also influences the

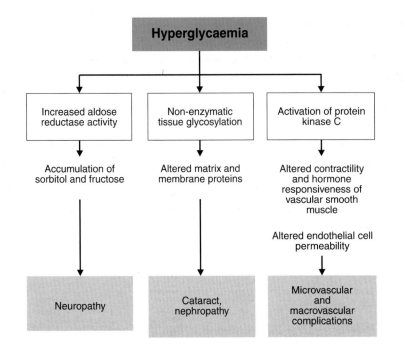

Key points

Macrovascular complications of diabetes

▲ Atherosclerosis in cerebral circulation and carotid arteries causes TIA or stroke
▲ Atherosclerosis in coronary circulation: causes angina or myocardial infarction
▲ Peripheral vascular disease: atherosclerosis in lower limbs causes intermittent claudication, ulceration, gangrene

Figure 23.5 Long-term metabolic effects of hyperglycaemia. Three metabolic pathways are implicated in the long-term tissue damage associated with hyperglycaemia. These are increased aldose reductase activity, protein glycosylation and increased activity of a subform of protein kinase C in vascular smooth muscle and endothelial cells. (Adapted from Porte, D. and Schwartz, M.W. (1996) *Science*, **272**, 699–700.)

Doppler ultrasound: the Doppler effect is a change in sound frequency (pitch) created by a moving object. The flow of blood in the arteries and veins has a similar effect and the sounds are detected by a transducer applied to the skin. Can detect decreased blood flow caused by partial arterial occlusion or by deep-vein thrombosis.

permeability of endothelial cells. These changes may affect the susceptibility of the blood vessels to damage by lipoprotein infiltration and free radicals (Figure 23.5).

Macrovascular disease

Diabetes is a risk factor for the development of atherosclerosis (see Chapter 20). Stroke, CHD and peripheral vascular disease are 2–5 times more common in people who have diabetes than in the general population.

Peripheral vascular disease

Peripheral vascular disease is very often a contributory factor in **diabetic foot** (pain, ulceration, gangrene and infection). These conditions often arise from the combination of vascular disease and neuropathy (see below) in diabetic patients. The presence of peripheral vascular disease is evident as pain in the leg muscles (claudication), the feet are cold and foot pulses are weak or absent. Poor blood supply to the feet often results in a wasted appearance with brittle nails. Doppler ultrasound of the foot can help to assess any reduction in arterial blood flow caused by diabetes-associated atherosclerosis.

The ischaemia results in death of tissue, usually in the distal ends of the

toes. The dead tissues are painless and appear dry and black. This is **dry gangrene**, and may separate from healthy tissue spontaneously. **Wet gangrene** is due to superimposition of infection on tissue ischaemia. Infection by anaerobic organisms results in a foul smell, and requires emergency treatment.

Microvascular disease

Good diabetic control significantly reduces the risk of microvascular disease

Microvascular disease results from diabetic damage to small blood vessels. The mechanism of damage is unclear, although the condition is characterised by a thickening of the capillary basement membrane. This probably involves a number of biochemical mechanisms including glycosylation of basement membrane proteins, damage by excessive generation of free radicals and alterations to platelet and blood clotting functions. The frequency of microvascular complications and neuropathy in Type I diabetes has been examined in the EURODIAB IDDM Complications Study (Stephenson and Fuller, 1994).

Retinopathy

Diabetic retinopathy is a leading cause of blindness

All people who have diabetes are at risk of developing retinopathy. The likelihood of developing the condition increases with the duration of the diabetes (Figure 23.6) but is also influenced by the age at which diabetes is first diagnosed. Retinopathy takes longer to develop in people with type I diabetes. For example, a subject with type I diabetes diagnosed at the age of 10 might develop retinopathy by 30 years of age; a 55-year-old diagnosed with type II diabetes might develop retinopathy by the age of 60. The pathological changes in the eyes develop in two main stages, eventually leading to ischaemia of the retinal cells and blindness.

In most patients an early-stage **background retinopathy** develops, which does not significantly impair vision but which can progress to **maculopathy** or **proliferative retinopathy**. Maculopathy tends to affect the older person with type II diabetes, whereas proliferative retinopathy occurs more commonly in type I. Both conditions are caused by damage to retinal blood vessels and ischaemia of the retina. Unless recognised and treated at an early stage both maculopathy and proliferative retinopathy eventually cause blindness.

Background retinopathy

Background retinopathy can exist for many years before progressing to a proliferative phase

Background retinopathy affects the small blood vessels in the retina. The mechanisms of damage are unclear, but the result is that the small blood vessels have abnormally fragile walls and tend to leak. The leaked fluid can accumulate in the layers of the retina, especially around the macula (causing maculopathy). In some areas the capillaries become closed, causing ischaemia to the retina.

Maculopathy

Blindness is caused by hard exudates or oedema, which directly affect the macula

The accumulation of fluid around the macula and subsequent damage is referred to as maculopathy. Macular oedema initially becomes evident as a deterioration in visual acuity but can cause blindness unless it is detected and

treated early. The walls of the blood vessels in the fluid-filled area become fragile and dilated, forming tiny outward pouches called **microaneurysms**. These are susceptible to haemorrhage. Although usually self-limiting, haemorrhages on the macula can severely impair vision and discrete yellow–white patches may occur in rings around the leaking blood vessels, coalescing to form **hard exudates**. Their presence on the macula causes blindness.

Proliferative retinopathy

The response to ischaemia and retinal damage is proliferation of blood vessels: hence the term proliferative retinopathy (Plate 10). Unfortunately, the new blood vessels are abnormal, have very thin walls, and grow on the surface of the retina rather than underneath it. They have a tendency to bleed. A sudden, major, haemorrhage can fill all the space inside the globe, causing a marked reduction in, or complete loss of, vision. This may clear but will be followed by repeated episodes of bleeding. The region becomes scarred and retinal detachment may occur, leading to total, irreversible blindness.

Macula: site of high-resolution colour vision.

Retina: light-receptive layer at the back of the eye. Photosensitive cells called rods and cones translate light focused on the surface of the retina into nerve impulses.

Retinopathy: damage to the retina, often caused by long-standing diabetes.

New blood vessels bleed, form scars and cause the retina to become detached

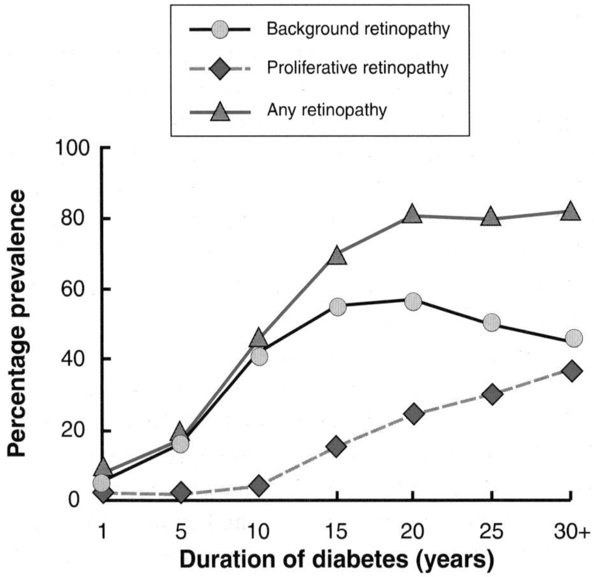

Figure 23.6 Retinopathy in type I diabetes. The likelihood of retinopathy increases with the duration of diabetes. At first the condition is only mild (background retinopathy) but this evolves into the more serious proliferative retinopathy. Any retinopathy is the sum of background and peripheral retinopathy. (Data from EURODIAB IDDM Complications Study, 1994.)

EURODIAB

▲ Cross-sectional study of 3250 type I diabetics in 26 European centres

▲ Stratified random sample of patients aged 15–60 years who attended a diabetes clinic

▲ Mean duration of diabetes 14.7 years

▲ Glycosylated haemoglobin levels normal in 16% of patients

▲ Urinary albumin excretion raised in 30.6% of patients

▲ Prevalence of retinopathy 46%

▲ Postural hypotension seen in 5.9%

▲ Abnormally variable heart rate in 20%

▲ Severe hypoglycaemia during past 12 months 32.2%

▲ 8.6% admitted to hospital for ketoacidosis in previous 12 months

▲ Microvascular and acute complications related to duration of diabetes and glycaemic control

Treatment of retinopathy

Background retinopathy does not require treatment but should be monitored closely so that progression to maculopathy or proliferative retinopathy can be treated by laser photocoagulation, which aims to abolish the proliferated new

Cataract: cloudiness and thickening of the lens of the eye. Occurs with advancing age, infection, trauma and diabetes.

Laser photocoagulation: use of a thermal laser to cause heat coagulation of tissues. The laser beam is focused onto the retina through a contact lens. Laser-induced burns are used to block off the proliferating blood vessels. This stops further leakage. Vision may not be improved, but disease progression is stopped and blindness prevented.

> *Cataracts are the most common eye problem in people with diabetes*

> *Nephropathy is the most significant cause of deaths in people with diabetes*

Glomerular filtration rate: a measure of kidney function. Can be accurately measured by clearance of a substance that is solely excreted by the kidney and is not reabsorbed by the kidney tubules. These criteria are met by endogenous creatinine. The creatinine clearance test measures blood and urine creatinine levels over a 12- or 24-hour period.

Microalbuminuria: urinary excretion of albumin above the normal, but below the level associated with clinical nephropathy. There are a variety of laboratory and test-strip methods for detecting microalbuminuria but measurements should be made on pooled or repeat samples since there is substantial diurnal variation in the excretion of albumin.

Myopia: short-sightedness. A refractive error of the lens, causing objects to be focused in front of the retina, rather than on it.

blood vessels. Damage to the retina is not treatable.

Screening for retinopathy

The aim of screening for retinopathy is to detect changes early so that laser treatment can be given before permanent visual impairment occurs. Screening should be performed annually and if a diabetic woman becomes pregnant (progression of retinopathy can be very rapid during pregnancy). Patients identified as having preproliferative background retinopathy with early maculopathy should be referred to an eye clinic and monitored every 6 months.

Cataract

Cataracts result from the glycosylation of lens proteins. Age-related cataracts occur even in the absence of diabetes, but appear earlier in people who have the disease (Chapter 9). Cataracts often cause gradual deterioration in vision and increasing myopia, although occasionally vision is disturbed little.

Nephropathy

Clinical nephropathy develops in about 30% of patients with type I diabetes and is related to the duration of the diabetes (Figure 23.7). Although it does not affect such a high *proportion* of patients with type II disease, the actual *numbers* of people affected are greater because this type of diabetes is more common. The onset of nephropathy is typically within 10–20 years of the initial diagnosis, affecting people with type I diabetes before the age of 40; patients with type II disease usually develop symptoms after the age of 60. The time to onset of nephropathy often appears shorter in patients with type II disease, because the diabetes itself is often recognised late. Treatment of hypertension and good glycaemic control slows the progression of kidney disease.

The early stage of the disease is characterised by kidney enlargement, a high glomerular filtration rate and **microalbuminuria**. Many people with diabetes exhibit these early signs, but not all go on to develop overt nephropathy.

Later stages are characterised by **macroproteinuria**, a lowered glomerular filtration rate and raised serum creatinine levels. Once patients reach this stage progression to renal failure is inevitable, if cardiovascular disease does not intervene first. The progression of microalbuminuria is closely associated with increased blood pressure and inadequacy of blood glucose control. The transition from early nephropathy to overt disease may be slowed or sometimes stopped by use of antihypertensive drugs, particularly the ACE inhibitors. In patients with overt nephropathy the decline in renal function can be slowed, but not reversed, by this form of treatment.

Patients who progress to renal failure will require peritoneal dialysis or transplantation.

The advantage of peritoneal dialysis for the diabetic patient is that insulin can be administered with the dialysis fluid, thereby obviating the need for injections. Patients are unsuitable for peritoneal dialysis if they have an

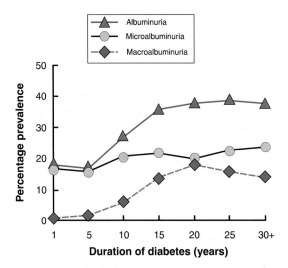

Figure 23.7 Albuminuria in type I diabetes. The prevalence of albuminuria is related to the duration of diabetes. The condition first becomes evident by the presence of very small amounts of albumin in the urine, but the condition can evolve into the more ominous macroalbuminuria, which often ends in renal failure. Albuminuria is the sum of microalbuminuria and macroalbuminuria. (Data from the EURODIAB IDDM Complications Study, 1994.)

> **▲ Key points**
>
> **Diabetic nephropathy**
>
> ▲ Initial kidney enlargement, increased glomerular filtration rate, microalbuminuria
> ▲ Can lead to overt nephropathy and albuminuria
> ▲ Progression can be slowed by good glycaemic control and control of hypertension with ACE inhibitors
> ▲ Renal failure treated by peritoneal dialysis or kidney transplant

Creatinine: a breakdown product of muscle creatine and creatine phosphate. Normally present in blood and urine, the amount produced is proportional to muscle mass. Loss of kidney function causes increase in blood creatinine levels.

Macroproteinuria: excess of protein in urine caused by damage to glomerular filter. Screened by reagent strip (dipstick) analysis of random urine sample. Positive results should be followed by a 24-hour urine sample. Normal amount of protein in urine is below 0.2 g in 24 hours.

Peritoneal dialysis: removal of urea, creatinine, potassium and other dangerous metabolites from the blood. Requires fitting, under general anaesthesia, of a pliable plastic cannula into the peritoneal cavity. The cannula is used to infuse sterile electrolyte solution into the peritoneal cavity. Blood metabolites diffuse from the capillaries through the peritoneal membrane into the electrolyte solution by osmosis. The fluid must be repeatedly changed. Can be self-administered.

abdominal fistula, stoma or drain. Diabetics are not excluded from the kidney transplant programme in the UK, but the availability of donor organs is a problem.

Much can be done to minimise the risk of renal complications, and part of the St Vincent declaration includes recommendations for the screening, monitoring and treatment of microalbuminuria. All patients with type I diabetes over the age of 12 years who have been diagnosed for at least 5 years should be screened annually for albumin in their urine and patients with type II diabetes should be tested annually from the time of diagnosis. Because of the association of microalbuminuria with other microvascular and macrovascular complications it is also recommended that patients are regularly checked for glycosylated haemoglobin (see below), blood pressure, serum lipids and serum creatinine.

Neuropathy

Neuropathy arises in the diabetic patient because of degeneration of the axons and nerve demyelination. The neuropathy may be of only one nerve (for example, neuropathy of the sixth or third cranial nerves causes palsy of the eyelid) or may extend to a generalised symmetrical involvement of peripheral nerves.

Most people who have had diabetes for longer than 5 years will have some evidence of neuropathy. The most common form is **chronic sensory neuropathy**. People with this form of neuropathy usually complain of numbness or a prickling or tingling sensation in the toes or feet. Eventually sensation in

Neuropathy is the most common long-term complication of diabetes

Charcot joints, neuropathic arthropathy: joints damaged by trauma, arising from loss of protective pain sensation.

Schwann cell: Component of peripheral nerves responsible for formation of the myelin protective sheath.

Vasa nervosum: blood vessels supplying the nerves.

the feet is lost, leading to the complications of foot ulceration, gangrene and Charcot joints. These complications are most common in older patients with type II diabetes, but can be found at any age and with any type of diabetes. The condition may be extremely painful, and is one of the most disabling complications of diabetes. Neuropathy can also occur as **autonomic neuropathy,** typically affecting nerves of the bladder, sexual organs, heart and gastrointestinal tract. A rare disorder is **acute neuropathy,** giving rise to shooting or burning pains in the feet and legs, typically worse at night. It is usually reversible in 3–12 months with good glycaemic control.

The nerve damage was believed to be primarily caused by occlusion of the vasa nervosum, and for this reason diabetic neuropathy is often classified as a microvascular disease. This may be the case for isolated nerve lesions but the more diffuse and symmetrical nature of some common forms suggests a metabolic cause.

The nerve damage (degeneration of the axons and a loss of myelin) is now thought to be initiated by high local concentrations of sorbitol and fructose. Many cells, including Schwann cells, contain the enzyme aldose reductase, which, in conditions of high blood glucose, converts glucose to sorbitol. This is in turn converted to fructose. These sugars cause structural and functional damage to the nerve, impairing the conduction of nerve impulses (Figure 23.8).

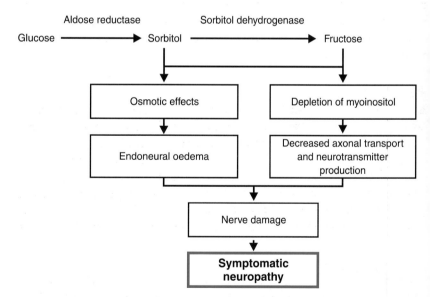

Figure 23.8 Metabolic nerve damage in diabetes. When the normal physiological pathways of glucose are saturated there is an increase in tissue glycosylation and disposal by the sorbitol pathway. The accumulation of sorbitol has an osmotic effect which could injure nerves. Accumulation of fructose and sorbitol is accompanied by depletion of myoinositol, a component of membrane phospholipids involved in neurotransmitter synthesis and nerve conduction. Symptomatic neuropathy arises from the combination of nerve damage and disruption to nerve conduction.

Foot problems

Diabetic foot can be caused by neuropathy or peripheral vascular disease. The neuropathic foot is usually painless, warm to the touch and has easily felt pulses. Problems are caused by the lack of sensation in the foot; ulcers can be produced by ill-fitting footwear without the patient realising what is happening (Plate 11). Regular examination and proper attention to foot care are essential. The patient must be advised on the most appropriate footwear and should regularly visit a chiropodist. Once ulceration has occurred the area becomes susceptible to infection and early antibiotic intervention is essential. The combination of ischaemia, infection and neuropathy can cause extensive damage to the tissues, which then become gangrenous. Amputation of the foot may be necessary.

> *Over 50% of non-traumatic amputations performed in the UK are to treat diabetic foot problems*

Autonomic nervous system

Involvement of the autonomic nervous system in diabetes is very often asymptomatic, and is detected by tests of autonomic function (for example, measurement of heart rate responses to deep breathing, sitting and standing, and pupillary reflex). However, autonomic system neuropathy can be the cause of death because loss of functional nerves in the heart initially causes postural hypotension, tachycardia and painless ischaemia or infarction; the absence of pain means that the heart condition is unrecognised and untreated. One of the most common autonomic neuropathies occurs in the nerves of the stomach and gut. This causes diarrhoea and constipation, present in up to 25% of people with diabetes (Figure 23.9).

Postural hypotension: normally blood pressure rises as a person stands up because of the increase in venous return as the veins are constricted. Postural hypotension is a common cause of dizziness and falls in older people. A decrease in systolic blood pressure of 30 mmHg or more is strongly suggestive of autonomic neuropathy.

Pupillary reflex: response of the pupils to light.

Tachycardia: rapid heart rate, caused by anxiety, stress, infection, thyroid disease and diabetic neuropathy.

Erectile impotence

Impotence affects up to 30% of men with diabetes, usually in combination with other features of neuropathy or peripheral vascular disease. Libido is usually preserved, but morning erections or erections with a full bladder are not possible. In common with erectile impotence in non-diabetic men, psychogenic problems may also be a cause. Some treatments may help to produce and maintain erection: use of a vacuum-forming pump to produce an erection (a tight rubber band is then placed around the base of the penis to maintain the erection), papaverine injection or a surgically inserted prosthesis.

Urinary retention

Involvement of the autonomic nervous system in diabetes can cause **neurogenic bladder**, a symptom of which is bladder paralysis, caused by a loss of the normal ability of the nerves to respond to pressure as the bladder fills. This causes **urinary retention**, which predisposes for urinary tract infections. The initial presentation is a painless swelling of the lower abdomen.

Treatment of neuropathy

There is no specific treatment for diabetic neuropathy, although many of the symptoms can be controlled. The main priority is to control the diabetes. The

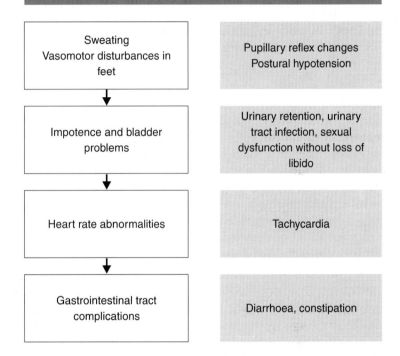

Figure 23.9 Effect of long-standing diabetes on the autonomic nervous system. Diabetic neuropathy of autonomic nerves is first noticeable as sweating during and after meals. Asymptomatic nerve involvement can be assessed by measuring blood pressure and resting pupillary reflexes. The condition progresses by involvement of nerves supplying the bladder, sexual organs, heart and gastrointestinal tract.

painful acute neuropathy often disappears over several months, but more chronic forms that develop later in the course of the disease can be resistant to all forms of therapy. Pain relief is another goal of treatment but because neuropathy can persist for months the addictive narcotics should be avoided. People with painful neuropathy often suffer from depression, anxiety and insomnia. The depression passes as the neuropathy subsides, but some people may need antidepressants.

Infections

People whose diabetes is well controlled are no more at risk of infection than

the general population. However, poorly controlled diabetes is associated with infections, usually of the skin, urinary tract and lungs. The activity of inflammatory cells that would normally control infection is impaired at high blood glucose levels. Staphylococcal, streptococcal and candidal infections are common. Staphylococcal infections cause boils, abscesses and carbuncles. Streptococcal infection often arises from cracks in the skin and is seen as cellulitis – a hot, painful, shiny red lesion which causes swelling of the local lymph glands. *Candida* usually infects the skin folds, typically in the toe webs, groin and genitals.

Infection can cause loss of glycaemic control. For the duration of the infection patients with type I diabetes may need to increase their insulin dose, while non-insulin-dependent patients might need insulin injections.

Skin and joints

Changes occur in the skin and joints of diabetic subjects, probably due to vascular changes and the glycosylation of structural connective tissue proteins. These changes can lead to joint contraction, causing stiffness and slight swelling of the hands.

Diabetes in pregnancy

At one time about 50% of pregnancies in diabetic women ended in death of the fetus. The situation in developed countries has been transformed by improved diabetic, obstetric and paediatric care, and the chances of delivering a normal healthy baby are similar to those of non-diabetic mothers. Optimal glycaemic control during pregnancy is vitally important and, in a planned pregnancy, should be commenced before conception. The aim is to achieve blood glucose or HbA$_1$ levels (see below) within the normal range. To help achieve this the patient should perform daily home blood glucose tests. The dose of insulin required usually increases substantially during pregnancy.

Poor glycaemic control in the first trimester is associated with increased risk of congenital malformations, usually of the cardiovascular and nervous systems. An ultrasound scan should be performed early in pregnancy to establish the exact gestational age and to detect any major fetal abnormalities.

The aim is for the baby to be born by normal vaginal delivery at term. Insulin and glucose are given by intravenous infusion during delivery, maintaining blood glucose levels at 3–6 mmol/l. After delivery, when the mother wants to take food, the pre-pregnancy insulin injection regime is restarted.

Diagnosis

The early stages of both type I and type II diabetes are asymptomatic. Blood glucose values have been specified by the WHO for the fasting state and 2 hours after ingestion of a standard glucose load in an oral glucose tolerance

---

Review question 1

Mr D (67 years old) is obese, has led a sedentary lifestyle for many years, has a family history of diabetes and was diagnosed as having type II diabetes when he was 60. His condition can be controlled by diet, although he does not strictly adhere to the recommended diet. He experienced a tingling sensation in his right foot for 2–3 months, but the foot has now become painful. The other foot has felt slightly numb.

- What is the explanation for these symptoms?
- How might the original diagnosis of diabetes have been made?
- What investigations would now be useful?
- What can be done about his condition?

The diagnosis of diabetes is based on determination of blood glucose concentration

Glycosylated haemoglobin (HbA₁): a stable complex of haemoglobin and glucose. Once formed, the complex lasts the entire life of the red cell (about 120 days). Measurement gives an indication of the effectiveness of glycaemic control over the previous month or two.

> *Estimation of glycosylated haemoglobin is used to monitor diabetic patients*

> *It is important to control hypertension and obesity as well as hyperglycaemia in people who have diabetes*

> *The principle of control in type I diabetes is to regulate blood glucose by balancing diet, exercise and insulin*

Oral glucose tolerance test: can be used to confirm diabetes mellitus in a person who has elevated blood glucose levels in random samples. The peak glucose level is achieved 30–60 minutes after ingestion of 75 g glucose. The blood sugar should return to fasting levels in 3 hours. The test is performed in the morning after an overnight fast.

test. The glucose tolerance test is not routinely used in practice and patients with symptoms are classified as diabetic if they have a random venous plasma glucose level higher than 11 mmol/l, or a fasting value of 7.8 mmol/l or more.

Blood glucose estimations can initially be performed with test strips, but confirmation should always be undertaken by a dedicated biochemistry laboratory.

Glycosuria (the presence of glucose in urine) can be checked by sensitive glucose-specific dipstick methods. The condition is not specific for diabetes, but indicates the need for further investigation.

A further consequence of diabetes is the **glycosylation of haemoglobin**. The measurement of glycosylated haemoglobin (also known as haemoglobin A_1 or HBA₁) indicates how effective the glycaemic control was in the previous 2 or 3 months. Measurement of HBA₁ is not intended as a diagnostic test but serves a monitoring purpose – levels can reach 20% of total haemoglobin in poorly controlled diabetic subjects, compared with 3–5% in people without diabetes.

Treatment

The aim of treatment is to maintain blood glucose levels within the normal range; **normoglycaemia** (Figure 23.10). This will relieve the acute symptoms of diabetes, and in the longer term should minimise the impact of microvascular and macrovascular complications. Normoglycaemia is usually unattainable, and treatments are optimised for each individual. The cornerstone of therapy is diet; alone or in combination with oral hypoglycaemic agents or insulin. Changes in exercise and smoking habits are advisable to reduce hypertension and hyperlipidaemia and hence the risk of long-term complications.

Type I diabetes

All patients with type I diabetes require insulin to control their hyperglycaemia. People with type II diabetes that does not respond to dietary control or treatment with hypoglycaemic agents may also need insulin. A number of insulin preparations are now available, purified from the pancreatic extracts of animals (porcine and bovine insulin), or prepared using recombinant DNA technology (human insulin).

The absorption characteristics of insulin can be modified either by increasing the particle size (crystals rather than amorphous) or by complexing the insulin with zinc or protamine. **Neutral,** or **soluble** insulin is very quick acting and has the shortest duration of effect. It must be injected subcutaneously 20 minutes before a meal. **Isophane** insulin is a complex of insulin with salmon or trout protamine. This has a slower onset of action, and can usually be injected subcutaneously twice daily, although patients vary in their responses. Various 'cocktail' preparations of neutral and isophane insulins allow optimal tailoring of the insulin to the patient's response. **Lente** and **ultralente** insulins are

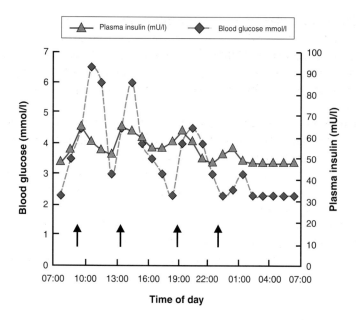

Figure 23.10 Normal blood glucose and insulin levels. In people without diabetes blood glucose levels are maintained within the range 2.5–7.5 mmol/l, regardless of how much is consumed. Insulin is secreted continually and increases in response to food intake. Arrows indicate meals taken.

prepared from amorphous or crystalline insulin and zinc. These preparations have the slowest onset of action.

Most people with type I diabetes inject their insulin subcutaneously using a syringe and vial system. Pen injection systems are becoming more popular and offer greater convenience and acceptability. They are more appropriate for older people who have poor eyesight or problems with manual dexterity, and help to promote greater dosage accuracy in children and teenagers.

Insulin is normally injected into the thigh, abdominal wall, upper arm or buttock. The injection site should be varied to prevent thickening of the subcutaneous tissues, which can cause impaired and erratic absorption. Insulin infusion pumps may be used to provide a continuous supply of insulin subcutaneously but these are rarely used in the UK. The management of ketoacidosis may require intravenous administration of insulin, but this route is not normally used for long-term control of hyperglycaemia.

Patients can usually manage their diabetes with twice-daily insulin injections. Those with type II diabetes retain some capacity to manufacture their own insulin and can be maintained using one of the slow-acting preparations once daily if they need insulin. The usual regime is to inject 20 minutes before breakfast and 20 minutes before the evening meal. The type of insulin used can be chosen to compensate for differences in activity levels during the day and night. Short-acting insulins, used in multiple injection regimes, are suitable for control during the day. A medium or long-term preparation is administered at bedtime. The doses used are derived empirically,

Bovine (cow) insulin: more slowly absorbed following subcutaneous injection and has a longer duration of action than other insulin types. Differs from human insulin by three amino acids.

Human insulin: produced by recombinant DNA technology using *E. coli*. Does not have substantial benefits over porcine insulin. It is still slightly antigenic, probably because of minor chemical changes during purification and storage.

Insulin infusion pump, continuous subcutaneous insulin infusion: a battery-operated pump provides a continuous basal supply of insulin with boosts before meals. The pump is worn on a belt or in a pocket. Insulin is delivered via a long plastic tube to a needle placed in the skin of the thigh or abdomen. The needle and tubing are usually replaced every 3–4 days. Provides very tight control of blood glucose levels.

Porcine (pig) insulin: structurally more similar to human insulin and less likely to cause an antibody reaction. Differs from human insulin by one amino acid. Porcine insulin can be chemically modified so that it is structurally identical to human insulin.

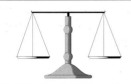

taking into account the person's age, weight and daily routine and the need to avoid hyperglycaemia and hypoglycaemia.

Complete normoglycaemia is not attainable with the use of insulin, probably because of the variability in absorption, the imperfections of the various insulins and the route of administration (into the systemic circulation rather than into the portal circulation that occurs naturally). Self-monitoring of blood glucose levels is an important part of management, and regular screening of blood and urine gives information on other prognostic factors (see below). A further important aspect in control is patient compliance with diet and other lifestyle risk factors.

The stabilisation of blood glucose levels in diabetes involves the establishment of a routine. By forward planning, account can be made for large changes, for example, increasing the insulin dose to allow for a larger meal or decreasing the dose before physical activity.

The Diabetes Control and Complications Trial (1993) has demonstrated that careful control of blood glucose levels can substantially reduce the risk of microvascular complications in patients with type I diabetes. In this trial patients without, or with only mild, retinopathy were randomised either to continue conventional insulin treatment (one or two insulin injections daily) or to intensive treatment aimed at achieving normoglycaemia using an external insulin pump or three or more insulin injections daily. The mean age of the patients at the outset of the trial was 27 years, and the follow-up period was 6.5 years.

In the patients who received intensive insulin therapy there were impressive gains in delaying the onset or slowing the progression of diabetic retinopathy, nephropathy and neuropathy. There were also indications that the risk of macrovascular complications could be reduced, as demonstrated by reduced hypercholesterolaemia in the group receiving intensive therapy. Because of the young age of the patients it is too soon to say whether this will translate into reductions in the incidence of macrovascular disease or in survival benefit. There are also doubts whether the compliance necessary to achieve such tight glycaemic control will be consistently maintained by most patients.

Type II diabetes

Although the DCCT trial was confined to patients with type I diabetes, there is no reason to suppose that the improvement in prospects for patients with good glycaemic control should be any different for those with type II disease. A clinical trial in type II diabetes (UK Prospective Diabetes Study Group, 1991) is currently under way. Until the results are known, prudence and common sense would dictate that good compliance with dietary control and other forms of treatment should lead to a healthier and longer life.

Dietary control
The aims of dietary control are to reduce hyperglycaemia and correct obesity. Obesity is the major obstacle to successful treatment, particularly as about

75% of newly diagnosed patients are obese. Obesity increases insulin resistance. Weight loss can improve blood glucose and lipid levels and reduce blood pressure. The most effective means of losing weight is to reduce the intake of fatty foods: metabolism of fat favours triglyceride deposition in adipose tissue and therefore obesity.

Regular physical exercise can improve sensitivity to insulin and reduce blood glucose levels. It may also improve blood pressure and blood lipid profiles to reduce not only the impact of type II diabetes but also that of obesity and the likelihood of subsequent macrovascular complications. Patients should be evaluated for cardiovascular and microvascular (neuropathy, diabetic foot, proliferative retinopathy) disease before undertaking any exercise programme. Daily exercise of 30 minutes brisk walking is recommended.

The current recommendations are to take a high proportion of complex carbohydrate (55–60% of total calories). This is most effectively achieved by replacing high-fat foods with complex carbohydrates that have a low glycaemic index: this usually means starchy foods and cereals such as pasta and rice.

> *The cornerstone of treatment in type II diabetes is dietary control*

Hypoglycaemic agents

Dietary control undoubtedly works for some patients, and those that respond have an improved life expectancy. However, many people have difficulty in permanently changing their diet and drugs are available for patients in whom dietary measures have failed to control the disease by stimulating the pancreatic production of insulin. The most widely used drugs are **sulphonylureas** (glibenclamide, gliclazide, glipizide), and the **biguanide** drug metformin. Also available are the α-**glucosidase inhibitor** acarbose, and the thiazolidinedione drug troglitazone.

> *Drug therapy should be used only when dietary control fails*

Sulphonylureas

The sulphonylureas work by increasing the sensitivity of the pancreatic β-cells to glucose, so that more insulin is released. This is accompanied by an increase in tissue sensitivity to insulin. The main difference between the different sulphonylureas is their duration of action. Side-effects (including nausea, vomiting and skin rash) are usually only mild and disappear when the patient stops taking the drugs. However, a serious side-effect is hypoglycaemia. This is more likely to occur with a long-acting agent in older patients who have inadequate carbohydrate intake and kidney or liver dysfunction (these organs are the routes of drug elimination). Some patients experience weight gain, rendering the drugs inappropriate for use, particularly if he or she is already obese.

Metformin

The mechanism of action of metformin is poorly understood but its effect is to lower blood glucose, probably by inhibiting intestinal glucose absorption and production of glucose by the liver. The drug does not cause hypoglycaemia or weight gain but some patients cannot tolerate it and others experience

▲ **Key points**

Non-pharmacological measures for controlling type II diabetes

▲ Diet – reduce fat consumption, replace fat-derived by carbohydrate-derived calories, complex carbohydrate and dietary fibre to minimise blood glucose surge
▲ Decrease salt intake
▲ Decrease alcohol intake
▲ Take exercise
▲ Reduce weight
▲ Stop smoking

Amylase: hydrolyses polysaccharides to smaller carbohydrate units, including disaccharides.

Maltase: breaks down the disaccharide maltose to glucose.

Sucrase: breaks down sucrose to glucose and fructose.

gastrointestinal disturbances such as anorexia, nausea, diarrhoea and abdominal discomfort. These disturbances can be controlled by reducing the dose.

The use of metformin after failure of dietary control usually results in a fall of 2–3 mmol/l in fasting and postprandial blood glucose levels. The drug is effective in both obese and non-obese patients. The contraindications are pregnancy and renal impairment, even if only mild.

Acarbose

The α-glucosidase inhibitor acarbose inhibits the intestinal enzymes amylase, sucrase and maltase, reducing the gastrointestinal absorption of glucose. Many patients cannot tolerate the side-effects of flatulence, diarrhoea and abdominal pain.

Thiazolidinediones

A new group of drugs, the thiazolidinediones, reduces insulin resistance and allows more glucose to be taken up from the blood into the peripheral tissues. One of these drugs, troglitazone, has been shown to reduce both blood glucose and insulin levels in patients with type II diabetes. It may also prevent the development of type II diabetes in obese adults by reducing blood glucose and insulin levels.

Insulin

Up to 30% of patients with type II diabetes do not respond well to oral hypoglycaemic agents. These patients are described as 'secondary failures' and need treatment with insulin. Often patients are very unwilling to start insulin treatment but the result is often a considerable improvement in well-being.

Prevention of long-term complications of diabetes

The risk of long-term complications is minimised by tight glycaemic control and proper attention to lifestyle risk factors such as diet, smoking and alcohol consumption (Figure 23.11). Although these measures undoubtedly extend life expectancy the microvascular and macrovascular complications are still responsible for most premature deaths in people with diabetes. New drug therapies in clinical trials may help prevent long-term complications such as neuropathy.

One such approach is to use aldose reductase inhibitors to inhibit the production of the sorbitol and fructose that are probably significant factors in nerve damage. A further approach using aminoguanidine has been shown in animal studies to reduce protein glycosylation, which again leads to tissue damage. Much of the damage of neuropathy is mediated by the body's immune system and inflammatory reactions. There could, therefore, be some scope for limiting the damage by inhibiting various mediators of inflammation. It may also be possible to stimulate nerve regeneration by use of nerve growth factors.

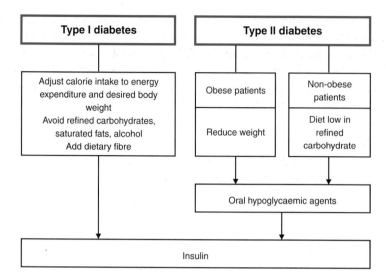

Figure 23.11 Control of diabetes. The control of type I diabetes is based on achieving a balance between energy intake (diet), energy expenditure (exercise) and insulin. The control of type II diabetes is based on dietary control and, if necessary, weight reduction. Medical treatments are available for patients in whom dietary control fails. Oral hypoglycaemic agents are usually adequate, although insulin control can also be used.

Monitoring of diabetes

The control and monitoring of diabetic patients can be tailored to meet individual needs and expectations. For example, the older patient with type II diabetes and co-existent severe disease such as malignancy or heart failure may be more comfortably managed with a once-daily insulin injection before breakfast, rather than strict diet. The aim of treatment in this case is to avoid the symptoms such as tiredness, weight loss and polyuria which affect the person's daily quality of life. Monitoring for glycosuria by urine tests will probably suffice. In contrast, a younger person with type I diabetes who is in good health would be advised to aim for more precise control by injection at least twice daily in order to delay or avoid later complications.

Monitoring takes two forms: self-monitoring by the patient and periodic (usually annual) medical surveillance. The insulin-dependent patient may initially monitor their own glucose levels daily using skinprick blood. Blood monitoring can be reduced to several times a week once the insulin regimen is established. Annual checks at a diabetes clinic include measurement of blood HBA_1 and total cholesterol. A full lipid screen should be undertaken if previous levels were abnormal. Urine creatinine and, ideally, urine microalbumin should also be checked. The injection sites, eyes, legs and feet should also be examined, together with blood pressure and cardiological and neurological function.

An important aspect of diabetes control is patient education, because patients will need to take responsibility for their treatment. Some diabetes centres incorporate a knowledge checklist at the annual appointment. Patients should

be asked about current medication and frequency of monitoring and the importance of foot care and attention to other risk factors such as smoking and alcohol consumption emphasised.

ANSWERS TO REVIEW QUESTIONS

Question 1

What is the explanation for Mr D's symptoms? The most probable explanation is symmetrical diabetic neuropathy, caused by nerve damage and possibly worsened by peripheral vascular disease.

How might the original diagnosis of diabetes have been made? Mr D could well have been asymptomatic at the time of the original diagnosis and initially investigated for diabetes because of his age, his obesity and sedentary lifestyle and his family history of diabetes. Screening can be done simply by taking capillary (fingerprick) blood and measuring glucose with a test strip. Elevated results on two or more random occasions should be confirmed by laboratory measurement of a fasting venous blood sample. Levels above 7.8 mmol/l are sufficient to confirm a diagnosis of diabetes.

What investigations would now be useful? A thorough examination of the patient, with particular emphasis on the cardiovascular and neurological systems. His eyes and feet should be closely examined, using Doppler ultrasound for the feet.

What can be done about his condition? The most important intervention is proper foot care. The feet can be injured because the patient no longer feels pain there. The feet should be inspected daily for signs of pressure spots or trauma caused by a foreign object in the shoe. A further (and necessary) objective is to reduce weight using a diet adapted to the patient. A dietary history of the times and types of meals should be taken together with details of family, social or religious circumstances. Saturated fats should be replaced by non-saturated fats and complex carbohydrate.

Probably the next logical step is to prescribe an oral hypoglycaemic agent. Exercise should be encouraged, but in view of the patient's current foot problems this should be approached with some care. With proper vigilance, gentle exercise, perhaps swimming, could be undertaken.

References

Diabetes Control and Complications Trial Research Group (1993) The effect of intensive treatment of diabetes on the development and progression of long-term complications in insulin-dependent diabetes mellitus. *N. Engl. J. Med.*, **339**, 977–86.

Stephenson, J. and Fuller, J.H., on behalf of the EURODIAB IDDDM Complications Study Group (1994) Microvascular and acute complications in IDDM patients: The EURODIAB IDDM Complications Study. *Diabetologica*, **37**, 278–85.

UK Prospective Diabetes Study Group (1991) UK Prospective Diabetes Study (UKPDS). VIII. Study design, progress and performance. *Diabetologica*, **34**, 877–90.

World Health Organization Europe and European Region of International Diabetes Federation (1989) *The St Vincent Declaration*, WHO Europe and European Region of IDF, Copenhagen.

Further reading

Atkinson, M.A. and Maclaren, N.K. (1994) The pathogenesis of insulin-dependent diabetes mellitus. *N. Engl. J. Med.*, **331**, 1428–36.

Nathan, D.M. (1993) Long-term complications of diabetes mellitus. *N. Engl. J. Med.*, **328**, 1676–85.

Pickup, J.C. and Williams, G. (eds) (1991) *Textbook of Diabetes*, Blackwell Scientific Publications, Oxford.

Watkins, P.J. (1993) *ABC of Diabetes*, 3rd edn, BMJ Publishing Group, London.

Williams, G. (1994) Management of non-insulin-dependent diabetes mellitus. *Lancet*, **343**, 95–100.

Yki-Jarvinen H. (1994) Pathogenesis of non-insulin-dependent diabetes mellitus. *Lancet*, **343**, 91–95.

24   Asthma

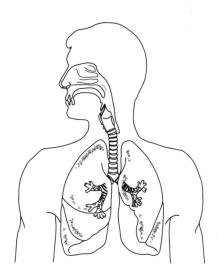

Pre-test

- **Is everybody equally prone to asthma or are particular groups of people more susceptible to the disease?**
- **When is asthma most likely to become apparent?**
- **What causes asthma? Are there any factors in the environment which can initiate the disease?**
- **Is asthma easy to diagnose? What tests might be employed to determine if someone has the condition?**
- **What treatments are available for asthma?**

Asthma is the most common chronic disease that affects both children and adults. The prevalence of the condition has increased, but it is not clear why. A possible reason is changes in living conditions that increase exposures to the house dust mite. Cigarette smoke and poor air quality worsen the symptoms of asthma.

The condition is characterised by reversible airways obstruction causing breathlessness, cough or wheeze. In acute attacks the main reason for airways obstruction is bronchoconstriction, caused by the action of histamine released from mast cells on bronchial smooth muscle. Other significant factors are inflammatory changes in the airways mucosa which stimulate mucus production, epithelial shedding and swelling.

Therapy is based on preventing symptoms by controlling the underlying inflammation and on relieving symptoms. Inflammation can be reduced by corticosteroids (inhaled or oral) and acute symptoms controlled with bronchodilators.

Aims of this chapter

By the end of this chapter you will have increased your knowledge of:

◆ The prevalence of asthma
◆ The role of genetic and environmental factors
◆ The pathological processes involved in asthma
◆ How asthma can be diagnosed and treated

In addition, this chapter will help you to:

◆ Discuss the factors that may have increased the prevalence of asthma
◆ Identify the factors which trigger an asthma attack
◆ Describe how cellular processes influence airway function and responsiveness
◆ Discuss the different roles of bronchodilators and anti-inflammatory agents in asthma therapy

Introduction

Asthma is the most common chronic disease in developed countries and appears to be increasing in prevalence. In the UK about 3 million people have asthma, including more than 750 000 children, and about 2000 people die from the disease each year. Many of these deaths could probably have been prevented had the severity of the condition been recognised.

There is substantial variation in the geographical distribution of asthma: it is virtually unknown among Eskimos and Papuans, but affects half the population of the tiny and isolated South Atlantic island of Tristan da Cunha. This is attributed to the presence of asthma in some of the original settlers. Although not directly inherited, the condition does tend to run in families. Children are more likely to have the condition if their parents are affected. Asthma often appears in association with hay fever (allergic rhinitis) and dermatitis (including eczema): predisposition to this triad of conditions is referred to as **atopy**. An American study conducted in the early 1980s revealed that up to 20% of people have one, or a combination, of these conditions.

Asthma is usually defined on the basis of clinical symptoms and tests of airway function. The classical stereotype of asthma, based on the three concepts of **variable airflow obstruction, bronchial hyperreactivity** and **airways inflammation,** is relatively easy to identify, but it can be difficult to distinguish the disease from other forms of airways obstruction. Airflow obstruction occurs in the small airways and is responsible for recurrent symptoms of breathlessness, cough and wheeze. It is caused by the combination of bronchospasm and mucosal swelling and mucus plugging. Exposure to allergens induces a chronic low-grade inflammation of the airways wall as well as stimulating acute episodes of bronchospasm. The limitation to air flow in asthma is usually reversible, spontaneously or with treatment.

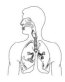

Reversible episodes of airways obstruction, with symptoms of breathlessness, cough or wheeze, are typical of asthma

Asthma is more likely to occur in children whose parents have an allergic disorder

Bronchospasm: smooth muscle contraction of the airway wall, which in asthma is triggered by allergens or irritants.

Epidemiology

Chronic obstructive airways (pulmonary) disease (COAD, COPD): describes conditions in which there are chronic limitations to airflow, caused by narrowing of the airways (chronic bronchitis) or loss of elastic recoil in the lungs (emphysema).

Because of variations in diagnostic criteria many epidemiological surveys are based on a questionnaire design that categorises asthma as wheezy breathlessness. Clearly, this could include a range of other respiratory conditions (viral infections, for example). The prevalence of asthma also follows seasonal variations, and for this reason prevalence data are usually collected over 12 months. Most surveys of school children indicate that the prevalence of wheezing in a 12-month period is 10–15%. Between 30 and 50% of these children have received a clinical diagnosis of asthma. In adults the diagnosis and the prevalence data very much depend on the distinction between asthma and chronic obstructive airways disease (COAD).

Data from the UK suggest that about 30% of adults of 40–70 years suffer chronic respiratory symptoms (cough, phlegm, breathlessness or wheeze). A reversibility of symptoms consistent with asthma is estimated to be present in 4% of men and 3% of women. Successive surveys in children and young adults suggest that the prevalence of asthma and wheezing illnesses has increased, as have the other forms of atopy.

With increasing age many wheezers cease to have symptoms, although adults who had more severe wheezing as children are more likely to continue to have symptoms. There is evidence that underlying physiological and pathological abnormalities persist in some asthmatics even though they may not have had symptoms for some time. The clinical and epidemiological evidence suggests that chronic asthma which persists into or develops during adult life often leads to later chronic obstructive airways disease.

Deaths from asthma are rare in children, accounting for just over 1% of total childhood deaths. Thereafter the risk of death increases exponentially with age (Figure 24.1) although the data for older subjects are less reliable because of possible misclassification with other respiratory diseases. In the UK the current trends in mortality rates are largely reassuring, but there has been a small increase in the number of deaths in young adults.

There is considerable international variation in the mortality rates – for example, in recent years roughly three times as many people die from asthma in New Zealand as in the UK. The trends have also changed with time. During the 1960s an epidemic of asthma deaths in the UK and a number of other countries correlated with increased use of high-dose isoprenaline aerosol inhalers. In New Zealand a further epidemic was seen in the late 1970s (Figure 24.2) which also has been ascribed to the introduction of a new bronchodilator therapy (see below).

Use of health services for asthma

Hospital admissions for asthma, particularly children, have increased markedly over the last 20 years. In the UK between 1979 and 1989 the overall number of hospital admissions for asthma tripled. These trends probably reflect changes in the prevalence and severity of the disease, together with changes in

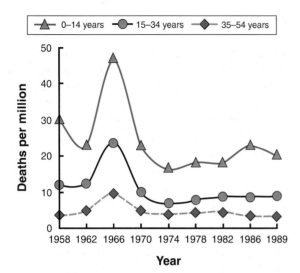

Figure 24.1 Deaths from asthma, England and Wales, 1958–1989. Deaths from asthma increase with the age of the patient. There was a marked increase in deaths from asthma in the 1960s. This has been ascribed to the introduction of high-dose isoprenaline inhalers. The trend since the mid 1970s has been a small increase in deaths in adults. (Adapted from Anderson, H.R. (1992) *Br. J Hosp. Med.*, **47**, 99–104.)

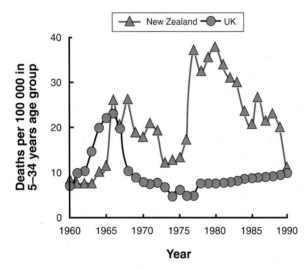

Figure 24.2 There was a substantial increase in the number of asthma deaths during the mid 1960s in both the UK and New Zealand. In New Zealand there was a further peak in the late 1970s. (Data from Rees and Price, 1995.)

management towards more specialised hospital care. The number of general practitioner consultations and prescriptions given for asthma has increased markedly.

Why has the prevalence of asthma increased?

The prevalence of asthma in most developed countries has increased over the last 30 years. This increase has been ascribed to poor air quality. While air pollution from industrial sources and domestic coal-burning has become less severe during this period, the contribution of vehicle emissions to adverse air quality has been unrelenting.

However, the evidence is conflicting. Observations that asthma (and atopy) is usually more common in urban areas support the argument that pollution has caused the increase but the increase in asthma has occurred at a time when general atmospheric pollution has fallen. The number of cases has increased in Fiji and northern Chile, where pollution is not a problem; the prevalence is lower in Leipzig, which has relatively high levels of air pollution, than in Munich, where air pollution is not such a problem; similarly, the prevalence of childhood asthma is very low in Papua New Guinea, despite very high levels of particulate air pollution.

In the domestic environment the use of aerosol sprays, such as air-fresheners, deodorants, hairsprays and polish, which could contain trigger agents for asthma, has increased. Warmer, better insulated living conditions could increase exposure to house dust mites and pet fur. It is difficult to see how exposure to other environmental agents, such as pollens, could have changed over time, unless related to specific crops.

High doses of β_2 adrenoceptor agonists are an important risk factor for death from asthma

Paradoxically, some of the drugs used to treat asthma have been blamed for contributing to an increase in the number of deaths from the disease. One class of drugs, the β_2 adrenoceptor agonists, is used to open up the airways during an asthma attack. These are being given in larger and more frequent doses. Over the years the types of bronchodilators available have changed. The increase in deaths from asthma which occurred in the 1960s was ascribed to a new high-dose preparation of isoprenaline, a relatively non-selective β_1 and β_2 adrenoceptor agonist. Deaths in the UK fell when the over-the-counter preparation was withdrawn. A second epidemic in New Zealand in the late 1970s followed the introduction of fenoterol. This drug rapidly achieved a high market share and was again marketed as a high-dose preparation. This epidemic also improved once the drug was withdrawn.

In the UK the use of bronchodilators has doubled in the past 10 years but the increase in deaths from asthma has been very much smaller. Other countries have experienced substantial increases in the prevalence of asthma, but these increases do not correlate with the introduction of new bronchodilators. No other causes have been positively identified.

Bronchodilators might cause adverse effects in a number of ways:

- Because they dilate (widen) the airways, the overall exposure to allergens might actually be increased
- The drugs might make the mucus produced by the lungs more sticky
- It is possible that the drugs become less effective over time, or interfere with corticosteroids, which are commonly prescribed at the same time to deal with inflammation. Alternatively, bronchodilators might simply mask

the need for anti-inflammatory treatment

- At high doses some β_2 adrenoceptor agonists lose their selectivity for β_2 receptors in the airways smooth muscle and will bind to β_1 receptors elsewhere. This can cause an increase in heart rate and tremor. Although serious dysrhythmias in younger people are extremely uncommon there will be many older asthma patients who have heart conditions or who take other drugs which might predispose them to dysrhythmias. It is therefore feasible that high dose bronchodilators could contribute to a small number of deaths from heart conditions. This still does not explain the increased number of deaths in New Zealand, which were mostly in young people.

Do β_2 adrenoceptor agonists cause, rather than prevent, some asthma deaths?

Point	Counterpoint
An epidemic of deaths from asthma in the 1960s in the UK and other countries corresponds to the availability of high-dose isoprenaline	Asthma epidemics were seen before the widespread use of inhaled β_2 agonists. Some countries escaped the epidemic of deaths from asthma despite the availability of inhaled β_2 agonists
An epidemic of deaths from asthma was seen in New Zealand after the introduction of fenoterol	The deaths in New Zealand were also associated with other drugs (theophylline and prednisolone)
Tolerance to β_2 agonists causes a deterioration in asthma, which leads to increasing size and frequency of doses	Most studies show no worsening effect on asthma control. There is no plausible explanation why β_2 agonists should worsen asthma
An incidence of serious adverse effects in one in 8000 patients taking β_2 agonists would account for nearly half of all deaths from asthma in the UK	Use of β_2 agonists in large doses is more common in patients with more severe disease, who are more likely to die anyway

(Tattersfield, A.E. (1994) *BMJ*, 309, 794–5)

(Fuller, R.W. (1994) *BMJ*, 309, 795–6)

Author's view

The β_2 adrenoceptor agonists effectively control symptoms in the vast majority of asthma sufferers. Sustained use in high doses is an important risk factor for death from asthma. Over-reliance on these drugs is therefore unwise and it is more appropriate to reserve their use for relief of an asthma attack. The β_2 adrenoceptor agonists treat the symptoms rather than the

cause of the disease, and there is now a move towards use of steroid inhalers with the aim of controlling the underlying inflammation. Poor asthma control should not be managed by simply increasing the dose or frequency of β_2 agonists.

Causes and trigger factors in asthma

The main cause of asthma is probably an allergy to the house dust mite, but symptoms can be triggered by other factors

The symptoms of asthma are caused by aberrant responses of cells in the airways wall to external agents. The condition is initiated by an **allergen** which stimulates IgE production and a cascade of inflammatory and other responses (see below) to produce chronic inflammation in the walls of the airways. The principal cause of asthma is sensitisation to the house dust mite.

An asthma attack (with airways obstruction) can be induced by a variety of **trigger factors**. These include further exposure to the original allergen(s), exposure to respiratory tract irritants such as sulphur dioxide, infections, or exposure to certain drugs or chemicals encountered occupationally. Trigger factors are usually obvious in children but can be more difficult to identify in adults.

House dust mites

Among the most common trigger factors are allergens associated with the house dust mite *Dermatophagoides pteronyssinus*. The mite lives on human skin scales and other detritus in the domestic environment and is almost universally present in bedding, carpets and soft furnishings. Skin tests (see below) show that most asthmatic children are sensitive to the house dust mite. Two antigens appear to be involved: one derived from proteolytic enzymes secreted from the digestive tract and found in faecal pellets (called Der p1), and the other found in the faecal pellets and bodies of the mites.

Epidemiological studies correlate the frequency of asthma with the prevalence of house dust mites. Some parts of the world are inhospitable to mites because of a cold climate or high altitude, and asthma is uncommon. The symptoms usually improve when someone with asthma moves from an environment of high mite exposure to one of low exposure (for example to the Swiss Alps).

Food allergy

Food, especially eggs and milk, can trigger an asthmatic reaction, but food allergies are more likely to cause gastrointestinal disturbances or eczema. Food additives such as sulphite (a preservative) and tartrazine (a colouring agent) are trigger factors in only a small minority of patients.

Seasonal variation

Seasonal variation in the frequency of symptoms and deaths is probably related to exposure to pollen, irritants in polluted air and infections. A common cause of seasonal asthma is an allergy to grass pollen (present in June and July). In children and young adults the increase in admissions and deaths in the autumn has been attributed to sudden fall in ambient temperature, an increase in house dust mites, dissemination of respiratory infections on return to school, and presence of autumn allergens (principally fungal spores). In older people asthma becomes more troublesome in the winter and is probably caused by associated respiratory disease. In tropical countries symptoms become more common almost invariably during the rainy season.

Pets

Furry animals, notably cats, can cause an asthmatic attack. Perhaps surprisingly, this is because of exposure not to their fur but to their saliva, which remains on the fur after preening. Parents should be cautious about introducing a new pet into the household if a child has asthma. Removal of the pet may improve symptoms but the emotional distress this might cause the child could worsen symptoms.

Emotional disturbance

It is generally believed that emotional disturbances do not cause asthma but can provoke or worsen bronchoconstriction or reduce the effectiveness of bronchodilator therapy. In some people an initiating allergen or irritant cannot be traced and symptoms are brought on by stress.

Occupational allergens

Substances in the working environment are responsible for about 15% of asthma cases. In the UK occupational asthma is now recognised as an industrial disease for which disablement benefit can be claimed. Over 300 causes of occupational asthma have been identified, usually involving exposures to animals or certain chemicals. The common feature is that exposure must be to an inhaled agent.

Chemical allergens include isocyanates (used to make polyurethane foam and some paints), platinum salts, epoxy resin curing agents, hardening agents found in paint and proteolytic enzymes used in detergents. Dusts arising from the storage of grain and milling of flour, and wood dusts can also trigger asthma. Pharmaceutical workers involved in the production of antibiotics can develop occupational asthma, but much more commonly become sensitive to aspirin and related drugs. Many people continue to suffer symptoms even when the exposure has stopped.

Longitudinal studies of workers exposed to respiratory allergens suggest

Adrenoceptors: render cells responsive to noradrenaline released from sympathetic nerve endings, or adrenaline released from the adrenal medulla. Noradrenaline binds to α and β_1 receptors, whereas adrenaline mostly binds with β_2 receptors. Receptors are present in organs such as the heart (β_1) and peripheral vasculature (β_2).

β_2 Adrenoceptor agonists: bind to the β_2 receptors and cause bronchial dilation by relaxing smooth muscle in the wall of the airway.

Agonists: substances that bind to receptors and produce a response.

that sensitisation usually occurs within 2 years of new employment. Exposure to respiratory irritants at the same time (by smoking for example) increases the risk of sensitisation.

Drug-induced asthma

Drugs which induce asthma attacks include non-selective β-adrenoceptor blockers and prostaglandin synthetase inhibitors (aspirin and its derivatives). β adrenoceptors are antagonists that promote bronchospasm by blocking the β_2 receptors in smooth muscle. The β adrenoceptor blockers are most commonly prescribed to control hypertension and angina (Chapter 12). Even the β adrenoceptor blockers in eye drops (used to treat glaucoma) can initiate an attack. Selective β_1 adrenoceptor blockers are believed to pose slightly less risk but can still be dangerous in high doses. It is therefore recommended that, if possible, asthmatics should avoid this group of drugs altogether.

Aspirin and related NSAIDs (such as ibuprofen) may cause severe bronchoconstriction in susceptible individuals. Aspirin inhibits prostaglandin synthetase, which normally converts arachidonic acid to prostaglandins. When this pathway is blocked an alternative mechanism increases the production of leukotrienes that cause bronchoconstriction (see Chapter 4). More than 15% of the adult asthma population are sensitive to aspirin.

Air pollution

Air pollution does not cause asthma but can make symptoms worse

The role of air pollution as a causative factor in asthma is controversial. Airborne components could act on the lung tissue in two ways, either by damaging the epithelium and rendering it more sensitive to allergens or by causing further damage to tissue that has already been affected by allergens. Pollutants that are believed to enhance the effects of certain allergens include ozone, sulphur dioxide and acid aerosols. There is no doubt that high concentrations of particulates, arising from diesel emissions, contribute to the symptoms of asthma.

The impact of ozone is less certain. This is the most common air pollutant in the summer in Europe and north America. The limit for ozone in the UK is currently 50 parts per billion, averaged over 8 hours (see Chapter 5). Peak concentrations regularly exceed 110 parts per billion, causing a slight fall in lung function in both people who have asthma and those who do not. Children appear to be more sensitive than adults, but symptoms do not usually develop until much higher ozone concentrations are reached. Interpreting the effects of ozone is complicated because high levels in summer are usually accompanied by an increase in the pollen count, both of which also increase in fine sunny weather.

Smoking

Smoking exacerbates asthma: irritants in cigarette smoke damage the

respiratory lining and contribute to inflammation. It may also exert more subtle effects. The increased prevalence of asthma in the UK has coincided with increased rates of smoking, particularly among young women. Smoking during pregnancy increases the IgE concentrations in cord blood and is a consistent risk factor for neonatal respiratory disease. IgE stimulates the release of histamine from mast cells, which causes constriction of bronchial smooth muscle (see below). In adults, smoking increases blood IgE levels and is believed to accelerate the age-related decline in respiratory function. There is also evidence that childhood exposure to passive smoking is detrimental to respiratory function and growth.

Exercise

Exercise is a common trigger factor of symptoms, particularly in children who have relatively mild asthma. It is the change in temperature and drying of the airways which provokes an attack rather than exercise itself. Hence outdoor exercise in the cold is more likely to precipitate an attack than swimming in a warm indoor pool. Exercise-induced asthma can be avoided by dosing with a bronchodilator before exercising.

Genetic influences

Given the frequency of asthma in certain families a genetic contribution to the disease is probable. A gene on chromosome 11, which codes for an IgE receptor, is associated with some (but not all) families with atopy. Other genes are probably also involved, almost certainly including those encoding the HLA system.

It is not known why atopy is manifest in different ways (as asthma, hay fever or eczema, singly or in combination) and why the disorder sometimes skips generations. Studies show that concordance for asthma is about 19% in monozygotic twins, compared with about 5% for dizygotic twins. A difference of this magnitude clearly suggests that genetic factors determine predisposition for asthma. The mode of inheritance is not well understood: the condition could be inherited as an autosomal dominant gene with incomplete penetrance (which would explain why the disease sometimes skips generations) or as a combination of dominant or recessive genes.

The condition is probably caused by a combination of genetic and environmental factors; although some people have a genetic predisposition not all will encounter the necessary environmental agent. Studies in less developed countries have shown that rural people who migrate to urban areas are more likely to develop asthma. These people must already have genetic susceptibility, but the necessary environmental agent is encountered only when they move elsewhere.

▲ Key points

Trigger factors for asthma

- ▲ Allergens: pollens, moulds, house dust mite, animal saliva or urine, bacteria
- ▲ Cold, dry air
- ▲ Exercise
- ▲ Viral respiratory infections
- ▲ Psychological stimulus (stress, anxiety)
- ▲ Drugs (e.g. aspirin, ibuprofen and other prostaglandin synthetase inhibitors, β adrenoceptor blockers)
- ▲ Industrial chemicals (e.g. isocyanates, epoxy resins, aluminium, hair sprays, penicillin, cimetidine)
- ▲ Other industrial agents (e.g. wood or grain dust, solder, cotton dust, grain weevils, mites)

Pathological changes in asthma

The main features of asthma arise from the activities of histamine, other mediators of inflammation and cytotoxic proteins released by inflammatory cells in the mucosa. The histological features (Figure 24.3) include:

- Mucous gland hypertrophy, leading to excessive production of mucus and plugging of the airway lumen
- Inflammation, causing epithelial damage, scarring and persistent narrowing of the lumen
- Mucosal oedema and impaired mucociliary clearance
- Enlargement of bronchial smooth muscle

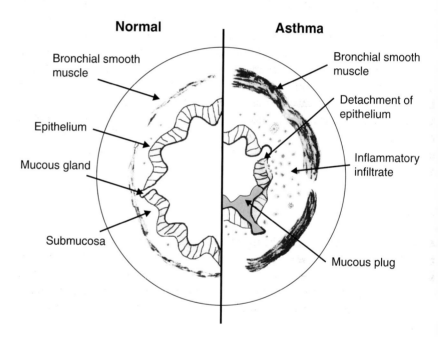

Figure 24.3 Histological changes in asthma. The bronchial wall comprises an epithelial lining (mucosa), submucosal connective tissue and a layer of smooth muscle. In asthma the lumen is narrowed by inflammation, oedema in the wall and blockage by mucus. Inflammation and external irritants also damage the epithelium, which may detach. There is hyperactivity and hypertrophy of the bronchial smooth muscle. The inflammatory infiltrate contains mast cells, eosinophils, neutrophils, macrophages and lymphocytes.

The respiratory system changes are initiated by an allergic reaction. The allergen stimulates the production of IgE by plasma cells. These antibodies attach to mast cells, stimulating the release of **histamine**. Histamine stimulates the release of mucus, contraction of bronchial smooth muscle and dilation of blood vessels.

The allergic reaction in asthma is preceded by a sensitisation phase (Figure 24.4). Sensitisation depends on genetic susceptibility and exposure to relevant agents. In a non-sensitised individual, exposure to very large quantities of an allergen does not provoke symptoms. In contrast, extremely small (picogram) amounts of allergen are sufficient to cause symptoms in people who have become sensitised. Measurement of allergen-specific IgE in the blood, and skin testing with common antigens (see below), can be used to determine whether sensitisation has taken place.

The first descriptions of the pathological changes in asthma relied on post-mortem examination of the lung tissue in people who had died from **status asthmaticus**. This condition is characterised by occlusion of large segments of the airways with mucus, plasma proteins and cell debris. The bronchial walls show oedema, a dense eosinophil infiltrate and loss of epithelium.

Fibreoptic bronchoscopy has enabled sampling of the respiratory mucosa at milder stages of the disease. The mucosa in all asthma patients is abnormal, showing infiltration by inflammatory cells (eosinophils, lymphocytes and, to a lesser extent, neutrophils) together with mast cells at various stages of degranulation. It is unusual to see large numbers of eosinophils in most other inflammatory diseases and it has been suggested that these cells play a central role in the pathogenesis of asthma. The number of eosinophils found in sputum or blood corresponds with the severity of the disease, and may be reduced by corticosteroid therapy.

> *Primary sensitisation occurs before an allergen has a clinical effect*

> ▲ **Key points**
>
> **Pathological changes in asthma**
>
> ▲ Hypertrophy and hyperplasia of bronchial smooth muscle
> ▲ Mucous gland hypertrophy
> ▲ Excessive mucus production
> ▲ Infiltration of inflammatory cells
> ▲ Damaged epithelium
> ▲ Mucosal oedema
> ▲ Impaired mucociliary clearance

Eosinophils

Eosinophils contribute to the inflammatory response by releasing a range of inflammatory mediators, including platelet-activating factor, leukotrienes, histamines and cytokines. Some of the proteins released by eosinophils (major basic protein, eosinophil cationic protein and eosinophil-derived neurotoxin) are directly toxic to airways epithelium and are probably largely responsible for epithelial shedding.

Eosinophils are also responsible for the release of membrane-derived phospholipid mediators. It is believed that these influence contraction of bronchial smooth muscle, permeability of small blood vessels (contributing to oedema) and excessive secretion of mucus (Figure 24.5).

Mast cells

Mast cells release histamine and various chemotactic factors from storage cells in the cell cytoplasm in response to the IgE binding to receptors on their surface.

One of the effects of histamine of particular relevance to asthma is that it triggers rapid bronchoconstriction. It also causes vasodilation and increases vascular permeability, assisting inflammatory cells to arrive at the site. Other chemotactic factors from mast cell granules attract macrophages, eosinophils and neutrophils into the mucosa and lumen.

> *Eosinophils are some of the major proinflammatory cells involved in the pathogenesis of asthma*

Cytokines: soluble protein mediators, produced by leukocytes and other cells that orchestrate the recruitment, differentiation and activation of specific cells in the inflammatory response and tissue repair.

Eosinophils: phagocytic cells rich in cytoplasmic granules which contain peroxidase enzymes and basic proteins. When activated, the cells generate large amounts of active oxygen metabolites which can kill large extracellular parasites.

Status asthmaticus: severe, acute condition that does not respond to drug therapy. Can cause death from respiratory insufficiency.

Mast cells: components of many normal tissues, particularly the connective tissues surrounding blood vessels. Contain cytoplasmic granules that store histamine and heparin.

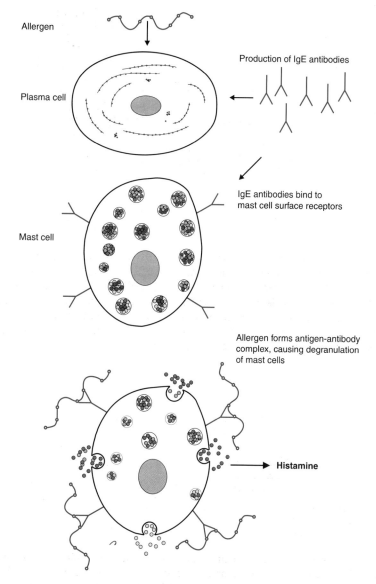

Allergen

Production of IgE antibodies

Plasma cell

IgE antibodies bind to mast cell surface receptors

Mast cell

Allergen forms antigen-antibody complex, causing degranulation of mast cells

Histamine

Figure 24.4 Allergic reaction in asthma. In an initial sensitisation stage an allergen (e.g. house mite dust or pollen) stimulates the production of IgE by plasma cells. This binds to mast cells which are located in many body tissues, particularly in connective tissues around blood vessels. Further contact with the allergen produces a cross-linked antigen-antibody complex on the surface of the mast cells. This triggers the release of histamine and other cytokines from mast cell granules. Histamine stimulates dilation of blood vessels, contraction of smooth muscle in the bronchioles and production of mucus in the airways. Together, these changes restrict air flow, making breathing difficult.

The activation of mast cells does not end with release substances from storage granules. Newly synthesised cytokines are released that recruit and stimulate other cells of the inflammatory response and affect bronchial muscle. Most

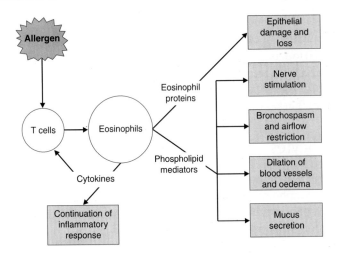

Figure 24.5 The role of eosinophils in asthma. Eosinophils are thought to play a central role in many of the underlying pathological processes in asthma. Eosinophil proteins are toxic to the epithelium and contribute to epithelial shedding. Irritants are more likely to stimulate underlying nerve receptors, causing bronchoconstriction, when the epithelium is damaged. A variety of phospholipid membrane-derived mediators influence smooth muscle contraction, blood vessel permeability and mucus production. Cytokines released by eosinophils ensure persistence of the inflammatory response.

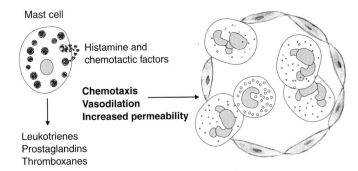

Figure 24.6 Mast cells in the inflammatory response. Substances released by activated mast cells contribute to the inflammatory response in asthma. Histamine and cytokines contribute to vasodilatation, increased capillary permeability and chemotaxis. Leukotrienes, prostaglandins and thromboxanes also contribute to these activities. The right-hand side of the diagram shows the migration of neutrophils and eosinophils through the blood vessel wall in response to mast cell factors.

notable among these are leukotriene B4 and various prostaglandins and thromboxanes (Figure 24.6).

Macrophages

Macrophages release prostaglandins, thromboxane and platelet activating factor, which appears to sustain bronchial hyperreactivity and cause respiratory

Macrophages: phagocytic cells derived from blood monocytes, which are present throughout the tissues.

T lymphocytes: play a role in all antigen-driven inflammatory responses. Divided into two major functional subgroups on the basis of cellular expression of surface antigens - CD4 (helper) or CD8 (suppressor).

Th1 cells: a subset of CD4 helper T lymphocytes which secrete IL-2, interferon-γ and TNF-β, but not IL 4, 5 or 6. Th1 cell products have the capacity to inhibit the growth of Th2 clones, and vice versa.

Th2 cells: secrete IL 4, 5 and 6 but not IL-2, interferon-γ or TNF-β.

capillaries to leak plasma. This increases mucosal oedema. It also facilitates the accumulation of eosinophils within the airways.

In addition to their well known antigen-presenting capabilities, macrophages have receptors for IgE and can release an array of inflammatory mediators. Of particular interest is their capacity to secrete IL-1 and GM-CSF (see below). These are important in amplifying the effector cell response.

Lymphocytes

Both B and T lymphocytes are involved in the allergic response of asthma. Mature B lymphocytes (plasma cells) are responsible for the production of IgE; T lymphocytes help to regulate B lymphocytes and other aspects of the inflammatory response by secreting lymphokines and cytokines. Production of IgE by the B cells is regulated by IL-4 (stimulates IgE synthesis) and interferon-γ (inhibits IgE synthesis), which are produced by Th1 cells. Other T lymphocyte products include IL-3, IL-5 and granulocyte-macrophage colony stimulating factor (GM-CSF), which regulate eosinophil production. Interleukins 3 and 4 are also important regulators of mast cell and basophil function.

Cytokines secreted by activated CD4 cells attract mast cells and eosinophils, causing inflammation of the bronchial mucosa.

Studies indicate that in asthmatic subjects there is an imbalance of Th2 cells over Th1. This could lead to increased production of IL-3, 4 and 5 and reduced production of the inhibitory interferon-γ. The net effect would be increased IgE synthesis and more frequent activation of mast cells and eosinophils (Figure 24.7).

Epithelium

Epithelial damage increases access of irritants and contributes to airway obstruction

The epithelium is the first line of defence against potentially damaging dusts, vapours, fumes and gases. Although it acts as a physical barrier it also has important homeostatic functions and influences events in the underlying submucosa.

The airways epithelium comprises ciliated, serous cells (which produce a watery secretion) and mucus-secreting goblet cells. Normally it presents an effective permeability barrier but damage allows increased entry of allergens, causes changes in fluid and mucus secretion and exposes the sensory nerves. The damaged cells release inflammatory mediators which attract inflammatory cells into the mucosa and stimulate their growth, differentiation and activation. The inflammatory cell reaction can cause further damage to the epithelium.

Mucus production

Mucus is produced as part of the defence mechanism to trap and clear particulate matter and irritants from the upper respiratory tract. In asthma

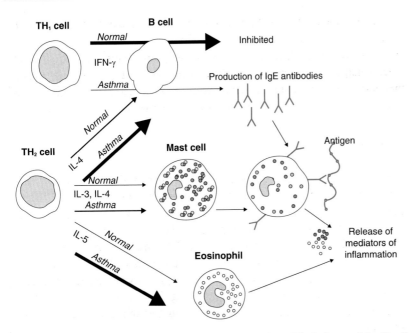

Figure 24.7 Mechanisms of allergic inflammation in asthma. The balance of the T-cell subtypes Th1 and Th2 is altered in favour of Th2 cells in people who have asthma. The Th1 cells produce interferon-γ, which suppresses IgE production by B cells. This inhibitory effect will be diminished in asthmatic subjects because Th1 cells are fewer. The increased number of Th2 cells will increase the production of IL-3, IL-4 and IL-5: IL-3 and IL-4 activate mast cells and IL-5 is chemotactic for eosinophils. In the presence of triggering antigen, eosinophils and mast cells release mediators of inflammation. These mediators affect blood vessels and mucus production and can amplify the response by attracting further inflammatory cells to the site. (Adapted from Johnston, S.L. and Holgate, S.T. (1991) *Br. J. Hosp. Med.*, **46**, 84–90.)

the size of the bronchial glands and goblet cells increases and they produce copious amounts of mucus, which becomes thickened by cell debris and plasma exudate. Ciliary clearance is inhibited, contributing to airway obstruction.

Oedema

A characteristic feature of asthma is oedema of the airway wall. Leakage of fluid from the blood vessels is probably stimulated by inflammatory mediators, some of which directly stimulate specific receptors on endothelial cells lining the post-capillary venules. In response, the endothelial cells contract, allowing leakage of plasma into the tissue (forming oedema) and out into the airway lumen (forming a plasma exudate). Oedema contributes to thickening of the airway wall and hence narrowing of the lumen. The exudate in the lumen is viscous because it contains plasma proteins and, with mucus, inhibits airflow. It has been suggested the outward flow of plasma across the mucosa contributes to epithelial shedding.

▲ **Key points**

Clinical symptoms of asthma

▲ Persistent cough
▲ Recurrent episodes of difficulty in breathing associated with wheezing
▲ Tightness of the chest, shortness of breath
▲ Acute severe asthma is life threatening: bronchospasm causes breathlessness and cardiac stress

Bronchoconstriction

Smooth muscle in the airways wall is innervated by parasympathetic nerves. The normal resting tone is maintained by the vagus nerve. The afferent system detects irritant chemical or mechanical stimuli by receptors immediately beneath the epithelial layer, and causes bronchoconstriction.

There is also evidence of an interaction between the afferent system and inflammatory cells. Some mediators of inflammation modify the release of neurotransmitters that cause bronchoconstriction. Neurotransmitters may influence the inflammatory response in the airway wall: a similar type of neurogenic inflammation is known to exist in the skin and gastrointestinal mucosa.

Clinical features and diagnosis of asthma

In most cases asthma attacks are mild and are triggered by easily recognisable factors. The features sought by the clinician are a strong personal or family history of atopy, exposure to allergens which precipitate attacks and a history of fluctuation in symptoms. Investigation of the condition is based on lung function tests. Skin tests may be used to identify extrinsic causes. The main diagnostic difficulty is in distinguishing asthma from COAD. It has been proposed that the distinction is made on the basis that symptoms of asthma may be reversed by bronchodilator drugs and corticosteroids. However, like asthma, COAD can be improved by oral corticosteroids, and bronchitis and emphysema may be reversible if caused by cigarette smoking. In the long term, reversibility of asthma can disappear.

Lung function tests

The simplest and quickest way to confirm variability in airway function is to measure the response to a short-acting bronchodilator such as a β adrenoceptor agonist. There will usually, but not necessarily, be a marked improvement in forced expiratory volume or peak expiratory flow in asthma. Reversibility is assessed by recording the best of three peak flow measurements, and then repeating the measurement 15–30 minutes after supervised inhalation of a bronchodilator.

A slower method is to evaluate the response of symptoms and airways function to oral or inhaled corticosteroids. Very often it takes 2–3 weeks of treatment before a response is obtained.

Peak flow metering is also used to monitor severity of asthma. Acute attacks are usually preceded by a gradual deterioration in control. This may not be noticed unless patients are encouraged to monitor airflow regularly with a mini peak flow meter. These are cheap to purchase and, although not the most accurate of devices, give reliable enough results for detecting trends over time.

Forced expiratory volume: the greatest amount of air exhaled in 1 second. Maximum inspiration is followed by forced expiration into a bellows spirometer. Expiration triggers a moving pen chart which measures and records volume against time.

Peak expiratory flow: the highest flow achieved in forced expiration, recorded as litres per second. Subjects are asked to breathe in fully and then to blow into a peak flow meter. The best of three measurements is recorded. There is a marked variation at different times of the day and measurements should be made on waking, during the afternoon and before going to bed.

Provocation tests

An alternative to measuring bronchodilator response is to try to provoke symptoms by exposing the patient to a trigger factor. The most commonly used method in the UK is an exercise test. It is usually used when other methods have failed to confirm the diagnosis (for example, asthma may be suspected but not seen when the patient is examined because of diurnal variation in symptoms).

Baseline peak flow is established before the exercise and the measurements repeated after 6 minutes of vigorous exercise. The exercise can be conducted on a treadmill, but an outdoor exercise such as running is better because breathing in cold dry air intensifies the response.

The characteristic response in asthma sufferers is a fall in peak flow of at least 15% within minutes of completing the exercise. Non-asthmatic people do not develop bronchoconstriction and, if anything, show a mild bronchodilatory response.

Other forms of challenge use non-specific agents such as inhalation of histamine or a specific agent to which the patient is believed to be sensitive. These tests are used only in special circumstances because the results can be unpredictable, causing a severe asthma attack, or reduction in symptom control lasting weeks or months. Challenges with specific allergens are usually reserved for investigation of occupational asthma.

Skin tests

A suspected allergen can be tested for its reaction in the skin. The agent is introduced into the superficial layer of the skin on the point of a needle. The test is painless. Most patients who have asthma produce a positive response to the common allergens such as house dust mites and pollens. A positive result is indicated by the production of a weal within 15 minutes of introducing the test substance. This result suggests that a specific IgE antibody is present and is an indicator of atopic tendency but does not necessarily mean that the patient has asthma – although it would be unusual for an agent which triggers an asthma attack not to produce a skin reaction.

Treatment

Treatment of asthma depends on clinical judgement of the severity of disease, taking into account the type and frequency of symptoms and physiological assessment of airways function. The frequency of drug use is an indication of how well the condition is controlled.

Treatment can be classified as drugs designed to relieve symptoms by opening the airways (bronchodilators) and those designed to prevent symptoms by controlling the underlying disease process (usually corticosteroids) (Table 24.1). The aim is to control the symptoms so that bronchodilators are hardly needed. Most patients will therefore require anti-inflammatory drugs. Because

---

▲ **Key points**

Investigation of asthma

▲ Lung function tests
▲ Forced expiratory volume, measured by spirometer
▲ Peak flow meter: measures maximum flow of air that can be forced during expiration
▲ Provocation tests: expose patient to suspected allergen factor or non-specific bronchoconstrictor
▲ Skin tests: allergens cause skin weals

Skin sensitivity to a particular allergen does not necessarily mean that it is responsible for asthma

---

The goal of treatment is to gain freedom from symptoms by reducing inflammation and dilating the airways

treatment must be self-managed patient education is an important aspect of asthma therapy: the differences between treatment of symptoms and regular maintenance therapies must be emphasised.

The treatments are used in the lowest doses possible in order to minimise short and long-term side effects. There are occasional difficulties in striking the correct balance because the severity of the disease has been under-estimated. Poorly controlled asthma is potentially life threatening.

Table 24.1 Drugs used to prevent or control symptoms of asthma

Type	Properties	Application
β2 Adrenoceptor agonists:	Stimulate β2 receptors in bronchial smooth muscle, causing bronchodilatation	
Fenoterol		Inhaled. Rapid onset of action. Now used at lower dose than previously recommended.
Salbutamol		Inhaled when required. Intravenous preparations also available
Salmeterol		Inhaled. Slow onset of action, but has long duration
Other bronchodilators:		
Cromoglycate	Prevents release of histamine from mast cells	Inhaled. Prophylactic agent, used before exercise. Useful in children with atopic asthma
Nedocromil	Similar properties to cromoglycate. May also have anti-inflammatory properties	Can be used as first-line therapy in mild asthma. Also used as an adjunct to corticosteroid therapy when control is poor
Methylxanthines:	Mechanisms of action unclear. May also have anti-inflammatory properties	
Aminophylline		Intravenous infusion in treatment of acute severe asthma
Theophylline		Oral. Therapeutic range close to toxic dose. May benefit children who cannot use inhalants. Also suitable for adults with nocturnal asthma
Ipratropium, oxitropium	Block cholinergic bronchoconstrictor effect of vagus nerve (muscarinic antagonist)	Inhaled. Effective in children and older patients with COAD

Corticosteroids:	Anti-inflammatory agents	Inhaled preparations. Drugs of choice in adults
Beclomethasone dipropionate, budesonide		Inhaled, metered dose inhaler or dry powder device. Should be used regularly even when patient feels well
Fluticasone propionate		Used at lower doses and has fewer systemic effects than beclomethasone or budesonide
Prednisolone		Oral preparation, usually used in a short course (14 days) after failure with other drugs. Some patients may need long-term therapy, but the goal is to return the patient to other drugs as soon as possible

Preventing symptoms

Two types of drug are used for preventing symptoms: non-steroids and steroids.

Cromoglycates and related drugs

The non-steroid drugs include sodium cromoglycate and nedocromil sodium. These effectively control asthma by inhibiting mast cells, eosinophils and the local nerve stimulation that causes bronchospasm and airflow restriction. The non-steroidal drug Intal (sodium cromoglycate) was used for many years, protecting against allergic or exercise-induced asthma attacks. It is now mainly used as a first-line treatment in children; adults with severe asthma being treated instead with inhaled corticosteroids. The cromoglycates are of no value in acute asthma.

Inhaled corticosteroids

Corticosteroids are believed to reduce the production of cytokines by most of the cells involved in the allergic response. This is evident in bronchial biopsies and in bronchoalveolar lavage fluid as a marked reduction in the number of epithelial and submucosal mast cells and eosinophils.

Corticosteroids control the underlying inflammatory process in asthma

Inhaled corticosteroids are particularly suitable for controlling chronic asthma in adults. They are also used to treat severe asthma in children. The preparations available include beclomethasone, budesonide and fluticasone propionate. All work by slowly reducing inflammation and mucus in the airways. High doses or prolonged treatment can suppress adrenal function and bone formation. It is believed by some that aggressive early treatment with steroids can reduce the likelihood of the illness continuing into adulthood, but this is not proven. High doses can slow down growth as well as causing the changes in the bones and adrenal glands.

Adrenaline: the substance naturally produced by the adrenal glands in situations of 'fight or flight'.

Oral steroid therapy

Oral corticosteroids are given if chronic symptoms persist. Their effects often last for months but do not give quick-acting symptom relief. Oral administration is associated with adverse effects such as fluid retention, adrenal suppression, Cushing's syndrome and increased susceptibility to infections (because of the immunosuppressive effect).

Relieving symptoms

One of the first treatments which became available to relieve the symptoms of asthma was adrenaline, a β adrenoceptor agonist. This relaxes the smooth muscles in the airways, allowing them to open wider so that breathing becomes easier. Adrenaline is relatively non-specific, short-acting and does not reduce the underlying inflammation. Adrenaline and isoprenaline have now been replaced by more specific preparations, such as salbutamol and terbutaline, which have fewer side-effects caused by cross-reaction with β_1 receptors.

β_2 Adrenoceptor agonists

Inhaled β_2 adrenoceptor agonists are still the mainstay of treatment in mild intermittent asthma. They relieve symptoms quickly and their effects last for several hours. It is not possible to eliminate side-effects completely and tachycardia or palpitations limit the doses that can be used. They are contraindicated in patients with a history of arrhythmia. The β_2 adrenoceptor agonists are used as required by the patient for the relief of breathlessness and wheezing, and may be the only treatment needed by some patients who have only infrequent symptoms. Other types of treatment should be considered if more than one dose daily is required.

Oral β_2 adrenoceptor agonists

These are available as longer-lasting oral preparations (bambuterol, for example). They are suitable for the relief of nocturnal asthma but are associated with more side-effects than the standard inhaled preparations. Longer-lasting inhaled preparations are now becoming available. Currently the longer-lasting preparations are recommended for use only in addition to inhaled corticosteroids: in spite of their prolonged effects they provide symptomatic relief only, and there is concern that anti-inflammatory therapy could be neglected.

Anticholinergic bronchodilators

Bronchial smooth muscle is stimulated by the efferent vagus nerve. This activity can be blocked by ipratropium or oxitropium bromide antagonists. These agents are most suitable for use in young children or older people with COAD. They are not as effective as the β_2 adrenoceptor agonists and so are usually administered to patients who have adverse effects to β_2 adrenoceptor agonists.

Methylxanthines

The methylxanthine drugs theophylline and aminophylline are effective bronchodilators and may also have anti-inflammatory activity. These have a narrow therapeutic dose range and a small dose increment can cause serious toxicity. A minority of patients experience nausea, diarrhoea, nervousness and headache at low doses. Larger doses are associated with persistent vomiting, insomnia, gastrointestinal bleeding and cardiac arrhythmias. Even so, many patients obtain a good therapeutic response without ill-effects at low doses. Drug clearance, and hence toxicity, is affected by other conditions such as congestive heart disease, COAD, viral pneumonia and concurrent therapy with other drugs.

Administration of asthma-controlling drugs

The preferred route of administration of the agents used to treat asthma is inhalation. This allows the drugs to be delivered directly to the airways in smaller doses and with fewer side-effects than systemic routes. Inhaled drugs have a faster onset of action. If chronic symptoms persist despite appropriate inhalation treatment then oral corticosteroids may be given. The aim is to give oral therapy in a short course and return the patient to inhaled bronchodilator therapy as soon as possible.

> *Inhalers deliver drugs direct to the airways*

Nebuliser: a machine that forces the drug through water or oxygen to make a fine mist that is easy to breathe in.

Several gadgets are available to dispense the drugs in aerosol form. The most common inhaler is a small canister from which the drug is released by pushing down a plunger. Auto-inhalers act in a similar way but release the drug as the person inhales.

A plastic container, or spacer, can be attached to the inhaler. This allows the drug to be breathed in more easily and ensures that none of it lands on the back of the throat. These tend be used for high-dose steroids, and by small children who may have trouble co-ordinating their breathing with an inhaler. A more recent development is powder inhalers which incorporate capsules of the drug in fine powder form. A nebuliser may be used if the asthma is particularly bad or if the sufferer is very young.

Chronic asthma

Chronic asthma is managed in a stepwise progression, reserving the more potent drugs for more severe symptoms (Figure 24.8). The first step is to ensure that the drugs are actually reaching their target by assessing the patient's inhaler technique, and if necessary changing the type of inhaler used. Because it is now understood that much of the disordered airway function in asthma is caused by inflammation there is a shift away from giving bronchodilators to using inhaled corticosteroids as first-line therapy in adults.

> *The aim of treatment is to reduce inflammation and dilate the airways*

The treatment of children depends on the frequency and severity of symptoms. Asthma is classed as mild if the symptoms appear less than once a month and are usually provoked by a viral respiratory tract infection. Mild asthma responds well to intermittent use of short-acting β_2 adrenoceptor

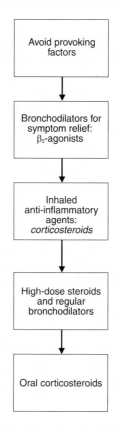

Figure 24.8 The treatment of chronic asthma in adults is tailored to the severity of symptoms. In some patients symptoms can be controlled by inhaling β_2 agonists (salbutamol, for example) alone when required. If the inhaler is required more than once a day, or if the patient has symptoms at night, the next step is to treat with inhaled corticosteroid (beclomethasone twice daily for example). Higher doses are used if symptoms persist. A second inhaled anti-inflammatory agent (sodium cromoglycate four times daily for example) might also be considered at this stage. A further bronchodilator (inhaled ipratropium bromide, oral slow-release β_2 agonists, or oral slow-release theophylline) can be added. Finally it may be necessary to stabilise the symptoms with oral corticosteroids. Contraindications to the use of all these drug types will apply to certain patients.

agonists. Lung function returns to normal between attacks.

Children with moderate asthma have symptoms several times a week, or an asthma attack more than once a month but less than once a week. These attacks tend to be triggered by viral infection, exposure to allergens or cigarette smoke, changes in climate and emotional upset. In these cases it is appropriate to add sodium cromoglycate to the bronchodilator therapy.

Severe asthma is characterised by symptoms on most days, often at night, but is relatively uncommon in children. It is treated with low-dose inhaled corticosteroids in addition to intermittent bronchodilator therapy. In very severe cases it may be necessary to increase the corticosteroid dose, add a long-acting β_2 agonist, theophylline, ipratropium bromide, or even to start on oral

prednisolone.

Another means of asthma control is to avoid precipitating factors. It is difficult to avoid specific allergens such as pollens and house mites, but it is possible to avoid cigarette smoke. This is not always easy, and ideally the person also needs to avoid passive smoking. Some studies have shown that vigorous attempts at removing house dust mites can bring about marked improvement. However, this can be very disruptive, involving eradicating mites from carpets with special high-powered vacuum cleaners, frequent laundering of bed linen and curtains, and literally freezing them to death by application of liquid nitrogen to mattresses and other surfaces.

Acute severe asthma

Acute severe asthma attacks (status asthmaticus) which are not controlled by the patient's usual medication are potentially life-threatening and most episodes require admission to hospital. Usually there is a history of worsening symptoms over several days but occasionally a severe attack occurs within minutes, without warning. Monitoring of bronchodilator use and home peak flow metering are helpful in warning of a deterioration in control.

> *People who have asthma should always be aware of how often they use their relievers*

The most common symptom of an acute attack is breathlessness. Moving about becomes difficult and there may be difficulties with eating and drinking. The patient finds it difficult to speak without gasping for breath between words. The severity of the attack is assessed by the general state of the patient, a rapid respiratory rate (above 25 breaths a minute) and increased pulse rate (above 110 beats a minute). Peak flow readings fall below 50% of best readings and in severe attacks may not be recordable.

Initial treatment comprises nebulised or intravenous β_2 agonist (usually salbutamol) or nebulised ipratropium bromide. Hypoxia is usual in a severe attack and supplemental oxygen may be necessary, usually in the ambulance on the way to hospital. Intravenous hydrocortisone or oral prednisolone is also given, preferably before the patient leaves home. Patients can be managed at home, depending on their response to the first nebuliser treatment. Observation must be continued for at least 30 minutes because severe asthma can quickly return. Any worsening of symptoms requires immediate hospital admission. If the patient improves then oral prednisolone and the regular bronchodilator should be continued, and the patient reassessed within 24 hours.

References

Rees, J. and Price, J. (1995) *ABC of Asthma*, 3rd edn, BMJ Publishing Group, London.

Further reading

Barnes, P.J. (1992) Asthma. *Br. Med. Bull.*, 48.

Holgate, S.T. (1993) Asthma: past, present and future. *Eur. Respir. J.*, **6**, 1507–20.

Rusznak, C., Devalia, J.L. and Davies, R.J. (1994) The impact of pollution on allergic disease. *Allergy*, **49**, 21–7.

Sporik, R., Chapman, M.D. and Platts-Mills, T.A.E. (1992) House dust mite exposure as a cause of asthma. *Clin. Exp. Allergy*, **22**, 897–906.

25 AIDS

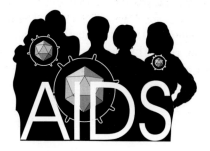

The acquired immune deficiency syndrome (AIDS) is caused by infection with the human immunodeficiency virus (HIV). Once AIDS develops life expectancy is very short, but the period between HIV infection and the onset of AIDS can be many years. Death is caused by immunosuppression, which leads to opportunistic infection and the development of malignancy. HIV follows two different patterns of viral transmission: in the less developed world infection is usually acquired through heterosexual intercourse; in developed countries HIV infection is more often seen in homosexual men and in people who have received blood or blood products contaminated with the virus – injecting drug users, haemophiliacs and people who have had blood transfusions. Heterosexual intercourse, particularly if the partner comes from abroad, is bisexual or has been infected by contaminated blood or blood products, also carries a risk of transmission.

The delay between infection with HIV and the onset of AIDS can be a decade or more. Once infected, individuals usually remain infected for life, and can pass their infection on to others, even while in the asymptomatic stage. Infection can be detected in this asymptomatic period by antibody testing. The main presenting conditions that characterise the onset of AIDS are *Pneumocystis carinii* pneumonia and Kaposi's sarcoma. Other conditions, such as primary CNS lymphoma, are more common in AIDS sufferers.

The main treatments for HIV infection and AIDS are aimed at controlling replication of the virus. The first drug that had any demonstrable efficacy against HIV was the reverse transcriptase inhibitor zidovudine. Other antiviral agents are now available; these appear to be more effective when used in combination, usually with zidovudine. Drugs with activities against a protease enzyme needed for viral replication (the protease inhibitors) are even more potent and can reduce the load of virus in the blood to undetectable levels. Although it is possible to delay the onset of AIDS and to improve survival for patients with AIDS, no treatment can yet cure the disease. Once AIDS develops antibiotics are given to control the opportunistic infections that beset all patients. Research is aimed at developing a vaccine against the virus, although a number of theoretical and practical problems suggest that even if such a vaccine becomes available it will not be entirely successful in stopping the AIDS epidemic.

Pre-test

- **What are the symptoms of HIV infection?**
- **What is the distinction between HIV infection and AIDS?**
- **Who is likely to suffer from AIDS?**
- **Why is AIDS invariably fatal?**
- **What diseases do people with AIDS die from?**
- **How is HIV infection diagnosed?**
- **Is there any treatment for HIV infection and AIDS?**
- **What measures can be taken to prevent the spread of HIV infection?**

Retrovirus: an RNA virus which replicates inside cells by forming a complementary strand of genetic material using reverse transcriptase.

Aims of this chapter

By the end of this chapter you will have increased your knowledge of:
◆ The characteristics of the human immunodeficiency virus (HIV)
◆ How HIV is acquired and transmitted
◆ How the transition from HIV infection to AIDS is recognised

In addition, this chapter will help you to:
◆ Describe how the spread of HIV differs in developed and less developed countries
◆ Understand how HIV infection can be prevented
◆ Discuss the pathological changes that lead to the development of AIDS-related infections and malignancies
◆ Discuss the approaches for treating HIV-infected people

Introduction

AIDS is at present invariably fatal, but progression of HIV infection can be delayed by antiviral drugs

There is usually a long incubation period before the appearance of AIDS

Many people are unaware that they are HIV positive, but they can infect others

The acquired immunodeficiency syndrome (AIDS) is characterised by opportunistic infections and cancers that are invariably fatal. The syndrome is caused by infection with the human immunodeficiency virus (HIV). This retrovirus invades the helper T cells (T4 cells), which co-ordinate a variety of essential immunological functions. Their loss results in progressive impairment of the immune response.

In infected individuals the virus will be present in most body fluids, and transmission to other individuals is through contact with cells and virus in these body fluids. The most important mode of transmission is through sexual intercourse, but HIV can also be transmitted through blood or transplanted organs and tissues, from an infected mother to her fetus, and by breast feeding. HIV has been identified in cerebrospinal fluid and in brain tissue and is believed to have been carried there by circulating monocytes.

The infection may remain silent for many years, without producing any specific clinical symptoms. Within a few weeks of infection antibodies to the virus can be detected by a blood test. At this point the person is said to have **seroconverted**. The timescale for further progression to loss of immune system functions varies from a few months to years: some cases have taken 15 years or more.

Even in the asymptomatic stages an HIV-infected person can transmit the virus to others. Because of the long interval between seroconversion and the development of overt AIDS there is uncertainty over whether HIV infection invariably develops into AIDS. Between 70 and 100% of HIV-infected people eventually develop the disease, but from experience with some other viral infections it would not be surprising if a minority remain as asymptomatic carriers.

The story of AIDS to date is one of unremitting tragedy. In addition to having to cope with their illness, many of the first AIDS patients had to face indifference, fear and hostility of people in the medical and 'caring' professions.

This resulted from homophobic attitudes, a feeling that patients brought their plight upon themselves, and fear that the disease might be generally contagious. The situation gradually changed as political pressure by patients and their families, and those involved in the gay scene, began to be exerted. The death, in 1985, of the film star Rock Hudson received widespread publicity and aroused public awareness of the problems faced by people with HIV – and that this disease could be a threat to the general population.

People with AIDS face the complete disintegration of their life and imminent death: the average period of 2 years from diagnosis to death is punctuated by repeated hospitalisation. This usually means that the person is no longer able to cope with their job. People with AIDS may lose their insurance benefits and may have to sell their homes in order to pay for treatments. The economic and social costs are huge, both for the patient and the community.

In less developed countries the situation is even more desperate. The much higher prevalence of the disease (caused by heterosexual transmission) has decimated families and promoted collapse of the rural economy. Often no-one is left to farm the crops or look after orphaned children – who themselves have acquired the virus from their mothers. In some areas whole communities have simply disappeared.

The discovery of AIDS

At the end of 1979, in New York and Los Angeles, a mysterious illness became apparent in which young men presented with swollen glands, high fever and fatigue that did not respond to treatment. No known cause was apparent, and the only common denominator was that all the men were homosexual. It had already been noted in San Francisco that young homosexual men were susceptible to contracting amoebic dysentery. The usual annual incidence of amoebic dysentery in that city was about ten cases a year, confined to people who had travelled to areas of the world with poor sanitation, such as India and Mexico. By the mid 1970s the incidence of amoebic dysentery had increased to over 1000 cases a year, mostly in homosexual young men. This increase corresponded to an increase in the population of gay men in San Francisco, which stemmed from the social and sexual revolution that took place in the 1960s. As a result of this change in attitudes the laws prohibiting homosexuality in many American states were repealed.

In the USA homosexuals began to congregate and live together openly. Most notable of these communities were the Castro district of San Francisco, and Fire Island, New York, which became a summer idyll for young gay men. Part of the gay lifestyle was a 'bath-house' culture – these venues were used for sexual liaisons with multiple partners. It was not uncommon for one gay man to have encounters with hundreds of different men in a year. Never before had so many men had sex with other men who themselves were promiscuous. Not surprisingly, these young men often had a long history of sexually transmitted diseases (STDs), such as non-specific urethritis, gonorrhoea, hepatitis B, herpes simplex, venereal warts, cytomegalovirus, Epstein–Barr viral infections and syphilis, as well as hepatitis A, shigella and amoebic infections (Table 25.1).

Table 25.1   Infections common in homosexual men (excluding HIV)

Disease	Causative organism	Mode of transmission	Characteristics and symptoms
Amoebic dysentery	*Entamoeba histolytica*	Ingestion of contaminated food or person-to-person contact	Mild intermittent diarrhoea with abdominal discomfort, progressing to bloody diarrhoea with mucus. The organism can penetrate the colonic mucosa, spread to the liver via the portal circulation, leading to hepatitis and liver abscesses. Invasive form can be fatal
Gonorrhoea	*Neisseria gonorrhoeae*	Sexual intercourse	Infects epithelium of the urogenital tract, rectum, pharynx and conjunctiva. In men infection usually causes urethritis, painful urination or urethral discharge. (Women have vaginal discharge, painful urination and intermenstrual bleeding but can remain asymptomatic)
Hepatitis A	Hepatitis A virus	Faecal–oral route	Most common cause of viral hepatitis. Initial symptoms are fever, malaise and anorexia, followed by acute hepatitis and jaundice. Patients usually recover fully
Hepatitis B	Hepatitis B virus	Sexual intercourse; also transmitted by blood and saliva	Chronic liver disease caused by an immunological reaction to the virus. Five patterns of clinical response: acute self-limiting hepatitis, from which patients fully recover; fulminant acute hepatitis (rare) causing massive necrosis of liver cells; chronic hepatitis, which may lead to cirrhosis; an asymptomatic carrier state; a subclinical asymptomatic infection,

			which may progress to chronic hepatitis
Hepatitis C	Hepatitis C virus	Exposure to unscreened blood and blood products	Mild 'flu-like' illness in acute phase. Causes mild jaundice in some patients. About 50% of patients go on to develop chronic liver disease. Can lead to cirrhosis and liver cancer. Extrahepatic disease includes arthritis, anaemia and neurological complications
Herpes genitalis	Herpes simplex virus type 1 or 2	Sexual intercourse, contact with oral lesions	Type 1 infection is more typically associated with sores on the lips. Genital herpes characterised by multiple blisters on the glans penis, and may be accompanied by initial symptoms of malaise, fever and headache. Rectal infection leads to proctitis. The virus can establish latency in the dorsal root ganglia and recurrent attacks can be expected from this source after the initial infection. Clinical symptoms are more severe in HIV infected patients and recurrences are likely to be more frequent
Shigellosis	*Shigella* spp.	Faecal–oral route	Acute self-limiting intestinal infection. Onset of fever, malaise, abdominal pain and watery diarrhoea, which may become bloody
Syphilis	*Treponema pallidum*	Sexual intercourse; organism enters the body through breaks in the squamous or columnar epithelium of the reproductive tract or rectum	Primary lesion consists of a firm, painless, inflammatory nodule or chancre. The organism disseminates through the lymphatics and bloodstream to involve the liver, cardiovascular system, testes, bone and brain, causing

			inflammation and necrotic gummas in these tissues. Good prognosis if treated early
Urethritis	Usually *Neisseria* or *Chlamydia*	Sexual intercourse	Discharge from the urethra, painful urination and penile discomfort

The sudden appearance of **Pneumocystis** *pneumonia and Kaposi's sarcoma was the first sign that a new epidemic was under way*

By the end of 1979 more ominous symptoms appeared – dark spots on the skin of the arms, face or trunk, which were diagnosed as **Kaposi's sarcoma**. This is a rare form of skin cancer that had previously been seen only in old men, usually of Mediterranean origin. Some men were also presenting with night fevers, swollen glands and fungal infections of the fingernails and mouth. Even more surprising was the appearance of ***Pneumocystis carinii* pneumonia**: this pneumonia had rarely been seen – and was unheard of in young people unless they were immunosuppressed (transplant recipients).

The appearance of *Pneumocystis carinii* pneumonia gave the first real clues as to what was happening. This condition is treated with pentamidine isothionate. Distribution of this drug in the USA is controlled by the Centers for Disease Control (CDC). Until 1980 there had never been a request for its use in a person who did not have a transplant, or had cancer, and was immunosuppressed. Suddenly, there was an increase in requests from centres in New York, San Francisco and Los Angeles to treat gay men with *Pneumocystis carinii* pneumonia.

The first victims of the new epidemic were young homosexual men

The previous association of this pneumonia only with immunosuppressed individuals led one group of investigators to examine the blood of a few patients who had died from it. The investigations revealed a cellular immunodeficiency (depletion of T4 lymphocytes) that had not been previously described. Publication of these findings led to yet more cases of the disease being reported to the CDC as physicians became aware that they were not dealing with an isolated case. Since all the cases were in gay men, the condition became known as 'gay-related immune deficiency' (GRID). By the end of June 1981, 199 cases of GRID had been reported and 73 of these men were dead.

A concerted investigation followed into how this deficiency was acquired and spread. First, a case-control study was conducted of homosexual men with Kaposi's sarcoma and *Pneumocystis carinii* pneumonia. It was suspected that some aspect of the gay lifestyle must predispose towards development of this disease and so a questionnaire was used to elicit information on history of STDs, sexual practices, number of partners, use of legal and illegal drugs and use of sexual stimulants such as amyl nitrite ('poppers'). The most significant difference that emerged between men with the disease and the unaffected controls was that affected men had more sexual partners.

The second investigation used was to trace sexual contacts. In a small series of patients in Los Angeles and New York a common contact had been diagnosed with Kaposi's sarcoma. This man gave details of his other sexual contacts –

who were by now scattered throughout the world. Many of the contacts had shared experiences on Fire Island in the summer of 1976. Contact tracing revealed that the disease most probably involved an infectious agent, which was transmitted by homosexual intercourse.

Injecting drug users then started to fall ill with symptoms similar to those of GRID. Both men and women were affected, regardless of their sexuality. Reports followed from Florida that some Hawaiian immigrants were showing symptoms similar to those of GRID, but these people were neither homosexuals nor drug abusers. Then, in Miami, three haemophiliacs who were previously healthy, were heterosexual and did not abuse drugs became ill with *Pneumocystis carinii* pneumonia. The controlled distribution of pentamidine proved useful in tracing haemophiliacs who had been treated for this pneumonia. Two people who had received blood transfusions also became ill. Together these cases scotched one 'fact' about the disease – that anal sex between men was the only mode of transmission.

The cases in drug abusers (through the sharing of needles), haemophiliacs and transfusion recipients signified that the infectious agent had to be carried in the blood. This posed an unprecedented problem for the blood transfusion service because there was no means of detecting anything wrong with the blood, but the service has a responsibility to ensure that patients are not harmed by blood or blood products. The factor VIII used by haemophiliacs caused a particularly difficult problem: one dose is purified from the pooled blood of up to 2000 donors. The irony is that some of the most committed blood donors are homosexuals. The first response was one of 'wait and see', since it was considered that the disease was so rare that the benefits easily outweighed the risks.

The immediate priority was to isolate the infectious agent and characterise its molecular biology – then to develop methods of blood screening, definitive diagnosis and effective treatments. No organism was immediately obvious so it was assumed that the agent was most probably a virus. The first objectives, to identify the agent and develop a test for it, were rapidly fulfilled. Unfortunately an effective treatment strategy continues to be elusive.

One finding that resulted from HIV testing was that the African disease called 'slim' was the same as that caused by HIV in homosexuals, drug users, haemophiliacs and transfusion recipients in other parts of the world. The African cases emphatically did not fall into these risk categories, and so it was recognised that the disease can be transmitted through heterosexual intercourse. Accordingly the disease received the name by which it is now known: the acquired immunodeficiency syndrome (AIDS).

The discovery of HIV

The retrovirus known as human T lymphocyte virus (HTLV) has the ability to replicate itself within human T lymphocytes, and can cause a type of leukaemia. At the National Institute of Health laboratories near Washington Robert Gallo (who already had a considerable reputation as the discoverer of

There came a growing realisation that GRID was not confined to homosexuals

Pneumocystis *pneumonia was reported in haemophiliacs and people who had received blood transfusions*

Haemophilia: inherited coagulation disorder caused by deficiency of blood clotting factor. Most common types are haemophilia A (factor VIII deficiency), haemophilia B (factor IX deficiency) and von Willebrand's disease (factor VIII deficiency with defective platelet function, abnormal factor VIII:vWF).

Until HIV, the only virus known to replicate inside T cells was HTLV

ELISA (enzyme-linked immunosorbent assay): test used for the detection of a variety of proteins. Wells of microtitre plates are coated with antigen. The patient's serum is applied and any antibody present specific to that antigen will bind. A second layer of anti-human antibody, previously conjugated to an enzyme (alkaline phosphatase, for example), is then applied. Binding of the whole complex is revealed by visualisation of the enzyme in a substrate-coloured product reaction. The concentration of patient's antibody is estimated by spectrophotometric measurement of the colour intensity.

Reverse transcriptase: an enzyme that enables the synthesis of DNA from RNA. This is a reversal of the normal sequence of transcription in mammalian cells, in which DNA is used as a template to produce RNA.

human retroviruses and extensive experience of working with human T lymphocytes) formed the hypothesis that the blood-borne AIDS agent might also be a retrovirus because of the characteristic depletion of T lymphocytes seen in AIDS.

The search for a virus was also taken up by Luc Montagnier at the Pasteur Institute in Paris. Cell cultures derived from a lymph node biopsy of a patient with AIDS were tested for the presence of reverse transcriptase, the 'signature' enzyme of a retrovirus. This was detected by the French group, but work in Washington was hampered by the fact that the cell cultures soon died, a property that was not characteristic of HTLV. Eventually both groups succeeded in culturing the virus, and this enabled work on a test for the virus to begin.

The test, based on the ELISA principle, relies on detecting antibodies in blood, rather than the virus itself. It enables a diagnosis of HIV infection to be made at the asymptomatic stage and also allows blood intended for transfusion to be screened. So far, identification of HIV infection at the asymptomatic stage has done little to help the person affected, although he or she can take steps to avoid infecting others. It was hoped that treatment with antiretroviral agents at the asymptomatic stage might stop the progression to AIDS, but this at best this can only be delayed.

Characteristics of HIV

> *HIV is a slow-acting virus able to reproduce itself using the genetic material of host cells*

Two types of HIV are capable of causing AIDS: HIV-1 and HIV-2. The latter is more prevalent in West Africa, but is spreading into West African communities in London and other large cities. In common with all retroviruses, HIV contains structural core and envelope proteins together with the crucial **reverse transcriptase** that allows it to replicate inside the cells it has infected. Two types of envelope proteins have been identified: a transmembrane protein called gp41 and an outer protein called gp120. The gp41 transmembrane protein appears to be important in cell fusion and the gp120 outer protein contains sites that allow the virus to bind with target cells. The core protein is known as p24.

> *HIV binds with cells that express the CD4+ antigen and other membrane cofactors*

The principal target cells are the T lymphocytes that bear a cell surface marker antigen known as CD4+. The virus binds to this antigen by sites in gp120. Other cells that bear the CD4+ antigen can also be infected with HIV; these include blood monocytes and tissue macrophages, dendritic cells and Langerhan's cells.

Binding to the CD4+ receptor is not the only requirement for entry of the virus into a target cell. An additional cofactor is needed to permit the virus and host cell membranes to fuse. A putative cofactor (**fusin**) has now been identified (Feng *et al.*, 1996). Antibodies to fusin have been shown to block the infection of susceptible cells by HIV. Another secondary receptor on CD4+ cells, a chemokine receptor known as CCR5, is probably also involved in the initial infection of T lymphocytes by HIV. The discovery of fusin opens a further avenue for the development of new therapies: drugs that block binding of the virus to a necessary cofactor could render cells invulnerable to infection.

The leading candidates would be drugs that mimic the activities of the chemokines RANTES, MIP-1α and MIP-1β. These chemokines have been shown to suppress the ability of HIV to infect cells, presumably by binding with the necessary secondary receptors. A similar approach (blocking the CD4+ receptor itself) has been tried but unfortunately causes immunosuppression. If the interaction with cofactors were specific for particular virus subtypes blocking of one cofactor might not completely compromise the function of the host cell.

Following binding to the CD4+ receptor virus is taken into the cell. Viral DNA is synthesised by reverse transcriptase and spliced into the host cell DNA. From this further RNA transcripts are produced using the host cell's replicative enzymes and these are translated into the viral proteins, which are assembled and transported to the cell surface. The virus particles bud off from the cell membrane, acquiring portions of the cell membrane for their own coating as they do so. The virus is then free to bind with new cells (Figure 25.1).

> Chemokines: a family of about 20 structurally related peptides with leukocyte activation and chemotactic activity. The various peptides differ in their effects on neutrophils, monocytes, lymphocytes, basophils and eosinophils. For example, MIP-1α is chemotactic for B lymphocytes and activated CD8+ cells, whereas MIP-1β is chemotactic for CD4+ cells. RANTES, MIP-1α and MIP-1β bind to a common receptor.

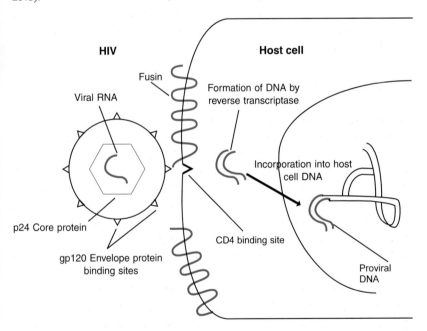

Figure 25.1 Mechanism of HIV infection. HIV enters the cell by binding with the CD4+ receptors on the host cell surface, using sites present within its envelope coating protein. Viral (gp41) and cellular (e.g. fusin) cofactors are probably also required for the fusion of virus and the host cell membranes. The virus particle is internalised, whereupon it loses its coating. Viral RNA is converted to double-stranded DNA by virally encoded reverse transcriptase. This DNA is spliced into the host cell genome.

Ultimately, HIV kills the cells it infects, although the precise mechanisms by which it does so remain unclear. Some destruction is probably mediated by the host immune response to the viral antigens. The devastating consequences of CD4+ lymphocyte depletion arise from their pivotal role in controlling the

> *HIV destroys the body's immune defence system*

immune response: it affects all other immune system components and functions.

Although free HIV is shed from cells, patients are permanently infected because of the proviral DNA that has been inserted into their genome. Whenever a cell divides the virus will be replicated. In its free state the virus is accessible to other components of the immune system and can be removed from the blood by antibody and cell mediated responses. It therefore seems likely that viral transmission is through infected cells (that is, by cells carrying the proviral DNA).

HIV is transmitted by contact with infected body fluids at vulnerable sites

Part of the function of the lymphocyte target cells is to migrate through tissues to mount a localised immune response. This means that the virus is disseminated with the lymphocytes and, of particular relevance to the ways in which HIV can be transmitted, finds its way into body fluids and secretions, particularly blood, semen and milk. The viral load in other body fluids is usually lower: viral particles and lymphocytes can be found in endocervical mucus or saliva, but are extremely rare in urine, sweat or tears. It is therefore no coincidence that the main modes of HIV transmission are contact with body fluid, such as would occur in sexual intercourse, the introduction of blood or blood products and from mother to child.

The rectum is a very thin barrier. It can be penetrated by virus and lymphocytes, presenting a relatively easy route for transmission. Although the vaginal wall has a very much thicker stratified squamous epithelium, the cervical canal is less thick and hence heterosexual vaginal intercourse represents a risk. Skin has a thick stratified squamous epithelium which is further protected by a covering of keratin, making it a formidable barrier against the passage of HIV or HIV-infected lymphocytes.

In all sites the transmission of HIV is much easier if the epithelium is damaged. The presence of other sexually transmitted diseases (such as genital herpes) that result in sores or other lesions will facilitate transfer, both into and out of the body (sores will produce exudate containing HIV-infected lymphocytes). Other host conditions, such as malnutrition and reduced immunity, could also increase vulnerability to HIV infection.

Background information: Cellular components of the immune system

The immune system works by the recognition of antigens, commonly glycoproteins on the surfaces of cells, bacteria and viruses. When a foreign antigen is recognised by cells of the immune system the usual response is that **antibodies** are produced by the B lymphocytes. The antibody will bind specifically to its target antigen, and when this antigen–antibody complex is produced a cascade of other components is activated which results in the complex being removed by macrophage activity. The immunity involving antigen–antibody reactions is called **humoral immunity**. The B cells normally comprise 25% of the lymphocyte population.

The cells that are involved in the recognition of antigens are collectively known as antigen-presenting cells and usually have very long cytoplasmic processes. For this reason they are called **dendritic cells**. Dendritic cells in the lymph nodes and spleen are able to trap antigens circulating in the lymph and blood, presenting the antigenic information to neighbouring lymphocytes. Several different types of lymphocytes are involved.

The immune system is regulated by the activities of T lymphocytes (helper T cells and suppressor T cells), derived from the thymus. In common with all cells, T lymphocytes carry antigens on their surface. The helper cells carry an antigenic marker known as CD4+, the suppressor cells carry CD8+ antigens. As their name suggests, the T helper cells stimulate or provide help for B cells to produce antibodies. In contrast, suppressor T cells inhibit the B cells, so that less antibody is produced. Overall production of lymphocytes in the body is also controlled by T cells. A further class of T cells, cytotoxic or killer cells, are able to kill infected cells by direct contact. This direct response is known as **cell-mediated immunity**. The T cells are also able to influence the activities of neutrophils and macrophages.

Heterosexual and non-heterosexual transmission of HIV

In Africa HIV infection is much more likely to be acquired through heterosexual intercourse; in the USA and Europe infection is more likely to be associated with anal intercourse or injecting drug use. These differences can be explained by different viral subtypes, labelled A–H and O, and identified on the basis of HIV envelope and *gag* gene sequences. They differ in geographical distribution, subtypes A, C and D being more prevalent in sub-Saharan Africa, whereas the B subtype dominates in the USA and Europe. Subtype C dominates in India and E in Thailand (Table 25.2).

It is believed that Langerhan's cells, present in oral and genital mucosal surfaces, but absent in rectal mucosa, are a primary target for some HIV subtypes, as evidenced by the fact that some HIV subtypes grow much more efficiently in cultures of Langerhan's cells than others. For example, subtype E (mainly associated with heterosexual transmission) grows well in Langerhan's cells but subtype B (isolated from homosexuals) grows less well. It is therefore likely that non-B HIV-1 subtypes are transmitted heterosexually through attachment to and replication within Langerhan's cells. The B subtype does not attach or replicate as well in Langerhan's cells and therefore must be introduced into the body beyond the epithelial surface (at a site of damage for instance). The rectal mucosa presents much less of a barrier for this, and contaminated needles effectively bypass all physical barriers.

It is still not known why non-B subtypes have not spread to the USA and Europe to cause significant heterosexual transmission of AIDS. It is unlikely, in this era of rapid and accessible travel, that Europeans and Americans have

Geographical differences in transmission of HIV can be explained by differences in viral subtype

Infectivity of HIV subtypes may depend on their affinity for Langerhan's cells

Langerhan's cells: cells with extensive cytoplasmic processes, present in skin, oral and genital mucosa. They are very efficient in presenting antigens to other cells of the immune system.

Table 25.2 Prevalence and transmission of HIV subtypes

Subtype	Main population	Main mode of transmission*
A	Sub-Saharan Africa	Heterosexual
B	USA, Europe, Caribbean, South America, Thailand, Japan	Non-heterosexual
C	Sub-Saharan Africa, India	Heterosexual
D	Sub-Saharan Africa	Heterosexual
E	Thailand, Japan, India	Heterosexual
F	Romania, Brazil, Zaire	Heterosexual
G	West Africa	Heterosexual
H	West Africa, Taiwan	Heterosexual
O	West Africa	Heterosexual

*Transmission modes are not exclusive, for example subtype B virus can also be transmitted heterosexually.

not been exposed to the subtypes prevalent in Africa and Thailand. The other biological and behavioural risk factors that must be involved, and their mode of action, remain purely speculative.

Mechanisms of preventing HIV transmission are based on denying lymphocyte access to the host cells by creating a barrier (for example a condom can prevent exposure of vaginal, rectal or oral mucosa to infected semen). Research is currently under way to formulate gels or creams that can be applied topically to form a local barrier. These are likely to contain sulphated polysaccharides, which have been shown *in vitro* to prevent adhesion of HIV-infected cells to epithelium. Sulphated polysaccharides are easily extracted from many plant and animal sources (they are already widely used in foods and cosmetics) and could be an inexpensive and safe method of inhibiting viral transmission by cell contact.

Vertical transmission of HIV

Nearly all HIV infections in children are acquired by vertical (mother to infant) transmission. In parts of Africa 15–45% of infants born to infected women are also infected. Transmission can occur in pregnancy, during delivery or by breast feeding. Transmission is more likely if the woman has symptoms of immunodeficiency.

A significant factor appears to be length of time between fetal membrane rupture and delivery. The Women and Infants Transmission Study, undertaken at centres in the USA and Puerto Rico (Landesman *et al.*, 1996), found that the rate of HIV-1 transmission was 25% among mothers in whom the membranes ruptured more than 4 hours before delivery but only 14% if the membranes ruptured less than 4 hours before delivery. This difference in transmission rate was independent of the mode of delivery.

A previous study, The European Collaborative Study (1994) showed that transmission rates were reduced if the baby had been born by caesarean section (11.7% compared with 17.6% of babies born by vaginal delivery). In this study some 80% of caesarean sections were performed in women in whom the membranes remained intact, suggesting that the crucial factor is membrane rupture rather than the mode of delivery.

Despite this, it is possible that some infections are acquired by exposure during delivery to HIV in cervical–vaginal secretions in the birth canal. One way to reduce this risk might be to cleanse the birth canal with an antiviral agent immediately before delivery. This approach has been attempted in Malawi (Biggar *et al.*, 1996) using a cotton wool pad soaked in 0.25% chlorhexidine. The HIV transmission rate in the intervention group (505 HIV-positive women) was 27%, compared to 28% in 477 untreated women. It was concluded that either exposure in the birth canal is not a significant risk factor or the intervention was inappropriate. A more effective intervention for reducing vertical transmission of HIV is treatment of the pregnant woman and newborn baby with zidovudine (see below). Unfortunately, cost considerations dictate that this is unlikely to be a realistic option in less developed countries.

> *The risk of vertical HIV transmission is strongly influenced by the duration of fetal membrane rupture before delivery*

Epidemiology

Global statistics

Statistics for AIDS are regularly collated and reported by the World Health Organization from records supplied by member organisations in each country. The data are usually presented as the cumulative number of cases. Inevitably, there are substantial differences in the accuracy of diagnosis and recording in different parts of the world. It is assumed that there is significant under-diagnosis and under-reporting in the less developed countries and hence estimates are based on the known distribution, spread and penetration of the disease. Although 50% of reported AIDS cases are from the developed countries, it is estimated that 80% of cases actually occur in less developed countries.

The prevalence of HIV infection is somewhat higher than that of AIDS because of the time lag between infection and onset of symptoms. For mid-1993, the cumulative number of AIDS cases throughout the world was estimated at more than 2.5 million and the cumulative number of HIV infections in excess of 13 million (Figure 25.2). The highest estimated

Review question 1

Explain why HIV cannot be caught by casual contact (for example by being sneezed on or from touching other people).

Pandemic: an epidemic over a large region.

prevalence of HIV infection is in sub-Saharan Africa. Other areas where the epidemic is spreading rapidly include India and Thailand.

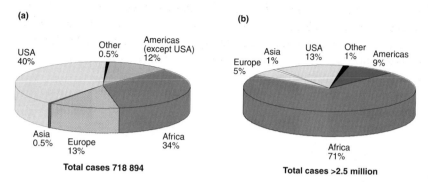

(a)

USA 40%

Other 0.5%

Americas (except USA) 12%

Asia 0.5%

Europe 13%

Africa 34%

Total cases 718 894

(b)

Europe 5%

Asia 1%

USA 13%

Other 1%

Americas 9%

Africa 71%

Total cases >2.5 million

Figure 25.2 Cumulative cases of AIDS in adults and children, mid 1993. (a) Reported cases; (b) estimated actual numbers. By far the greatest burden of AIDS is in Africa, but this is not indicated by the number of reported cases. Medical resources are in pitifully short supply in many areas of Africa and this, together with people's own knowledge of the hopelessness of their plight, means that the majority of cases are never recorded. (Source: WHO, 1993.)

The overall prevalence of adult HIV infection in sub-Saharan Africa is estimated at 15–20% (1992 figures). It is also estimated that one in three children born to HIV-positive women in this area are infected. Most of these children are unlikely to survive beyond 5 years. Uninfected children are likely to become orphans because their parents die from AIDS. It is now believed that AIDS is the second most common cause of death (after diarrhoea) in children under 5 in this part of the world.

In the developed world the AIDS epidemic has stabilised, but in other areas the pandemic grows unabated. The only hope for the less developed countries is through scientific advances made in the developed countries. Fear has been expressed that if the problem is 'hidden away' in Africa this task will be less urgent. Nonetheless, AIDS is expected to remain a serious problem in the developed countries for the foreseeable future, and containment of the disease in the developed countries will primarily depend on the degree of spread into the heterosexual population. In the USA and some European countries newly reported cases of AIDS are increasing most rapidly in heterosexuals.

UK statistics

In the UK, the number of cases of AIDS and HIV reported is based on voluntary confidential records that are returned by clinicians, microbiologists, or doctors at haemophilia centres. Data on the prevalence of HIV in women are obtained by anonymous unlinked antenatal blood testing (in this the source of a positive sample cannot be traced) to provide a measure of the spread and progression of HIV in the heterosexual population.

A total of 9865 cases of AIDS had been reported by the end of September 1994 (reporting began in 1982), including 175 children under the age of 15 years. The total number of HIV-infected people recorded since testing began in 1984 to the end of September 1994 was 22 851, of whom 3084 were women (Figure 25.3). There is a significant geographical variation in the distribution of HIV and AIDS, the highest prevalence being in London and other metropolitan areas.

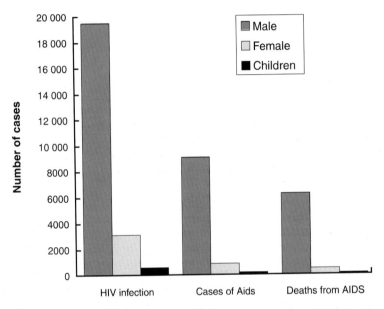

Figure 25.3 Cumulative cases of HIV and AIDS in men, women and children in the UK. The recording period for AIDS in children in January 1982 to July 1994, for AIDS in males and females (including children) January 1982 to September 1994 and for HIV infection November 1984 to September 1994. In the UK the prevalence of HIV and AIDS is greater in men. Childhood disease is acquired primarily by vertical transmission. (Source: *Communicable Disease Report* 1994, **4**, 199–202.)

Most cases (40–80%) of AIDS in the UK are attributed to exposure to infection through sexual intercourse between men (highest in the London area). Infection through heterosexual exposure accounts for 7–24% of cases, mostly in people who had sexual intercourse with someone from, or who has lived in, a country where the major route of HIV-1 transmission is through heterosexual intercourse. Infections acquired by injecting drug use account for 3–36% of cases (highest in Scotland). Most infections in children (nearly 80%) were acquired through mother to infant transmission, the remainder by transfer of HIV-infected blood or tissue (Figure 25.4). This is very different from the pattern seen in Africa, where the disease is predominantly transmitted by heterosexual intercourse.

In the UK about 2500 new cases of HIV infection are reported annually. A significant fall in the number of new cases reported in 1987 and 1990 was seen,

Key points

Exposure factors in HIV transmission

▲ Sexual intercourse between men

▲ Sexual intercourse between men and women with a high-risk partner (injecting drug user, someone infected by blood factor treatment or blood transfusion, or a woman who has had intercourse with a bisexual man)

▲ Heterosexual intercourse with a partner from, or who has lived in, an area where the major route of HIV-1 transmission is through heterosexual intercourse

▲ Injecting drug use

▲ Mother to infant

▲ Blood or tissue transfer (e.g. transfusion)

▲ Blood factor treatment (e.g. for haemophilia)

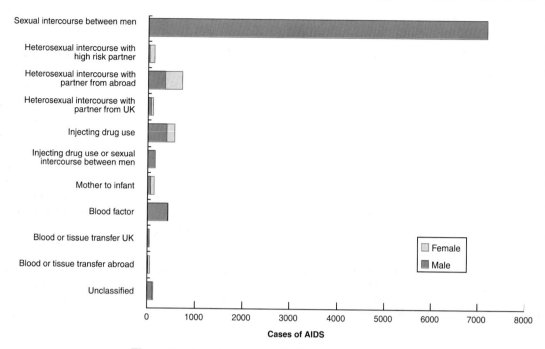

Figure 25.4 Cumulative cases of AIDS in the UK (to end September 1994) in men and women. The patterns of exposure and infection in the UK are similar to those seen in other parts of Europe and North America; the disease primarily affects homosexual men, injecting drug users and haemophiliacs. (Source: *Communicable Disease Report* 1994, **4**, 199–202.)

which may reflect the substantial media campaign in 1986–1987. Unfortunately, after being 'scared' into safe sex or abstinence, some people in high-risk categories may become complacent as time passes and revert to their old lifestyle (Figure 25.5).

Patterns of HIV infection in the USA

In the large metropolitan areas of the USA about 50% of new HIV infections are transmitted through injecting drug use, 25% are acquired through heterosexual intercourse (of which 70–80% are in women) and 25% through homosexual intercourse. The largest increase in the rate of infection has occurred in African American and Hispanic populations.

Symptoms and clinical definition of AIDS

Infection with HIV proceeds in four clinical phases. **Seroconversion** takes place in a median time of 2 months after infection. About 50% of patients develop flu-like symptoms at this time. There then follows an **asymptomatic incubation period** during which HIV antibodies are detectable in the blood,

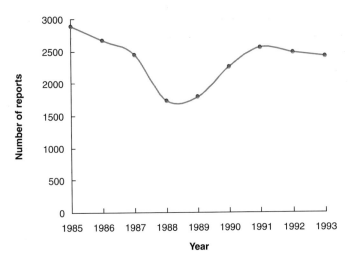

Figure 25.5 The incidence of HIV infection in the UK has declined. This was particularly apparent in 1987–1990, presumably as people realised the importance of safe sex and avoidance of other risky behaviours. There is still much that needs to be done. (Source: Communicable Disease Surveillance Centre.)

increased numbers of CD8 cells are directed against viral antigens and numbers of CD4 cells remain within the normal range. Some symptoms relating to a loss of immune regulation may become evident, such as a worsening of pre-existing psoriasis (Figure 25.6). The next phase is often referred to as **AIDS-related complex** (ARC), and is considered to be the precursor stage for full-blown AIDS. The signs and symptoms of ARC are generalised lymphadenopathy, fever, weight loss, hairy leukoplakia, recurrent oral candidiasis, anaemia, bleeding disorders, kidney failure and some neurological abnormalities. In the ARC there is an increased susceptibility to infections, which usually become severe. For example, herpes simplex infection in a normal person would cause a self-limiting vesicular eruption, but in ARC the lesions become florid, ulcerating and persistent. Superficial fungal infections become more frequent, and infections with *Salmonella* and *Haemophilus* are severe. In women, gynaecological problems such as pelvic inflammatory disease and candidiasis are more common. There is also an increased susceptibility to infection by human papillomavirus (HPV), leading to cervical neoplastic (CIN) changes (see Chapter 16). Ultimately patients go on to develop the more serious complications associated with **full-blown AIDS**. The presenting complaints vary widely, but are very often due to opportunistic infection. Certain conditions that arise in HIV-infected people are used to define the transition to full-blown AIDS.

The original 1982 definition of AIDS used by the CDC was based on the occurrence of indicator infections and malignant states that reflected the underlying cellular immunodeficiency. These **AIDS-defining conditions** include Kaposi's sarcoma and pneumonia resulting from *Pneumocystis carinii*

Candidiasis: mucosal infection ('thrush') of the oropharynx or vulvovaginal regions by the fungal organism *Candida albicans*.

Hairy leukoplakia: white patches on the oral mucosa with a 'hairy' or corrugated surface. Caused by thickening of the epithelium and excess production of keratin. Lesions may be infected with HPV and Epstein–Barr virus as well as HIV.

Lymphadenopathy: enlargement of the lymph nodes.

Pelvic inflammatory disease: an infection that begins in the vulva or vagina but spreads upwards to involve the entire genital tract. Causes pelvic pain and menstrual abnormalities. Complications include peritonitis, intestinal obstruction, bacteraemia and infertility. Gonococcal infections are the most common culprits.

▲ **Key points**

AIDS-defining conditions

▲ SLIM disease — weight loss, body wasting, weakness, chronic diarrhoea and persistent cough
▲ *Pneumocystis carinii* pneumonia
▲ Kaposi's sarcoma
▲ High-grade non-Hodgkin's B-cell lymphoma
▲ AIDS-related dementia
▲ AIDS-related complex

infection. Before the identification and spread of AIDS these conditions were very rare and affected only well defined patient groups such as older people or those on immunosuppressant therapy.

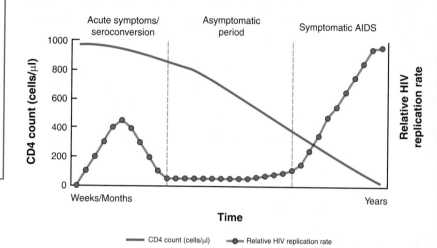

Figure 25.6 Natural history of HIV infection. Viral replication proceeds rapidly in the first few weeks. Eventually the host mounts an antibody response that is adequate to suppress HIV replication. However, because HIV infects cells of the immune system the capacity to sustain this response indefinitely is compromised as infected CD4 cells lose function and die. After a median time of 10 years the CD4 count falls below 200 cells/μl, at which stage the infected individual becomes susceptible to the development of serious opportunistic infections and malignancy. (Adapted from Kessler, H.H., Bick, J.A., Pottage, J.C. Jr and Benson, C.A. (1992) *Dis. Mon.*, **38**, 633–90.)

Death usually occurs within 2 years of diagnosis of an AIDS-defining condition

Following the discovery of HIV and the development of serological tests to detect the production of antibodies the concept of seropositivity was added to the definition. By 1987 other indicator conditions such as encephalopathy and wasting disease had become recognised.

In recognition of the clinical importance of lymphocyte depletion in the production of the disease, a depressed T4 lymphocyte count was added to the definition of the syndrome. It was also recognised that pulmonary tuberculosis, recurrent pneumonia and invasive cervical cancer are manifest in some patients with AIDS. Taking account of these factors the CDC produced a classification that has been used for epidemiological surveillance purposes in all American states since 1993 (CDC, 1993).

Eventual death from AIDS is slow and painful, often involving several infectious, degenerative or malignant diseases. These conditions may occur sequentially or be present in combination. In the early stages periods of remission occur, but these become shorter and less frequent as lymphocytes become disabled and infections take over.

Progression of HIV infection

There is evidence that not everyone exposed to the virus becomes infected and some babies who test positively for HIV infection at birth subsequently test as negative (most of these can be explained by clearance of maternal HIV antibodies from the blood but in a very small minority there was evidence of genuine infection).

Adults are infected with HIV for life, but individuals vary in the time taken for progression to AIDS. Some homosexual men with a well documented history of seroconversion have remained free of AIDS for 14 years, and they might never develop AIDS. The reasons why these men have such a lengthy and stable course of HIV infection are not fully elucidated, although several contributory factors are likely:

- The viral strain
- Genetic susceptibility
- Immune response
- Lifestyle practices
- Antiretroviral therapy

> *HIV infection in adults is permanent, but may take many years to progress to AIDS*

▲ **Key points**

Clinical categories of HIV infection

▲ All categories include documented HIV infection

Category A:
▲ Limited to adolescents or adults with asymptomatic or acute HIV infection or history of acute HIV infection and/or persistent generalised lymphadenopathy
▲ CD4+ T-lymphocyte count 500 cells/µl or more

Category B:
▲ Limited to adolescents or adults with symptomatic conditions that are attributable to HIV infection or are indicative of a defect in cell-mediated immunity or have a clinical course or require management that is complicated by HIV infection
▲ Conditions include, but are not limited to, persistent oral or vulvovaginal candidiasis, cervical neoplasia (CIN II or III), oral leukoplakia, herpes zoster involving at least two episodes, listeriosis, pelvic inflammatory disease, peripheral neuropathy. Category C conditions are excluded
▲ CD4+ T-lymphocyte count 200–499 cells/µl

Category C:
▲ Presence of AIDS-defining disease (e.g. PCP, Kaposi's sarcoma)
▲ CD4+ T-lymphocyte count below 200 cells/µl
Data from: CDC, 1993

An important genetic factor appears to be inheritance of the gene for the CCR5 receptor, involved in the initial binding of HIV to lymphocytes (see pp. 764–5). People who have two mutant copies of the gene appear to progress to AIDS more slowly than people who have two copies of the normal gene.

Cohort studies in the USA and Europe have shown that the proportion of 'non-progressors' (usually defined as remaining AIDS-free for 7 years or more and with a CD4 cell count above 500/μl) is 5–10% of the infected population. The CD4 cell count is the most important criterion for identifying non-progressors, as the median time from seroconversion to a fall in the CD4 count below the 500 cells/μl threshold (patient remains asymptomatic) is less than 2 years, whereas the median time from seroconversion to (symptomatic) AIDS is 10 years.

> *Early changes in cell markers are predictive of the subsequent disease course*

Progression to AIDS appears to be independent of age, race, gender, mode of infection, past history of STDs, lifetime number of sexual partners, frequency of sexual activity or use of recreational drugs. Despite having relatively high CD4 counts, the immunological profile of non-progressors is not entirely normal, and there are other early markers such as high numbers of CD8 cells and cytotoxic T lymphocytes that appear to influence subsequent disease course.

The value of lifestyle changes after seroconversion in delaying progression to AIDS is unknown (there is some evidence that good nutritional status slows the rate of progression). The early changes in cell markers are much more important determinants of subsequent clinical course and changes in lifestyle once seroconversion has been confirmed do not markedly influence the outcome.

The CD8 lymphocytes are able to suppress HIV infection of cultured cells, possibly by the secretion of chemokines which may block the fusin and other secondary receptors.

Opportunistic infections in HIV-infected patients

All HIV-infected patients will acquire opportunistic infections once their CD4 levels fall. Very often the infection comprises reactivation of a previously acquired infection that has remained latent. Some infections (for example tuberculosis) occur early in the disease when immunosuppression is only mild but when the immunodeficiency becomes severe even poorly pathogenic organisms (for example protozoa) become a problem and are very difficult to treat (Figure 25.7). The most common infection is by *Pneumocystis carinii*, and PCP is often the principal presenting clinical condition in AIDS. Other protozoan infections encountered are toxoplasmosis, cryptosporidiosis and microsporidiosis.

Pneumocystis carinii pneumonia

This is a prime cause of death in AIDS. However, the monitoring of HIV-infected individuals has enabled prophylactic antibiotic treatment to be introduced, with the consequence that PCP now comprises a smaller proportion of the initial AIDS-defining conditions. With improved survival resulting from the early treatment of the infection the more unusual conditions such as

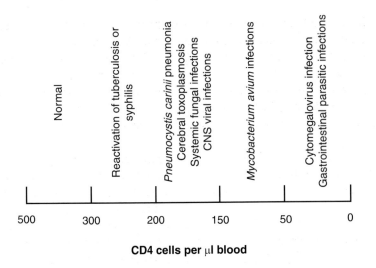

Figure 25.7 Opportunistic infections in HIV-positive individuals. Low CD4 counts in HIV infection increase the risk of opportunistic infections, beginning with reactivation of previously acquired infections such as tuberculosis and syphilis. As the CD4 count falls further the normally less pathogenic organisms become more problematic.

non-Hodgkin's lymphoma and primary CNS lymphoma are becoming more common in AIDS.

The symptoms of PCP are persistent, non-productive cough, shortness of breath and fever. The organism can also cause systemic infection. Treatment should be initiated as soon as possible, with nebulised pentamidine or co-trimoxazole. Prophylactic treatment is increasingly used, particularly in patients whose CD4 counts fall below 200 cells/µl. Only the nebulised form of pentamidine is effective in the prevention of lung infection.

Toxoplasmosis

Toxoplasmosis in AIDS is usually reactivation of a previously acquired infection. The organism most commonly causes encephalitis and cerebral abscesses. Treatment, with pyrimethamine in combination with sulphonamide drugs, is usually successful in controlling the condition but does not eradicate the organism responsible. Lifelong maintenance doses are required to prevent relapse.

Cryptosporidiosis

In people with a normal immune response *Cryptosporidium parvum* can cause a self-limiting acute diarrhoea. However in immunocompromised individuals the diarrhoea is severe and may be associated with abdominal pain, nausea

Keratoconjunctivitis: inflammation of the conjunctiva, near the cornea.

and vomiting. No agents are effective against this organism: rehydration and other supportive therapies are all that can be offered.

Microsporidiosis

The most commonly encountered microsporidial infection in humans is *Enterocytozoon bieneusi*. This organism usually infects the small intestine but lung infections have been reported in patients with AIDS. Other microsporidial protozoans cause keratoconjunctivitis. Microsporidiosis is now the most common cause of diarrhoea in AIDS (with a prevalence of about 40%) in the UK and USA, and furthers weight loss in these patients by malabsorption.

Tuberculosis

Tuberculosis is endemic in many of the countries now facing the spread of HIV. Some individuals with tuberculosis are able to contain the infection by an active immune response. When this becomes compromised by HIV infection the original tuberculosis is reactivated. There is also evidence that people with HIV can acquire tuberculosis.

The pattern of disease in immunosuppressed patients is different from that usually seen, with a greater likelihood of extrapulmonary and disseminated disease. The infection usually responds to the normal treatment, although multidrug resistance can occur. Treatment is not curative and lifelong maintenance therapy with isoniazid is required.

Disseminated *Mycobacterium avium* complex

Disseminated *Mycobacterium avium* complex disease (MAC) is becoming increasingly common. It causes lymphadenitis, pulmonary lesions and disseminated disease. Infection is associated with poor survival prospects and the condition is debilitating. About 20% of patients die in the first 12 weeks of treatment; median survival is about 7 months. The condition can be treated with clarithromycin or azithromycin but there is a high frequency of side-effects which necessitate withdrawal of the drug (in about 35% of patients) and treatment failure (50%) because of the development of drug resistance.

Viral infections

Cytomegalovirus infections are common in HIV-infected patients, particularly in the later stages of the disease. The usual problems are retinitis and colitis, although oesophagitis, encephalitis and pneumonia also occur. Treatment with the antiviral agents ganciclovir or foscarnet often halts the symptoms but does not completely eradicate the virus responsible and hence it may recur. Recurrent cytomegalovirus retinitis leads to blindness.

Herpes simplex infections are exacerbated in people with HIV. Therapy

(with acyclovir) is effective although recurrences are frequent. Occasionally resistant herpes strains are encountered, but these may respond to foscarnet.

Papovavirus infection can cause a demyelinating disease of the cerebral white matter. The clinical features are of progressive neurological or intellectual impairment. No specific treatment is available for this condition.

Fungal infections

The principal fungal infections that become problematic in HIV infection are *Cryptococcus* and *Candida*. Cryptococcus is a cause of HIV-associated meningitis, pneumonia and disseminated infection. It is treated with intravenous amphotericin B or fluconazole, although the organism is not usually eradicated and continued therapy with fluconazole will be required.

Infection of the oropharyngeal, oesophageal and vulvovaginal mucous membranes by *Candida* is frequent in HIV-infected patients. Treatment is usually with systemic antifungal agents.

AIDS and cancer

One of the features of AIDS is the development of certain cancers that are rarely seen in healthy people. The first cancer to be recognised in AIDS was Kaposi's sarcoma, but primary CNS lymphomas, high-grade B-cell lymphomas and atypical Hodgkin's disease are also seen more frequently in AIDS patients than in the general population. A feature of all the AIDS-associated cancers is that they follow a much more aggressive course and respond less well to treatment than in individuals without HIV infection.

To some extent AIDS-associated cancers probably result from immunodeficiency caused by HIV infection: Kaposi's sarcoma and non-Hodgkin's lymphomas are also associated with other congenital and acquired immune deficiencies. The immunocompromised state is thought to enhance the acquisition and pathogenicity of other viruses with oncogenic potential, such as HPV and Epstein–Barr virus.

Kaposi's sarcoma

Before the AIDS epidemic this type of tumour was principally confined to men over the age of 50, in whom it appeared as a localised nodular blue or purple tumour on the lower extremities, and usually followed a slow and benign course.

Kaposi's sarcoma is now much more commonly seen in patients with AIDS; since the start of the epidemic in the USA more than 24 000 cases have been reported to the CDC. Most of these cases are in homosexual or bisexual men of average age 34 years. At the beginning of the AIDS epidemic 35–40% of cases had Kaposi's sarcoma, but the incidence appears to have fallen to about 14% of all reported AIDS cases.

▲ **Key points**

AIDS and cancer

AIDS-defining conditions:
▲ Kaposi's sarcoma
▲ High-grade non-Hodgkin's B-cell lymphoma
▲ Primary CNS lymphoma

Other associations:
▲ Intermediate grade non-Hodgkin's B-cell lymphoma
▲ Hodgkin's disease
▲ Non-Hodgkin's T-cell lymphomas
▲ Cervical neoplasia
▲ Anal cancer

Burkitt's lymphoma: very common tumour in some parts of Africa, but also occurs sporadically in non-endemic areas. Mostly found in children and young adults and involves the maxilla or mandible. The bowel, retroperitoneum and ovaries are more likely to be involved in non-African cases of the tumour.

Non-Hodgkin's lymphoma: non-tender local or general lymphadenopathy. Originates in lymph nodes or lymphoid tissues in the oropharynx, skin, gut and bone marrow. May eventually spread to spleen, bone marrow and liver, producing features akin to leukaemia in the peripheral blood. Classified on the basis of cell of origin, determined by morphology and cell surface markers.

It is now believed that a virus known as Kaposi's sarcoma-associated herpesvirus (KSHV) is primarily responsible for the production of Kaposi's sarcoma. This virus is present in nearly all Kaposi's sarcoma lesions both in the presence and absence of HIV co-infection. Presumably, HIV infection and consequent immunosuppression render an individual more susceptible to infection by KSHV.

The clinical presentation of Kaposi's sarcoma in AIDS is different from that of the classical syndrome seen in older men. In AIDS the tumour is much more widespread and follows a rapidly progressive course to involve almost every organ, except the brain. The distribution of the tumours in the skin is also different, involving the trunk, arms, head and neck and only occasionally the lower extremities.

The histological features of AIDS-related Kaposi's sarcoma are similar to those of the classical disease – the principal difference being the extent of the disease. The tumour is believed to be derived from lymphatic endothelium and hence the number of thin-walled vessels in the dermis increases. This proliferation is accompanied by presence of scattered spindle-shaped cells and an inflammatory infiltrate.

The treatment of Kaposi's sarcoma involves surgical excision, cryothermy or injection of the cytotoxic drug vincristine into the lesion. In some areas, such as the face, hands, feet, oral cavity and anus, use of X-rays may be more appropriate. Patients with widespread Kaposi's sarcoma may be treated with single or combined systemic chemotherapy.

Non-Hodgkin's lymphoma

The relative risk of non-Hodgkin's lymphoma in HIV infection is 60–100 times that of the general population. High-grade B-cell lymphomas in HIV-infected people are classified as an AIDS-defining condition. The disease is seen earlier in HIV infection (mean age 38 years) than in the uninfected general population (mean age 56 years).

In some cases the lymphoma remains silent but usually presents with malaise and fever or a rapidly enlarging mass. The disease is usually advanced at the time of diagnosis (stage III or IV). Cancers at sites other than the lymph nodes (such as the CNS, bone marrow, gastrointestinal tract and liver) are more common in HIV-infected patients.

The prognosis for the HIV-positive patient with non-Hodgkin's lymphoma is much worse (median survival only 5 months) than that of patients without immunodeficiency. Treatment with cytotoxic agents is less effective and results in further immunological impairment and risk of opportunistic infection.

The main risk factor for the development of lymphoma is the presence of Epstein–Barr virus. The association between this virus and B-cell lymphoma is well known; for example virtually all cases of Burkitt's lymphoma in Africa are associated with the virus. Epstein–Barr infections are common in all populations, causing glandular fever (infectious mononucleosis) but when the individual is immunosuppressed it is more likely to be oncogenic.

Primary CNS lymphoma

Up to 2% of all individuals with HIV are likely to develop primary CNS lymphoma. This is in contrast to the general population, in whom brain tumours are rare (1–2% of all necropsies), and of these only 1–2% are caused by primary lymphoma.

Patients with HIV-related primary lymphoma usually present with a cognitive or focal neurological defect, seizures or headache. The diagnosis is often difficult because AIDS is also associated with other nervous system diseases, such as toxoplasmosis, which have similar symptoms. These are indistinguishable by CT scanning, and definitive diagnosis requires a brain biopsy. The course of primary CNS lymphoma in AIDS is very rapid and survival beyond a few months would not be expected, even with treatment. The treatment for this group of patients is usually radiotherapy.

Hodgkin's disease

Other malignant conditions are associated with HIV infection but are not considered as AIDS indicators, although their presentation is often unusual. One of these is Hodgkin's disease. Usually the age incidence of this condition is bimodal, with a peak in early adulthood, followed by a plateau, and then a further peak in old age. In AIDS-associated disease the incidence between 35 and 49 years is much higher. The stage of presentation is also different, with more patients presenting with stage III or IV disease (83% compared with 40% in the non HIV-infected population). Disease is also seen in unusual extranodal sites such as the CNS, gastrointestinal tract and skin.

Patients with HIV respond to conventional chemotherapy for Hodgkin's disease but the mortality rate is high because of opportunistic infection. Median survival ranges from 8 to 15 months.

Cervical neoplasia

The incidence of cervical neoplasia (see Chapter 16) is greater in women with HIV. One cross-sectional study showed that the prevalence of neoplasia (CIN I, II or III) was 40% in women infected with HIV, compared with only 6% of women in an HIV-negative control group (Branca *et al.*, 1995). This observation may reflect differences in lifestyle, such as number of sexual partners or injecting drug use, but is more likely to be a consequence of HIV-induced immunosuppression. The loss of cell-mediated immunity probably facilitates infection by HPV and the induction or progression of HPV-induced cervical neoplasia.

Loss of cell-mediated immunity following HIV infection is thought to facilitate the progression of concomitant HPV infection; hence the increase in HPV-induced neoplasia.

Hodgkin's lymphoma: usually arises in a single lymph node or chain of nodes. Distinguished from non-Hodgkin's lymphoma by the presence of distinctive Reed–Sternberg giant cells, with systemic symptoms including fever.

Lymphoma: malignancy of lymphoid origin (derived from lymphocytes or histiocytes and their precursors or derivatives). All types are lethal unless treated, usually with cytotoxic drugs.

Encephalitis: inflammation of the brain. May be focal with abscess formation or diffuse, causing only occasional cell death.

Meningitis: inflammation of the meninges (membranes surrounding the brain) and subarachnoid space. Most commonly caused by infection, but also by chemical agents or tumour infiltration.

Anal cancer

Rates of anal cancer in both men and women have dramatically increased in the USA and Europe. The reasons for this are unclear but may reflect changes in sexual habits and exposure to HPV. Among men, a history of homosexual activity, presumably involving receptive anal intercourse, is recognised as a strong risk factor. A higher incidence of anal cancer has been observed in HIV-infected homosexual men, which probably reflects concomitant or sequential acquisition of HIV and HPV. Infection with HIV probably results in reduced immunity to HPV. In common with cervical cancer, anal cancer is preceded by morphologically distinguishable precancerous lesions and is probably preventable.

Nervous system involvement

Infection with HIV has several manifestations in the nervous system. Some arise from the primary HIV infection itself but others are caused by the immunosuppressive effects of the virus. The most common neurological complications in AIDS are meningitis, AIDS–dementia complex, encephalitis and primary malignant lymphoma. Patients are also at increased risk of cerebrovascular disease.

Meningitis

A lymphocytic meningitis develops in some patients around the time of seroconversion; usually they recover spontaneously. The chronic meningitis that can be produced in response to HIV infection itself, or is caused by infection with fungi (for example *Cryptococcus neoformans* or *Aspergillus*), tuberculosis or bacteria such as *Escherichia coli* is much more serious. Treatment is often difficult or unsuccessful.

AIDS–dementia complex

The AIDS–dementia complex is believed to be caused by primary HIV infection of the nervous system. It has clinical elements of intellectual impairment, behavioural, and motor changes. The condition is progressive and usually fatal.

Encephalitis

This is characterised by the presence of inflammatory and multinucleated giant cells, usually in the white matter, basal ganglia and brainstem. The most typical causative agents are herpes simplex, *Toxoplasma* and cytomegalovirus. The encephalitis is often severe and fatal.

Diagnosis of HIV infection and investigation of AIDS symptoms

The most commonly used test for HIV relies on the detection of IgG to the gp12 viral envelope protein. All IgG antibodies cross the placenta, and hence a baby born to an HIV-positive mother will also be HIV-positive, regardless of whether HIV is actually present. The maternal antibody is gradually lost during the first 18 months of life, and so the test is a more reliable indicator of infection in a child after this period. In adults up to 3 months may elapse between the initial infection and the production of antibodies, during which time the test results will be negative.

Viral antigen (p24) and antibodies to this antigen can be detected in the blood shortly after infection. The viral antigen usually disappears 8–10 weeks after exposure. These markers are therefore useful for the detection of very recent exposure.

Skin lesions

The diagnosis of Kaposi's sarcoma is made by histological examination of a skin biopsy. The appearances are of spindle-shaped cells, intracellular clefts and extravasated blood cells.

Respiratory symptoms

Usually chest radiography, sputum cytology and possibly histological examination of a bronchial biopsy will be performed. In addition to excluding non-HIV-related illness the opportunistic agent must be identified. The most common cause of respiratory dysfunction in HIV-related illness is *Pneumocystis carinii*. Other less common causes are concomitant cytomegalovirus and fungal infections and Kaposi's sarcoma.

Radiography

The chest radiograph may be normal in the early stages of *Pneumocystis carinii* infection. The usual appearance is of a perihilar haze. This can progress to a diffuse symmetrical shadowing in the mid and lower zones. Radiographic appearances in cytomegalovirus infection may be similar, although reticular shadowing extending to the periphery of the lung field is more common. In Kaposi's sarcoma the radiographic abnormalities are more likely to be unilateral or nodular than diffuse.

Sputum analysis

Pneumocystis carinii can identified by cytological staining and sputum culture. However, this is not a definitive test and produces a large number of false-negative results.

Bronchoscopy: direct inspection of the larynx, trachea and bronchi through a metal bronchoscope or flexible fibreoptic instrument. A catheter brush or biopsy forceps can be passed through the instrument to obtain bronchial secretions or small tissue samples.

Bronchoscopy, bronchial lavage, open lung biopsy

These methods are used to obtain cell or tissue samples for cytological or histological examination. Bronchial lavage is the least invasive and has a 90% sensitivity for *Pneumocystis carinii*; it is less reliable for the diagnosis of cytomegalovirus or Kaposi's sarcoma. Bronchoscopy and biopsy are more reliable and are usually associated with low morbidity and mortality. Occasionally an open lung biopsy may be needed to detect Kaposi's sarcoma, cytomegalovirus or some fungal organisms. The response to treatment is sometimes used as a diagnostic tool when initial tests are inconclusive and immediate therapy is required.

Gastrointestinal symptoms

Many HIV-positive patients experience diarrhoea. This usually prompts investigation to identify possible infectious or malignant causes. Enteric organisms causing diarrhoea can be identified in stool specimens. Endoscopy with biopsy and culture may also be used. Kaposi's sarcoma and lymphomas usually appear as patchy ulceration with submucosal haemorrhage.

Oesophageal candidiasis is also common and can be seen by endoscopy as a flat superficial exudate or as a raised 'cottage cheese' lesion with deep ulceration. Cytomegalovirus or herpes simplex oesophagitis are diagnosed by biopsy and culture.

Treatment

Treatments for AIDS fall into three categories:
1. Those targeted at preventing replication of the virus
2. Those aimed at prophylaxis or control of AIDS-related infections and malignancies
3. Those aimed at restoring lost immune function by stimulating immune system cellular constituents

The problems surrounding the treatment of HIV and AIDS are both technological and economic. The technological problems concern the general ineffectiveness of drug treatments to combat viral infections and the changing nature of the virus because of mutation. Given the research effort currently under way, together with fundamental advances in molecular biology, treatment prospects could be expected to improve in the next 10 or 20 years. It is the economic problems that are more likely to be insurmountable. As one commentator has put it, even if a cure for AIDS was no more than a glass of dirty water, it would still be beyond the reach of many sufferers in Africa.

Antiviral therapy

A number of antiretroviral agents are available that work by inhibiting reverse transcriptase. These include zidovudine (azidothymidine, AZT) didanosine

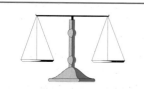

CONCORDE

Immediate vs. delayed administration of zidovudine

▲ Non-pregnant symptom-free adults with HIV infection

▲ Randomisation into immediate group, given zidovudine (AZT)

▲ Deferred group to be given AZT only after onset of AIDS or AIDS-related complex

▲ 25% of deferred group were given AZT (non-blinded) after low CD4 counts

▲ Median follow-up 3.3 years

▲ No statistically significant differences in survival or disease progression between the two groups

Data from: Concorde Coordinating Committee, 1994.

and dideoxycytidine (zalcitabine).

Zidovudine inhibits the reverse transcriptase enzyme that HIV uses to incorporate itself and replicate within the genome of the human cell, slowing the synthesis of proviral DNA. The first randomised clinical trial of the agent in individuals with AIDS or advanced AIDS-related complex demonstrated a significant reduction in mortality and frequency of opportunistic infections over an average follow-up time of 4 months (Fischl *et al.*, 1987). The main effect is a transient rise in CD4 lymphocytes and a fall in blood levels of p24 viral core antigen. This is often reflected in a marked improvement in the general condition of the patient. Unfortunately HIV resistance can develop in patients with advanced disease who have been on therapy for longer than 6 months.

The side-effects of zidovudine treatment are usually nausea, vomiting, malaise and headaches. These can be managed by dose reduction. A common toxic effect is bone marrow suppression, particularly involving the red blood cell line. Adverse reactions are more frequent in patients with advanced disease.

It was hoped that initiation of therapy soon after a person is diagnosed as having HIV would delay disease progression and improve survival. This was tested in the Concorde clinical trial (see p. 784), but no significant differences in survival or disease progression were seen in those given immediate zidovudine treatment compared with those whose treatment was deferred until the onset of AIDS or AIDS-related complex, or who were treated on the basis of low CD4 counts. There were some improvements in CD4 counts in the individuals treated earlier, but this was not translated into any clinical benefit. The follow-up period in the trial was 3 years, during which time 172 of the 1749 participants had died (22 from unrelated causes). Longer follow-up could still reveal differences in disease or survival prospects.

The optimal time for starting zidovudine treatment remains unclear, and the gains in limiting disease progression by early treatment have to be balanced against drug toxicity and its impact on quality of life. However, one asymptomatic group that could benefit substantially from early zidovudine treatment is pregnant women and their offspring – there is evidence that this reduces vertical transmission of HIV.

In a double-blind randomised trial, the Paediatric AIDS Clinical Trials Study Group (ACTG) compared the results of giving zidovudine to the mother during pregnancy and to the newborn infant with placebo (Connor *et al.*, 1994). A marked reduction in HIV-infected infants was seen in the group treated with the antiretroviral agent. These results are so encouraging that the clinical trial had to be interrupted so that the benefits could be made available to all HIV-infected pregnant women.

There are, however, some unanswered questions. Because the trial was limited to women with only mild or moderate immunosuppression it is not known how effective treatment would be in women with more advanced disease (the risk of vertical HIV transmission is higher with advanced disease). It is also not known whether there is any benefit to be gained by giving zidovudine to women who have previously been treated with the drug: it is likely in this

> *There is no advantage in starting zidovudine therapy in men and non-pregnant women who do not yet have symptoms of AIDS*

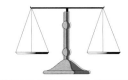

ACTG (076 protocol)

Administration of zidovudine during pregnancy and in the newborn vs. placebo

▲ Double-blind randomised trial in women who had not previously received zidovudine during pregnancy

▲ All women had CD4 counts above 200 cells/μl

▲ Drug or placebo given for a median 11 weeks before birth (range 0–26 weeks)

▲ Treatment continued during delivery, and in newborn for 6 weeks

▲ Total of 409 women gave birth to 415 live babies (205 women in group receiving zidovudine)

▲ Babies were not breast fed

▲ In group receiving zidovudine 13 (8.3%) HIV-infected infants were born; compared with 40 (25.5%) in group receiving placebo

▲ Risk of mother-to-infant HIV transmission reduced by two-thirds

Data from: Connor et al., 1994.

situation that the virus will be zidovudine resistant. Further information on the stage at which treatment might be most effective would also be useful, since many HIV-infected women do not receive antenatal care.

Combination and sequential use of antiretroviral agents

Second-line antiretroviral therapies can be offered to patients who develop adverse reactions to zidovudine or who become drug resistant. The two agents available are didanosine and zalcitabine. Didanosine is associated with the side-effects of painful neuritis and pancreatitis. Unlike zidovudine therapy, bone marrow toxicity is rare but HIV becomes resistant to the drug by mutations that cause changes to reverse transcriptase.

Clinical trials of didanosine and zalcitabine therapies have revealed that their effectiveness depends on whether the patient had been previously treated with zidovudine. For example, the AIDS Clinical Trials Group (Collier *et al*., 1996) compared a combination of zidovudine and zalcitabine with zalcitabine alone or zidovudine alone in patients who had previously been treated with zidovudine. No marked differences in outcome were seen, except that in a small group of patients (with CD4 counts higher than 150 cells/μl) the combined treatments offered an advantage in terms of clinical progression.

Combination retroviral therapy is most useful in patients who have not been previously treated with zidovudine

Similar results were seen in the Delta 2 trial, which compared combinations of zidovudine, didanosine and zalcitabine with zidovudine alone in patients with HIV, AIDS or AIDS-related complex. When randomised for treatment at the beginning of the trial 17% of patients already had AIDS or AIDS-related complex; the remainder had a CD4 count below 350 cells/μl and had already taken zidovudine for at least 3 months. Much more promising results were produced in the Delta 1 trial (Choo, 1995), which randomised patients not previously treated with zidovudine to the same treatment combination (12% of patients had AIDS or AIDS-related complex at randomisation). The median follow-up in both trials was 26 months (Figure 25.8).

A new category of drugs for treating HIV infection has been developed that block the activity of a protease enzyme needed for viral replication. These **protease inhibitors** (ritonavir, indinavir, saquinavir), are currently undergoing clinical trials and some encouraging results have already been forthcoming. The inhibitors effectively reduce the load of virus in the bloodstream, which in turn appears to influence the eventual outcome (Figure 25.9).

Protease inhibitors can reduce the HIV load in the body, prolong life and reduce complications

In a randomised placebo-controlled clinical trial conducted among over 1000 advanced AIDS patients world-wide (reported by Cohen, 1996 and Richman, 1996), ritonavir reduced mortality by about 50% in patients treated for up to 7 months (13% of patients died or developed a new AIDS-related illness, compared with 27% of patients who received placebo). All patients had CD4 counts below 100 cells/μl blood (normal CD4 counts are above 600) and most participants had also taken other anti-HIV drugs. The viral load was reduced by a factor of about six during the 4 months of the trial.

Another trial compared indinavir with the reverse transcriptase inhibitors

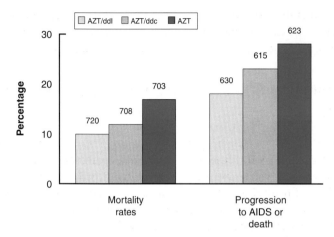

Figure 25.8 Delta 1 trial of combination therapy in HIV-infected patients. Combination therapy appears effective provided that patients have not been previously treated with zidovudine. The most effective combination for slowing the progression of HIV to AIDS, and mortality from AIDS, appears to be zidovudine with didanosine (AZT/ddl). (Data from Choo, 1995.)

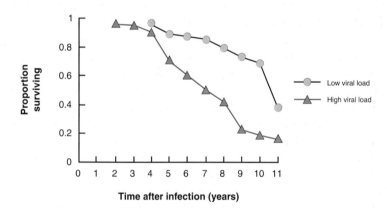

Figure 25.9 HIV load and survival. The survival prospects of HIV-infected patients is influenced by the baseline viral load, independently of the starting CD4 counts which were virtually identical (in the normal range) for both groups. High viral load is more than 10 190 copies of HIV RNA/ml blood; low load is below 10 190 copies/ml. (Adapted from Cohen, 1996.)

zidovudine and lamivudine (reported by Cohen, 1996 and Richman, 1996). Nearly 100 patients were split into three treatment groups: indinavir alone, zidovudine with lamivudine, or all three drugs. At the beginning of the trial all the patients had a high viral load (in excess of 20 000 copies of HIV RNA/ml blood). After 6 months the viral load had fallen to undetectable levels in the large majority of patients who had received all three drugs. At the time of writing the trial had not continued long enough to see whether the response translates into improved clinical outcome. In addition, undetectable virus in

the blood does not necessarily signify that all virus infection has been cleared from the body. A possible problem is that the HIV protease gene may mutate to cause drug resistance. The drugs appear fairly well tolerated, although 13% of patients in the ritonavir trial dropped out because of nausea, diarrhoea, vomiting and fatigue.

Prophylaxis of HIV-related infections

Prophylactic treatments can be used to prevent opportunistic infections in patients with AIDS or AIDS-related complex

The most common life-threatening opportunistic infection in AIDS patients is PCP. It is now recognised from the results of prospective studies that vulnerability to this infection markedly increases when the patient's CD4 count falls below 220 cells/μl. This finding offers a well defined circumstance in which prophylactic treatment can be initiated, and indeed since the late 1980s it is now the standard care protocol for HIV-infected patients.

As a result there has been a marked decline in the incidence of PCP as an AIDS-defining disease. The agents most frequently used are pentamidine (aerosol) or oral trimethoprim-sulphamethoxazole. The latter is more effective and is widely accepted as the regimen of choice for patients who can tolerate it. It is also active against other opportunistic infections such as toxoplasmosis and certain bacteria including *Staphylococcus aureus*, *Haemophilus influenzae*, *Streptococcus pneumoniae* and *Salmonella*. Adverse reactions include fever, rash, nausea, vomiting and bone marrow suppression.

The success of this prophylaxis has resulted in extension of the concept to other AIDS-related pathogens: toxoplasmosis, *M. avium* and *M. tuberculosis*. Studies to date have yielded encouraging results in preventing diseases caused by these pathogens in HIV-infected patients, and a strategy for multiple opportunistic pathogen prophylaxis is evolving. Undoubtedly these interventions will increase survival of HIV-infected patients, but will also change the clinical course so that malignancies become more common as the AIDS-defining illnesses and ultimate causes of death. There are also issues concerning compliance with the large number of drugs that need to be taken, adverse drug interactions and the potential for encouraging the emergence of resistant organisms.

Attempts have also been made to stimulate the immune system in HIV-infected individuals. One group of agents currently under consideration are the interferons, which have antiviral properties and are able to modulate the immune response.

Development of a vaccine against HIV

In common with many other viruses (for example those causing the common cold) HIV mutates readily, making development of a vaccine against the virus extremely difficult. A further problem is that the production of a vaccine against the virus is no guarantee of success – after all, patients mount an antibody response against the virus but this is ineffective. This is because the virus is

transmitted directly from one cell to another and hence remains 'hidden' from antibodies present in body fluids. The virus also arrives within the body already wrapped within a cell.

Protection might be given by enhancing cell-mediated immunity rather than by stimulating antibody production. Cell-mediated responses to HIV may be the reason why some people who are at particular risk of acquiring infection remain disease free. It is necessary therefore to find ways of enhancing cell-mediated responses. This can be achieved with vaccination, using a very low dose. Any vaccine would probably be a 'cocktail', with activities against the principal virus mutations, but considerable technical problems need to be overcome in its development. Even if vaccines do become available it is unlikely that they would offer 100% protection and it will still be necessary to take the appropriate lifestyle precautions against infection.

So far more than 20 candidate vaccines are in various phases of evaluation in both uninfected people and in those with asymptomatic HIV infection. In patients already infected with HIV the hope is that the vaccine will further stimulate the immune system. One vaccine, comprising gp160 (the outer viral coat protein) manufactured by recombinant DNA technology, has been given to both healthy volunteers and people with asymptomatic infection. It has produced a limited immune response in the healthy volunteers and has slowed the decline in CD4 cell counts compared with controls given placebo (in 10 months follow up). Whether the limited immune response produced in the healthy volunteers actually affords any protection against HIV cannot be determined (this would require deliberate HIV infection) and therefore animal studies must be used.

Animal research directed towards understanding the molecular biology of HIV and the production of vaccines has been hindered because the virus is not pathogenic in many species. Rhesus monkeys may be infected with HIV-2 and with a related virus, called SIV. Research is now under way to compare the infective and pathogenic potential of HIV and SIV isolates in these monkeys with a view to developing a vaccine. So far, a vaccine consisting of recombinant SIV genetic material has been shown to provide protection in animals subsequently challenged with the complete virus.

Strategies for the prevention of HIV infection

In most developed countries the initial strategy for preventing HIV infection used extensive media campaigns targeted at the general population. This was at least partly based on the assumption that HIV infection would spread rapidly into the heterosexual population. This has not occurred in the UK, and efforts have been retargeted to those groups at special risk – homosexual and bisexual men, injecting drug users and their sexual partners, male or female. In addition fundamental changes have been made to the handling of blood and tissue products, comprising virus screening, heat treatment where possible and substitution with recombinant DNA products.

Review question 2

What can be done to reduce the risk of vertical HIV transmission?

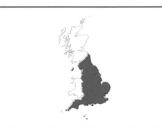

HEALTH OF THE NATION

Targets for HIV/AIDS and sexual health

▲ Reduce the incidence of gonorrhoea among men and women aged 15–64 by at least 20% by 1995 (from 61 new cases per 100 000 population in 1990 to no more than 49)

▲ Reduce the rate of conceptions among girls under 16 by at least 50% by the year 2000 (from 9.5 per 1000 girls aged 13–15 in 1989 to no more than 4.8)

▲ Reduce the percentage of injecting drug abusers who report having shared injecting equipment in the previous 4 weeks by at least 50% by 1997 and a further 50% by 2000 (from 20% in 1990 to no more than 5%)

In the UK the strategy for preventing AIDS forms part of the overall programme for improving sexual health. The principal aim is the prevention of STDs such as gonorrhoea, because these infections are acquired in a similar fashion to HIV and increase the susceptibility for HIV infection. A further aim is to reduce the number of drug users who share needles and syringes. This would have some impact on the transmission of hepatitis B and HIV infections, in both homosexual and heterosexual populations.

The objectives are to:

- Reduce the incidence of HIV infection
- Reduce the incidence of other sexually transmitted diseases
- Further develop and strengthen disease monitoring and surveillance
- Provide effective services for the diagnosis and treatment of HIV and other sexually transmitted diseases
- Reduce the number of unwanted pregnancies
- Ensure the provision of effective family planning services for those who want them

At the local community level this translates into actions aimed at ensuring that:

- Young people receive appropriate education concerning HIV and AIDS, the hazards of drug use, and the best environment for exploring relationships and sexual experience
- Condoms, lubricant and clean injecting equipment are freely available to those who need them
- Prevention work is developed and integrated within the primary health team
- Information, support and resources are available to those within the criminal justice system
- Services are developed to promote and protect the health of people who are already infected

More work is aimed at identifying the sexual health needs of patients attending genitourinary clinics. This would include giving advice on the prevention of transmission of STDs generally and on the use of contact tracing to bring high-risk partners into contact with appropriate health care professionals. Outreach work is also conducted in the places where men meet in order to make sexual contacts – public toilets, saunas, clubs and pubs.

Adequate counselling is also needed. This should be provided before the test for HIV is undertaken, and informed consent to the test must be obtained before blood is taken. It will be necessary to discuss the reasons for testing, regardless of whether the request for testing was initiated by the patient or by health care personnel. It may also be appropriate to offer screening for other infections such as hepatitis B. It must be emphasised that the test is not for AIDS but for HIV infection, and that there is a 'window period' before infection becomes evident.

The implications of a positive result are profound. Perhaps the least of these is that the person could face difficulties in obtaining life insurance or, in countries with insurance-based health care systems, sufficient cover for care

when the condition eventually progresses to AIDS. The patient will show the psychological effects of anger, guilt and denial, and personal relationships will be affected. Although confidentiality of testing must be assured, a positive result will mean that any sexual contacts of an HIV-positive person will also be at risk. It is not surprising that many personal relationships break up after a positive test result.

How safe is 'safe' sex?

Heterosexual intercourse

On a world-wide basis the vast majority of cases of AIDS are acquired through sexual intercourse between men and women. There is almost universal agreement that the best way of avoiding AIDS is abstinence from sex, or to remain in a monogamous relationship with an uninfected partner. Human relationships being what they are, these suggestions are impractical for many people. The next best course, therefore, is to engage in 'safe sex'. This essentially means that a condom should be used during oral and penetrative sex. Prospective studies have shown that consistent condom use is virtually 100% effective in preventing seroconversion in heterosexuals of whom one partner is known to be HIV-positive. Condom use is less effective in preventing anal transmission of HIV because the risk of condom failure is greater and transmission is easier during this form of sexual contact. There are problems with the supply, cost and acceptability of using condoms. In a prospective study of heterosexual couples, nearly 50% continued to have unprotected sex despite repeated counselling. More than 10% of the uninfected partners will become infected within 2 years.

In African countries the risks of acquiring HIV through heterosexual intercourse are similar for both the man and the woman. In other countries, however, the risk is greater for the woman, possibly due the larger mucosal surface that could be exposed to the virus and the greater duration of exposure from semen deposited in the vagina and cervical canal.

Condoms offer the best physical barrier to HIV

The choice of other contraceptives can also modify the risk of acquiring HIV. Other barrier methods, such as the diaphragm and the female condom, have not been extensively evaluated. Tests have demonstrated that the female condom does present an effective physical barrier to HIV, and therefore there is no reason (in theory) why it should be any more or less effective than the male condom. The diaphragm may offer less protection because it covers only the cervix. Although the cervix is probably the most susceptible area for HIV transmission, exposure of the vagina alone can result in HIV infection. The spermicide nonoxynol-9 is active against a variety of bacterial and fungal agents: it is also active *in vitro* against HIV. However, studies conducted in high-risk populations (such as prostitutes) so far do not support a protective role for the spermicide, and it is possible that nonoxynol-9 enhances HIV transmission by causing vaginal irritation. Similarly, there are fears that endometrial trauma induced by an intrauterine device (IUD) could also increase the risk of transmission above that for a woman who engages in

intercourse without contraceptive protection. The epidemiological studies available are not conclusive, but tend to support this hypothesis. In any case, the IUD is not generally recommended for women with multiple sexual partners because of its association with pelvic inflammatory disease.

Other contraceptive methods, such as oral contraceptives and tubal ligation, offer no protection because they present no physical barrier, but there is also no reason to expect that these methods would exacerbate the risk. Although vasectomy reduces the sperm content of the ejaculate, leukocytes and HIV may persist and therefore the method should not be relied on to prevent viral transmission. In short, methods that are effective in preventing pregnancy are not necessarily effective in preventing the acquisition of HIV or any other STDs.

> *Other STDs are important cofactors in facilitating the transmission of HIV-1*

Homosexual practices

The probability of encountering HIV increases with the number of sexual partners. The type of sexual practice also determines the exposure of vulnerable sites (particularly mucosa) to infected body fluids and hence the likelihood of HIV acquisition. The greatest risk is attached to unprotected receptive anal intercourse. Susceptibility to infection increases further in the presence of an ulcerative STD (for example herpes simplex).

Until recently, receptive orogenital sex was generally regarded as 'safe' but there have been reports of seroconversion in individuals who deny having engaged in receptive anogenital intercourse. Insertive anogenital intercourse and insertive orogenital sex are less risky – the greatest danger is to the receptive partner. Most homosexual men engage in both insertive and receptive practices.

The main health education message for gay men is to avoid anogenital intercourse. If this restriction is unacceptable a condom will give some protection. Although there is a risk attached to orogenital sex, this is comparatively small and consequently many people concerned with health education prefer to use a less forceful message for this kind of activity, fearing that a 'ban' on everything will encourage a return to anogenital intercourse. The small risk attached to orogenital sex will be further reduced by condom use.

Review question 3

What advice would you give to enable people to protect themselves against HIV infection?

ANSWERS TO REVIEW QUESTIONS

Question 1

Explain why HIV is not contagious by casual contact

The answer to this question lies in the requirement for HIV to replicate within lymphocytes. These find their way into body fluids, which would then contain both infected lymphocytes and free virus particles. Blood and semen have a much higher viral load than nasal secretions, saliva and urine. Other factors that influence transmission are the accessibility of body surfaces and, probably, the duration of contact. Free virus does not survive very long in the general

environment and there is little chance of transmission from outside sources. Accessibility is improved by breaches in epithelium due to injury or other infections (particularly STDs). Deposition of HIV and infected lymphocytes in the rectum or vagina is an excellent way of prolonging contact, as is direct injection. It is impossible to acquire HIV by shaking hands, hugging, drinking from the same cup, being sneezed or coughed on or using public toilets.

What can be done to reduce the risk of vertical HIV transmission?   **Question 2**

At present the most effective means of limiting the vertical transmission of HIV is to treat the woman during pregnancy and the baby in the first few weeks of life with zidovudine. This presumes that the mother is aware of her HIV status or is willing to be tested, that she has access to the health care system and that resources are available for treatment. These criteria are not likely to apply to less developed countries – even in the USA the provision of HIV screening, counselling and treatment in pregnancy is extremely patchy. In some, but not all, American states laws require that HIV testing is offered to pregnant women. Even when test results are positive a substantial proportion of women decline treatment.

Another approach is to limit exposure of the baby to infected cervical and vaginal secretions during the birth. One trial in which the birth canal was regularly swabbed with chlorhexidine (an agent shown to have anti-HIV activity) before birth demonstrated no marked reduction in the rate of vertical transmission (Biggar *et al.*, 1996). It may be that transmission at this stage is relatively unimportant, or that the regimen used was ineffective.

Any procedure in which the fetal membranes are ruptured more than 4 hours before delivery, or the placement of an internal fetal scalp electrode, is likely to increase the risk of vertical transmission.

Some babies probably acquire HIV from the mother's milk; therefore HIV-infected mothers should not breast feed. In the less developed countries this advice may be difficult to apply, even if the mother's HIV status is known, because of the cost and availability of formula milk and clean water.

What advice would you give to ensure that people can protect themselves   **Question 3**
against HIV infection?

The main precautions to be taken involve the nature of sexual activity and the use of injecting drugs. Screening has greatly reduced the risk of contracting HIV by blood transfusion or use of blood products. However, the sexual partners of people who are infected remain at risk.

People who have been and remain in monogamous sexual relationships are virtually risk-free of HIV infection. In new sexual relationships barrier methods that prevent the exchange of potentially infectious body fluids are effective if used consistently. Studies have shown that regular condom use is effective, but other methods of contraception such as vaginal diaphragms or cervical

caps that prevent sperm (and lymphocytes) reaching the uterus probably give only limited protection.

Needles or sharp instruments contaminated with the blood of another person should not be handled.

Homosexual men should avoid anal sex and should use condoms during other sexual activities. Homosexual or heterosexual intercourse should be avoided with any person who injects drugs, or who engages in the purchase or sale of sexual favours. Women should avoid intercourse with bisexual men.

Casual sex should be avoided: the principal means of avoiding HIV infection is by building caring and trusting relationships.

References

Biggar, R.J., Miotti, P.G., Taha, E.T. *et al.* (1996) Perinatal intervention trial in Africa: effect of a birth canal cleansing intervention to prevent HIV transmission. *Lancet*, **347**, 1647–50.

Branca, M., Delfino, A., Rossi, E. *et al.* (1995) Cervical intraepithelial neoplasia and human papillomavirus related lesions of the genital tract in HIV positive and negative women. *Eur. J. Gynaecol. Oncol.*, **16**, 410–17.

Centre for Disease Control (1992) 1993 revised classification system for HIV infection and expanded surveillance case definition for AIDS among adolescents and adults. *MMWR*, **41**, December, 1–11.

Choo, V. (1995) Combination superior to zidovidine in Delta trial. *Lancet*, **346**, 895.

Cohen, J. (1996) Results on new AIDS drugs begin cautious optimism. *Science*, **271**, 755–6.

Collier, A.C., Coombs, R.W., Schoenfeld, D.A. *et al.* (1996) Retreatment of human immunodeficiency virus infection with saquinavir, zidovudine and zalcitabine. AIDS Clinical Trials Group. *N. Engl. J. Med.*, **334**, 1011–17.

Concorde Coordinating Committee (1994) Concorde: MRC/ANRS randomised double-blind controlled trial of immediate and deferred zidovudine in symptom-free HIV infection. *Lancet*, **343**, 871–81.

Connor, E.M., Sperling, R.S., Gelber, R. *et al.* (1994) Reduction of maternal-infant transmission of human immunodeficiency virus type 1 with zidovudine treatment. *N. Engl. J. Med.*, **331**, 1173–80.

European Collaborative Study (1994) Caesarean section and risk of vertical transmission of HIV-1 infection. *Lancet*, **343**, 1464–7.

Feng, Y., Broder, C.C., Kennedy, P.E. and Berger, E.A. (1996) HIV-1 entry cofactor: functional cloning of a seven-transmembrane, G protein-coupled receptor. *Science*, **272**, 872–7.

Fischl, M.A., Richman, D.D., Grieko, M.H. *et al.* and the AZT Collaborative Working Group (1987) The efficacy of azidothymidine (AZT) in the treatment of participants with AIDS and AIDS-related complex: a double-blind, placebo-controlled trial. *N. Engl. J. Med.*, **317**, 185–91.

Landesman, S.H., Kalish, L.A., Burns, D.N. *et al.* (1996) Obstetrical factors and

the transmission of human deficiency virus type 1 from mother to child. The Women and Infants Transmission Study. *N. Engl. J. Med.*, **334**, 1617–23.
Richman, D.D. (1996) HIV therapeutics. *Science*, **272**, 1886–8.

Further reading

General
Barter, G., Barton, S. and Gazzard, B. (1993) *HIV and AIDS – Your Questions Answered*, Churchill Livingstone, Edinburgh.

Epidemiology
Barnett, T. and Blaikie, P. (1992) *AIDS in Africa: Its Present and Future Impact*, Belhaven Press, London.
Chin, J., Remenyi, M., Morrison, F. and Bulatao, R. (1992) The global epidemiology of the HIV/AIDS pandemic and its projected demographic impact in Africa. *World Health Stat. Q.*, **45**, 220–7.
Easterbrook, P.J. (1994) Non-progression in HIV infection. *AIDS*, 8, 1179–82.

Virology
Phillips, D.M. (1994) The role of cell-to-cell transmission in HIV infection. *AIDS*, **8**, 719–31.

HIV and malignancy
Safai, B., Diaz, B. and Schwartz, J. (1992) Malignant neoplasms associated with human immunodeficiency virus infection. *CA Cancer J. Clin.*, **42**, 74–94.

Therapy
Decker, C.F. and Masu, H. (1994) Current status of prophylaxis for opportunistic infections in HIV-infected patients. *AIDS*, **8**, 11–20.
Hirsch, M.S. and D'Aquila, R.T. (1993) Therapy for human immunodeficiency virus infection. *N. Engl. J. Med.*, **328**, 1686–95.
Sande, M.A., Carpenter, C.C.J., Cobbs, C.G. *et al.* (1993) Antiretroviral therapy for adult HIV-infected patients: recommendations from state-of-the-art conference. *JAMA*, **270**, 2583–9.
Various authors (1996) The new face of AIDS. *Science*, **272**, 1876–90.

26   Alzheimer's disease

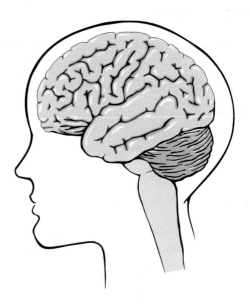

Alzheimer's disease is the principal cause of dementia. Most cases are seen in older people, but an early-onset form can be inherited. The cause of Alzheimer's disease remains uncertain but there is evidence for both genetic and environmental influences. The genetic predisposition is believed to involve genes controlling the production of amyloid precursor protein. Over-expression or mutation of these genes may explain the excessive deposition of amyloid that is found in the brain in Alzheimer's disease. Variants of the apolipoprotein E gene have been identified in individuals with late-onset disease.

The pathological features of Alzheimer's disease are degeneration and loss of neurons in cortical areas of the brain. Neuronal damage and death are evident as neurofibrillary tangles within the neurons, and by plaques outside them. These changes are not easily identifiable during life, and are confirmed only at *post mortem*.

Much has been done to determine the composition and derivation of the plaques and neurofibrillary tangles in Alzheimer's disease. An early stage in the disease process appears to be the deposition of amyloid plaques. This may be followed by the appearance of plaques containing filamentous material derived from neurons. The severity of the mental deterioration in Alzheimer's disease appears to be related to the number and complexity of the plaques and neurofibrillary tangles.

At present there is no cure for Alzheimer's disease, most treatments being aimed at alleviating some of its effects (such as depression). Some new drug therapies are aimed at conserving neurotransmitter function in the brain but at best these treatments only slow down the progress of the disease. It may be possible in the future to interfere with the processes of plaque formation, and so arrest the disease.

Pre-test

- **Can anyone get Alzheimer's disease or are any particular groups of people more susceptible than others?**
- **When is Alzheimer's disease most likely to become apparent?**
- **What causes Alzheimer's disease?**
- **Are there any factors in the environment which can initiate the disease?**
- **Is Alzheimer's disease easy to diagnose?**
- **What tests might be employed to determine if someone has the condition?**
- **Is there any treatment for Alzheimer's disease?**

Aims of this chapter

By the end of this chapter you will have increased your knowledge of:
◆ What dementia is and how common it is in the UK
◆ The various causes of dementia and the main changes that take place in the brain
◆ How Alzheimer's disease is diagnosed
◆ The current and proposed treatments for Alzheimer's disease

In addition, this chapter will help you to:
◆ Distinguish between normal ageing changes of the brain and the pathologies of dementia
◆ Comprehend recent advances in understanding the genetic basis of Alzheimer's disease
◆ Assess the contribution of environmental factors to Alzheimer's disease
◆ Describe the current difficulties in diagnosing dementia and how diagnosis might improve in the future

Amyloid: an abnormal fibrillar protein deposited outside cells. Usually associated with disease, particularly in sites of chronic inflammation or malignancy. There are different types of amyloid deposit, varying in composition depending on site or disease association. The deposits are formed from circulating or locally produced protein precursors which are abnormal in structure or concentration. Some amyloid deposits are a consequence of ageing.

Dementia: a generalised and progressive impairment of mental ability that interferes with normal social and occupational activities.

Introduction

Alzheimer's disease was first described in 1906 by the Bavarian psychiatrist Alois Alzheimer. He presented the case of a 51-year-old woman who suffered primarily from unaccountable paranoia, memory loss, disorientation, depression, hallucinations and, eventually, profound dementia. The disease is the most common cause of dementia. Patients ultimately lose all sense of time, place and purpose.

The disease is caused by degeneration and death of neurons in cortical areas of the brain. The dead or dying neurons produce numerous senile plaques and neurofibrillary tangles, which can be seen by microscopic examination of brain tissues. Because of the amount of tissue required to estimate the plaques and tangles in the brain, laboratory investigations are restricted to confirming the disease after the patient is dead. In life, the diagnosis is made by testing mental function and by excluding other causes of dementia such as brain infarct.

There is no known cause or cure for Alzheimer's disease. Some of the alterations seen in the brain are, to a lesser extent, also seen in the ageing brain. It has been postulated that the disease is an acceleration of the ageing process but there is evidence that environmental factors such as head injury, exposure to aluminium and viral infection combine with a genetic predisposition for the disease in some people to produce a degenerative process which is distinct from normal ageing of the brain.

Epidemiological studies have suggested that exposure to aluminium may be important in initiating the disease. This has been substantiated by the finding of aluminium in the cerebral plaques and tangles. Most cases of Alzheimer's disease are sporadic: a family history of the disease is not necessary. However, some inherited disorders account for a minority of cases. These include Down's syndrome. Many of the plaques in the brain contain amyloid, and a gene for amyloid precursor protein has been identified on the long arm

Alzheimer's disease is a form of dementia with no known cure

Alzheimer's disease can affect anybody

of chromosome 21: abnormalities of this chromosome also account for Down's syndrome. It is possible that the amyloid plaques arise through over-expression of this gene.

Symptoms of Alzheimer-type dementia

Down's syndrome: chromosomal abnormality characterised by mental retardation and physical features of small stature, slanting eyes, flat facial profile, thick tongue and broad neck. Caused by alteration in chromosome number (extra copy of chromosome 21) or structural abnormality involving chromosome 21.

The main symptoms of Alzheimer's disease are progressive **amnesia** (loss of recent memory), **aphasia** (difficulty in using or understanding words), **apraxia** (difficulty in carrying out familiar movements and tasks) and **agnosia** (difficulty in recognising people and objects). In the early stages of the disease the symptoms may not cause undue concern, presenting as the kind of lapse that we all make, such as forgetting a name or how to spell a word. Patients often exhibit lack of emotional response and poor time-keeping. Visuospatial and perceptual problems are fairly common. Other effects include depression, restlessness, anxiety and fatigue.

Long-term memory usually remains intact and for this reason people with dementia tend to dwell in the past. The patient can be stimulated by referring to old photographs or by playing music, bringing back happy memories and reducing anxiety. Patients become confused by unfamiliar surroundings and are helped by being allowed to live as normal a life as possible in their own home.

However, a stage is reached at which a patient can no longer cope with the activities of daily living and their safety is jeopardised. The memory lapses become more frequent and ultimately the patient cannot remember what they were doing even a few minutes ago. They no longer recognise people and places and lose their purpose in life as virtually all the higher brain functions are lost. Mood changes are common, with a tendency towards depression and irritation. Patients may become anxious and aggressive. They will often wander aimlessly around the house, become restless at night or search the streets for a childhood home. The stress on carers is enormous as it becomes difficult to leave the patient alone for more than a few minutes. For these reasons many patients become institutionalised.

The effects of the disease can be devastating for both the patient and their immediate family – it has been referred to as a 'living bereavement' as the patient ceases to recognise their close family and friends. Communication becomes a problem in the later stages; patients are unable to talk clearly or to understand what is being said to them. Incontinence is common and patients often become chair-bound or bedridden. The rate of progression varies, but patients usually die within a decade of the original diagnosis, often as a result of viral pneumonia.

Other causes of dementia

▲   **Key points**

Features of Alzheimer's disease

▲ Alzheimer's disease is the most common cause of dementia, mostly affecting people over the age of 60

▲ The disease arises from an irreversible loss of brain cells, and cannot be halted

▲ Symptoms: progressive loss of higher mental function, affecting the ability to remember, learn, think and reason

Alzheimer's disease accounts for about 50% of cases of dementia. Another common type of dementia (accounting for about 20% of cases) is **multiple infarct dementia,** caused by a series of small strokes. A further 15% of cases

are caused by a combination of multiple strokes and Alzheimer's disease. A minority of patients with Parkinson's disease develop dementia, usually in the late stages of the disease (Figure 26.1). Other less common causes include thyroid disease, chronic infections of the nervous system, AIDS, subdural haematoma, occult hydrocephalus, Huntington's disease, Creutzfeldt–Jakob disease, Pick's disease and brain tumours.

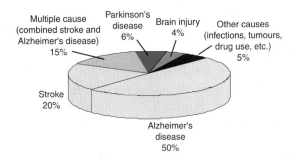

Figure 26.1 Causes of dementia. Most dementias are irreversible and progressive. However, some types are reversible if the cause is reversible (e.g. subdural haematoma, vitamin B$_{12}$ deficiency, some infections and brain tumours).

Creutzfeldt–Jakob disease: rapidly progressive dementia characterised by accumulation of a modified cell membrane protein termed prion protein. Histologically the brain tissue is vacuolated (spongiform encephalopathy). Similar to kuru in humans, scrapie in sheep and bovine spongiform encephalopathy (BSE).

Huntington's disease: an autosomal dominant single-gene disorder. Below the age of 30, affected individuals are usually asymptomatic. A progressive loss of motor co-ordination follows, leading to twitching of the limbs and muscles of the face. As the disease progresses, depression, schizophrenia, and personality changes are common, as well as dementia. There is no cure.

Hydrocephalus: increased volume of cerebrospinal fluid, with expansion of the cerebral ventricles. Usually caused by obstruction (e.g. tumour, haemorrhage).

Case study

Mrs Brown is 78 years old and lives alone in her own house. Her husband died 15 years ago. She has a daughter who visits daily. She does not suffer from hypertension, diabetes or any other known metabolic disturbance and there is no history of transient ischaemic attack or stroke in her or her family. At her last check-up by her general practitioner 1 year ago she was not found to be suffering from any major illnesses, although her daughter had noticed slight memory loss and uncharacteristic behaviour.

Over the past year Mrs Brown has found it increasingly difficult to remember the names of people around her and would often forget to pay her bills. She gradually withdrew from her usual social life and would not visit friends or go out of the house alone. Recently she began to neglect her appearance, nearly always wearing the same clothes. Mrs Brown started to make frequent references to her husband and of things they did together. She was often found sitting by the window waiting for him, and would become angry with her daughter whom she accused of lying and trying to upset her by saying that he was dead. She also irritated her daughter by repeatedly asking a question only moments after being provided with an answer.

Her present admission to an elderly care unit was precipitated when the daughter had arrived to find the house unlocked and her mother missing. The police were called, and eventually Mrs Brown was found in her night-clothes a few miles from home, in a very agitated condition because she could not find her husband.

The assessment of this history was that Mrs Brown was probably suffering from dementia. Various tests of memory, intelligence and powers of observation were conducted over the next few days. These confirmed widespread

Review question 1

What is the progression of symptoms in Alzheimer's disease?

intellectual impairment consistent with dementia. The next stage was to identify the cause of the dementia. Blood tests, urinalysis, chest radiography and ECG were all within normal limits but electroencephalography (EEG) was slow. These tests effectively ruled out metabolic disturbances, infection and multiple strokes. In the absence of other known causes, the history of gradual memory deterioration and changes in behaviour and function, together with impaired intellectual ability indicated that the dementia was most likely to be of the Alzheimer type.

Epidemiology

Alzheimer's disease is most commonly seen in older people

It has been difficult to assess the prevalence of Alzheimer's disease because the diagnostic criteria are not always reliable. Nonetheless both the figures for dementias as a whole and the separate figures for Alzheimer's disease reveal a marked increase with age. All forms of dementia are rare in individuals under 45 years of age; where it does occur the people affected are more likely to have a genetic predisposition such as Down's syndrome or to have the reversible forms associated with infection or drug abuse.

In the UK, one in five people over the age of 80 has dementia

In people over 60 the proportion of people with dementia can approach 10%; this means that in the UK about 500 000 people are affected. As longevity and the proportion of older people in the population increase the prevalence of Alzheimer's disease and other dementias is likely to increase further. In various American studies the prevalence of Alzheimer's disease has been estimated at 0.5–3.0% for people between 65 and 74 years, 4–19% for those of 75–84 years and 13–48% in people of 84 years and older (Figure 26.2).

Electroencephalography (EEG): uses scalp electrodes to record the spontaneous electrical activity of the brain. Brain-wave rhythms are recorded as traces on moving paper, with some changes in pattern characteristic of conditions such as seizure disorders, tumours, strokes, head trauma or nervous system infections.

Pick's disease: a rare degenerative brain disease of unknown cause that usually begins between the age of 50 and 60 years. Women are affected twice as frequently as men. Neuronal loss is most severe in the outer layers of the cortex, particularly in the frontal and temporal lobes. Unlike Alzheimer's disease, neurons in the parietal lobe are spared. Some surviving neurons exhibit characteristic oval inclusions known as Pick bodies.

Subdural haematoma: development of blood clots in the subdural space, below the dura and arachnoid (membranes covering the surface of the brain). Usually caused by head injury, sometimes with minimal trauma.

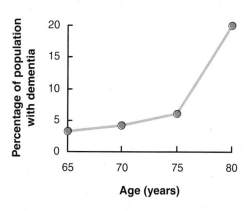

Figure 26.2 Prevalence of dementia in the UK. About 5% of the population over the age of 65 develop Alzheimer's disease; this increases to over 20% of those over 80 years.

Alzheimer's disease is the most common reason for admission to nursing homes. In the older population the disease is the fourth most common cause of death, after heart attacks, cancers and strokes.

Aetiology

Genetic predisposition

At one time it was believed that most cases of Alzheimer's disease occurred sporadically because the disease is so common in later life. This may be the case, but evidence has now accumulated for the involvement of genetic factors in both early-onset and late-onset forms of the disease (Figure 26.3).

Most cases of Alzheimer's disease occur in people with no family history of the disease

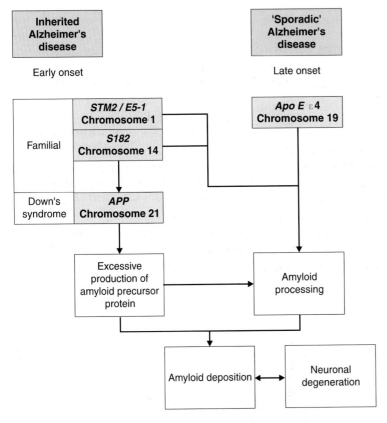

Figure 26.3 Genetic alterations in Alzheimer's disease. Early-onset disease is caused by mutations to genes in chromosomes 1, 14 or 21. The chromosome 1 and 14 genes probably influence the processing of amyloid to an insoluble fibrillar form, which is deposited extracellularly in the brain. Extra copies or mutation of the amyloid precursor protein gene in chromosome 21 probably cause excess production of the protein. Many patients with the late-onset form of Alzheimer's disease are heterozygous or homozygous for the *apoE ε4* allele. These genes could be expressed in the neurons themselves, or by other cells. The *apoE* gene product may influence processing of amyloid precursor protein. Deposition of insoluble amyloid in the brain may act as a catalyst for further neuronal degeneration.

The familial, early-onset form is inherited in an autosomal dominant fashion. The majority of patients with Down's syndrome who survive beyond

Alterations in chromosome 21 are seen in Down's syndrome and some inherited cases of Alzheimer's disease

the age of 50 develop Alzheimer's disease. These apparently disparate groups of patients are connected by alterations affecting chromosome 21, which contains a gene for **amyloid precursor protein** (the *APP* gene). The protein is normally present across all membranes and is believed to play a role in maintaining membrane stability or possibly as a membrane receptor. People with Down's syndrome have an extra copy of this chromosome. Extra copies of the gene may mean that the protein is produced in excessive quantities. Similarly, mutations to the gene may cause its over-expression. In these instances the amyloid material may become deposited as insoluble β-amyloid in the brain.

Early-onset Alzheimer's disease

In the inherited forms of the disease, mutations to chromosome 14 are more common than defects in chromosome 21

Genetic linkage studies have established a further genetic abnormality associated with the early-onset familial form of the disease linked to markers in the middle of the long arm of chromosome 14. Most early-onset families so far studied have displayed this linkage, regardless of mutations in the gene for amyloid precursor protein on chromosome 21. The relevant gene has been cloned and belongs to a class of **presenilin** genes, so named because of their association with premature senility. Various mutations in the gene have been identified in affected family members with early-onset disease. No such mutations have been detected in unaffected family members who were beyond the age of early-onset disease or in a large series of unrelated controls. The precise functions of the gene, termed *S182* (also named presenilin 1 or PS1), and its protein product are unclear.

Amazingly, the closest structural resemblance of the product to any other known protein is with a protein found in the sperm of the roundworm. The roundworm protein appears to be involved in intracellular transport and interactions with fibrillar proteins. This is not far removed from processes in Alzheimer's disease involving the deposition of β-amyloid (see below). It is possible that the human protein influences the metabolism or processing of amyloid precursor protein and, when the gene is mutated, leads to deposition of abnormal β-amyloid. If this is not the case it throws into question the whole hypothesis of the role of amyloid as a causative factor in Alzheimer's disease. The deposition of β-amyloid may be a mere byproduct of cellular degeneration. The next research imperatives will be to identify any further mutations in this gene and to unravel its functions.

Mutation in another gene – *STM2/E5-1* (also named presenilin 2 or PS2), on chromosome 1 – is associated with familial Alzheimer's disease. This gene, like *APP* and *S182*, is inherited in an autosomal dominant manner. It belongs to the same gene family as *S182* and both are thought to code for transmembrane proteins. It is possible that *STM2/E5-1* and *S182* encode different subunits of the same receptor complex. The reports of these two genes followed each other within the space of 1 month in 1995 (Levy-Lahad *et al.*, 1995; Rogaev *et al.*, 1995; Sherrington *et al.*, 1995). Given this rapid rate of progress it is probable that rather more will be known about these genes and indeed more genes may have been identified by the time this book is in print.

▲ **Key points**

Genetics of early-onset Alzheimer's disease

- ▲ A minority of cases are inherited in an autosomal dominant manner
- ▲ Alzheimer-type dementia is common in older patients with Down's syndrome
- ▲ Some cases are probably caused by over-expression of chromosome 21 genes coding for amyloid precursor protein
- ▲ Activity of amyloid precursor protein gene may be controlled by presenilin S182 gene on chromosome 14
- ▲ Most cases of early-onset disease have mutations in chromosome 14
- ▲ STM2/E5-1 (presenilin) genes on chromosome 1 probably encode (with S182?) a transmembrane receptor complex

Late-onset Alzheimer's disease

There is now evidence to suggest that there is an underlying abnormality in the much more common, and seemingly sporadic, late-onset Alzheimer's disease. A common variant of the apolipoprotein E (*apoE ε4*) gene may confer increased susceptibility for late-onset disease. About 25% of the population of the world are heterozygous for the *apoE ε4* allele (present on chromosome 19), and a further 2–3% are homozygous. A homozygote has up to a 90% risk of developing Alzheimer's disease. The degree of risk is much less for heterozygotes, but the frequency of this gene could do much to explain the frequency of late-onset Alzheimer's disease.

Apolipoprotein E (apoE) is involved in lipid metabolism in the brain, and plays a part in regeneration of the peripheral and central nervous systems after injury. It has been found in association with both the neurofibrillary plaques and the tangles of Alzheimer's disease, particularly those containing amyloid. It is thus possible that apoE ε4 is involved in the inappropriate deposition of insoluble β-amyloid plaque. Future drug therapy for Alzheimer's disease could be based on blocking the interaction between apoE and the amyloid proteins, thereby preventing the formation of the potentially damaging plaques.

There is some evidence that another *apoE* allele, *apoE ε2*, may protect against the development of Alzheimer's disease. It is believed that the ε2 isoform of apoE may bind less strongly to amyloid protein. Studies of neuropathologically confirmed cases of Alzheimer's disease have revealed that this gene variant is less common than expected.

One outcome of the apoE ε4 linkage with the many cases of late-onset Alzheimer's disease is that it may at last be possible to identify people at risk through genetic screening. However, until preventive measures can be identified, or treatments made available, many people would probably prefer not to know that they carry the *apoE ε4* gene.

Environmental risk factors

Several environmental factors have been suggested as possible causes of sporadic Alzheimer's disease: chemical toxins, disordered mineral metabolism, head injury and viral infections. The damage to nerve cells by viral infection may be direct, or indirect through some sort of allergic reaction. However, no virus has yet been positively identified in relation to Alzheimer's disease.

Many environmental toxins, particularly lead and aluminium, are known to damage nerve cells, and it is possible that these could build up in the neurons and ultimately bring about the degenerative changes characteristic of the disease. The possible role of aluminium has aroused much interest, although the evidence is inconclusive.

Some people may be more at risk than others because they are less able to metabolise and neutralise toxic agents. Using probe drugs it has been shown that some metabolic pathways in the brain are impaired in Alzheimer's disease. At present it is uncertain whether these metabolic deficiencies cause the disease

---

People with the gene for apoE ε4 are at greater risk of developing Alzheimer's disease

▲ Key points

Genetics of late-onset Alzheimer's disease

▲ Most cases of Alzheimer's disease are sporadic, with risk increasing with age

▲ Many 'sporadic' cases are now believed to occur in people with the gene for apoE ε4

▲ Homozygotes for apoE ε4 have a high risk of developing Alzheimer's disease (2–3% of the population)

Apolipoprotein E: a protein carrier normally involved in the transport and clearance of lipids as plasma lipoproteins. There are three common genetic variants, producing single amino acid substitutions in the final protein. This affects the functional capacity of the protein to bind lipid. People with the apoE ε4 form have raised levels of plasma cholesterol and triglycerides, and increased risk of CHD.

Alzheimer's disease may be triggered by environmental factors

Epidemiological and neuropathological evidence implicates aluminium as a causative factor

Patients with Alzheimer's disease have an impaired capacity to metabolise toxic agents

or are the result of neuronal degeneration.

Aluminium

A number of lines of evidence implicate aluminium as a causative factor in various types of dementia, but the evidence linking aluminium to Alzheimer's disease is weak.

> *Dialysis patients treated with aluminium salts may suffer symptoms of dementia*

The toxicity of aluminium became apparent when some patients with renal failure who had been treated with dialysis fluids containing aluminium developed symptoms of dementia, anaemia and osteomalacia. Similar complications arose after oral aluminium preparations (employed to prevent the accumulation of calcium phosphate deposits in the tissues of patients undergoing dialysis) were used as phosphate binders. Because aluminium is excreted by the kidneys, individuals with impaired renal function are more likely to accumulate aluminium, especially in the bones and brain.

> *Most aluminium is taken into the body through the diet but very little is absorbed*

In normal individuals the question of whether aluminium can accumulate in sufficient quantities from normal environmental sources is controversial. Most of the aluminium taken into the body through food and water passes through the intestine without being absorbed: the daily urinary excretion of aluminium is only 0.02–0.05 mg. A small amount may be inhaled, particularly as occupational exposure to aluminium in the metal-working industries.

Epidemiology

Several epidemiological studies have linked the prevalence of Alzheimer's disease to levels of aluminium in the water supply. One British study (Martyn *et al.*, 1989) demonstrated that the risk of Alzheimer's disease was increased by 50% in areas where the concentration of aluminium in drinking water exceeded 0.11 mg/l (the current EU directive specifies an acceptable limit of 0.2 mg/l). High concentrations of aluminium in water and some clustering of dementia cases have been found in Northumberland, Tyne and Wear, Durham, Devon and Cornwall.

> *Some studies show more cases of Alzheimer's disease in areas where the water supply contains high levels of aluminium*

Another type of dementia (amyotrophic lateral sclerosis–parkinsonism dementia complex) has been reported in areas where the water supply contains very high levels of aluminium, such as on the Pacific island of Guam and the Japanese island Kii. In this condition aluminium accumulates within neurons.

Amyotrophic lateral sclerosis, motor neuron disease: a progressive neurodegenerative disease causing paralysis. Motor neurons are lost from the cortex, brainstem and spinal cord. Begins with a mild weakness in one limb, progresses to severe paralysis with loss of swallowing and respiration.

A further line of evidence comes from the experience with people undergoing dialysis. These patients were at risk of developing encephalopathy and brain damage when they were treated in areas where the concentration of aluminium in tap water was high, or when the dialysate contained high levels of added aluminium.

Encephalopathy: any disturbance of cerebral function.

Experimental data

Deposits of aluminium within neurofibrillary tangles and senile plaques have been found in patients with Alzheimer's disease. The experimental administration of aluminium or its salts by intracerebral or subcutaneous

> *The plaques and tangles of Alzheimer's disease contain aluminium*

injection causes encephalopathy, and the production of aluminium-containing neurofibrillary tangles.

Aluminium has been shown to cause aggregation *in vitro* of neuronal cytoskeletal proteins, including neurofilament and microtubule-associated proteins. The addition of aluminium to the culture medium of neuroblastoma cells also induces the aggregation of neurofilament proteins.

> *Experiments show that aluminium induces changes in neurons*

In animals exposed intranasally to aluminium salts the aluminium is absorbed into the brain. It is noteworthy that the sites of the earliest lesions of Alzheimer's disease are the amygdala and hippocampus, which are connected to the olfactory bulbs and tracts.

> *Damage to the neurons may arise through the inhalation of aluminium pollutants in air*

Evidence against aluminium

Epidemiology

Not all epidemiological studies support a link between high concentrations of aluminium and dementia. There are a number of methodological problems in establishing a link.

> *There are problems in ascertaining exposure to aluminium and in establishing the true frequency of Alzheimer's disease*

1. Exposure to aluminium is difficult to assess accurately and there are inconsistencies in the data from different water authorities on aluminium concentrations. Aluminium salts may be added as part of the purification procedure, and the amounts required will alter depending on the degree of water contamination. There may be substantial seasonal variations in aluminium concentration as well as changes in water purification practice.
2. Alzheimer's disease tends to be under-reported and misdiagnosed, and some areas of the country may have better diagnostic facilities (for example availability of MRI and CT scanners which can more accurately pinpoint the cause of dementia) than others.
3. The family history of affected individuals (a known risk factor for early-onset Alzheimer's disease) has not always been taken into account.

Notwithstanding the difficulties in establishing exposure to aluminium in the water, the most important source of aluminium is the diet. Approximately 10–25 mg of aluminium are ingested each day: 1 kg of food typically contains about 20 mg (compared with the limit of 0.2 mg/l in water). The richest sources of aluminium are in processed and baked foods in which emulsifying, anti-caking, bleaching and raising agents are used. Tea leaves and brewed tea contain high levels of aluminium. Similarly, the widespread use of antacids that contain aluminium for the treatment of dyspepsia means that intake far exceeds the levels of aluminium in drinking water, but this is not known to be associated with dementia.

> *Most aluminium is taken into the body through the diet*

The clinical picture of Alzheimer's disease is different from those cases in which encephalopathy was induced by exposure to aluminium. In the dialysis patients reported above, the encephalopathy bore a greater resemblance to epilepsy than dementia, although mental deterioration did follow. In addition, the patients developed anaemia and osteomalacia, which does not happen in Alzheimer's disease. Moreover, aluminium absorption in these dialysis patients

> *The symptoms produced by exposure to large amounts of aluminium are not identical to those of Alzheimer's disease*

Chelating agent: a chemical that forms a stable complex with some metals and other ions, forming a ring structure around the ion. One of the most common chelating agents is EDTA, used as an anticoagulant (by binding with calcium ions) in blood samples for laboratory analysis. Chelating agents have a therapeutic potential if they can be used to eliminate deposits of toxic metals from the tissues.

The brain pathology produced by aluminium is not identical to that of Alzheimer's disease

Review question 2

What are the known risk factors for Alzheimer's disease?

did not appear to cause the plaques and tangles in the brain that are characteristic of Alzheimer's disease. If detected early enough, the symptoms in affected dialysis patients are reversible, either by changing the dialysis regime or by eliminating the aluminium with chelating agents. Alzheimer's disease is not reversed or substantially arrested by the use of chelating agents, and is always fatal.

Similarly, the clinical picture of patients in Guam (see above) shares only some features with Alzheimer's disease, and showed additional features of parkinsonism and motor paralysis.

Experimental data

The distribution and morphology of the neurofibrillary tangles produced by aluminium injection are different from the tangles seen in Alzheimer's disease. Furthermore, aluminium has been found in the senile plaques and tangles of functionally normal older people. Why should aluminium cause dementia in some people but not in others? It is possible that the presence of aluminium is purely a coincidental finding and has nothing to do with neuronal degeneration and consequent dementia.

Aluminium and Alzheimer's disease

Point	Counterpoint
Aluminium is present in neuritic plaques and neurofibrillary tangles	Plaques and tangles containing aluminium are also seen in mentally normal older people
Injection of aluminium in animals causes formation of neurofibrillary tangles and symptoms of encephalopathy	Plaques and tangles induced experimentally by aluminium injection are morphologically different from those seen in Alzheimer's disease
Clustering of cases in areas with high aluminium concentration in water	Epidemiological studies related to water concentrations of aluminium are problematic because of seasonal variation in aluminium levels and larger sources of aluminium in food
Encephalopathy in dialysis patients caused by aluminium	Dialysis-associated encephalopathy is more like epilepsy than dementia. Unlike Alzheimer's disease, dialysis-induced aluminium neurotoxicity is potentially reversible
Encephalopathy with features of dementia in Guam caused by ingestion of aluminium	Guam-type dementia has distinctive clinical features

Author's view

The role of aluminium in Alzheimer's disease has not been proven conclusively, and it is unlikely that aluminium could ever be regarded as a single cause of the disease – it would be in combination with other factors such as genetic susceptibility or the over-production of amyloid by other mechanisms.

Amyloid metabolism is a crucial component of the underlying pathological process. Several genes are involved in amyloid metabolism although little is known about how these genes work and what environmental factors, if any, could influence their activities. The possibility remains that aberrant amyloid production can be initiated by damage to the neurons.

Neuronal damage could be caused by aluminium, but viral infection or other neurotoxic agents (lead for example) could also cause the problem. In common with other multifactorial diseases, the risk of developing sporadic Alzheimer's disease is influenced by the person's own genetic susceptibility and the presence or absence of other predisposing factors.

Smoking

Smoking appears to exert some protection against the development of Alzheimer's disease and Parkinson's disease, in contrast to its effects elsewhere in the body. Anecdotal evidence suggests that smoking helps people to concentrate. Nicotine is known to be addictive, probably due to changes in brain neurotransmitter function and receptor activity. Nicotine acts on acetylcholine receptors, increasing nerve cell activity (of particular relevance in Alzheimer's disease). It also triggers the release of dopamine (important in Parkinson's disease). It might be possible to exploit these effects by developing drugs which have an effect similar to that of nicotine, without having to resort to smoking.

Some forms of dementia are less common in smokers

Pathology

The gross anatomy of the brain is altered in Alzheimer's disease, with an increase in the size of the fluid-filled cavities and widening of the sulci. These appearances can be evaluated by CT scans, but to a lesser extent they are also features of the aged brain in functionally normal people. The most distinctive changes of Alzheimer's disease occur at the cellular level, with the appearance of neurofibrillary tangles and senile plaques.

Background information: The brain

The principal cells of the brain are the **neurons** (nerve cells), which form interconnecting networks with the capability of detecting, analysing and integrating information generated from sensory stimuli. These cells consist

of a **cell body** containing the nucleus, with very long processes which are of two types: a single **axon** together with one or more **dendrites** (Figure 26.4). The dendrites are highly branched tapering processes which receive information from neighbouring neurons at their junction or **synapse**. Together the axon and dendrites are referred to as **neurites**.

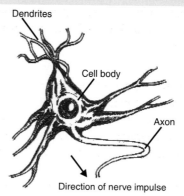

Figure 26.4.

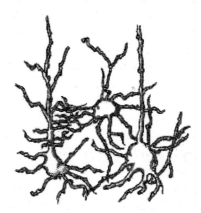

Figure 26.5 Neurons are organised into extensive networks of about 100 billion cells linked through their highly branched axons and dendrites, giving rise to intelligence, creativity, emotion, consciousness and memory.

The nerve impulse consists of an electrical signal that can be modified in the cell body of the neuron as required. The electrical impulse is transmitted via the axon to other neurons, muscles or glands. The axons can stretch over great distances before they make connection with other neurons or target cells.

The neurons are supported by a group of cells called **neuroglia**; these cells participate in neural nutrition and in defence and repair mechanisms of the brain. There are several types of cells in the neuroglia group: oligodendrocytes, astrocytes, microglia and ependymal cells. The **oligodendrocytes** are responsible for the myelination of the nerve cells

axons in the brain (this acts like an insulating coat). The **astrocytes** are highly branched cells which occupy most of the interneuronal spaces. They give physical support to the neurons and are involved in neuronal nutrition: many of the astrocyte cell processes connect with small blood vessels. The **microglia** are small cells with fine highly branched processes and transform into large phagocytic cells in response to tissue damage. The **ependymal cells** line the ventricles and are involved in the production and circulation of the cerebrospinal fluid.

Composition of normal neurons
The structure of axons and dendrites is maintained by a cytoskeletal framework, the principal cytoskeletal components of which are the **neurofilaments** and the **microtubules**, which differ in protein composition. The distribution of these proteins varies according to their location within the neuron.

Neurofilaments are present in both the neuronal cell body and the axon. Microtubules contain two main classes of proteins: **tubulin** and **microtubule-associated proteins** (MAPs). Tubulin is evenly distributed between the neuronal cell body and the axon, but the distribution of the MAPs varies. A high molecular weight protein, designated MAP-2, is present only in the neuronal cell body and the dendrites. A series of smaller proteins (**tau proteins**) are present in greatest concentration in the axons and facilitate rapid transport along the axon.

Functional areas of the brain
Most memory resides in the **cerebral cortex**. Memory for recent events is held in the **medial temporal lobe** and the **thalamus**, parts of the limbic system. The conscious review of short-term memory often brings about the transfer of information to a form called recent memory, which can last for several days. This store is located in a portion of the temporal lobe called the **hippocampus**. Long-term memory is processed in large diffuse areas in both hemispheres of the cerebral cortex.

Motor functions are controlled from the cortical areas of the frontal lobes, and impulses from pyramid-shaped neurons in this area travel downward through the brainstem into the spinal cord.

Sensory areas are found in several lobes of the **cerebrum**, these neurons interpreting incoming impulses from the various sensory receptors. This processing gives rise to feelings and sensations such as temperature, touch and pain.

Neuronal processing takes place in the cortex of the brain. Although this area is only about 2 mm thick its surface area is extensively enlarged by the folds in the surface of the brain known as **sulci**. Particularly deep sulci divide the brain into different anatomical areas: the **frontal, temporal, parietal** and **occipital** lobes (Figure 26.6).

▲ Key points

Filament composition of normal neurons

▲ Nerve cell processes, or neurites, are composed of an axon and numerous dendrites

▲ Internal structural integrity of neurons is maintained by cytoskeletal network of two types of filaments – neurofilaments and microtubules

▲ Microtubules are composed of tubulin and microtubule-associated proteins (MAPs)

▲ Tau protein is an MAP present in greatest concentration in the axon

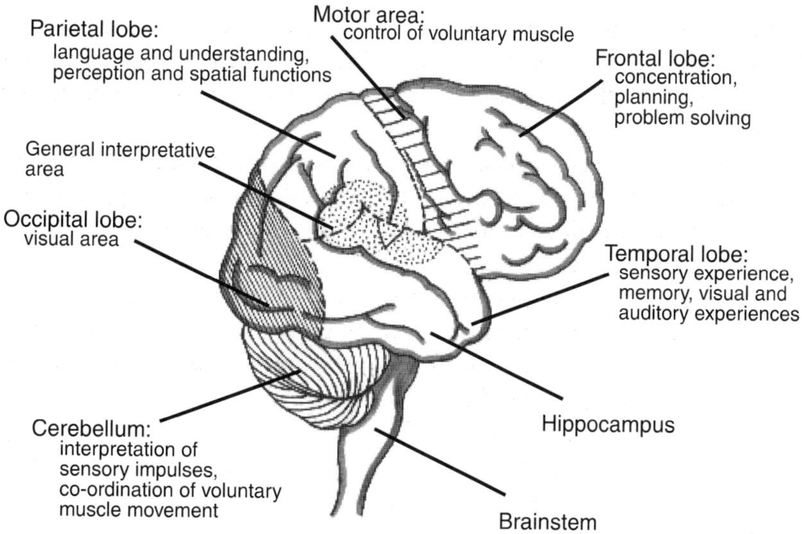

Figure 26.6 Functional areas of the brain.

Plaques and tangles

Alzheimer's disease is characterised by the presence of large numbers of senile plaques and neurofibrillary tangles in the brain

The plaques and tangles are usually present in the hippocampus, and in the temporal and parietal cortex. The tangles are usually seen actually inside the neurons and they can be regarded as evidence that the neurons have undergone degeneration. The plaques are seen outside the neurons and some are probably made up of debris from neurons that have died (Figure 26.7).

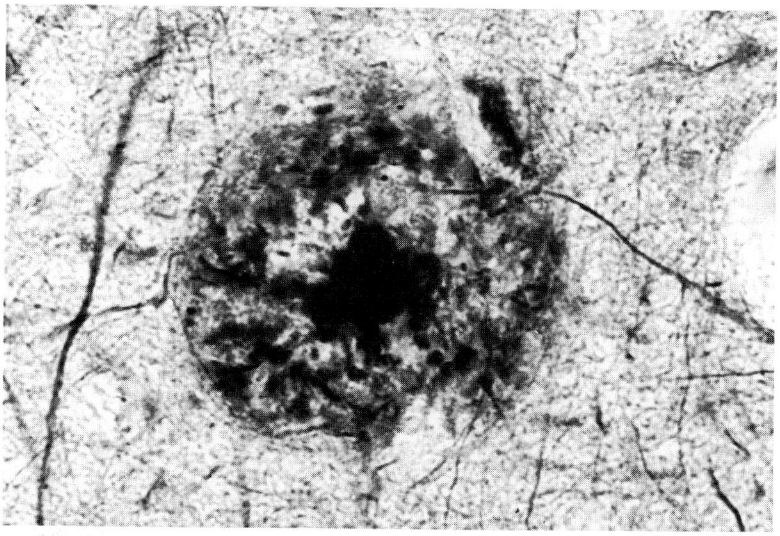

Figure 26.7 Senile plaque. Silver-stained histological preparation of brain tissue in Alzheimer's disease. (From: Burns, A., Levy, R. *Dementia*, published by Chapman & Hall, London, 1994.)

Plaques and tangles are not unique to Alzheimer's disease; they are also found in the brains of functionally normal individuals, particularly as they get older. The main difference is that far more are seen in the brain in Alzheimer's disease.

Alzheimer's disease is not an inevitable consequence of ageing

The pattern of neuronal degeneration is also different. One of the areas of the brain most severely affected in Alzheimer's disease is the hippocampus. Loss of neurons in this particular area of the hippocampus is rare in the normally ageing brain.

The composition of the plaques and tangles has been the subject of intensive study. The tangles have a fibrillar structure (hence the name neurofibrillary tangles). They differ from normal neurofilaments and microtubules in appearance and composition (Figure 26.8).

The plaques take a number of different forms, some of which certainly contain material derived from neurons, but others contain an unusual fibrous carbohydrate–protein complex known as amyloid.

Neurofibrillary tangles

Neurofibrillary tangles are found in a variety of diseases, including Alzheimer's disease, post-encephalitic parkinsonism, and the Guam amyotrophic lateral sclerosis–parkinsonism dementia complex. The tangles are primarily located intracellularly and consist of filamentous material within the axon of the neuron. They are highly insoluble, and persist in the brain even after the neuron has died. Hence, a small population of extra-neuronal neurofibrillary tangles can be seen in severely affected areas of the brain in Alzheimer's disease. As these were derived from once viable neurons they are referred to as 'tombstone' or 'ghost' tangles marking the site of the original neuron. These tombstone tangles sometimes contain β-amyloid.

Most tangles are seen within neurons, but some may be seen outside, presumably marking the spot where a neuron has died

By electron microscopy the neurofibrillary tangles are seen to consist of **paired helical filaments**, which differ from the normal neurofilaments and microtubules in the neuron. Their chemical composition has been difficult to elucidate and it has been variously suggested that they comprise collapsed cytoskeletal filaments, amyloid or even a novel protein.

Neurofibrillary tangles contain paired helical filaments

One method of elucidating the composition is simply to see what antibodies will attach to it. Such studies have shown a number of antigenic determinants, corresponding to a high-molecular-weight protein derived from neurofilaments, to microtubule-associated proteins and to tau proteins. The presence of tau in the paired helical filaments may be particularly important in that none may be left for its normal association with the microtubules. As a result the affected nerve cells degenerate and die, ultimately producing the symptoms of dementia.

Paired helical filaments contain material derived from neurofilaments and microtubules

Paired helical filaments also contain **ubiquitin**, a protein common to all nucleated cells. This protein has been identified in association with other types of cell inclusion bodies, such as the Lewy body of Parkinson's disease and the Mallory body of alcoholic liver disease. All of these can be considered as forms of chronic degenerative disease, and the inclusions (including neurofibrillary tangles) could result from a specific protective mechanism

within the cell designed to combat stressful stimuli.

(a)   **(b)**

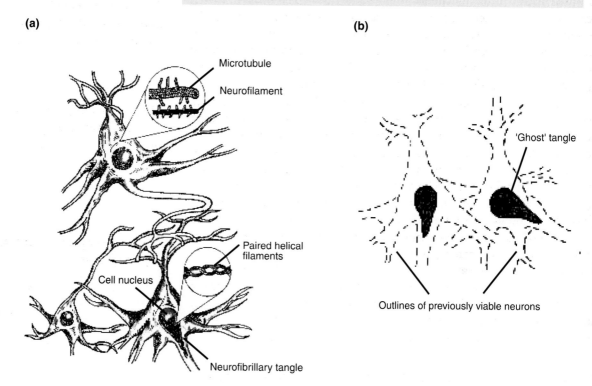

Figure 26.8 Neurofibrillary tangles. (a) Top: the normal neuron contains microtubules and neurofilaments which ensure structural integrity and allow the neuron to carry out its functions; bottom: in Alzheimer's disease there are large numbers of degenerate neurons, characterised by neurofibrillary tangles in the cell body and axon. The tangles are composed of paired helical filaments which are morphologically and biochemically distinct from the microtubules and neurofilaments of the normal neuron. (b) Eventually some neurons die, leaving behind the neurofibrillary elements known as 'ghost' tangles.

Senile plaques

> *Senile plaques are complex structures which can contain both neuronal and non-neuronal elements*

The several classes of senile plaques differ in their composition. All types display a filamentous structure and may also contain material that has been deposited extracellularly, such as aluminium silicates. The main differences lie in whether the plaques contain elements derived from neurons (neuritic plaques) or contain amyloid without the neuritic elements (amyloid plaques).

Neuritic plaques contain degenerated and abnormal neuronal components, including paired helical filaments. One type consists of an amyloid core surrounded by a corona of dystrophic neurites and amyloid-containing filaments. Other neuritic plaques lack the amyloid core. **Amyloid plaques** contain the amyloid core but no neuronal structures.

Amyloid

Amyloid can be found in the brain around blood vessels (cerebrovascular deposits) or as extracellular plaques. The composition of the amyloid deposits differs in these two sites. Almost all amyloid deposits elsewhere in the body, including cerebrovascular deposits, contain a protein known as amyloid P component, which is a normal constituent of blood plasma, but the amyloid plaques of Alzheimer's disease do not contain this component.

> *Amyloid is deposited in the brain around blood vessels and as extracellular plaques*

The principal component of both types of amyloid deposit in the brain is a small protein known either as β-**amyloid** or **A4 amyloid**. A gene on chromosome 21 gene encodes for the much larger **amyloid precursor protein** and it is believed that β-amyloid is derived from this. The function of amyloid precursor protein is uncertain. It shows some resemblance to a cell-surface receptor protein, but there is also evidence that it is secreted by cells and has growth-regulatory activity. In the brain, amyloid precursor protein is produced by neurons, microglia, astrocytes and choroid plexus cells.

> *The β-amyloid of the plaques is derived from a larger amyloid precursor protein*

The amyloid of age-related senile plaques and amyloid in the corona of neuritic plaques differ in composition. Some neuritic plaques contain amyloid precursor protein, which is co-distributed with the neurofilament and tau proteins. This suggests that the neuron itself secreted the amyloid precursor protein and that the various neuritic elements became entrapped within the amyloid when the neuron died. Most other plaques contain β-amyloid, and the original amyloid precursor protein is missing, as are the neuritic elements.

> *A minority of plaques contain amyloid precursor protein*

What is the significance of the different amyloid types in the plaques?

The difference in amyloid composition of neuritic and amyloid plaques has been exploited as a means of differentiating between the plaques of Alzheimer's disease and those that are merely age-related. The neuritic plaques which contain amyloid precursor protein in their coronas are associated with the severe mental deterioration of Alzheimer's disease. The large subset of senile plaques which contain β-amyloid, but which are totally devoid of amyloid precursor protein and neuritic elements, are probably age-related plaques.

> *Neuritic plaques are associated with dementia*

In Alzheimer's disease, plaques containing amyloid are present in the brain cortex, the basal ganglia, brainstem, cerebellum and spinal cord. The plaques may be the only morphological abnormality present, or may be surrounded by abnormal neurons and by a proliferation of neuroglia (these represent the 'scar tissue' of the brain).

What is the relationship between the plaques and the tangles?

Many extracellular plaques do not apparently contain neuritic tangles. This raises a question about the sequence of morphological abnormalities in Alzheimer's disease: does the amyloid appear first as extracellular plaques and then become surrounded by neurites, or does amyloid deposition occur after the neuron degenerates? Recent studies in young and old patients with Down's syndrome suggest that the sequence starts with a diffuse plaque

> *Alzheimer's disease may be initiated by abnormal production of amyloid*

containing only β-amyloid. Many aged and non-demented Down's syndrome patients have numerous β-amyloid plaques, but few neurofibrillary tangles.

In patients with Alzheimer's disease the degree of mental impairment appears to correlate progressively with the number and complexity of the plaques and the presence of neurofibrillary tangles. Plaques containing only amyloid are more common in individuals in whom mental impairment is only slight, whereas neuritic plaques, bearing paired helical filaments, seem to be associated with severe mental deterioration.

Alzheimer's disease may be exacerbated by the abnormal production of amyloid protein

It may be, therefore, that the initial event is abnormal production of amyloid protein, caused either by toxic damage to the neurons (in the sporadic cases of Alzheimer's disease) or by aberrant gene activation (in Down's syndrome and inherited Alzheimer's disease) (Figure 26.9). The presence of amyloid deposits as plaques causes the surrounding neurons to degenerate and die. It is possible that amyloid toxicity leads to generation of free radicals (see Chapter 4), thereby creating a chain reaction in which more and more neurons are affected. The neurofibrillary tangles are produced in the process of neuronal degeneration, and when the neuron dies the various neurofibril and amyloid proteins are precipitated as plaques.

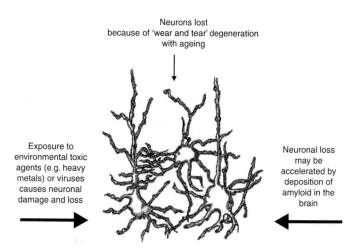

Neurons lost because of 'wear and tear' degeneration with ageing

Exposure to environmental toxic agents (e.g. heavy metals) or viruses causes neuronal damage and loss

Neuronal loss may be accelerated by deposition of amyloid in the brain

Figure 26.9 Possible mechanisms of neuronal degeneration and loss. In the functionally normal individual there is a small progressive decline in neuronal status with age. This loss may be exacerbated by exposure to environmental neurotoxic agents. In the inherited form of the disease, and in patients with Down's syndrome, the initial damage to neurons may be mediated by deposition of amyloid in the brain.

Neuronal regeneration and repair

Some neurons attempt to regenerate after they have been injured

A further morphological change seen in Alzheimer's disease, known as **neuronal sprouting**, probably occurs in response to neuronal damage. The sprouting consists of meshworks of curly fibres, called **neuropil threads**, which emanate from the body and dendrites of cortical neurons. Their presence is probably an attempt to regenerate and restore the functions lost by the damaged

Deposits in the brain

Deposit	Site	Composition	Significance
β-Amyloid	Initially deposited in perivascular sites	Component of neurofibrillary tangles and plaques in both Alzheimer's disease and ageing brain	Derived from amyloid precursor protein encoded by chromosome 21. May cause neuronal damage and initiate degeneration
Aluminium	Associated with plaques and tangles		May cause neuronal damage and initiate degeneration
Neurofibrillary tangles	Mainly as intracellular deposits in neurons	Abnormal composition: contain paired helical filaments	Marker of neuronal degeneration
Plaques	Extracellular deposits	May contain neuronal and non-neuronal material: neuritic plaques consist of abnormal neurites, sometimes surrounding an amyloid core; amyloid plaques contain β-amyloid but no neuronal structures	Neuritic plaques; marker of neuronal death Amyloid plaques; may initiate neuronal degeneration or may arise as a consequence of degeneration
Neuropil threads		Constituent of neurons	Marker of neuronal attempt at regeneration
Lewy bodies	Intracellular deposits in neurons		Marker of neuronal degeneration in Parkinson's disease

neurons by making new connections with adjacent cells.

Another response is to fill the neuronal space that has been lost through cell death by proliferation of **neuroglia** (the 'scar tissue' of the brain). Before the influx of neuroglia, damaged neurons and cell debris must be removed. This function is carried out by specialised brain cells called **microglia**, and is akin to the inflammatory process in other parts of the body. In common with inflammation elsewhere, the process can cause further damage because of the uncontrolled release of proteolytic enzymes. It is believed that the microglia, in carrying out their role of digesting and removing dead neurons, initiate

Further damage to neurons may arise through the repair process

Review question 4

How does the pathology of Alzheimer's disease differ from the normal ageing processes of the brain?

damage to surrounding viable neurons. The plaques of Alzheimer's disease are often seen surrounded by both neuroglia and microglia.

Neurotransmitters

The result of the cell damage and death that take place in Alzheimer's disease is a progressive loss of cognitive function. This is caused by the degeneration and death of neurons and the consequent disruption to neural networks and neurotransmission. Many neurotransmitter systems are affected by the cell damage in Alzheimer's disease, but the cholinergic system (see Chapter 27) is probably affected the most. Loss of acetylcholine correlates with increased numbers of plaques and a decline in mental test scores.

Diagnosis

Plaques and tangles can be evaluated in the brain only after the patient has died

The morphological changes in the brain which accompany Alzheimer's disease can be adequately evaluated only after the patient dies. Consequently the diagnosis must be made on clinical grounds only. In specialist centres, where clinicians have a reasonable experience of seeing patients with dementia, Alzheimer's disease is diagnosed accurately by careful application of evaluation protocols.

During life, the diagnosis of Alzheimer's disease mainly relies on clinical evaluation

The diagnosis of Alzheimer's disease is based on assessment of the patient's behaviour, memory and other cognitive functions. This can be supported by EEG, CT and functional imaging of the brain. These tests, together with laboratory investigations, are useful for excluding other causes of dementia.

Much of the assessment of Alzheimer's disease patients is by means of psychometric testing. This encompasses observation of the patient by a trained person, use of rating scales and tests of memory and cognitive performance.

Review question 3

What pathological changes occur in the brain in Alzheimer's disease?

Intelligence scales

Examples of the kinds of tests used to assess patients with suspected dementia are the Wechsler Adult Intelligence Scales. These are in two parts: a verbal scale which measures memory, application of language and mental arithmetic problems (Table 26.1), and a performance scale which measures non-verbal problem-solving skills (Table 26.2).

Patients with Alzheimer's disease do badly in tests which rely on recent learning and memory recall

In these tests 50% of the population achieve an average score of 100. About 10% of the population achieve scores greater than 120. Mentally retarded people score below 70. In patients with Alzheimer's disease the most significant finding is not the overall IQ score but the pattern of strengths and weaknesses in the various tests. The least impairment is found with the information and vocabulary tests, but performance is poor with respect to digit symbol and block design. Performance is best in tests which assess information acquired in the past. Conversely, performance is poor in tests which rely on the acquisition of new knowledge or skills. About 50% of people with Alzheimer's

Table 26.1 Wechsler Verbal Scale

Mental function	Test method
Information	General knowledge questions
Digit span	Memorising numbers for a few seconds
Vocabulary	Defining the meaning of words
Arithmetic	Solving mental arithmetic problems
Comprehension	Knowing the reasons for social conventions
Similarities	Explaining the way in which two things are alike

Table 26.2 Wechsler Performance Scale

Function	Test method
Picture completion	Finding the missing parts of incomplete pictures
Picture arrangement	Ordering a series of cartoon pictures to make a story
Block design	Making abstract patterns from blocks
Object assembly	Solving jigsaw puzzles
Digit symbol	Rapidly writing abstract symbols beneath numbers with which they go

Table 26.3 Wechsler Memory Scale

Memory parameter	Test method
Personal and current information	Giving information about oneself and people in the news
Orientation	Knowing the date and place
Mental control	Counting backwards, counting in multiples of three, knowing the alphabet
Logical memory	Recalling the ideas in two written passages
Memory span	Holding numbers in memory for a few seconds
Visual reproduction	Drawing simple geometric figures from memory
Association learning	Learning word associations so that when one word is given by the tester the other is recalled

Review question 5

How is Alzheimer's disease diagnosed?

disease demonstrate this pattern, compared with less than 1% of the non-demented older population.

A further test is based on memory. The Wechsler Memory Scale comprises seven tests covering different aspects of memory (Table 26.3).

This scale was originally devised about 40 years ago when there was very little understanding of normal memory processes and disorders. A more recent development, computerised testing, has the advantage of tailoring the questions to suit a person's ability. At present, however, many older people are unfamiliar with computers (which could affect their performance) and may also have problems with vision, hearing or movement.

Laboratory investigation

During life, laboratory investigations are of use in excluding the other causes of dementia

The examination of blood and CSF may be useful in ruling out chronic infections such as cryptococcal meningitis and syphilis as causes of dementia. Amyloid proteins can be identified in the CSF but this is not a reliable diagnostic marker for Alzheimer's disease.

There is no reliable peripheral marker for Alzheimer's disease in either the blood or the CSF. Decreased levels of amyloid precursor proteins in CSF of patients with Alzheimer's disease appeared to be correlated with the mental status of the patients. These changes were not as marked in functionally normal older people. Unfortunately, there is some overlap in the values from the two groups, which limits the usefulness of measuring the level of amyloid precursor in CSF as a diagnostic or predictive test. It is tempting to speculate that in the pathogenesis of Alzheimer's disease, amyloid precursor protein is sequestered in the plaques and cerebrovascular deposits, rather than finding its way into the CSF.

Another possible peripheral marker is the iron-binding protein melantransferrin, also known as p97. This protein is involved in the cellular uptake of iron and is present in microglia, the inflammatory cells that surround amyloid plaques in the brains of people with Alzheimer's disease. A small study has shown that concentrations of the protein are elevated in the blood and CSF of Alzheimer's disease patients compared with healthy controls. Further work needs to be carried out in larger groups of patients and control populations but the results show that the protein has some potential as a biochemical marker for identifying and monitoring the onset and progression of Alzheimer's disease. The findings also suggest the possibility that disruption to iron metabolism may somehow be involved in the pathogenesis of the disease.

Currently, most laboratory investigations are undertaken *post mortem* for confirmatory purposes. They involve the application of traditional histological staining methods and immunohistochemical demonstration techniques.

Single photon emission tomography (SPECT): allows functional imaging of the brain, distinct from the structural images obtained by CT or MRI. Tracers are labelled with iodine-23 or technetium-99m which cross the blood–brain barrier and become trapped in the brain in a distribution proportional to regional blood flow. Gamma rays (photons) emitted by the radiotracer are detected by a rotating gamma camera, or multiple detectors placed around the head. The data are processed to give three-dimensional images of the regional blood flow. The technique is relatively inexpensive and becoming widely available.

Imaging methods

The use of CT or MRI confirms the presence of cortical atrophy and may exclude other lesions such as brain tumours. Functional imaging is a useful adjunct to clinical assessment for making the diagnosis. The most widely

Review question 6

Is the diagnosis of Alzheimer's disease reliable? What are the other possible causes of dementia?

available investigation is single photon emission tomography (SPECT), which gives a three-dimensional image of regional cerebral blood flow. In Alzheimer's disease a characteristic pattern is produced by a bilateral deficit in regional blood flow in the parietal and temporal lobes, adjacent to the occipital lobes.

Treatment

At present there is no effective treatment for Alzheimer's disease. Drug treatments are given mainly to alleviate symptoms such as depression and anxiety. Vasodilators are also employed to increase the blood supply to the brain: these have mild effects in increasing alertness and decreasing confusion. Drugs have been designed to correct the more fundamental defects in Alzheimer's disease, such as neurotransmitter deficiency, but the results have been very disappointing. The damage in the brain has already been done, and neurons have been lost, so these treatments can do nothing to reverse the disease. At best, what can be hoped for is to arrest its progress.

No drug reverses or stops the progression of Alzheimer's disease

It was hoped that the neurotransmitter deficit could be compensated by drug therapy, in a fashion similar to that used to treat Parkinson's disease with the dopamine precursor L-dopa (see Chapter 27). Precursor loading with the acetylcholine precursors choline or lecithin has been attempted in Alzheimer's disease patients but without success.

Some drugs are aimed at preserving brain neurotransmitters

An alternative approach is to conserve acetylcholine using acetylcholinesterase inhibitors. One such agent is tetrahydroaminoacridine (Tacrine). Initial trials of the drug were promising: patients showed some improvement in mental test parameters. More extensive and rigorous trials have revealed substantial variations in individual responses, and there is a possible complication of liver damage. At best, the drug produces some improvement in the ability to carry out simple tasks, roughly corresponding to the deterioration that might have occurred over 6–12 months. It does nothing to arrest the disease process itself. Tacrine has been approved for the palliative treatment of Alzheimer's disease in the USA and France, but has been refused a product licence in the UK.

A further approach is aimed at removing aluminium deposits in the brain using a chelating agent (desferrioxamine). The rate of deterioration might be slowed slightly by this treatment, but in most patients the drug appears to have no effect.

Another approach is to reduce the amount of aluminium in the brain

The microglial response in Alzheimer's disease which removes the dead or degenerating neurons may damage surrounding healthy neurons. Because the reaction is very similar to inflammation it is possible that the microglial cells will respond to anti-inflammatory drugs such as aspirin. It appears that sufferers of rheumatoid arthritis, who routinely take anti-inflammatory drugs, exhibit a lower frequency of Alzheimer's disease. Trials are under way to see whether anti-inflammatory agents (such as indomethacin) can help people with Alzheimer's disease.

It may be helpful to limit the inflammatory response in Alzheimer's disease

A fundamental part of the pathogenesis of Alzheimer's disease is the aberrant production of amyloid proteins which initiates plaque formation. The amyloid

Future developments in drug therapy may be directed towards blocking amyloid production

Review question 7

What treatments are available for Alzheimer's disease?

deposits may be toxic to neurons. If the production of these plaques could be prevented, much of the neuronal damage in Alzheimer's disease could be avoided. A future strategy for drug therapy, therefore, will be to develop drugs that interfere with amyloid production, perhaps by inhibiting the enzymes necessary to split β-amyloid from its precursor protein. However, at present it is not possible to predict who will develop sporadic Alzheimer's disease and preventive measures will be impossible to implement, unless applied to everybody.

▲ **Key points**

Drug therapies for Alzheimer's disease

Agent	Mode of action
Choline, lecithin	Precursor loading: attempt to correct neurotransmitter deficit
Tacrine	Anticholinesterase: attempt to conserve neurotransmitter
Desferrioxamine	Chelating agent: attempt to remove aluminium from the brain
Indomethacin	Anti-inflammatory drug: attempt to reduce neuronal damage by microglial activity
Neuroprotective agents	Potential therapy: it may be possible to design drugs that interfere with proteolytic breakdown of amyloid precursor protein

---

ANSWERS TO REVIEW QUESTIONS

Question 1

What is the progression of symptoms in Alzheimer's disease?

- Progressive loss of short-term memory (amnesia)
- Disorientation in time and place, for example by getting lost in unfamiliar and, in later stages of the disease, familiar surroundings
- Loss of recognition (agnosia), for example of close friends and family.
- Changes in personality and loss of judgement
- Deterioration of language functions (aphasia)
- Loss of intellect and problem-solving ability
- Everyday tasks are disrupted because the patient forgets what they are doing part way through the task
- Motor function is usually unaffected, except in terminal phases of the disease, or when complicated by Parkinson's disease or other neurological disorders
- Changes are often rapid

- Late stages may be accompanied by aggressive behaviour, impaired ability to use and understand language

What are the known risk factors for Alzheimer's disease?

Question 2

- Age
- A family history of early-onset disease
- People with Down's syndrome are susceptible to the disease after 35 years of age
- Some individuals with Alzheimer's disease show impaired capacity to metabolise certain drugs and neurotoxic agents; it is not known whether this has put them at risk of developing Alzheimer's disease, or whether the metabolic changes are consequent to the disease
- Exposure to aluminium has been suggested as a risk factor for the disease, but the evidence is inconclusive
- Carrier of apoE ε4 gene alleles

What pathological changes occur in the brain in Alzheimer's disease?

Question 3

- Senile plaques and neuritic plaques are deposited extracellularly. These plaques differ according to their content of amyloid and cytoskeletal elements derived from neurons
- Neurofibrillary tangles are present within degenerating neurons. These contain paired helical filaments, which are not believed to be a constituent of normally functioning myelinated nerve cells. They may be abnormally synthesised proteins, or normal cytoskeletal filaments that have been modified and degraded by degenerative processes in the neuron
- Perivascular amyloid deposits are seen
- Surviving neurons may show shrinkage and loss of processes (neurites). In some areas the damaged neurons may attempt to recover function by dendritic sprouting; this can be seen as neuropil threads
- Neurofibrillary tangles and extracellular plaques in the brain are markers of neuronal degeneration and death respectively. A consequence of the lost neuronal activity is a reduction in brain neurotransmitters. This mainly affects the acetylcholine-secreting neurons projecting from the basal forebrain to the hippocampus and various areas of the cortex. Acetylcholine is one of the neurotransmitters by which neurons convey signals to each other.

How does the pathology of Alzheimer's disease differ from the normal ageing processes of the brain?

Question 4

The principal difference is quantitative: plaques and tangles in the brain are also seen in the normal elderly brain, but there are proportionately many more

in Alzheimer's disease. Degeneration of neurons also takes place in normal ageing, and where neurons survive their cell bodies and neurites may atrophy. A further sign of ageing is the appearance of pigmented granules containing lipofuscin in the neuronal cytoplasm. This pigment is believed to be derived from the incomplete digestion of redundant membrane-bound cellular organelles.

There are also differences in the amyloid content of the plaques – some neuritic plaques contain a portion of amyloid precursor protein not seen in age-related plaques.

Question 5

How is Alzheimer's disease diagnosed?

There is no specific marker for the disease and diagnosis is usually based on clinical evaluation and elimination of other causes of dementia.

Psychometric tests of cognitive function and observation of the associated psychiatric and neurological symptoms are used. CT scans, EEG measurements, functional imaging, and laboratory investigations support the clinical examination and are helpful for eliminating other causes of dementia.

Question 6

Is the diagnosis of Alzheimer's disease reliable? What are the other possibilities?

In experienced hands the accuracy of the diagnosis on clinical grounds approaches 80%. After death, a definitive diagnosis of Alzheimer's disease can be made by examining the brain for excessive deposits of senile and neuritic plaques, and neurofibrillary tangles.

It is necessary to exclude other causes of dementia, including:
- Multi-infarct stroke
- Parkinson's disease
- Brain injury
- Brain tumours and infections
- Medications
- Chronic alcoholism
- Vitamin B_{12} deficiency

Question 7

What treatments are available for Alzheimer's disease?

As yet, no treatment will prevent or arrest the course of the disease and therapy is aimed at minimising the effects of associated conditions such as depression or anxiety. Inhibition of cholinesterase activity (the enzyme that degrades acetylcholine) may preserve the amount of neurotransmitter available. Trials of the drug Tacrine (tetrahydroaminoacridine) have already been started, but to date the responses have been variable.

A different strategy assumes that aluminium reaching the brain initiates or

maintains the neuronal damage, and that removal of aluminium from the brain will result in some functional improvement. Trials with an agent which will isolate aluminium by chelation have been undertaken but only marginal improvement has been seen in a few patients.

Future therapy may be directed at inhibiting the enzymes that liberate β-amyloid from its precursor protein, thus inhibiting the deposition of perivascular amyloid and plaque formation. Deposition of amyloid in the brain is believed by some to initiate inflammatory and neurotoxic responses, ultimately leading to neuronal death. No drug is currently available which would interfere with these actions.

References

Levy-Lahad, E., Wasco, W., Pookay, P. et al. (1995) Candidate gene for the chromosome 1 familial Alzheimer's disease locus. *Science*, **269**, 973–7.

Martyn, C.N., Osmond, C., Edwardson, J.A. et al. (1989) Geographical relation between Alzheimer's disease and aluminium in the drinking water. *Lancet*, **i**, 59–62.

Rogaev, E.I., Sherrington, R. and Roagev, E.A. (1995) Familial Alzheimer's disease in kindreds with missense mutations in a gene on chromosome 1 related to Alzheimer's disease type 3 gene. *Nature*, **379**, 775–8.

Sherrington, R., Rogaev, E.I., Liang, Y. et al. (1995) Cloning of a gene bearing mis-sense mutations in early-onset familial Alzheimer's disease. *Nature*, **375**, 754–60.

Further reading

Cutler, N.R., Gottfies, C.G. and Siegfried, K. (1995) *Alzheimer's Disease*, John Wiley, Chichester.

Davis, K.L. and Powchik, P. (1995) Tacrine. *Lancet*, **345**, 625–30.

Jacques, A. (1988) *Understanding Dementia*, Churchill Livingstone, Edinburgh.

Mera, S.L. (1991) Aluminium, amyloid, and Alzheimer's disease. *Med. Lab. Sci.*, **48**, 283–95.

Selkoe, D. (1986) The importance of altered structural proteins to the pathogenesis of Alzheimer's disease. *Neurobiol. Aging*, **7**, 400–13.

Selkoe, D.J. (1992) Aging brain, aging mind. *Sci. Am.*, **267**, 97–103.

Sherrard, D.J. (1991) Aluminium – much ado about something. *N. Engl. J. Med.*, **324**, 558–9.

27 Parkinson's disease

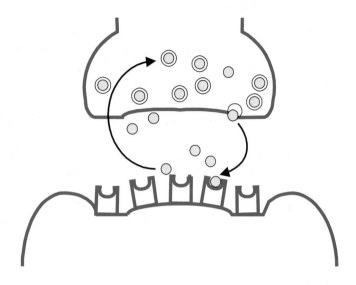

Parkinson's disease is a movement disorder caused by selective degeneration of motor neurons. This degeneration causes loss of the dopamine-containing neurons. Dopamine is a neurotransmitter involved in control of motor function and its deficiency leads to a complex of symptoms comprising slowness of movement, difficulty in initiating and ending movement, tremor and rigidity.

There is no cure for Parkinson's disease, but the neurotransmitter imbalance can to some extent be corrected by administration of drugs. The principal agent used is L-dopa, a dopamine precursor which is transported across the blood–brain barrier, taken up by neurons and then converted to dopamine. Unfortunately this drug does nothing to arrest the process of neuronal degeneration and patients eventually become unresponsive to it. Other agents are available to supplement dopamine or correct the imbalance with other neurotransmitters, but none gives a response as effective as L-dopa.

Pre-test

• **What are the main symptoms of Parkinson's disease?**
• **Who is most likely to develop the disease?**
• **What causes Parkinson's disease?**
• **Is Parkinson's disease easy to diagnose?**
• **What treatments are available?**
• **Is there any known cure for the disease?**
• **Can Parkinson's disease be prevented?**

Aims of this chapter

By the end of this chapter you will have increased your knowledge of:
◆ What Parkinson's disease is and how common the condition is in the UK
◆ The main changes that take place in the brain in Parkinson's disease
◆ How Parkinson's disease is diagnosed and treated

In addition, this chapter will help you to:
◆ Describe the symptoms of Parkinson's disease in relation to changes in the brain
◆ Discuss the aetiology of Parkinson's disease and the ways in which Parkinson-like diseases contribute to our understanding of the disease process
◆ Discuss the problems of diagnosis of Parkinson's disease
◆ Discuss the rationale behind and application of treatments for Parkinson's disease

Introduction

Parkinson's disease was described by James Parkinson in 1817 as a 'shaking palsy'. Essentially the disease presents as disturbances in motor function caused by neuronal degeneration in the motor centres of the brain, particularly the **substantia nigra**. The loss of neurotransmitters, particularly dopamine, affects motor function.

One of the main strategies for treating Parkinson's disease is to replace or conserve as much dopamine in the brain as possible. This treatment, using the dopamine precursor L-dopa, almost always improves symptoms but ultimately does not stop the progress of the disease.

Parkinson's disease is a disorder of motor function caused by neuronal degeneration

Symptoms

Disturbances of motor function in Parkinson's disease are manifest in a number of ways (Figure 27.1).

Parkinson's disease is characterised by a triad of symptoms: tremor, bradykinesia and rigidity

Principal features

The most obvious feature is an uncontrollable **tremor**, which is often worse in one side and usually seen in the arm and hand, at a frequency of 4–6 beats per second. The tremor is commonly referred to as a 'pill-rolling' tremor as it resembles a rotary action, with rhythmic movement of the thumb backwards and forwards on the palm of the hand. It is more difficult to control when the patient is stressed or emotional, but diminishes during movement and in sleep. Some patients do not present with tremor but it usually develops during the course of the disease. A minority of patients never develop tremor.

Conscious movements may be very slow (**bradykinesia**) and difficult to initiate or stop, causing difficulties with walking and getting out of chairs and

Substantia nigra: a region in the upper part of the brainstem. The area gets its name because it contains the brown/black pigment melanin.

Akinesia: loss of movement, often used to describe the disability of initiating movement in Parkinson's disease.

Bradykinesia: a slowing of movement.

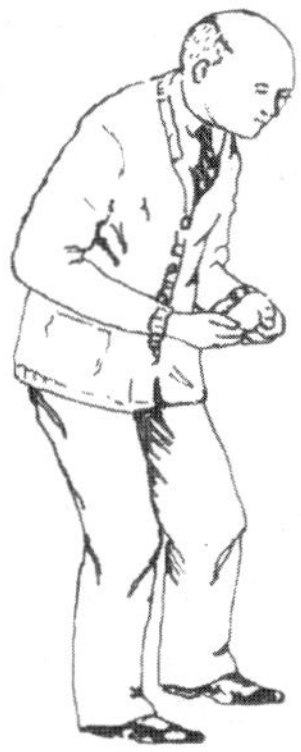

Mask-like expressionless
face, often with drooling

Bent posture

'Pin-rolling' tremor of
hands

Stiff, shuffling gait

Figure 27.1 Clinical features of Parkinson's disease. (Adapted from Lindsay, K.W., Bone, I. and Callander, R. *Neurology and Neurosurgery Illustrated*, 2nd edn. Published by Churchill Livingstone, Edinburgh, 1991.)

bed. The patient walks with very short steps in a shuffling movement. A great deal of concentration is required to stop the movement, which the patient finds particularly frustrating because he or she is aware of what to do but is physically unable to do it. The difficulty in initiating movement means that the patient appears in a 'frozen' state (**akinesia**).

Rigidity usually, but not in all cases, affects the large muscle groups in the limbs. It is caused by increased muscle tone (the muscles are in a continuous state of slight contraction). The rigidity takes a peculiar and characteristic form known as 'cogwheel', especially on rotation of the passive wrist or elbow. This stiffness is often accompanied by pain, and patients suffer from an aching discomfort in the shoulder and back as result of the stooped posture that develops. In the later stages of the disease the tongue may be affected and drooling often occurs.

Other signs of Parkinson's disease are an altered gait, stooped posture and expressionless (mask-like) facial features.

Secondary features

Secondary symptoms include depression, constipation, speech difficulties and dizziness. Patients become depressed because of frustration with the physical disability and as a result of chemical imbalances in the brain. Constipation is caused by sluggish bowel muscles, poor peristalsis and the anticholinergic drugs used in treatment. The ability to speak requires co-ordination of muscles in the larynx, throat, tongue and nasal passages; as these muscles become affected speech becomes more difficult.

About 30% of patients with idiopathic Parkinson's disease suffer cognitive impairment. The signs are a slowness in thinking, with deficits in language, visuospatial processing and perception of motor functions, together with mild memory disturbance. This can amount to a mild dementia and resemble Alzheimer's disease.

Idiopathic: a disorder of unknown cause.

 Key points

Primary symptoms of Parkinson's disease

▲ Akinesia: lack of movement
▲ Tremor: rotary or 'pill-rolling' action at a frequency of 4–6 beats per second
▲ Bradykinesia: slowness of movement with difficulty in initiating and stopping movement
▲ Rigidity: 'cogwheel' type caused by increased muscle tone
▲ Tremor and rigidity are not invariably present

Some patients become rapidly disabled within a few years; others have a mild, faintly progressive disorder for many years requiring little treatment. Most fall between these two extremes, with the condition becoming more intrusive over a period of about 10 years.

Epidemiology

Parkinson's disease occurs in 1–2% of people over 70 years of age, with mean age of onset at about 55 years. Most cases are sporadic, but in 10–15% there is a family history of the disease. This could mean that there is a genetic component to the disease, but it could simply be that some family members are exposed to the same environmental agents.

The rate of disease concordance in identical twins is very similar to that in non-identical twins, although very rarely classical Parkinson's disease is inherited in an autosomal dominant fashion, with many cases in a single family. Genetic linkage studies have been carried out in one of these multicase families, and a genetic marker linked to the Parkinson's disease phenotype has been found on the long arm of chromosome 4. This discovery will aid the search for a Parkinson's disease gene, but at this stage it is impossible to say how important the putative gene on chromosome 4 would be in contributing to the more common idiopathic cases of the disease and how it interacts with other possible genetic and environmental factors.

Parkinson's disease is present throughout the world but is less common in China and Africa. No explanations for this discrepancy have been found, but differences in industrial pollution and pesticide use have been suggested as predisposing factors.

Aetiology

Neurotransmitters

A neuron communicates with other cells by generating electrical impulses, which travel like waves down the length of the axon until they reach the terminal portion, or synapse. At the synapse the electrical signal stimulates the release of **neurotransmitters**, which rapidly diffuse across the synaptic gap and bind to receptors on the dendritic membrane of the adjacent neuron.

There are thought to be about 50 different neurotransmitters. The most common are **glutamic acid**, **γ-aminobutyric acid** (GABA), **dopamine**, **serotonin**, **noradrenaline** and **acetylcholine**. Dopamine, acetylcholine and GABA are involved in motor functions, dopamine and acetylcholine having opposing effects in the striatum. The neuronal degeneration in Parkinson's disease leads to a deficiency of dopamine: in some cases only about 10% of the normal concentration remains. Cholinergic activity is relatively unaffected and hence there is an imbalance of acetylcholine over dopamine. The main aim of therapy is to restore dopamine levels, but the imbalance may be partially

Acetylcholine: neurotransmitter synthesised by small neurons in the striatum. Has an excitatory effect on motor functions. Deficiency leads to chorea.

γ-Aminobutyric acid (GABA): neurotransmitter synthesised by cells of the striatum and globus pallidum. Mainly inhibits nerve impulses. Depletion leads to convulsions and seizures. Deficiency (with acetylcholine) is associated with Huntington's disease.

Chorea: derived from the Greek, meaning 'dance'. Involuntary jerky movements of limbs and axial muscle groups interrupt voluntary movement – walking and eating unaided are impossible.

▲ Key points

Post-encephalitic parkinsonism

- ▲ Followed the influenza epidemic of 1914–1918
- ▲ After several years some survivors developed parkinsonism
- ▲ Symptoms developed at an earlier age than idiopathic Parkinson's disease
- ▲ Dopamine depletion in substantia nigra
- ▲ Neurofibrillary tangles, but not Lewy bodies, are present in neurons

redressed by inhibiting acetylcholine.

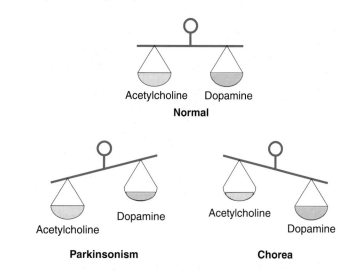

Figure 27.2 Neurotransmitter balance in Parkinson's disease and chorea. Normally the excitatory effect of acetylcholine and the inhibitory effect of dopamine are balanced. Dopamine depletion causes parkinsonism; an imbalance in favour of dopamine causes the movement disorder chorea.

Dopamine is produced in the presynaptic nerve terminals from the amino acid precursors **tyrosine** and **L-dopa** (levodopa; dihydroxyphenylalanine) by the enzymes tyrosine hydroxylase and dopa decarboxylase. Normally dopamine rapidly diffuses across the synapse and binds to specific receptors in the adjacent neuron. Excess amounts are taken up by the original neuron to be stored and reused, or degraded by monoamine oxidase B (MAO-B).

The cause of Parkinson's disease is unknown, although a number of other conditions of known cause are very similar. An example is post-encephalitic parkinsonism, acquired by some individuals as a sequel to the influenza epidemic of 1914–1918. Some people died in the acute phases of the disease with symptoms of viral encephalitis although some apparently recovered. Some of these survivors went on to develop symptoms of Parkinson's disease, but at an earlier age than is normally associated with idiopathic Parkinson's disease. In common with Parkinson's disease, dopamine is depleted in the neurons of the substantia nigra; in this case, however, the neuronal damage and subsequent degeneration are initiated by a viral agent. There are certain other differences between Parkinson's disease and post-encephalic parkinsonism: the virally induced disease is not as rapidly progressive as Parkinson's disease and the features of degeneration within the neurons themselves are neurofibrillary tangles, not the Lewy bodies characteristic of Parkinson's disease.

A major advance in our understanding of Parkinson's disease came unexpectedly with the unfortunate experiences of some young drug abusers in California. These people were exposed to a toxin, methyl-4-phenyl-1,2,3,6-tetrahydropyridine (MPTP), which was present as a contaminant in a 'designer'

A condition similar to Parkinson's disease was found in people who previously had viral encephalitis

Symptoms of Parkinson's disease can be induced by chemical toxins

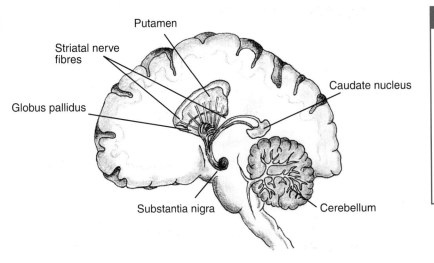

Figure 27.3 Dopaminergic pathways in the brain. The dopamine-producing nerve cell bodies are situated in the substantia nigra. The nerve bundles project into the striatum (comprising the putamen and caudate nucleus). Acetylcholinergic interneurons in the striatum modulate the activity of the dopaminergic neurons.

> ▲ **Key points**
>
> **Drug-induced parkinsonism**
>
> ▲ Contaminant of synthetic heroin (MPTP) causes parkinsonism
> ▲ Toxin selectively damages the substantia nigra
> ▲ Damage by MPTP in animals can be prevented by co-administration of MAO-B inhibitor

synthetic heroin. The result was a very rapid deterioration in motor function with all the classical symptoms of Parkinson's disease. This observation has made it possible to replicate parkinsonism in laboratory animals by administration of neurotoxic agents, and thereby to evaluate directly the changes that take place in the brain together with any responses to treatment.

In various brain cells MAO-B converts MPTP to the potent oxidative neurotoxin MPP$^+$ (1-methyl-4-phenyl pyridinium ion). This toxin is selectively taken up by the neurons of the substantia nigra, using the normal dopamine reuptake system. Once inside the neuron MPP$^+$ inhibits the essential mitochondrial respiratory chain, placing the neuron under oxidative stress and resulting in the degeneration and ultimate death of the neuron. When MPTP is given to laboratory animals the toxic effects to the neurons can be prevented by co-administering an inhibitor of MAO-B: this inhibitor is now used in the treatment of Parkinson's disease.

Chemical damage by MPTP can be prevented by a monoamine oxidase inhibitor

In the more common sporadic cases of the disease environmental factors may operate in a similar fashion, but far more subtly, perhaps with very low concentrations of toxic agents building up over many years. This makes isolation of any single factor or combination of factors which may multiply the risks very difficult. Other mechanisms that could contribute to neuronal damage include autoimmunity, increased concentrations of oxygen free radicals and disturbance in cell trophic factors, although there is little or no proof for any of these. For example, immunosuppressive therapy is of no benefit to patients with Parkinson's disease; similarly, vitamin E (which scavenges free radicals) has no effect on the progress of the disease.

Parkinson's disease itself might be initiated by environmental factors

Pathology

Parkinson's disease is one of several progressive degenerative disorders affecting the brain (Table 27.1). All of these diseases involve the loss of neuronal function, with symptoms varying with the part of the brain affected.

Review question 1

What pathological changes occur in the brain in Parkinson's disease?

Review question 2

How do the symptoms and pathology of Alzheimer's disease and Parkinson's disease differ?

Table 27.1   Degenerative diseases of the nervous system

Disease	Symptoms	Pathology	Cause
Parkinson's disease	Disturbed motor function	Degeneration and loss of pigmented neurons in substantial nigra. Dopamine depletion, although acetylcholine activity is relatively unaffected. Neuronal degeneration evident as Lewy bodies	Exposure to chemical or viral agents
Alzheimer's disease	Dementia	Cortical atrophy and widening of cerebral sulci. Degeneration and neuronal death evident as neurofibrillary tangles and neuritic plaques	Genetic predisposition in some individuals, environmental factors suspected
Huntington's disease	Disturbed motor function and dementia	Atrophy of caudate nucleus. Reductions in activity of acetylcholine and GABA, although dopamine activity is normal	Genetic: autosomal dominant
Pick's disease	Similar to Alzheimer's disease	Atrophy of frontal and temporal lobes. Neuronal degeneration evident as Pick bodies	Probably genetic

Because neurons are affected selectively, one or more functional systems may be affected while others are left intact. In general, when the neurons of the cerebral cortex are affected the most likely outcome is dementia. Where the degeneration is in the basal ganglia, the most likely outcome is a movement disorder. Degeneration and loss of the neurons in the basal ganglia cause depletion of dopamine and melanin. Melanin is produced by the oxidation of L-dopa and brain slices from the area are much paler than normal.

Characteristic cytoplasmic inclusions known as **Lewy bodies** (round or elongated bodies with a densely staining core, surrounded by a paler rim) are seen in neurons of the substantia nigra of Parkinson's patients. Under the electron microscope the core contains granular material and densely packed fine filaments, the filaments becoming more loosely packed at the rim.

Immunological studies have shown that the filaments contain neurofilament components, and in this respect they are not unlike the neurofibrillary tangles of Alzheimer's disease. They are not confined to the dopamine-producing cells of the substantia nigra but can also be seen in non-pigmented neurons of the hypothalamus and upper brainstem.

The severity of the motor syndrome in Parkinson's disease is related to the degree of dopamine deficiency. Up to 85% of dopaminergic neurons must be affected before clinical signs become apparent and it therefore follows that a preclinical stage of the disease may exist for many years. It has been suggested that environmental damage to the neurons is masked for several decades but becomes apparent later when ageing causes further attrition of neurons.

Other neuronal systems using noradrenaline, serotonin and GABA may also be affected in Parkinson's disease but these do not contribute to the classical motor symptoms of the disease. Cholinergic pathways are affected because dopamine pathways oppose their effect: a deficiency of dopamine may cause over-stimulation of cholinergic neurons in the striatum. Some non-striatal cholinergic cells may be lost, contributing to dementia.

Positron emission tomography (PET): used to visualise and monitor active metabolic processes. The patient is given an injection of a biologically active molecule (e.g. glucose or fluorodopa) labelled with a radioactive isotope. The radioisotopes are absorbed by the most active brain cells, which thus emit γ-rays. The γ-ray emission is analysed by a computer and converted to a coloured image

> *Neuronal loss causes dopamine deficiency and acetylcholine imbalance*

Diagnosis

The diagnosis of Parkinson's disease is based on the evaluation of clinical symptoms. Unfortunately the symptoms arise only after significant neuronal damage has occurred: the characteristic pathological changes can be properly evaluated only after the patient has died. Other than by using the specialised (and not widely available) positron emission tomography (PET) scanning there is no means of identifying the disease in asymptomatic patients but the use of PET scanning cannot be justified in asymptomatic people because it is invasive and expensive.

The two conditions most commonly confused with Parkinson's disease are **essential tremor** and **arteriosclerotic pseudoparkinsonism**. Essential tremor is usually inherited but often only becomes manifest in middle age or later. The tremor can be seen when the patient is sitting and is sometimes most obvious at the end of a movement. The main differences between essential tremor and Parkinson's disease are in the type and frequency of the tremor and the parts of the body affected: a slow vertical jaw tremor or leg movement is often seen in Parkinson's disease but not in essential tremor. Arteriosclerotic pseudoparkinsonism usually occurs in hypertensive older people. The distinctive feature of this disorder is that the upper half of the body is relatively unaffected. As in Parkinson's disease there may be difficulty in initiating and stopping movement, but this is largely confined to below the waist. The voice is well modulated and there is no deficit in facial expression or arm movement.

Several other neurological conditions may be mistaken for Parkinson's disease:

- The most common are caused by antipsychotic drugs used to treat mental illness such as schizophrenia. These drugs are almost exclusively dopamine

> *There is no laboratory test or marker which can be used to positively identify patients with Parkinson's disease*

▲ Key points

Common features of degenerative diseases of the nervous system

- ▲ Selective neuronal degeneration and cell death
- ▲ Neuronal degeneration seen as cytoplasmic inclusions (neurofibrillary tangles, Lewy bodies, Pick bodies)
- ▲ One or more functional systems may be affected, although others are left intact
- ▲ Selectivity in the brain leads to characteristic symptoms
- ▲ Brain areas usually affected symmetrically
- ▲ Progressive diseases associated with disability and poor survival

Wilson's disease: a rare inherited disorder of copper metabolism.

antagonists, blocking its action at the dopamine receptors. Withdrawal of the drug usually leads to a gradual disappearance of all symptoms

- Repeated small strokes can also give a picture similar to that of Parkinson's disease
- Wilson's disease may present with symptoms of parkinsonism in the young, but this is treatable by drugs which remove excess copper from the body

Virtually all patients with Parkinson's disease show some response to L-dopa; if they do not then they probably do not have the disease.

Several criteria are used to assess the severity of the disease. These include the evaluation of disabilities such as facial masking, speech impairment and difficulty in swallowing. In a later stage balance may be impaired. The disease can be severely disabling, and patients may need help with the normal activities of daily living, ultimately being confined to a wheelchair or bed.

Treatment

Because it is difficult to identify Parkinson's disease at an early asymptomatic stage the only therapeutic experience is with later stages of the disease. It may become possible to identify and treat the disease in its initial phase, with the aim of preventing further neuronal degeneration.

The aim of current treatments for Parkinson's disease is to replenish or mimic dopamine in the brain and to restore the balance with acetylcholine

The focus of current treatment is pharmaceutical management (Figure 27.4), although patients also need wide-ranging support from speech and language therapists, occupational therapists, physiotherapists, dieticians, social workers and psychologists.

Drug treatments

L-Dopa

Probably the most well known of the treatments for Parkinson's disease is L-dopa. Both the amino acid precursors of dopamine are able to cross the blood–brain barrier by a specific transport system. Dopamine itself is not taken up by this transport system and so will not cross the blood–brain barrier. It is also very quickly metabolised by peripheral tissues. Tyrosine hydroxylase acts as a rate-limiting step in the conversion of tyrosine to L-dopa (Figure 27.4), and therefore larger amounts of dopamine can be produced if this metabolic step is bypassed using L-dopa.

L-Dopa is also metabolised by cells in the liver and gut: this can be prevented by an enzyme inhibitor

The drug is usually given in conjunction with a **decarboxylase inhibitor** (this does not cross into the brain) to reduce its conversion into dopamine in the liver, conserving the amount of drug available for activity in the brain and allowing smaller doses to be given. This minimises the side-effects of nausea and vomiting, hypotension, hallucinations, depression, abnormal involuntary movements and the 'on/off' syndrome (see below). The decarboxylase inhibitors employed (carbidopa or benserazide) can be given as single preparations in combination with L-dopa.

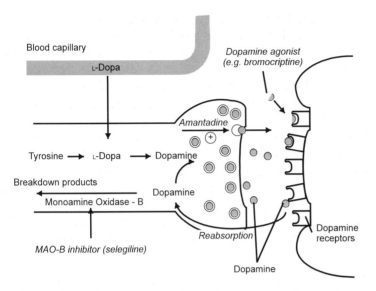

Blood capillary

L-Dopa

Tyrosine → L-Dopa → Dopamine

Breakdown products

Monoamine Oxidase - B

MAO-B inhibitor (selegiline)

Dopamine agonist
(e.g. bromocriptine)

Amantadine

Dopamine

Reabsorption

Dopamine
receptors

Dopamine

Figure 27.4 Action of therapeutic agents in Parkinson's disease. In normal neuronal metabolism tyrosine is converted to L-dopa and then to dopamine, which is stored in synaptic vesicles. On its release into the synapse dopamine binds to receptors on the surface of the post-synaptic neuron. L-Dopa given therapeutically will be taken up by dopaminergic neurons and converted to dopamine. Once the dopamine has bound to its receptor and 'fired' the next neuron it is reabsorbed and recycled or degraded by MAO-B. The MAO-B inhibitor selegiline prevents degradation, conserving dopamine supplies. Amantadine is believed to stimulate the release of dopamine from the synaptic vesicles. Dopamine agonists mimic the action of dopamine by binding to dopamine receptors. (Adapted from Webster, R.A. and Jordan, C.C. (eds) *Neurotransmitters, Drugs and Diseases*, published by Blackwell Scientific, Oxford, 1989.)

Generally, akinesia and rigidity respond well to dopaminergic therapy, but tremor is relatively less responsive. The use of L-dopa undoubtedly prolongs life expectancy and alleviates symptoms. Unfortunately it produces only symptomatic relief because it does not prevent the continued degeneration and death of the neurons and eventually patients will experience new symptoms. First there is a wearing-off effect, in which the symptoms can be controlled for only short periods of time. This problem is usually countered by increasing the dose and by shortening the duration between doses. With time the response to individual doses becomes unpredictable and the patient may switch from good symptomatic control to a sudden deterioration: this is referred to as the 'on/off' syndrome. In the 'off' state the patient is 'frozen'; the 'on' state is characterised by a marked improvement in mobility, although this is accompanied by dyskinesia or interrupted by dystonia. This syndrome is a consequence of the treatment itself.

There is some controversy over the optimal timing of L-dopa therapy. In younger patients (below 50 years) L-dopa is often reserved for the late stages of the disease. Excessive doses can lead to a number of psychotic conditions including insomnia and nightmares, altered sleep/waking cycles,

L-dopa does nothing to arrest the progress of the disease and eventually patients become unresponsive to treatment

Dyskinesia: irregular involuntary movements of face, lips and tongue, neck, trunk and limbs (in dopa-treated disease).

Dystonia: abnormal fixed posture caused by spasms of large trunk and limb muscles.

hallucinations, confusion, delusions, aggression and various other behaviour disorders.

Synthetic dopamine agonists

Rather than using the metabolic pathways of the neuron to produce dopamine, attempts have been made to mimic its action with synthetic agents. Two such agents, bromocriptine and pergolide, bind directly with dopamine receptors. The effectiveness of both agents is similar. They have longer half-lives in the body than L-dopa and therefore the gap between doses can be longer. Their toxic effects are similar to those of L-dopa, but the psychosis produced can be more severe. These agents are sometimes used in combination with L-dopa in an attempt to reduce dosage or to improve the therapeutic response when the wearing-off or on/off effects occur.

Amantadine

Amantadine therapy is mostly used in the early phases of the disease. Its precise mechanism of action is unclear but it is believed to stimulate the release of dopamine from its granular stores. Patients often show initial improvement but over time this declines, presumably as the finite dopamine reserves are depleted. The advantages of amantadine are that it is easy to administer and has only minimal side-effects. Although less potent than L-dopa, it is suitable for older patients who cannot tolerate L-dopa.

Monoamine oxidase B inhibitors

MAO-B inhibitors are potential protective agents

Monoamine oxidase B is normally involved in the breakdown of dopamine; its inhibition can be used to conserve the amount of dopamine available. An MAO-B inhibitor (such as selegiline) given in conjunction with L-dopa will extend the duration of symptom improvement.

Selegiline is also though to act as a neuroprotective agent and slow the progression of the disease, although exactly how it does this is not known. The drug may neutralise free radicals or activate other neurotropic agents and so aid regeneration of damaged neurons. The results of one clinical trial (Parkinson's Study Group, 1989) showed that the onset of disability requiring L-dopa therapy in patients with early-stage Parkinson's disease could be delayed by up to 9 months by administration of selegiline.

However, a lengthier trial (mean follow-up 5.6 years) conducted by the Parkinson's Research Group of the UK (Lees, 1995) has dampened enthusiasm for this drug. In this trial, early-stage Parkinson's disease patients who were not taking L-dopa were randomised to receive L-dopa or L-dopa and selegiline. Unexpectedly, the selegiline-treated group fared worse, with a 60% increase in mortality. However, those patients who took selegiline required much lower doses of L-dopa for symptom control, illustrating the dopamine-sparing effect of MAO-B inhibition. In future it might be possible to develop other agents that would effectively inhibit MAO-B and conserve dopamine without causing excessive deaths.

Anticholinergic agents

Reduced dopamine levels create an imbalance with acetylcholine in the striatum. Some drug therapies are aimed at restoring the balance by diminishing the action of acetylcholine to improve rigidity and tremor by decreasing the muscle tone.

Other treatments are aimed at modifying neurotransmitter balance by suppressing acetylcholine

The main drugs available in this category are benzhexol and orphenadrine, which have similar activities. These drugs are often given in the early stages of the disease but are not suitable for older patients because they may cause glaucoma or urinary retention and could induce or further impair memory loss.

▲ **Key points**

Drug treatment of Parkinson's disease

L-**Dopa:**
▲ Cornerstone of therapy; virtually all patients respond to therapy
▲ Reduces rigidity, bradykinesia, freezing and effects on posture; control of tremor is variable
▲ Does not arrest the disease; responses become unpredictable with time
▲ Co-administration with a peripheral decarboxylase inhibitor (carbidopa or benserazide) minimises extracerebral toxicity

L-**Dopa agonists:**
▲ Act directly on dopamine receptors
▲ Bromocriptine and pergolide are used in patients treated with L-dopa whose symptoms are fluctuating

Anticholinergic agents:
▲ Benzhexol and orphenadrine improve the balance between dopamine and acetylcholine
▲ Helps to control tremor but not rigidity or bradykinesia
▲ Side-effects include dry mouth, blurred vision, urinary retention, hallucinations, impaired memory

Amantadine:
▲ Helps to control rigidity and bradykinesia
▲ Believed to stimulate release of dopamine from granular stores in the neurons, weakly anticholinergic
▲ Side-effects (e.g. oedema, skin discoloration) are slight

Monoamine oxidase B inhibitors:
▲ Drug most used is selegiline
▲ Inhibits degradation of dopamine by MAO-B

Treatment regimens

Treatment regimens vary. In the early stages of the disease treatment will probably involve anticholinergic drugs, possibly with selegiline: L-dopa and decarboxylase inhibitors are more commonly reserved for treating established

Review question 3

Explain how L-dopa works in the treatment of Parkinson's disease.

A further therapeutic strategy is to implant dopamine-producing cells into the brain

Results of fetal grafting have been variable and the technique remains experimental

disease. Selegiline and anticholinergic drugs are also used at this stage. In severe disease L-dopa treatment may be modified to smaller, more frequent doses (combined with a decarboxylase inhibitor). Selegiline and low-dose bromocriptine may also be considered.

Transplantation

Two main sources of cells are used in transplantation: cultured cells from the adrenal medulla and fetal brain tissue. The adrenal medulla produces dopamine normally and auto-transplantation ensures that there will be no rejection problems. Unfortunately, this approach has suffered many postoperative complications and a high mortality rate. Post-mortem studies of people who have been treated in this way have indicated that very few viable graft cells survive.

The alternative approach of transplanting suspensions of fetal brain cells works in experiments with rodents and non-human primates, consistently showing graft survival, incorporation into neural networks and improvement of behavioural defects, but the history of the technique in humans has been more equivocal and, although initial improvements are noted, these do generally persist. Possible reasons for the variation in outcomes are that the optimal age and number of fetal cells are yet to be determined and that their viability is affected by frozen storage.

It is not clear whether immunosuppressive therapy after transplantation is needed because the blood–brain barrier could protect the graft from the host's immune system. However, cyclosporin immunosuppression is usually used before treatment and continued for some months thereafter.

The limited clinical trials so far conducted have involved treatment of idiopathic Parkinson's disease and parkinsonism induced by MPTP. The results have been variable but in a few patients there have been indications that graft tissue survives for several months; these patients have shown some improvement in motor functions and less reliance on L-dopa. It is still to be seen whether the survival of implanted cells and clinical improvement will be long-lasting and correlates with the improvement in clinical status. One means of doing this is to monitor brain activity and uptake of labelled dopa in the brain by PET. Although this method provides indirect evidence of graft survival the invasive procedure of implanting the cells could stimulate the surrounding brain cells non-specifically, causing neuronal sprouting (see Chapter 26) and increased dopaminergic activity.

In one study (of a patient who died 18 months after transplantation from an unrelated cause; Kordower *et al.*, 1995) there was evidence of graft survival, both histologically and on PET. The patient was controlled by medication and had to stop working. After transplantation, in two procedures using seven immunologically unrelated fetuses, the patient's drug dependence was reduced and the patient could independently perform activities of daily living. Histological examination of the brain confirmed the original diagnosis of Parkinson's disease and survival of the grafted tissue. The grafts were larger

than they were at the time of implantation, were highly vascularised and had become integrated into the surrounding tissue.

It remains unclear whether newly grafted tissue will succumb to whatever pathological processes initiated the condition. As yet no patient has become free of symptoms without medication. Additional surgical procedures, perhaps involving intracranial administration of growth factors, may need to be combined with fetal transplantation. The ethical issues involved in using tissue obtained from fetuses combined with the cost of the procedure make it unlikely that fetal transplantation could ever become available to the many thousands of patients who require treatment for Parkinson's disease.

Case study

Mr P is a 70-year old man who retired from his job as an accountant at the age of 63. He is white, and was born (and still lives) in an industrial city in the Midlands.

At the age of 60 Mr P's handwriting became untidy and he developed a slight tremor in his right hand. After investigation, he was considered to be in the early stages of Parkinson's disease. No treatment was initiated at this stage.

Mr P had suffered from no major illnesses and had kept fit by playing badminton regularly since his twenties. He regularly played darts at his local pub, where he would usually consume around three pints of beer in an evening (twice a week). He has never smoked.

Two years after the initial presentation, further symptoms of stiffness in his right arm and leg developed. Mr P suffered from muscular pain, and the tremor had become worse and was noticeable at rest. His handwriting had deteriorated noticeably. He was placed on medication.

- Is the patient typical of the age, gender and socioeconomic distribution of Parkinson's disease?
- What risk factors are usually associated with Parkinson's disease?
- What are the usual symptoms of Parkinson's disease?
- What other conditions might feature in a differential diagnosis?
- What tests can be used to confirm the diagnosis?
- What are the options for treatment?
- Comment on the current symptoms and describe any future problems that might arise.

ANSWERS TO REVIEW QUESTIONS

What pathological changes occur in the brain in Parkinson's disease?

Question 1

The key points are:
- Degeneration and loss of neurons in the substantia nigra of the brain
- Loss of pigmentation of the substantia nigra
- Reduced production of dopamine due to neuronal degeneration and loss,

and the resulting imbalance with cholinergic nerve pathways, causes the motor deficits of Parkinson's disease.

- Degenerate neurons are characterised by the presence of spherical inclusions called Lewy bodies, which are formed from aggregated neurofilaments

Question 2

How do the symptoms and pathology of Alzheimer's and Parkinson's disease differ?

Both Alzheimer's disease and Parkinson's disease are neurodegenerative conditions. Differences in presentation are due to differences in the areas of the brain that are affected. In Alzheimer's disease the neuronal degeneration and loss occur in the cortical areas of the brain, responsible for memory and cognitive functions. The symptoms of Parkinson's disease stem from a selective loss, mostly involving nigrostriatal neurons concerned with motor function.

In both diseases the initiating factors are unknown. Both are believed to involve genetic and environmental factors, and most cases of Alzheimer's disease probably involve some alteration in amyloid metabolism. The neuronal response to damage is different: in Alzheimer's disease neuronal degeneration is evident as neurofibrillary tangles, whereas Lewy bodies are found in Parkinson's disease.

Question 3

Explain how L-dopa works in the treatment of Parkinson's disease

The principle of L-dopa therapy is that of precursor loading. Surviving normal and degenerating neurons in the substantia nigra will, in the presence of physiologically excessive quantities of precursor, respond by synthesising dopamine.

Dopamine should not be given directly because it will not cross the blood–brain barrier. Much of the L-dopa given is degraded by tissues outside the brain but this breakdown can be inhibited by a peripheral decarboxylase inhibitor that does not cross the blood–brain barrier. This allows the dose of L-dopa to be reduced, so that the side-effects of nausea and vomiting are less likely.

Case study

Is the patient typical of the age, gender and socioeconomic distribution of Parkinson's disease? Yes. The disease generally develops between the ages of 50 and 80 years, with a mean age of onset of 55 years. It becomes more common with increasing age, and is very rare in people below 40. The disease is equally common in men and women and there are no distinctive socioeconomic differences.

What risk factors are usually associated with Parkinson's disease? There are no known risk factors associated with this disease. Most cases are sporadic, but there are some rare familial occurrences.

What are the usual symptoms of Parkinson's disease? The main symptoms include tremor, which is typically one-sided, and generally appears at rest. It occurs at a frequency of 4–6 times a second and is often referred to as 'pill-rolling'. Not all patients have a tremor. Other problems with movement are rigidity and bradykinesia. Rigidity is caused by the muscles being in a state of slight contraction, and movement is initiated in a jerky or 'cogwheel' fashion. Movement is very slow and tasks take a lot longer to complete. Other symptoms include disturbed balance, tiredness, depression, dribbling, constipation and confusion. Parkinson's disease is progressive and initially the symptoms are not handicapping. As the disease progresses the level of disability increases.

What other conditions might feature in a differential diagnosis? The most obvious would include stroke, Alzheimer's disease, multiple sclerosis and brain tumour or infection.

What tests can be used to confirm the diagnosis? In most cases diagnosis is made by clinical examination and exclusion of other possible causes. Response to L-dopa medication is a definitive indicator of parkinsonism. Other causes may be excluded by radiography, CT scanning, MRI and EEG. Loss of dopamine from the brain can be visualised by PET but this is not generally available as a diagnostic test.

What are the options for treatment? The metabolic precursor of dopamine, L-dopa, helps to correct the neuronal deficiency. This should be co-administered with a decarboxylase inhibitor (such as Sinemet), which lowers the dose requirement by inhibiting catabolism of L-dopa in the gut. Amantadine is sometimes useful in treating early, mild parkinsonism, or to augment the effects of L-dopa later in the course of the illness. Bromocriptine may be used in patients not stabilised by L-dopa.

Comment on the current symptoms and describe any future problems that might arise. Symptoms become much more difficult to control in advanced stages of the disease, with on/off fluctuations. All drug therapies produce side-effects such as nausea and psychological disturbance. As time goes by the disease becomes more debilitating, and it is likely that Mr P will eventually become bed-ridden.

References

Kordower, J.H., Freeman, T.B., Snow, B.J. *et al*. (1995) Neuropathological evidence of graft survival and striatal reinnervation after the transplantation of fetal mesencephalic tissue in a patient with Parkinson's disease. *N. Engl. J. Med.*, **332**, 1118–24.

Lees, A.J., on behalf of the Parkinson's Disease Research Group of the United Kingdom. (1995) Comparison of therapeutic effects and mortality data of levodopa and levodopa combined with selegiline in patients with early, mild Parkinson's disease. *Br. Med. J.*, **311**, 1602–2.

Parkinson's Study Group. (1989) Effect of deprenyl on the progression of disability in early Parkinson's disease. *N. Engl. J. Med.*, **321**, 1364–71.

Further reading

Calne, D.B. (1993) Treatment of Parkinson's disease. *N. Engl. J. Med.*, **329**, 1021–7.

Perry, E.K. (1991) Neurotransmitters and diseases of the brain. *Br. J. Hosp. Med.*, **45**, 73–83.

Quinn, N. (1995) Drug treatment of Parkinson's disease. *BMJ*, **310**, 575–7.

Quinn, N. (1995) Parkinsonism – recognition and differential diagnosis. *BMJ*, **310**, 447–52.

Williams, A. and Waring, R. (1993) The MPTP tale: pathway to the prevention of Parkinson's disease? *Br. J. Hosp. Med.*, **49**, 716–9.

Index